SYSTEMIC PATHOLOGY / THIRD EDITION

Volume 10 The Cardiovascular System
Part B: Acquired Diseases of the Heart

SYSTEMIC PATHOLOGY / THIRD EDITION

Emeritus Editor W. St C. Symmers

Volume Editors

M. C. Anderson **Female Reproductive System**
I. D. Ansell **Male Reproductive System**
M. E. Catto and A. J. Malcolm **Bone, Joints and Soft Tissues**
B. Corrin **The Lungs**
M. J. Davies and J. Mann **Cardiovascular System: Part B**
C. W. Elston and I. O. Ellis **Breasts**
I. Friedmann **Nose, Throat and Ears**
K. Henry and W. St C. Symmers **Thymus, Lymph Nodes, Spleen and Lymphatics**
P. D. Lewis **Endocrine System**
B. C. Morson **Alimentary Tract**
K. A. Porter, R. C. B. Pugh and I. D. Ansell **The Kidneys/The Urinary Tract**
W. B. Robertson **Cardiovascular System: Part A**
D. Weedon **The Skin**
R. O. Weller **Nervous System, Muscle and Eyes**
S. N. Wickramasinghe **Blood and Bone Marrow**
D. G. D. Wight **Liver, Biliary Tract and Pancreas**

For Churchill Livingstone
Publisher: Geoff Nutall
Copy Editor: Sukie Hunter
Indexer: Brian Armitage
Production Editor: Elspeth Masson
Production Controller: Nora Cameron
Designer: Sarah Cape
Marketing: Susan Jerdan-Taylor

SYSTEMIC PATHOLOGY / THIRD EDITION

Emeritus Editor W. St C. Symmers

Volume 10

The Cardiovascular System

Part B: Acquired Diseases of the Heart

EDITED BY

M.J. Davies MD FRCPath FRCP
British Heart Foundation Professor of Cardiovascular Pathology
St. George's Hospital Medical School
London, UK

and

Jessica M. Mann
Lecturer in Cardiovascular Pathology
St. George's Hospital Medical School
London, UK

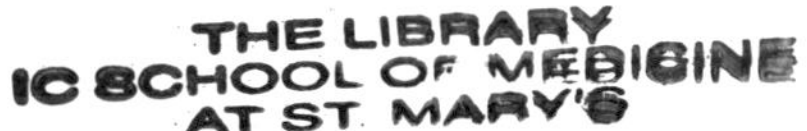

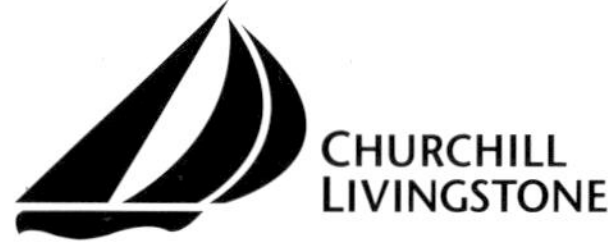

NEW YORK, EDINBURGH, LONDON, MADRID, MELBOURNE, SAN FRANCISCO. TOKYO 1995

CHURCHILL LIVINGSTONE
Medical Division of Pearson Professional Limited

Distributed in the United States of America by Churchill Livingstone Inc., 650 Avenue of the Americas, New York, N.Y. 10011, and by associated companies, branches and representatives throughout the world.

First published 1995

ISBN 0-443-04930-0

British Library Cataloguing in Publication Data
A catalogue record for this book is available from the British Library.

Library of Congress Cataloging in Publication Data
A catalog record for this book is available from the Library of Congress.

The publisher's policy is to use paper manufactured from sustainable forests

Printed in Hong Kong
NPC/01

Contents

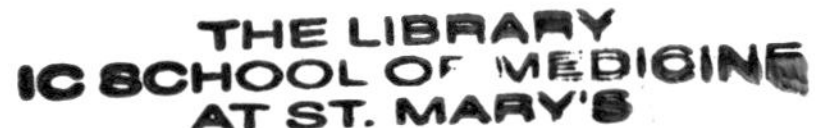

Preface

I have been particularly fortunate in my career as a full time cardiovascular pathologist to inherit a long tradition of the subspecialty at St. George's. This began with Sir Theo Crawford and continues in an unbroken line through W.B. Robertson, Donald Teare and Neville Woolf down to myself and Jessica Mann. Such a tradition could only develop alongside an expanding clinical service in cardiology. Both the clinical and pathological tradition could be said to begin with James Hope, Physician at St. George's Hospital in the 1830's, whose illustrations of valve lesions are instantly recognisable to us today. The development of modern cardiology at St. George's, however, began with Aubrey Leatham and Charles Drew and has culminated in the creation of a busy cardiothoracic service centre under John Parker in which there is a thriving cardiac transplant unit and a British Heart Foundation Department of Cardiological Sciences in which John Camm heads a team containing three other Professors — myself, Bill McKenna (Molecular Cardiology) and Christopher Spry (Cardiovascular Immunology).

All of this is important because it allows Jessica Mann and myself to write a book from our own experience covering a wide range of cardiovascular conditions. This includes atherogenesis, cardiomyopathies, post-surgical complications, valve disease and transplant work. The influence of Donald Teare continues and we have access through his successor Rufus Crompton to abundant forensic material. It is particularly appropriate that at St. George's, where Donald Teare first described the pathological appearances of hypertrophic cardiomyopathy, Bill McKenna is in the forefront of research on the molecular basis of the disease and members of the families originally studied by Donald Teare have been shown to have a gene for abnormal heavy chain myosin.

The book is aimed to be a practical guide to adult cardiovascular pathology for pathologists rather than clinicians. We have, however, tried to integrate the pathology to the clinical situation. There is no other purpose for pathology.

Congenital cardiovascular disease and the results of hypertension on the vascular tree have already been described by Robert Anderson, Anton Becker and W.B. Robertson in Part A of this book.

We have not attempted to provide an exhaustive list of references. In the past, a major role of books was to provide references — with the advent and wide availability of on-line computer searching this role is now redundant. Much of cardiovascular pathology is heavily dependent on macroscopic rather than microscopic examination and this is emphasised throughout. The book aims to show pathologists how to examine the heart practically. It is a book written by authors who practise the trade!

St. George's, London, UK, 1995 M.J.D.

1

Introduction to normal cardiac anatomy

GENERAL INTRODUCTION TO NORMAL ANATOMY

Part A of Volume 10 has dealt in detail with the structure of the normal heart. This introductory chapter re-emphasises certain salient points and relates cardiac structure to the current clinical methods of assessing the heart. Many clinical methods, including echocardiography and magnetic resonance, examine cross-sections of the heart in planes which are not instantly recognisable to most pathologists. Why should we, as pathologists, change our approach? The answer is that if we wish to correlate pathology to clinical findings we have no choice but to adapt. Another reason is that many of the clinical planes view the heart in a more physiological way and help in the understanding of valve function. The anatomy of the heart will be briefly explored in relation to both the conventional pathology approach and the new clinical approach.

Pericardium

The heart is suspended within a pericardial sac. The outer layer of the pericardium is a collagenous structure lined by the parietal layer of mesothelial cells while the visceral layer is simply a single layer of cells. The pericardial cavity is thus the space between the visceral and parietal pericardium — the two are contiguous around the aorta and pulmonary artery and around the pulmonary veins. The bulk of the ventricles and much of the atria are suspended freely in the sac — localised out-pouches of the sac pass behind the atrium (oblique sinus) and behind the aorta and pulmonary artery (transverse sinus).

Position of the heart

When viewed in situ after opening the pericardial sac anteriorly the right border of the heart is formed by the right atrium, and the inferior border by the right ventricle. Much of the anterior surface of the heart is formed by the right ventricle. The left ventricle forms the left border but relatively little projects on to the anterior surface. The tip of the left atrial appendage alone is visible. Thus the left ventricle and left atrium are essentially more posterior structures than either the right ventricle or atrium. After separation from the lungs by dividing the aorta and pulmonary trunk the heart can be placed with its posterior surface on a flat surface and rather more of the left ventricle can be seen from the front.

The pulmonary trunk lies in front of the aorta and the right ventricular outflow crosses the aortic root from right to left.

MORPHOLOGICAL FEATURES OF INDIVIDUAL CHAMBERS

Right and left ventricles

The normal right ventricle in both functional and anatomical terms has an inlet, an apical and an outflow component (Figs 1.1, 1.2). The inlet

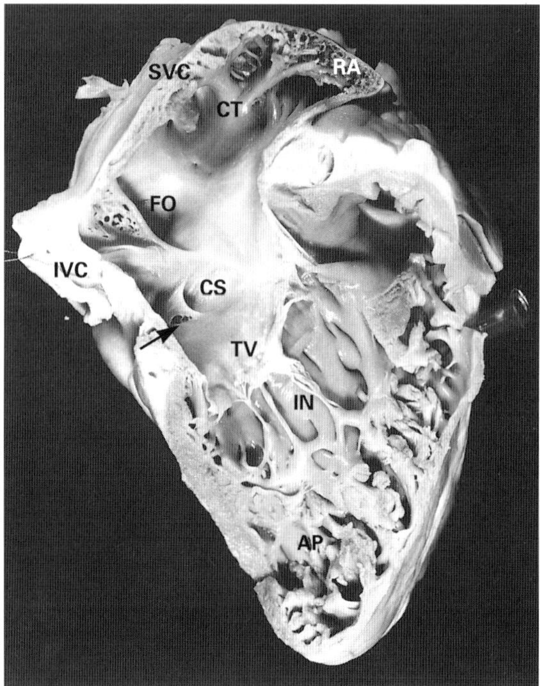

Fig. 1.1 Right atrial and right ventricular morphology. The lateral walls of the atrium and ventricle have been removed to view the interatrial and interventricular septum from the right. The septal cusp of the tricuspid valve (TV) is shown, with the inlet portion of the right ventricle (IN). The apical portion of the ventricle (AP) is heavily trabeculated. The coronary sinus (CS) entering the right atrium has a fenestrated valve (arrow). The inferior vena cava (IVC) also shows a fenestrated remnant of the valve of the sinus venosus. The right atrial appendage (RA) has a ridge surrounding its orifice. The foramen ovale (FO) is an oval depression with a membranous floor. The crista terminalis (CT) is the ridge surrounding the superior vena cava (SVC).

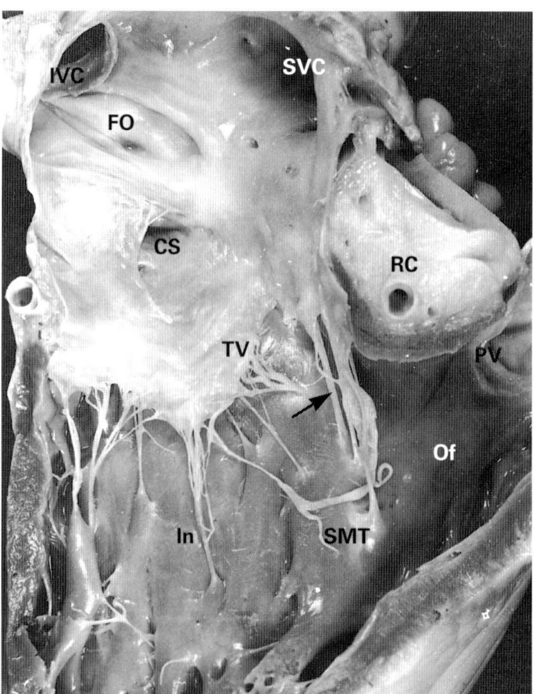

Fig. 1.2 Right atrial and right ventricular morphology. The interatrial and interventricular septum are viewed from the right side. The inflow portion of the ventricle (In) is separated from the outflow tract (Of) by the anterior cusp of the tricuspid valve (arrow). The tricuspid (TV) and pulmonary valves (PV) are not in continuity, being separated by a triangular ridge of muscle containing the first part of the right coronary artery (RC). The inflow and apical segments are also separated by a ridge of septal muscle, the septomarginal trabecula (SMT).

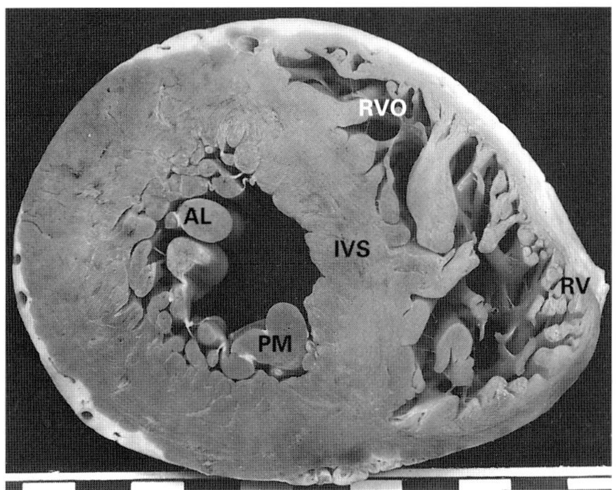

Fig. 1.3 Transverse section of the ventricles. The short axis transection of the ventricles at the mid point of the papillary muscles is a common view used in echocardiography to display ventricular shape. The interventricular septum (IVS) is an integral part of the circular shape of the left ventricular muscle. The more triangular right ventricle (RV) is attached to the septum. There are two major groups of mitral papillary muscles — anterolateral (AL) and posteromedial (PM). The right ventricular outflow (RVO) lies anteriorly and crosses from right to left.

portion lies between the tricuspid valve cusp insertions and the tips of the papillary muscles. The apical portion lies below this and surrounds the papillary muscles while the outflow portion runs up toward the pulmonary valve. The apical portion is very trabeculated while the outflow tract has a largely smooth endocardial surface. The anterior cusp of the tricuspid valve separates the inflow and outflow segments of the ventricle. The junction between the apical and outflow portions of the ventricle is often marked by a particularly prominent muscle bundle (septal band or septomarginal trabecula) and from this another muscle bundle crosses to reach the anterior papillary muscle and thus the free wall of the ventricle. This bundle (moderator band) carries the right bundle branch. In some species

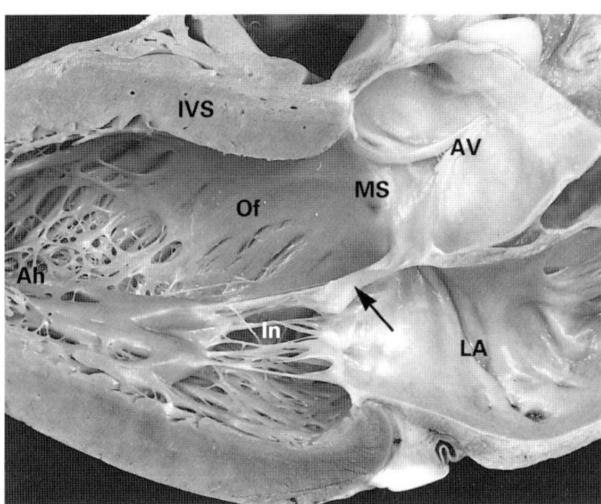

Fig. 1.4 Long axis section of the left atrium, mitral valve and left ventricular outflow tract. This long axis plane is widely used in echocardiography to study the aortic and mitral valves. The left atrium (LA) has a featureless internal surface. The left ventricle has an inlet portion (In), a trabeculated apical segment (Ap) and an outflow (Of) tract. The outflow tract is bounded on one side by the smooth endocardial surface of the muscular interventricular septum (IVS) and on the other by the anterior cusp of the mitral valve (arrow). Just below the aortic valve (AV) is the membranous interventricular septum (MS). The aortic (AV) and mitral valves (MV) are in continuity.

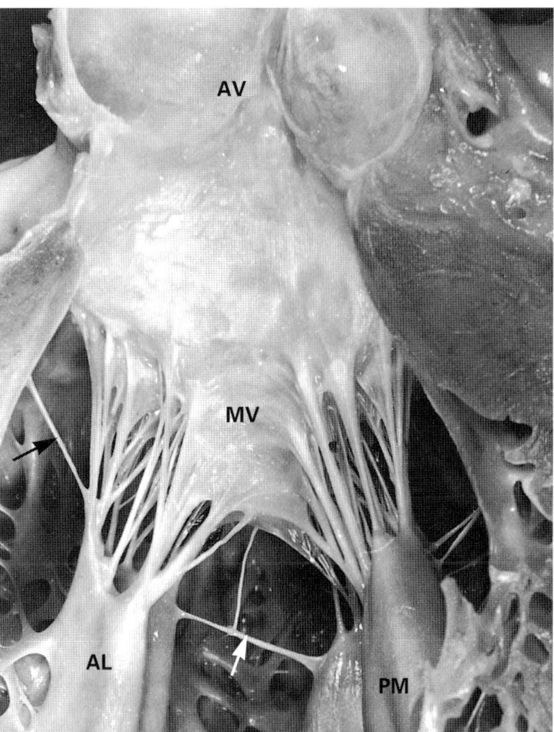

Fig. 1.5 Mitral/aortic continuity. The rough surface of the anterior cusp of the mitral valve (MV) has chordae inserted into it from both the anterolateral (AL) and posteromedial (PM) papillary muscles. The anterior cusp of the mitral valve is in direct continuity with the aortic valve (AV). Endocardial chords (arrows) join both the two papillary muscles and the papillary muscle to the ventricular septum. Such chords have no functional consequence but may cause puzzling echoes during echocardiography.

(e.g. pig) it is a bundle suspended across the ventricular cavity but in man it is usually a ridge.

The wall of the right ventricle is thin compared with the left and, viewed in short axis sections of the ventricles (Fig. 1.3), it is a triangular structure attached to the circular, thick-walled left ventricle.

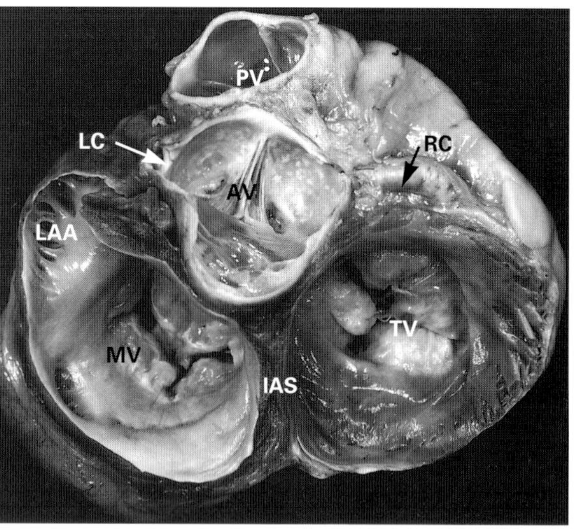

Fig. 1.6 Anatomical relations of the valves. The heart is viewed from above after removing the roof of both atria. The aortic root and valve (AV) lie centrally between the mitral and tricuspid valves (MV, TV). The pulmonary valve (PV) is anterior and slightly apart from the aortic root. The interatrial septum (IAS) and left atrial appendage (LAA) are just above the plane of the atrioventricular valve orifices. An en-face view of the aortic valve can also be obtained by echocardiography in life (RC: right coronary artery; LC: left coronary artery).

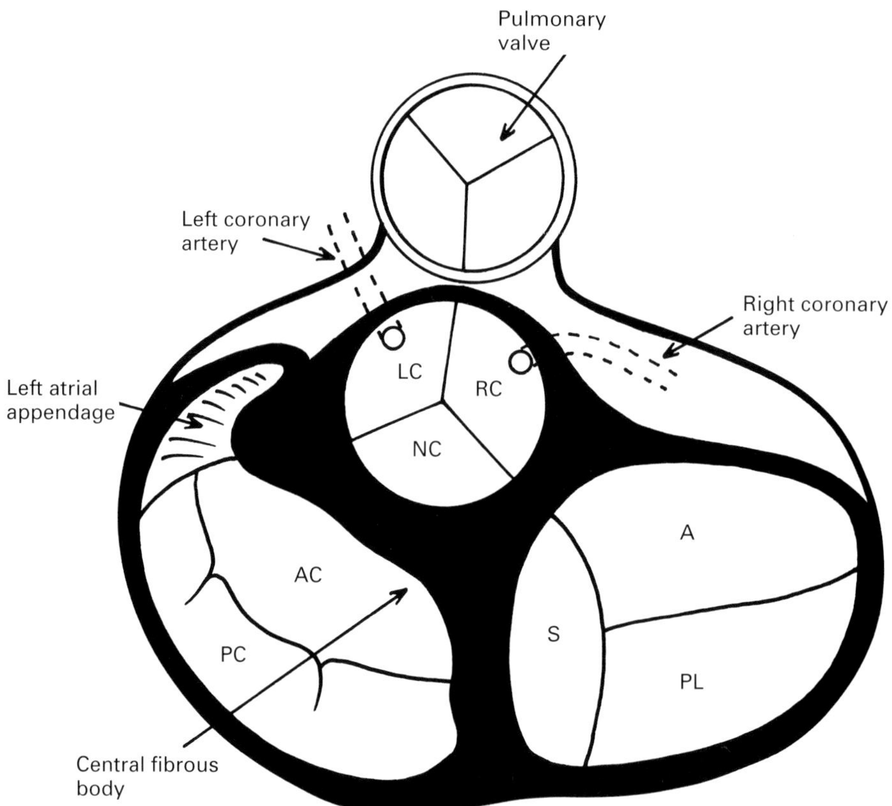

Fig. 1.7 Nomenclature of valve cusps. The central fibrous body ties together the aortic, mitral and tricuspid valves and is contiguous with the connective tissue in the rings to which the bases of the cusps are attached. The aortic cusps are usually named as right coronary (RC) and left coronary (LC), reflecting the origin of the coronary arteries from their respective sinuses. The third is the non-coronary (NC) cusp. The tricuspid valve has septal (S), anterior (A) and posterolateral (PL) cusps. The mitral valve has an anterior cusp (AC) and a posterior cusp (PC), often partially divided into three scallops.

In cross-section the right ventricular outflow can be seen to pass anteriorly across the left ventricle.

The normal left ventricle also has an inlet segment from the valve orifice to the tips of the papillary muscles, an apical segment containing the papillary muscles and an outflow tract (Fig. 1.4). The outflow tract is formed by the smooth endocardial surface of the interventricular septum and the anterior cusp of the mitral valve. The continuity of the anterior cusp of the mitral valve with the aortic valve is an important feature of the left side of the heart and contrasts with the right, where the pulmonary valve is not in continuity with any part of the tricuspid valve. Endocardial chords often cross the left ventricular cavity (Fig. 1.5). They may or may not contain fine branches of the conduction tissue.

Anatomical relations of the valves and cusp nomenclature

The heart has a dense fibrous central body to which the connective tissue of the valve apertures is attached. The pulmonary trunk lies anteriorly and slightly separate from the aortic valve and aortic root. The nomenclature of the valve cusps causes some terminological disagreement. Personally, we name the aortic valve cusps right and left coronary cusps, with a posterior non-coronary cusp. The simplest nomenclature for the mitral valve is anterior and posterior and for the tricuspid valve septal, anterior and postero-lateral (Figs 1.6, 1.7).

Right atrium

The normal right atrium has a smooth venous sinus component which receives both venae cavae and the coronary sinus. This is in continuity with the main bulk of the atrial chamber which lies above the orifice of the tricuspid valve. This main chamber (vestibule) has a septal wall and a lateral wall. Anteriorly the right atrium has a large, wide orifice triangular appendage. The septal surface has a number of key landmarks (Figs 1.1–1.2). There is a prominent oval shaped pit (fossa ovalis) opposite the orifice of the inferior vena cava. The floor of the pit is membranous and is often not fused to the main muscle mass of the interatrial septum around its whole circumference (Fig. 1.8). This allows a probe to be passed

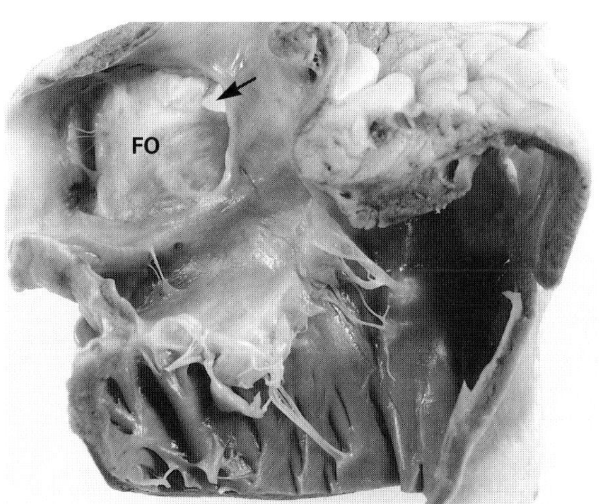

a)

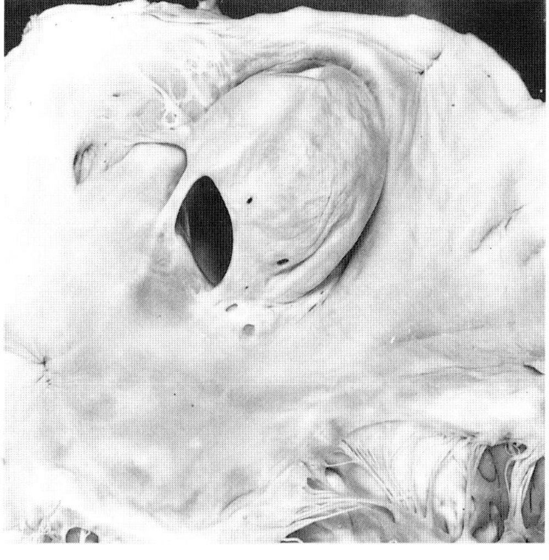

b)

Fig. 1.8a, b Morphology of the foramen ovale. The flap of the valve of the foramen ovale (FO) may not be totally fused to the atrial septum. This allows a probe to be passed or even a small clinically insignificant atrial septal defect to develop. In (**a**), viewed from the right atrium, there is a small defect (arrow) where the floor of the foramen ovale (FO) is not fused to the rim. In another heart (**b**), viewed from the left atrium, due to a rise in right atrial pressure following pulmonary hypertension and chronic lung disease a small atrial shunt developed through the defect and the flap of the foramen ballooned into the left atrium.

from the right to the left atrium, although in life the differential pressures in the atrium keep the foramen closed, preventing shunting of blood. The junction of the appendage with the venous component of the atrium is marked by a prominent crest (crista terminalis) from which the parallel trabeculae of the pectinate part of the atrium arise. Remnants of the inferior vena cava valve (Thebesian valve) often lie close to the orifice of the coronary sinus.

Left atrium

The internal structure of the left atrium is relatively simple and smooth (Fig. 1.9). Four pulmonary veins enter the vestibular portion. The lateral wall shows the flap valve of the fossa ovalis. The appendage is a tubular structure without a striking crest or ridge at its origin (Fig. 1.9).

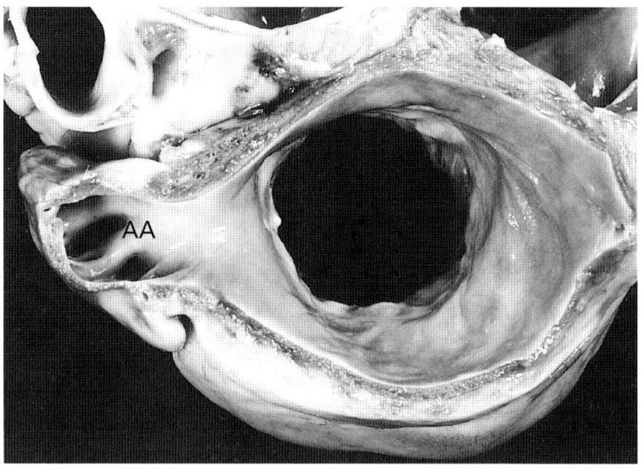

Fig. 1.9 Left atrial morphology. The mitral valve orifice is viewed from above after removing the roof of the atria. The valve is fully open, showing the large size of the mitral orifice in a normal heart. The wall of the left atrium is smooth and featureless apart from the opening of the atrial appendage (AA).

2

Atherosclerosis

INTRODUCTION

The largest cause of cardiac morbidity and mortality in the developed world today is ischaemic (coronary) heart disease. This is virtually all due to atherosclerosis (atheroma) and for this reason the disease justifies a chapter for itself.

There are inconsistencies in the definitions of atherosclerosis and arteriosclerosis. Some would use the term arteriosclerosis as a generic term for a wide range of arterial diseases including atherosclerosis. In this chapter atherosclerosis is defined as an intimal disease of large and medium (external diameter >2 mm) arteries in which the focal accumulation of lipid and smooth muscle proliferation produce lesions called plaques. In contrast, arteriosclerosis is a disease in which medial smooth muscle hypertrophy, and subsequently fibrosis with hyaline change, occur in the media of much smaller arteries. Both atherosclerosis and arteriosclerosis have age and hypertension as predisposing factors. Arteriosclerosis is considered in the companion part to this volume. The lay term 'hardening of the arteries' leads to further confusion and usually encompasses both arteriosclerosis and atherosclerosis.

THE PROCESS OF ATHEROSCLEROSIS

Atherosclerosis is a focal intimal disease of arteries which range in size from the aorta to the epicardial coronary arteries. Some vessels within this size range are, however, virtually spared, an example being the internal mammary arteries. The focal nature of the intimal disease is highlighted by the use of the term 'plaque' for each individual lesion. Every plaque has two major constituents which are present to a lesser or greater degree; these are lipid and the extracellular matrix proteins, predominantly collagen, produced by smooth muscle cells. The lipid may be extracellular or intracellular. The bulk of lipid-containing foam cells can be shown by immunohistochemistry to be of monocytic origin, but smooth muscle cells also contain some lipid droplets. The extracellular lipid is cholesterol in both a crystalline form and as cholesterol esters. Fatty acids and lipoproteins are also present. The intimal lipid is thought to largely originate through alterations in the lipoproteins which diffuse into the intima from the plasma across the intact endothelium.

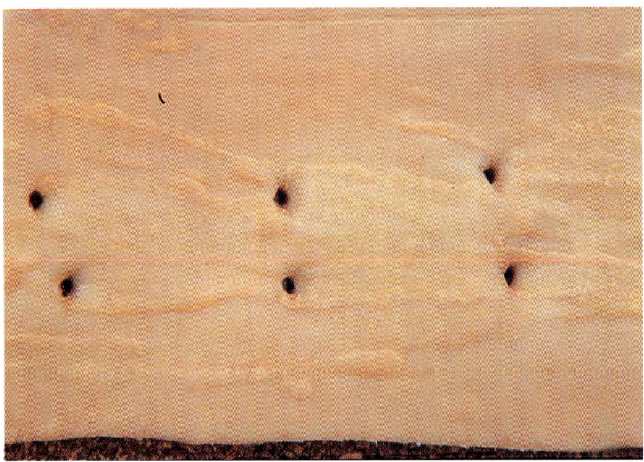

Fig. 2.1 Aortic fatty streaks. The intimal surface of the aorta of a male of 20 is viewed en face. Numerous linear flat yellow lesions are present. Some are related to the origin of the intercostal arteries occurring proximal to the flow dividing edges but many are not related to branches.

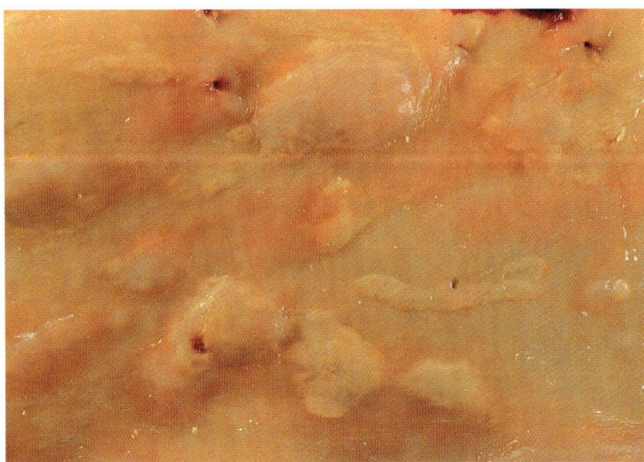

Fig. 2.2 Aortic advanced plaques. The intimal surface of the aorta of a male of 56 is viewed en face. There are a number of raised fibrolipid plaques which vary considerably in size. Some are yellow, others white in colour.

Smooth muscle cell proliferation in the intima is a general response to injury by the vessel wall, and as such occurs in atherosclerosis. Smooth muscle proliferation per se within a vessel is, however, not necessarily indicative of atherosclerosis. Many animal models of vessel wall injury exist in which endothelial denudation is caused by balloon injury. Intimal smooth muscle cell proliferation inevitably follows. These models simulate one component of the atherosclerotic process but do not recreate the human disease. Atherosclerosis cannot be dissociated from the presence of lipid in the arterial wall and is best regarded as an intimal injury in some way initiated by the lipid.

DEVELOPMENT AND MORPHOLOGY OF ATHEROSCLEROTIC PLAQUES

Studies of human atherosclerosis are dominated by descriptions of the plaques seen when arteries are opened and the intimal surface viewed en face (Figs 2.1–2.3).

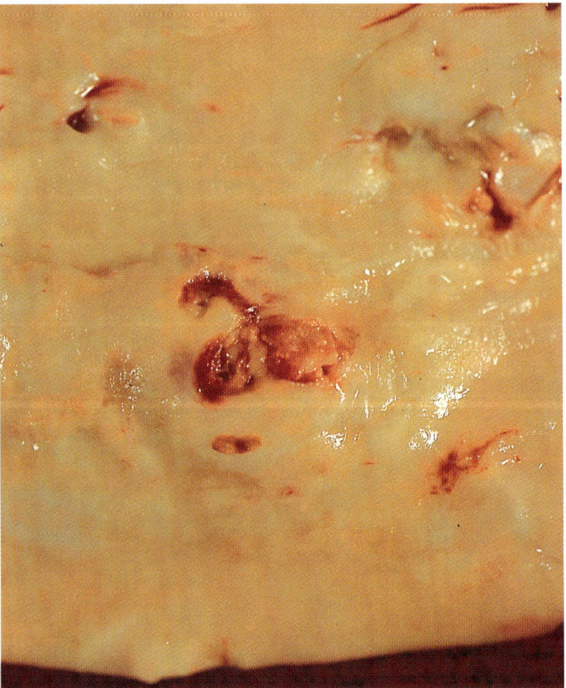

Fig. 2.3 Complicated aortic plaque. The surface of this raised fibrolipid plaque has undergone disruption and is covered by thrombus.

A major advance in the understanding of the evolution of human plaques has came from the work of Stary[1] on the aortas and coronary arteries of young subjects dying from non-vascular causes. Individuals were gathered in age cohorts, allowing identification of the time at which atherosclerotic plaques of a particular type first appear.

The study shows that all humans develop coronary artery intimal thickening at a young age. This thickening is accentuated at points of branching and involves a migration of smooth muscle cells into the intima from the media. Stary argues that this intimal colonisation is an adaptive intimal response and should not be regarded as atherosclerosis. It may however imply that there is a presensitisation to the development of atherosclerosis. The human coronary artery contrasts in this regard with smaller animals such as the rabbit in which the adult intima does not contain smooth muscle cells.

The development of plaques (Fig. 2.4) begins with the aggregation of lipid-filled macrophages at focal points within the intima. These lesions appear as flat yellow dots or streaks (Fig. 2.1) on

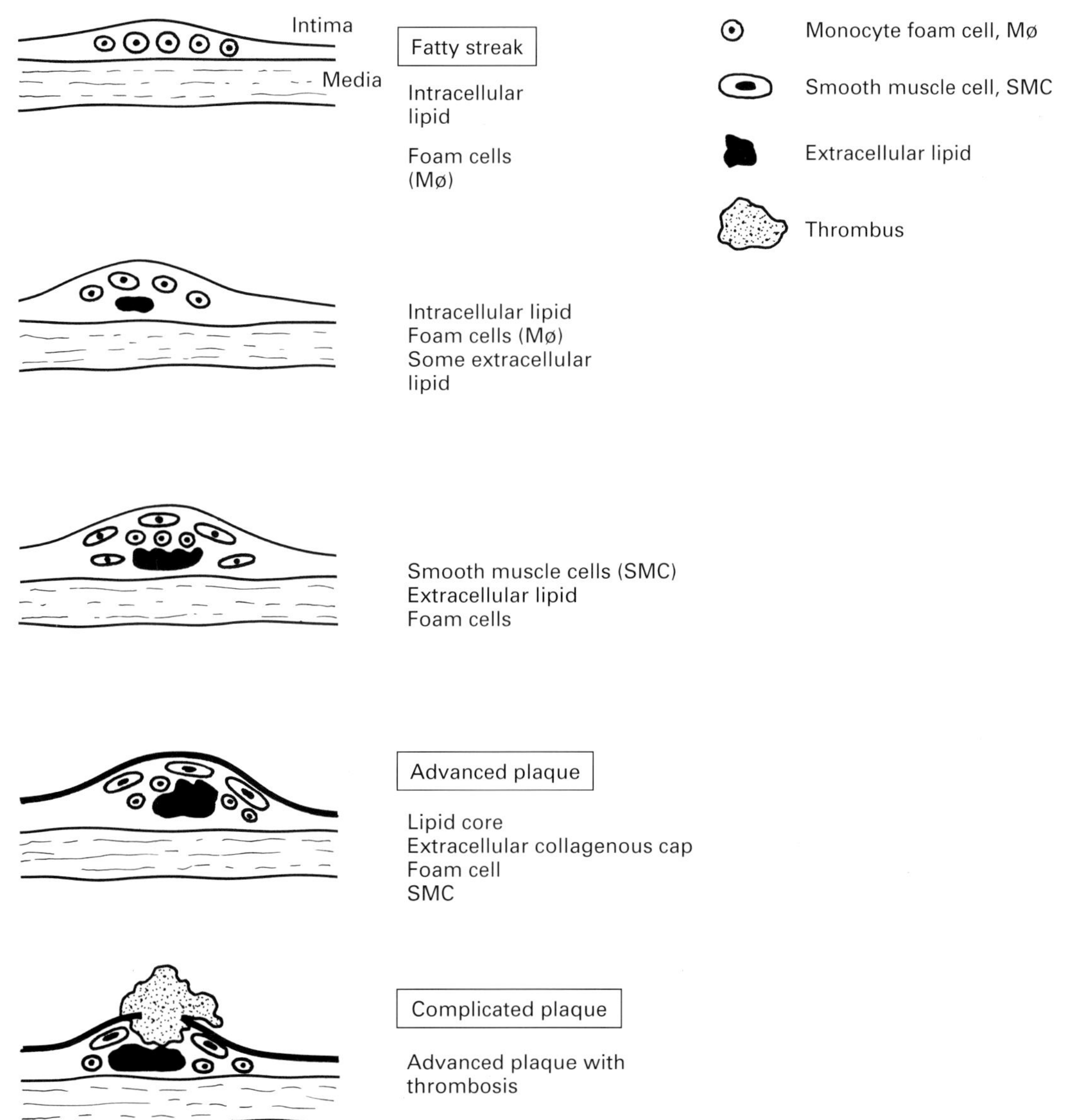

Fig. 2.4 Evolution of atherosclerotic plaques

the intima of the artery. Histological examination shows an accumulation of lipid-filled foam cells beneath an intact endothelium. Epidemiological evidence suggests that some fatty streaks remain static or even regress. Coronary fatty streaks are common in young individuals from geographic populations in which atherosclerosis in adults is virtually absent. Adults in such populations often have fewer fatty streaks than children from the same population; a fact taken to show that some fatty streaks vanish.[2]

Progression from the fatty streak stage is associated with the appearance of extracellular lipid. Smooth muscle proliferation now develops and encapsulates the extracellular lipid, separating it from the adaptive smooth muscle thickening in the intima and from the endothelial luminal surface. Collagen appears in larger and larger amounts, produced by the smooth muscle cells, the process culminating in an advanced or raised fibrolipid plaque.

When viewed macroscopically en face in the aorta the advanced plaque (Fig. 2.2) is elevated above the surface as an oval hump. Some advanced plaques are white, because they contain large amounts of collagen, others with a high lipid content appear yellow.

The lipid core (Fig. 2.5) of advanced plaques is composed of esterified and crystalline cholesterol, which is soft and can be extruded like toothpaste by pressure. The lipids in the core may well be semifluid at body temperature[3] and the term 'lipid pool' is sometimes used. The lipid core occupies anything from 5% to more than 70% of the overall volume of the plaque. The pultaceous nature of the core leads to the name atheroma itself (Greek *athero* = 'gruel').

Other forms of advanced plaque exist. Solid fibrous plaques do not contain a lipid core and the histological structure does not suggest one ever existed. These fibrous plaques contain predominantly smooth muscle cells. Another type of human plaque is the gelatinous lesion which is raised, semi-translucent and brown. No foam cells are present and it has an oedematous connective tissue stroma.[4] It may be the precursor of the entirely fibrous raised plaque.

There is a wide variation in composition of advanced plaques, even in one individual.[5] Some subjects have entirely fibrous plaques, some have entirely lipid-rich plaques, most individuals have a mixture. It is not known whether lipid-rich plaques evolve into purely fibrous plaques or vice versa.

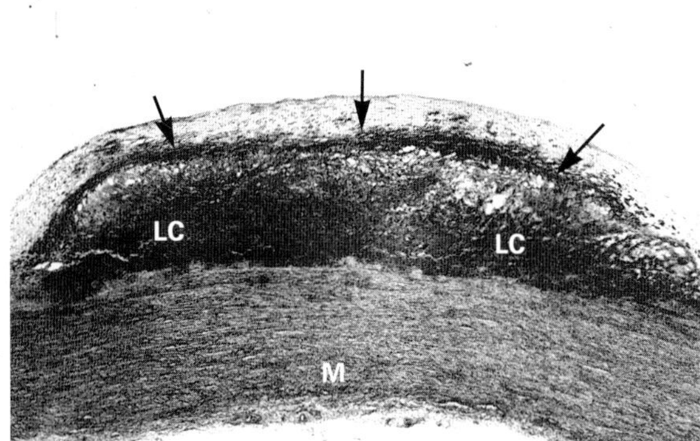

Fig. 2.5 Aortic raised advanced plaques. This histological cross-section of an advanced plaque shows a lipid-containing core (LC) with a well formed fibrous cap (arrow). The media (M) is normal.
Oil red 0 × 18

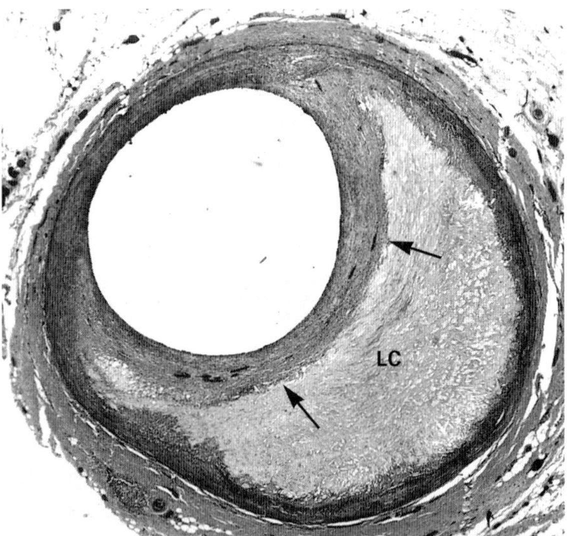

Fig. 2.6 Coronary artery advanced plaque. In this cross-section of a plaque from a coronary artery fixed by perfusion of the lumen at systolic pressure the lipid core (LC) is crescentic in shape and separated from the lumen by a fibrous cap (arrows).
Haematoxylin–eosin × 12

The lipid core of advanced plaques is encapsulated by connective tissue, predominantly collagen, and separated from the lumen of the artery by a fibrous cap containing smooth muscle cells (Fig. 2.6). The lipid core is also surrounded by lipid-filled macrophages (Fig. 2.7), particularly at the lateral margin of the core (Fig. 2.8).[6] The lipid core is thought to be formed by the death of lipid containing macrophages (Fig. 2.9) but some extracellular assembly of cholesterol from lipoproteins bound to proteoglycans may occur. Destruction of the plaque collagen by proteases to create a space within the connective matrix of the plaque, may also play a part in the creation of the lipid core.

In arteries which have been fixed by perfusion, at systemic pressures such as exist in life, the arterial lumen is round and the lipid core seen in

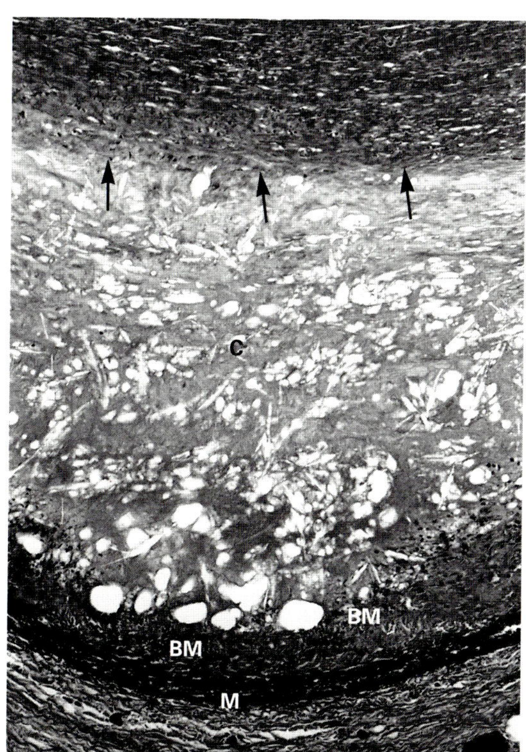

Fig. 2.7 Advanced plaque — histology. The section passes through the entire thickness of the plaque at its centre. The lipid core (C) is acellular and consists of lipid rich debris including cholesterol clefts. The cap (arrows) is made up of collagen and smooth muscle cells. At the base of the core separating the plaque from the media (M) is a basal layer of intimal smooth muscle cells (BM).
Haematoxylin–eosin × 15

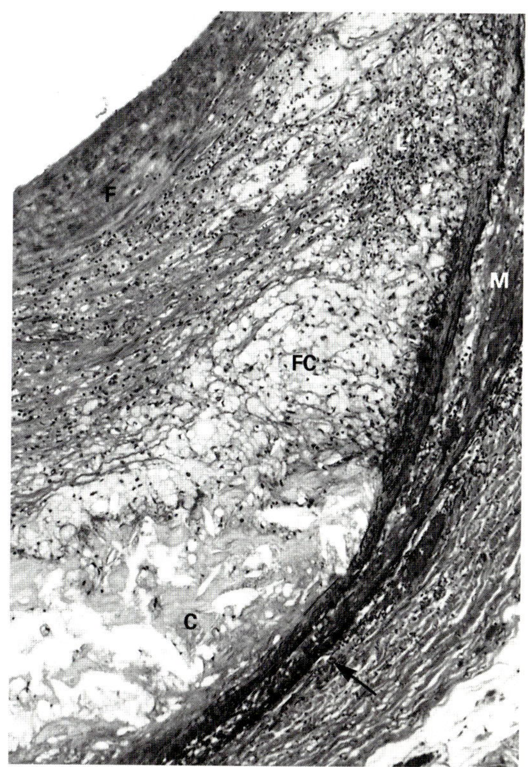

Fig. 2.8 Advanced plaque — histology. The section shows the peripheral area of the plaque (shoulder region). The lipid core (C) is surrounded by a layer of foam cells (FC). The fibrous cap (F) contains abundant smooth muscle cells. The media at the periphery of the plaque is thick (M) but becomes much thinner (arrow) behind the lipid core. The cells with small dark nuclei mixed with the foam cells in focal areas (L) are lymphocytes.
Haematoxylin–eosin × 38

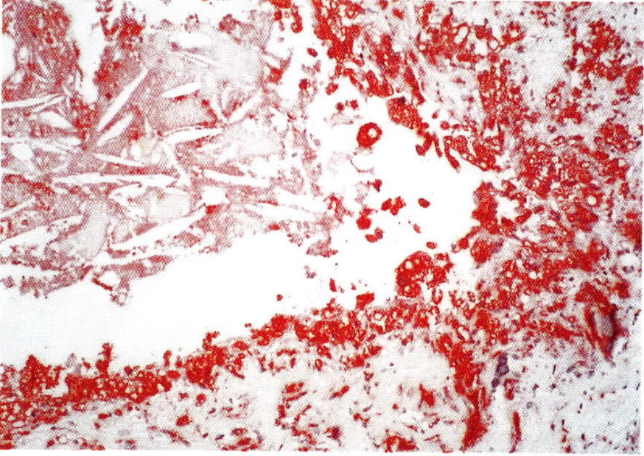

Fig. 2.9 Advanced plaque — lipid core. The edge of a lipid core is shown surrounded by foam cells staining red very strongly for CD68 (EBM11). There is also staining in the acellular lipid debris suggesting that death of macrophages has occurred.
Immunohistochemistry × 345

transverse section is crescentic in shape (Fig. 2.6). The fibrous cap separates lipid encapsulated within the intima from the arterial lumen. The lipid core is highly thrombogenic, containing collagen fragments and tissue factor produced by the macrophages.[7]

The raised fibrolipid or advanced plaque is the basis for the development of clinical symptoms. Epidemiological studies comparing geographic populations show that the proportion of the intima of the aorta and coronary arteries occupied by raised plaques at necropsy is directly related to the incidence of expressed ischaemic heart disease in that population.[8] The PDAY studies[9] show that populations with hyperlipidaemia, smoking and hypertension have more raised plaques than subjects without such risk factors. These results, confirming earlier results by the International Geographic Survey,[8] demonstrate that the increased risk of developing symptoms is in part mediated by the possession of more advanced plaques. Population data, however, obscures the fact that there are individuals who die because of the possession of a single plaque in a strategically important site.

The 'advanced' plaque does not necessarily cause stenosis or become visible angiographically in the coronary arteries. The importance of the advanced plaque is that it may either grow slowly and ultimately encroach on the lumen or become unstable, undergo thrombosis and produce acute obstruction. The two processes are not mutually exclusive and subclinical thrombosis may be an important component of plaque growth.

LOCALISATION OF PLAQUES

A striking feature of atherosclerosis is its focal distribution. In the low pressure pulmonary artery atherosclerosis does not develop without pulmonary hypertension.

The normal endothelial surface is a single layer of contiguous cells aligned with their long axis in the direction of blood flow. The rate of division is low and endothelial cells are long-lived. Endothelial cells are subjected to stretch in the circumferential direction, pressure at each systolic pulse and shear forces from blood flowing over their surface. Evidence in tissue and organ culture in vitro shows that altering these forces can radically alter endothelial cell metabolic activity and intercellular cytoskeleton composition.[10]

Both human and experimental atherosclerotic lesions show enhancement of plaque formation just proximal to branching points, with sparing of the flow dividing regions. This distribution corresponds to areas of low shear rate (atheroma-prone) and high shear rate (atheroma-protected). Shear rates refer to the velocity gradients between the layers of fluid in close proximity to the endothelial surface. In low-shear areas more prolonged contact between platelets and the endothelial surface occurs, putatively allowing time for receptor-mediated adhesion to develop. In contrast, in high-shear areas the contact times are reduced and there is a greater tendency for platelet disaggregation. The endothelial surface is however structurally intact in earliest stages of atherogenesis and platelet/endothelial reactions are not important in initiating atherosclerosis. There is good evidence, nevertheless, for functional abnormalities and altered flux of lipoproteins through the endothelium at points of low shear rate; in these areas LDL enters the intima in larger amounts and is retained longer within the intima, and monocyte adhesion is enhanced.

THE PATHOGENESIS OF ATHEROSCLEROSIS — ANIMAL MODELS

Models of atherosclerosis have inherent limitations but however have provided information about the initiation of atherosclerosis.[11] One fact is clear: only hyperlipidaemia in animals produces lesions with the characteristics of human plaques.

Animal models include those in which hyperlipidaemia is induced either by diet or by using strains in which there are genetic abnormalities of lipid metabolism. These include the Watanabe, the St Thomas' rabbits and the White Carneau pigeon. Dietary models are limited by the unphysiological nature of raising plasma lipids to very high levels over short periods. Rabbit atherosclerosis is characterised by diffuse infiltration of the intima with lipid-filled macrophages, and focal advanced plaques with lipid cores are not produced. In effect, giant or confluent fatty streaks can be induced by high fat diets within 12 weeks in rabbits. The validity of these models of human disease remains an open question. Porcine and primate models fed high-fat diets for longer periods induce plaques with a closer analogy to human disease.[12–14] Transgenic animals show the result of deleting, or enhancing, genes concerned in lipid metabolism in small rodents normally totally resistant to the development of atherosclerosis. Insertion of the Lp(a) gene, for example, leads to florid atherosclerosis in mice.[15]

Arterial lesions with the smooth muscle and collagenous component of atherosclerosis can also be induced by arterial injury. Most models use endothelial denuding injury produced internally by inflating an intravascular balloon. Local smooth muscle proliferation is produced and provides a means of studying one component of plaque formation. Even an inexperienced microscopist would have little difficulty in distinguishing the resulting lesion from a human plaque. When the balloon injury is carried out concurrently with high-fat diets, lipid is deposited within the injured segment and lesions which more closely resemble atherosclerotic plaques develop.[16]

The major lesson learned from the animal models concerns early plaque formation.[13,14,17] The first morphological event is the adhesion of monocytes to an intact endothelial surface. Migration between the endothelial cells to enter the intima follows. Within the intima monocytes ingest lipid and become lipid-filled macrophage foam cells. Endothelial denudation and exposure of subendothelial collagen does not occur in early atherogenesis, and adhesion of platelets to the vessel wall does not occur. The absence of morphological damage does not imply that there is no alteration in endothelial function.

Morphological studies in man suggest that the sequence of plaque initiation is identical to that observed in animal models. The earliest observed event is monocyte adhesion to an intact endothelium followed by their migration into the intima and the formation of lipid-filled foam cells.

Later in plaque formation lipid-filled macrophages cluster directly beneath the endothelial surface and breaks do appear within the endothelium.[17] Platelets can then attach to exposed intimal connective tissue matrix. Lipid-filled macrophages may recross the endothelium to enter the blood stream.[18]

PATHOGENESIS OF HUMAN ATHEROSCLEROSIS

Atherosclerosis is the result of intimal injury initiated in some way by lipid and followed by a set of cellular responses which involve monocytes, endothelial cells, smooth muscle cells and T lymphocytes. The responses have much in common with inflammatory responses elsewhere. A vast range of growth factors, cytokines and proteolytic enzymes are produced within the plaque by the macrophages activated by lipid. Smooth muscle proliferation can be regarded as the repair response to this inflammation.

Role of oxidised lipid and foam cell formation in atherogenesis

A major aspect of atherosclerosis is the intracellular accumulation of lipid within foam cells — so called because of the bubbly appearance in the cytoplasm after the fat is removed from the cell by solvents used in histological preparations. At a later stage in plaque development lipid appears as large extracellular conglomerates. The majority of the foam cells can be shown to be macrophages, derived from monocytes which had migrated into the intima.[6] This fact created a paradox because monocytes do not possess the normal LDL receptor and it was not known how the lipid could enter the cell.

The work of Steinberg and others[19,20] resolved this paradox. Plasma LDL undergoes oxidative modification within the intima to form a product which is avidly taken up by monocyte/macrophage cells by the scavenger receptor. Modified LDL is also a potent stimulus of an inflammatory reaction (Figs 2.10, 2.11).

LDL in contact with cells, and in particular endothelial cells, undergoes lipid peroxidation.[20] The mechanisms by which cells mediate this change are not entirely clear but both superoxide anion secretion and cellular lipoxygenases may be involved. The result is an LDL molecule 'seeded'

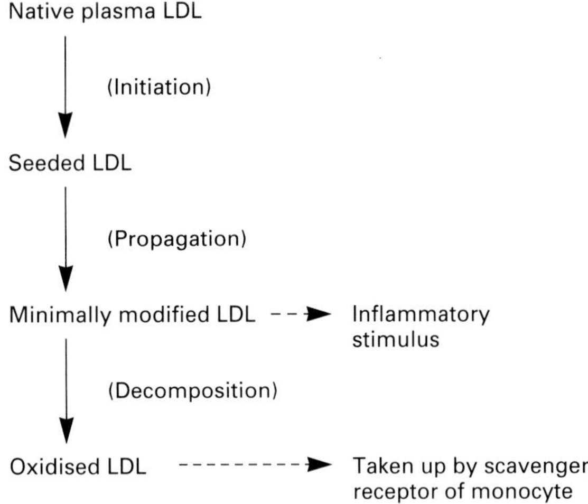

Fig. 2.10 Stages in the formation of oxidised lipid

with lipoperoxides. Once seeded a chain reaction catalysed by copper and iron can occur, leading to the formation of conjugated dienes. At this point aldehydes, ketones and modified fatty acids are produced. The sequence continues with the conjugation of aldehydes to apoprotein B and phospholipids, leading to an epitope readily recognised by a scavenger receptor on macrophages. These changes have been elucidated in vitro; there is good evidence that similar oxidation of LDL occurs within the human plaque,[20] and in rabbit atherosclerosis.[21]

Macrophage scavenger receptors mediate the uptake of a wide range of negatively charged particles and as their name suggests are probably normally concerned in removing cell debris. The receptors are strongly expressed in Kupffer cells and alveolar macrophages. Fortuitously, the receptor when expressed on macrophages in the intima allows the avid uptake of modified lipid.

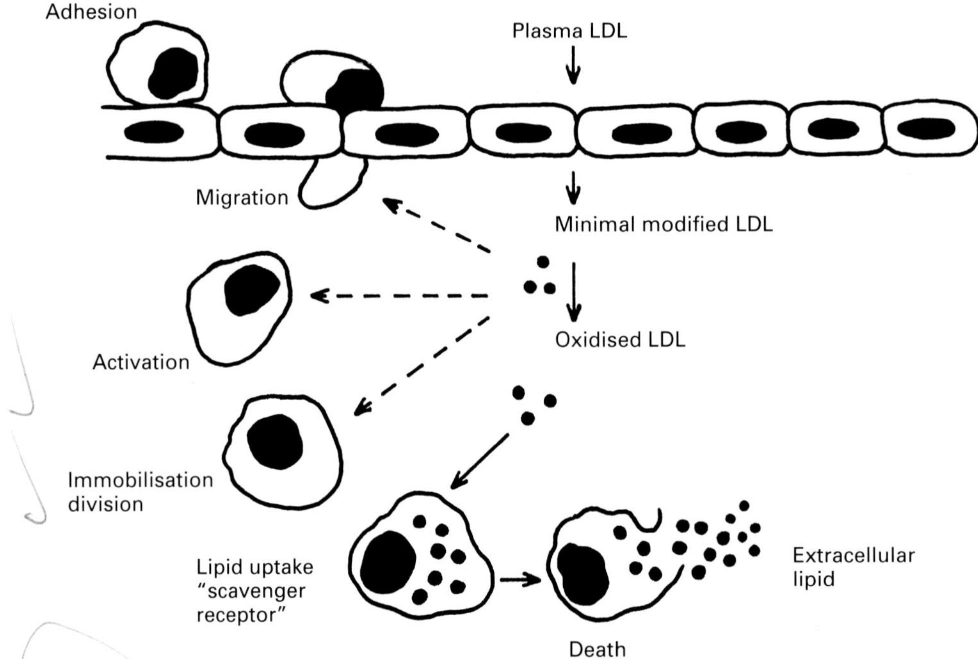

Fig. 2.11 Pathogenesis of atherosclerosis — foam cell formation. The modification of plasma LDL within the intima leads to recruitment of monocytes by migration across the intact endothelium. In the intima they are activated and begin to take up the modified LDL by a scavenger receptor. Later macrophage death releases oxidised lipid into the intima once more. The released lipid is often rich in crystalline cholesterol and now highly oxidised.

Two scavenger receptors are currently known;[22] both contain extracellular domains that form a triple-stranded helix with some similarities to the structure of collagen. Both receptors seem equally efficient at mediating the endocytosis of modified LDL and are expressed on macrophages in human plaques. The scavenger receptor is upregulated rather than downregulated by lipid uptake; thus the process continues until the cell is stuffed with lipid, forming the typical foam cell. Even at this end stage the foam cell is by no means effete and cytokine production, albeit at a lower level, may continue. Ultimately cell death occurs and the intracellular lipid is extruded into the extracellular space to form the lipid core. Oxidised lipid has been demonstrated to be present both in the foam cells and in the extracellular lipid pools of both human and animal atheroma.[20]

Before the generation of a modified LDL recognised by scavenger receptors there is the production of lipid hydroxides and the conversion of lecithin to lysolecithin. These products are themselves initiators of an inflammatory response, will activate monocytes, are cytotoxic and will immobilise monocytes. Monocytes which are activated either by these products or by ingesting lipid via the scavenger receptor have an enhanced production of cytokines such as tumour necrosis factor (TNF), interleukin I (ILI), monocyte chemotactic protein (MCP-I) and macrophage colony stimulating factor (MCSF).[23]

The view that lipid oxidation is the key to plaque initiation raises the question of where the process begins. It probably occurs within the vessel wall at the surface of endothelial cells. Monocytes also have the capacity to continue lipid oxidation and are probably responsible for further oxidation within the intima. It is uncertain whether there is any lipid oxidation in the normal intima or whether it is solely a pathological event developing at a focal point. It is likely that the more lipid which enters the intima and the longer it is retained, the more likely is oxidation to be initiated. It is also possible that, although significant degrees of oxidative modification of LDL in the plasma are prevented by circulating antioxidants, enough minor seeding may occur for the reaction to subsequently continue in sequestered microdomains within the intima. Protection against oxidation is conferred by the incorporation of Vitamins C, E and beta carotene into the LDL before it enters the intima, leading to the possibility that these substances may be antiatherogenic.

Inflammatory/immune mechanisms in atherogenesis

There is increasing realisation that inflammatory and/or immune mechanisms are involved in the development of the atherosclerotic plaque. The major evidence for this view is the close association of macrophages and T lymphocytes, both of which are present in large numbers in both the human and experimental animal atherosclerotic plaque.[24]

A key initial step is the adhesion of circulating monocytes to the intact endothelial surface.[25] This is mediated by the activation of endothelial cells to express adhesion molecules on their surface — for which circulating monocytes and T lymphocytes have specific ligands. Two main families of adhesion molecules are expressed on the endothelial cells of arteries. Of the two selectins, E-selectin is most likely to be that involved in monocyte adhesion. Of those adhesion molecules in the Ig group (so called because of structural similarities to the immunoglobulin molecule), VCAM-1 and ICAM-1 could each be responsible for monocyte or lymphocyte adhesion.[26]

Most endothelial adhesion molecules are not constitutively expressed but are induced by stimuli such as cytokines. The question is why are cytokines expressed before there is any morphological evidence of extracellular lipid in the intima. The answer seems to lie in the first products of lipid oxidation. Very minimally modified LDL and beta-VLDL both induce monocyte adhesion.[25]

Adhesion is followed by chemotactic migration of the monocytes through endothelial cell junctions. Monocyte chemotactic protein (MCP-1) is the most powerful chemoattractant and is released from endothelial cells, smooth muscle cells and monocytes following stimulation.[25] Other factors inducing monocyte chemotaxis include TNF-α and -β, complement fraction 5a, thrombin, glycosylation products found in diabetes, transforming growth factor beta (TGF-β) and platelet derived growth factor (PGDF). The whole complex process has been described in a three-step model of recruitment, attachment and migration.[27] In this process receptors and chemotactic factors combine in different ways to produce monocyte accumulation at the site of inflammation.

The role of T lymphocytes in the plaque remains uncertain. Analysis of the cell surface protein composition of such lymphocytes show that they are in the activated state and that both CD4 and CD8 cells can be detected.[24] Recent molecular genetic studies have, however, demonstrated that these T cells within plaques are very heterogeneous with regard to their immunological specificities.[27]

One function for such T lymphocytes is to moderate the inflammatory process, and in particular the monocyte. T cells produce interferon-γ which is a potent growth inhibitor for both endothelial and smooth muscle cells. Interferon-γ and tumour necrosis factor produced by macrophages and lymphocytes will down regulate the scavenger receptor on the macrophage. This would have the effect of inhibiting the formation of foam cells.

In the adventitia of the artery adjacent to atherosclerotic plaques large numbers of B lymphocytes and plasma cells accumulate. Their presence is thought to indicate an antibody response to antigens such as oxidised LDL in the plaque. Antibodies to oxidised LDL may appear in the plasma and have been used to predict the progression of clinical disease. Oxidised LDL/antibody complexes can be taken up by the F_c receptor of monocytes and provide a further mechanism for intracellular accumulation of lipid.

Smooth muscle proliferation in atherogenesis

A major component of plaque volume is the connective tissue matrix. The matrix, largely collagen in advanced plaques, is synthesised by smooth muscle cells. In animal models of atherogenesis an initial event, that of migration of smooth muscle cells into the intima from the media, is required, but in human arteries they are already present in the intima. Smooth muscle proliferation within plaques is controlled by growth factors produced by a number of sources.[28] Such growth factors (Table 2.1; Fig. 2.12), may be autocrine, i.e. produced by smooth muscle cells themselves, or paracrine, coming from activated macrophages, endothelial cells or T lymphocytes. To be effective, production of growth factors has to be matched by smooth muscle cells which have specific receptors for that particular factor. Smooth muscle cells exist either in a synthetic phenotype in which division is possible and extracellular matrix production predominates or in a contractile form in which division is suppressed and the intracellular content of contractile filaments such as actin is high. Medial smooth muscle is predominantly of the latter type. The initiation of division in smooth muscle cells is thought to involve a phenotypic change to the synthetic type,[29] although there is some evidence of the existence of a non-differentiated smooth muscle cell from which proliferating smooth muscle cells are derived in arterial injury. Platelet derived growth factor (PDGF) is the best characterised modulator of smooth muscle proliferation and has been shown to be produced within human plaques by both endothelial cells, smooth muscle cells and macrophages, but many other growth factors exist.[28]

Platelet derived growth factor (so called because it is stored in the alpha granules of the platelets) is a cationic dimeric protein with a molecular

Table 2.1 Control of smooth muscle activity in plaques

Cytokine/growth factor	Smooth muscle cell	
	Proliferation	Migration
Tumour necrosis factor		
TNF-α	+	
Transforming growth factor		
TGF-β	±	+
TGF-α	+	
Platelet derived growth factor		
PDGF	+	+
Interleukin-1		
IL-1	+	
Interferon-γ		
INF-γ	−	
Insulin growth factor-1		
IGF-1	+	+
Epidermal growth factor		
EGF	+	
Basic fibroblast growth factor		
BFGF	++	0

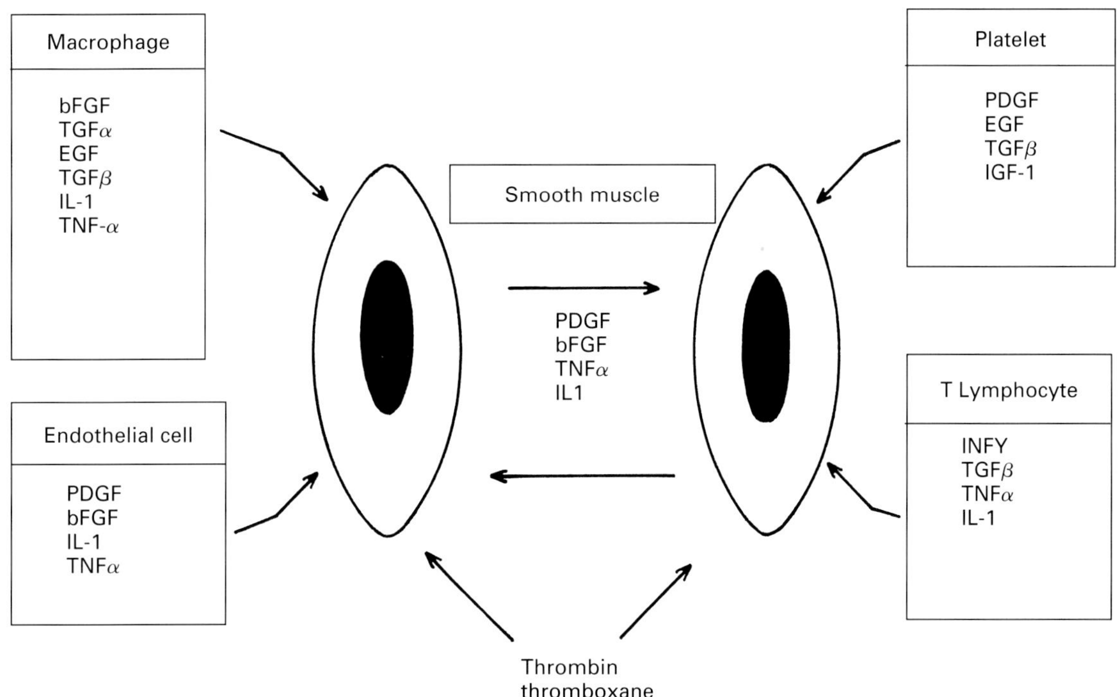

Fig. 2.12 Potential factors influencing smooth muscle proliferation. In the synthetic phenotype within the intima the smooth muscle cell is predominantly concerned with synthesis of connective tissue components but also produces autocrine growth factors (abbreviations as in Table 2.1).

weight of 28 000–32 000. It has two homologous polypeptide A and B chains which are encoded by genes on different chromosomes. PDGF binds with high affinity to receptors on smooth muscle cells and fibroblasts but not to endothelial cells. It acts as a competence growth factor, bringing the cells to which it binds out of the Go phase into the cell cycle, as well as being chemotactic for smooth muscle cells.[30]

Binding of PDGF to its surface receptor causes activation of the phosphatidylinositol pathway and activates the c-*myc* and c-*fos* proto-oncogenes. Differential expression of the two types of PDGF receptor, which can exist as AA, AB and BB forms, may control selective smooth muscle proliferation in different sites in the vessel wall.[28]

Among the other growth factors acting on smooth muscle cells in the arterial wall is transforming growth factor beta (TGF-β), produced by both macrophages and endothelial cells. This factor may be stimulatory or inhibitory, depending on the coexisting levels of other cytokines such as TNF and IL1. Acidic and basic fibroblast growth factors produced by macrophages are mitogens which actually enter the smooth muscle cell and stimulate mitogenesis. Insulin-like growth factors produced by smooth muscle cells are mitogenic for other smooth muscle cells which are already in the cell cycle (progression factors).

Intimal smooth muscle proliferation has largely been studied by balloon injury producing endothelial denudation. Such models in small animals have the limitation that an initial migration of the smooth muscle cells from the media must occur. This step may have no relevance to human coronary arteries, which already contain intimal smooth muscle. These animal models show that there is an initial burst of medial smooth muscle proliferation mediated by the release of fibroblast growth factor (FGF) from damaged smooth muscle cells. This response can be blocked by antibodies to FGF. PDGF is a weak mitogenic agent but a strong stimulus to migration which can be blocked by antibodies.[30] Insulin-like growth factors may also play a role in migration. Very little is known about the relative importance of these factors in intimal proliferation. In general smooth muscle cells derived from the intima have limited replication when compared with medial-derived cells. PDGF is a stimulus for division but inhibition with antibodies is poor. Gene transfer studies suggest that hyperexpression of basic FGF, PDGF-β and TGF-β all enhance intimal smooth muscle proliferation.

Fibrinogen and plaque growth

Fibrinogen, in common with plasma LDL, crosses the normal endothelium to enter the intima. At the sites of potential plaque formation more fibrinogen enters and is retained for a longer period. Within the plaque thrombin is generated by macrophage activity, leading to intraintimal fibrin deposition (Fig. 2.13). There is a balance between fibrin generation and degradation by plasmin with the plaque, and there is evidence of increasing deposition of fibrin in growing plaques.[31] Both thrombin and fibrin degradation products are potent stimulants of smooth muscle growth.

Calcification and atherosclerosis

Calcification either as nodular masses within areas of extracellular lipid or as plates of calcium within connective tissue at the base of the plaque is common and increases with age. There is no direct relation between the amount of calcium and the degree of stenosis. Coronary calcification detected during life will indicate that atheroma is present, nothing more.

The strong association of calcification with atherosclerosis has led to suggestions that it plays a major role in producing symptoms. Calcified tissue is not however a major component of additional plaque volume because it develops either within the lipid or collagen which are already in situ.

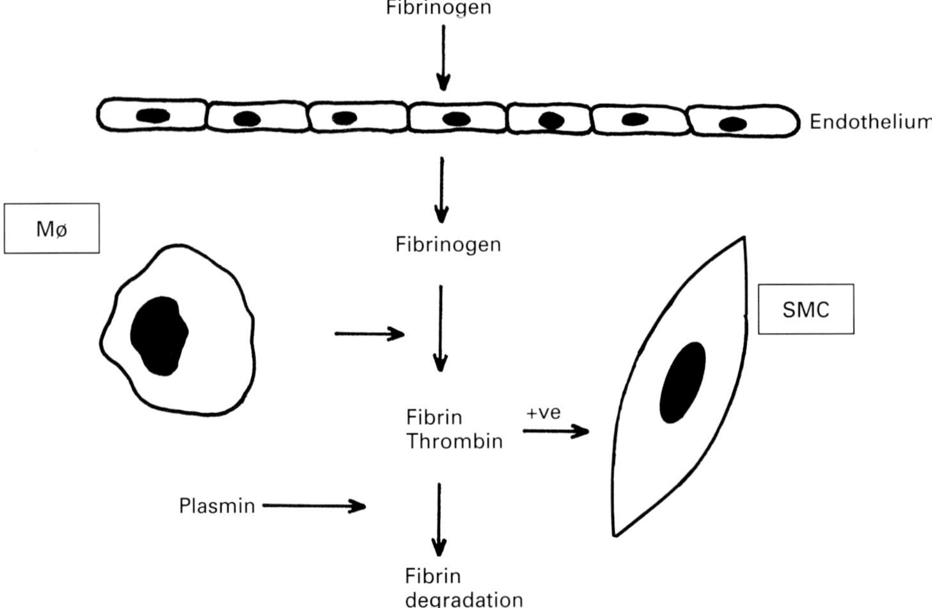

Fig. 2.13 Fibrinogen in plaque growth. Fibrinogen passes the intact endothelium to enter the intima. In the intima tissue factor activates coagulation, leading to fibrin formation. The complex of fibrin and thrombin is a potent stimulus for smooth muscle proliferation. Removal of fibrin by plasmin within the plaque may be an important protective mechanism against plaque growth.

Mechanism of calcification within plaques

In many tissues, including bone, extracellular vesicles (matrix vesicles) from disrupted cells form the nidus for calcification. The lipid core of plaques contains numerous such vesicles formed from disintegrating foam cells. Calcification is initiated by the deposition of crystalline hydroxyapatite; the first crystal then acts as a nucleus for further crystallisation even in the presence of physiological levels of calcium and phosphate. The initial deposition is aided by calcium binding lipids in the vesicle membrane and the action of phosphatases, which locally elevate PO_4 in the vicinity of the vesicle membrane.[32]

A further factor enhancing calcification in the core region is the local production within the plaque of a calcium binding protein rich in sialic acid, osteopontin.

The second form of calcification occurs in the collagen of the deeper layers of the intima and different mechanisms may be involved. A bone-related Gla protein, osteonectin, which binds calcium and hydroxyapatite to collagen, can be produced by smooth muscle cells and may play a role in initiating this deep intimal calcification.

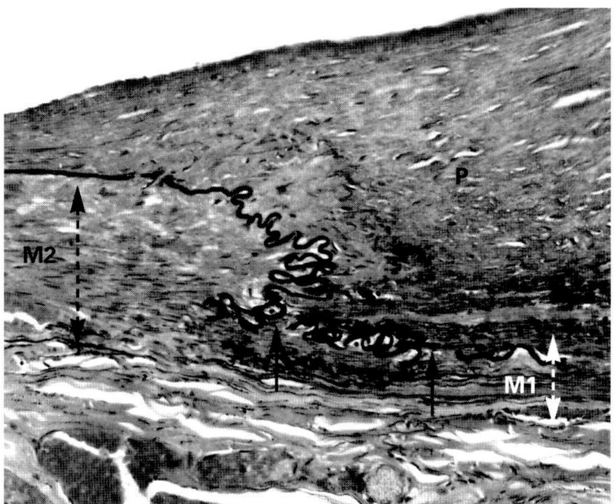

Fig. 2.14 Medial atrophy in atherosclerosis. Behind a large fibrous plaque (P) without a lipid core the internal elastic lamina has broken (arrows). The thickness of media behind the plaque (M1) is greatly reduced compared with that of the adjacent normal vessel wall (M2).

VASCULAR REMODELLING AND THE MEDIA IN ATHEROSCLEROSIS

The arterial media and thus the shape and external size of the vessel have a considerable capacity to remodel. As intimal atherosclerosis develops, the vessel wall adapts to preserve the lumen dimensions inevitably meaning that the external diameter of the vessel increases. Much of this adaptation is achieved by a rearrangement of medial smooth muscle. The work of Glagov[32] shows that the intima has to be increased by more than 40% of the original cross-sectional area of the vessel before this capacity of the arterial wall to accommodate the plaque is overcome.

Many advanced coronary plaques have a more fundamental local effect on the media immediately behind the lesion. The media undergoes atrophy and thinning with loss of medial smooth muscle cells; the result is that the plaque bulges outward rather than inward. The external outline of the vessel becomes eccentric, although the lumen remains circular in shape. In extreme cases the whole media is destroyed and the internal elastic lamina breaks down allowing the plaque to be extruded outward, preserving normal lumen dimensions (Fig. 2.14). Viewed from the adventitial surface atherosclerotic coronary arteries often show a very marked focal variation in external diameter. The result of both these processes, medial rearrangement and medial destruction, is that angiography will always underestimate the amount of intimal disease to a wide and unpredictable degree.[33] Many angiographically normal coronary arteries will contain advanced plaques.

In ectasia the increase in the external diameter of the artery is so excessive that even though atherosclerosis is present within the intima the lumen is enlarged rather than narrowed. Such ectatic segments may alternate with segments in which atherosclerotic narrowing has developed. At a morphological level two factors mark such ectatic segments: the diffuse involvement of the intima and an extreme degree of medial smooth muscle loss.

THE CLINICAL EXPRESSION OF CORONARY ATHEROSCLEROSIS

Clinical symptoms depend on four mechanisms (Table 2.2). The primary process of atherogenesis may increase the volume of one or more plaques so that they encroach on the lumen and become flow-limiting. Secondly, a plaque may enter an unstable phase and be complicated by the formation of a thrombus. This thrombus may itself encroach on or occlude the arterial lumen or break away, embolise and impact in smaller more distal vessels. Thirdly, although atherosclerosis is a focal disease it is associated with a generalised abnormality of vascular tone in affected arteries that favours vasoconstriction, often at inappropriate times such as during exercise. Finally, medial atrophy and destruction secondary to intimal atherosclerosis may lead to aneurysm formation. This aspect of atherosclerosis is of little consequence in coronary arterial disease but is of great importance in the aorta.[34] Many patients suffer combinations of all these mechanisms.

Table 2.2 Mechanisms of clinical expression in atherosclerosis

Mechanism	Clinical expression
Primary atherosclerosis Slow plaque growth Chronic reduction in lumen	Stable exertional angina Intermittent claudication
Acute obstruction to flow — thrombosis	Acute myocardial infarction Cerebral infarction Lower limb ischaemia
Thrombosis with distal emboli	Unstable angina Transient cerebral ischaemia Lower limb ischaemia
Variable stenosis — vasomotor tone variation	Stable angina with rest pain Variant angina
Medial destruction — aneurysm	Abdominal aortic aneurysm

Progression of human atherosclerosis

All autopsy studies are limited by being a 'snapshot' image of the state of the coronary arteries at one point in time. All that can be said is that because many arteries contain plaques at all stages of development new lesions are generated throughout life. One measure of disease progression is the number of acute ischaemic coronary events a patient develops over a period of time. More detailed information about the progression of coronary disease is derived from serial coronary angiography in subjects without acute events. Such studies are limited by the insensitivity of the technique for non-stenosing plaques. Nevertheless some valuable lessons have emerged.[35] In general, disease progress is slow and intermittent rather than a steady linear progression. Progression is largely due to the relatively sudden appearance of new angiographic lesions rather than the growth

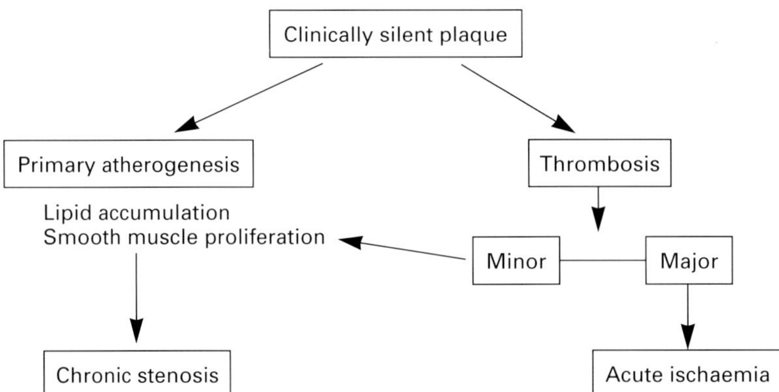

Fig. 2.15 Progression of atherosclerosis. The processes inherent in atherosclerosis (smooth muscle proliferation/lipid accumulation) can cause a plaque to grow to sufficient size to slowly obstruct the lumen. If an intermittent thrombotic episode is major it invokes acute symptoms. If a thrombotic episode is minor it is clinically silent but will stimulate smooth muscle proliferation and accelerate plaque growth.

of pre-existing lesions. High-grade and occluding lesions often develop in segments of artery previously judged to be normal. All these facts are in accord with the concept that sudden complications of plaques are a major cause of disease progression (Fig. 2.15).

Mechanisms of progression

The lipid accumulation and smooth muscle proliferation inherent in the primary process of atherosclerosis are themselves capable of slowly increasing plaque volume to a degree at which the lumen becomes compromised. Sudden increases in plaque volume that are responsible for angiographic progression are due to the incorporation of thrombus into the plaque. This process itself will invoke florid smooth muscle proliferation as a repair process (Fig. 2.15).

Causes of plaque thrombosis

Two different mechanisms (Fig. 2.16) are responsible for thrombosis on plaques.[36] Each process can cause at one extreme microscopic thrombi or at the other extreme thrombosis sufficient in size to occlude the lumen.

Superficial intimal injury causes denudation of the endothelial covering over the plaque. Subendothelial connective tissue matrix is exposed and platelet adhesion occurs on the surface of the plaque.

Superficial injury causes thrombi which range widely in size. At one extreme they are ultramicroscopic (Fig. 2.17). Loss of small areas of endothelial covering is very common over advanced plaques and the resulting thrombi are far too small to cause symptoms but may contribute to plaque growth. Somewhat larger mural thrombi result from more extensive endothelial loss and are associated with heavy infiltrate of the most superficial layers of the intima with foam cells (Fig. 2.18). Larger areas of denudation, particularly at points of high-grade stenosis in the smaller coronary arteries, may lead to thrombi of sufficient size to occlude the lumen (Fig. 2.19).

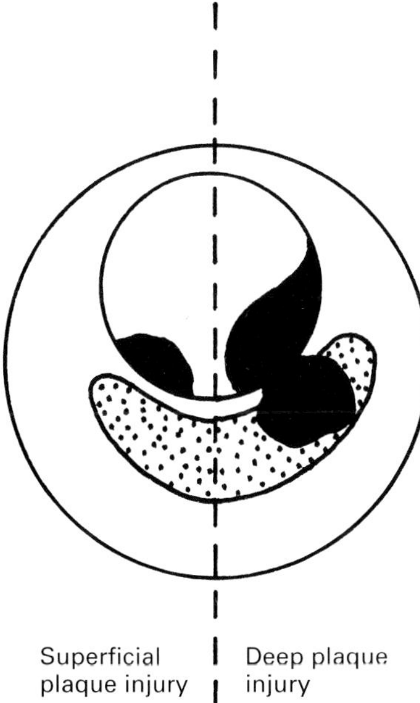

Fig. 2.16 Contrast between superficial and deep injury. In superficial injury thrombus is deposited on the surface of an otherwise intact plaque. Endothelial denudation is the major trigger. In deep injury the plaque is disrupted with a tear in the cap. There is a bilobed thrombus partly inside the plaque projecting into the lumen.

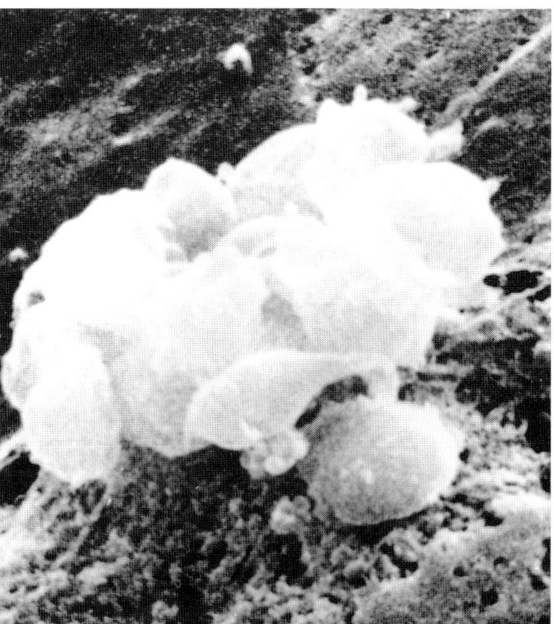

Fig. 2.17 Endothelial denudation in human atherosclerosis. In this human coronary artery prepared for scanning EM by perfused fixation a single endothelial cell has been lost over an advanced plaque. A small platelet thrombus has formed, confined to the area where the underlying matrix is exposed. Electronmicrograph × 3400

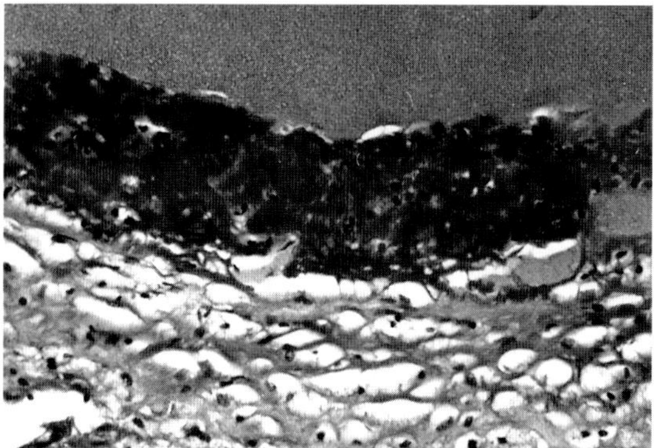

Fig. 2.18 Superficial intimal injury with thrombosis. There is a small mural thrombus on the intimal surface which is densely infiltrated by foam cells.
Haematoxylin–eosin × 150

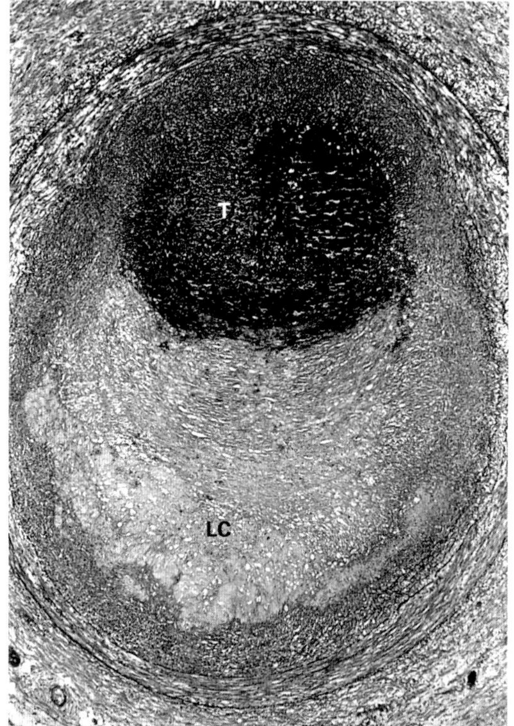

Fig. 2.19 Occluding thrombosis due to superficial injury. A small coronary artery shows a large plaque which is not disrupted and the lipid (LC) core is intact. Over the surface is an occluding thrombus (T).

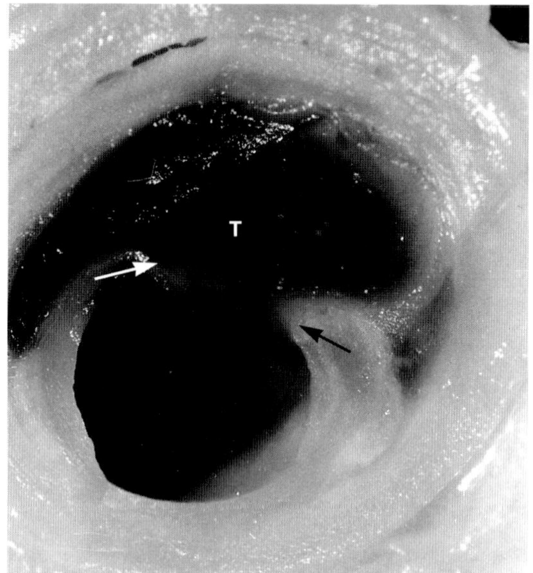

Fig. 2.20 Plaque disruption and thrombosis. The coronary artery has been perfuse-fixed and a cross-section is viewed under a dissecting microscope. A plaque has a tear in the cap (arrows) which has allowed blood to enter the lipid core. Thrombus formation (T) is almost confined to within the plaque itself.

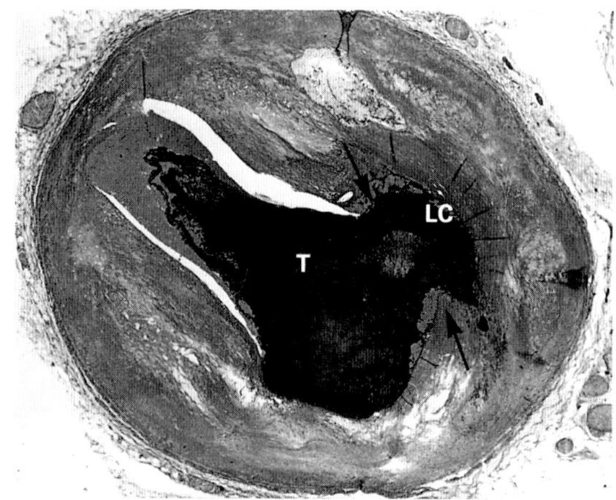

Fig. 2.21 Plaque disruption and thrombosis. In this histological cross section the plaque has a cap tear (arrows) and a mass of thrombus (T) which has its base in the lipid core (LC) projects out into the lumen of the artery.
Haematoxylin–eosin × 7.5

Deep intimal injury complicates an advanced plaque with a lipid core. The plaque cap tears, allowing blood from the lumen to enter the interior of the plaque itself. The core is a highly thrombogenic material containing lamellar lipid surfaces, tissue factor produced by macrophages and exposed collagen. Thrombus therefore forms within the plaque, expanding its volume and distorting its shape (Fig. 2.20). Subsequently thrombosis may extend into the lumen (Fig. 2.21) although this is by no means inevitable. This process of mechanical tearing apart of the plaque has gone by a variety of names, including plaque disruption, fissuring, rupture and ulceration. These different names reflect the fact that the magnitude of the tear ranges from 100–200 μm to many millimetres across.

Mechanisms of plaque disruption

Observational data from autopsies[37,38] show that the majority of plaques that undergo fissuring have a large lipid core, and it is into this core that the tear in the cap allows blood from the lumen to enter. The reasons for the vulnerability of plaques with a large lipid core has been explored by creating computer models of circumferential wall stress during systole.[39] Factors such as a core subtending a large arc of the vessel circumference, differing degrees of stiffness between the cap and adjacent intima, a thin cap and lack of internal collagenous support for the cap from within the core, all increase and concentrate stress on the cap itself. The point of maximum stress varies but is usually close to the insertion of the cap into the more normal vessel wall. This elevation and concentration of stress at focal points on the cap is essentially due to the fact that the soft core cannot carry a mechanical load during systole. The load has to be carried elsewhere, and falls on the cap.

A second approach has been to analyse plaque cap tissue obtained at autopsy.[40] Plaque caps show great variation in tensile strength, even after allowing for differences in cross-sectional area. Strong caps have the collagen arranged in an interweaving mesh while weak caps have collagen arranged in an open lattice containing foam cells.

A final approach has been to compare the composition, morphology and cell populations at autopsy of plaques that have or have not undergone disruption.[41] Plaques that have undergone disruption have a larger proportion of their volume occupied by extracellular lipid; values of over 40% are an indicator of vulnerable plaques. Plaques undergoing rupture also have a reduced collagen concentration in the cap, a decreased number of smooth muscle cells and an increased number of macrophages in the cap.

The vulnerability of lipid rich plaques for undergoing thrombosis has been confirmed by angioscopy[42] and intravascular ultrasound in living patients.[43]

Autopsy studies have shown that a smaller number of intimal tears occur in calcified plaques without a lipid core. Tears occur at the margins of plates of calcium and are probably related to shear stresses. Such tears may play a more important role in causing thrombosis in calcified ectatic arteries in old age.[44,45]

EVOLUTION OF CORONARY THROMBOSIS

Coronary thrombosis is a dynamic process and a series of repair processes are rapidly initiated within the vessel wall. Spontaneous lysis due to activation of plasminogen bound to fibrin is rapid and initiated by any tissue damage in the intima. If not removed by lysis, surface thrombi are rapidly organised to connective tissue and collagen and incorporated into the vessel wall. Thrombus invokes a rapid smooth muscle proliferative process; these cells invade the thrombus and ultimately replace it with collagen. This surface incorporation of small thrombi as a stimulus for intermittent plaque growth has been stressed by pathologists for many years, going back to Duguid in 1946. The main stimulus for smooth muscle proliferation may be thrombin bound to fibrin.

The repair processes following plaque disruption are more complex and the range of possible outcomes is wide (Fig. 2.22). Spontaneous fibrinolysis of thrombus within the lumen is responsible for transitions from occlusive to mural thrombus, and often to restoration of the lumen. If intraluminal thrombus is not removed by lysis it is invaded by endothelial cells and mesenchymal cells of the smooth muscle type. The thrombus is thus converted into a mass of collagenous tissue through which new vascular channels may develop. These multichannelled lumina thus represent the end stage of organisation of intraluminal thrombus.

Within the plaque itself, and at the site of cap tearing, smooth muscle proliferation is also

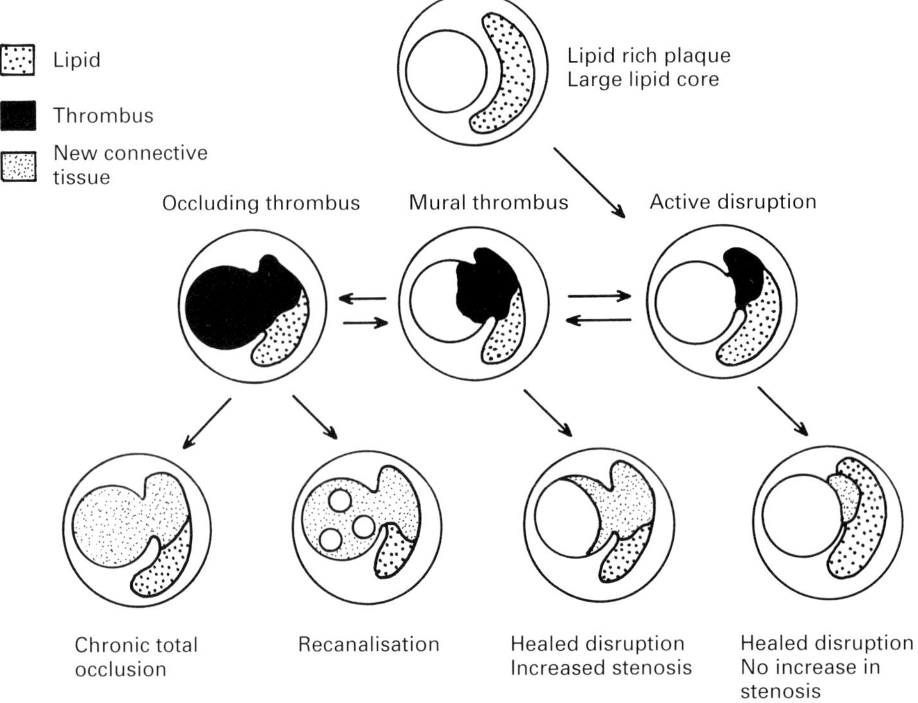

Fig. 2.22 Potential outcome of plaque disruption. Healing of an episode of disruption is dependent on lysis of thrombotic material and on smooth muscle proliferation with the production of new connective tissue.

induced. The repair fibrosis may or may not significantly encroach on the lumen.

Study of coronary arteries taken from control subjects, i.e. those who have coronary atherosclerosis but no history of ischaemic heart disease and who have died of accidental causes, shows that small episodes of plaque fissuring (Fig. 2.23) and resultant intraplaque thrombosis are not uncommon.[46] In subjects without diabetes or hypertension a small recent plaque fissure has been found in 8%, while in those with these risk factors the frequency rises to 16%. Such data indicate that plaque fissuring is integral to the progression of atherosclerosis and not simply a cause of acute ischaemia.

Once plaque fissures are seen to be a common complication in any subject with coronary atherosclerosis the question arises of why some episodes lead to clinical symptoms but others do not.[47]

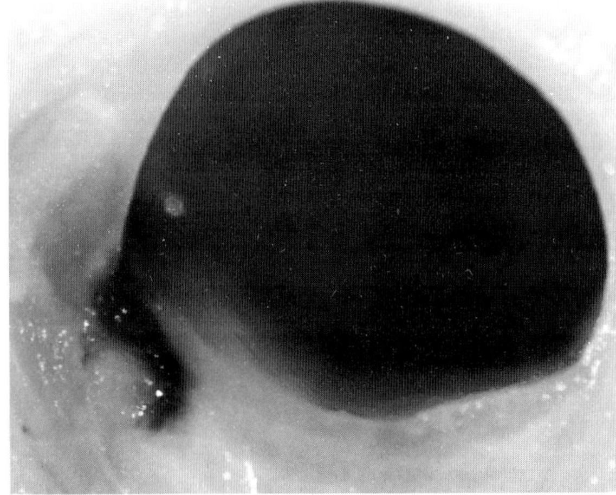

Fig. 2.23 Minor plaque disruption. In this perfused fixed coronary artery viewed under a dissecting microscope there is a small tear into the lateral margin of a plaque with some intraintimal thrombosis but no mural thrombus formation. Control subject dying of non-cardiac cause.

The major determinant of whether acute symptoms occur is whether intraluminal thrombus formation develops. Acute myocardial infarction is associated with thrombosis that, at least for a time, is occlusive; unstable angina is associated with mural, i.e. protruding but not occlusive, thrombi. The determinants of whether intraluminal thrombosis occurs are on one hand the strength of the stimulus for thrombosis. Major determinants of this aspect are the size of the tear, whether lipid core material is extruded, the degree of mechanical obstruction due to plaque distortion and local spasm reducing blood flow. On the other hand the propensity to thrombosis at the time in that particular individual is decided by the balance between the systemic thrombotic potential and systemic fibrinolytic activity.

REFERENCES

1. Stary H. Composition and classification of human atherosclerotic lesions. Virchows Archiv A Pathol Anat 1992; 421: 277–290.
2. Restrepo C, Tracy R. Variation in human aortic fatty streaks among geographic locations. Atherosclerosis 1975; 21: 179–193.
3. Lundberg B. Chemical composition and physical state of lipid deposits in atherosclerosis. Atherosclerosis 1985; 56: 93–110.
4. Smith E. Atherosclerotic lesions – an overview. In: Crepaldi G, Gotto A, Manzato E, ed. Atherosclerosis VIII. Amsterdam, Excerpta Medica, 1989: 13–19.
5. Hangartner J, Charleston A, Davies M, Thomas A. Morphological characteristics of clinically significant coronary artery stenosis in stable angina. Br Heart J 1986; 56: 501–508.
6. Aqel N, Ball R, Waldmann H, Mitchinson M. Identification of macrophages and smooth muscle cells in human atherosclerosis using monoclonal antibodies. J Pathol 1985; 146: 197–204.
7. Wilcox J, Smith S, Schwartz S, Gordon D. Localization of tissue factor in the normal vessel wall and atherosclerotic plaque. Proc Natl Acad Sci USA 1989; 86: 2839–2843.
8. Tejada C, Strong J, Montenegro M, Restrepo C, Solberg L. Distribution of aortic and coronary atherosclerosis by geographic location, race and sex. Lab Invest 1968; 18: 509–526.
9. PDAY Research G. Relationship of atherosclerosis in young men to serum lipoprotein, cholesterol concentrations and smoking. A preliminary report from the Pathological Determinants of Atherosclerosis in Youth Study. JAMA 1990; 264: 3018–3024.
10. Glagov S, Zarins C, Giddens D, Ku D. Mechanical factors in the pathogenesis, localization and evolution of atherosclerotic plaques. In: Camilleri J-P, Berry C, Fiessinger J-N, Bariety J, ed. Diseases of the Arterial Wall. Paris: Springer-Verlag, 1987: 217–239.
11. Ross R. The pathogenesis of atherosclerosis – an update. N Engl J Med 1986; 8: 488–500.
12. Small D. Progression and regression of atherosclerotic lesions. Arteriosclerosis 1988; 8: 103–129.
13. Faggiotto A, Ross R, Harker L. Studies of hypercholesterolaemia in the non-human primate. I. Changes that lead to fatty streak formation. Arteriosclerosis 1984; 4: 323–340.
14. Faggiotto A, Ross R. Studies of hypercholesterolaemia in non-human primates. II. Fatty streak conversion to fibrous plaque. Arteriosclerosis 1984; 4: 341–356.
15. Lawn R, Wade D, Hammer R, Chiesa G, Verstuyft J, Rubin E. Atherogenesis in transgenic mice expressing human apolipoprotein(a). Nature 1992; 360: 670–672.
16. Gellman J, Ezekowitz M, Sarembock I et al. Effect of lovastatin on intimal hyperplasia after balloon angioplasty: a study in an atherosclerotic hypercholesterolemic rabbit. J Am Coll Cardiol 1991; 17: 251–259.
17. Masuda J, Ross R. Atherogenesis during low level hypercholesterolaemia in the non-human primate. I. Fatty streak formation. Arteriosclerosis 1990; 10: 164–177.
18. Daoud A, Fritz I, Jarmolych J, Frank A. Role of macrophages in regression of atherosclerosis. Ann NY Acad Sci 1985; 454: 101–114.
19. Steinberg D, Parthasarathy S, Carew T, Khoo J, Witztum J. Beyond cholesterol. Modifications of low-density lipoprotein that increase its atherogenicity. N Engl J Med 1989; 320: 915–924.
20. Witztum J. Role of oxidised low density lipoprotein in atherogenesis. Br Heart J 1993; 69: S12–S18.
21. Yla-Herttuala S, Palinski W, Rosenfeld M, et al. Evidence for the presence of oxidatively modified low density lipoprotein in atherosclerotic lesions of rabbit and man. J Clin Invest 1989; 84; 1086–1095.
22. Naito M, Suzuki H, Mori T, Matsumoto A, Kodama T, Takahashi K. Coexpression of type I and type II human macrophage scavenger receptors in macrophages of various organs and foam cells in atherosclerotic lesions. Am J Pathol 1992; 141: 591–599.
23. Liao F, Berliner J, Mehrabian M. Minimally modified low density lipoprotein is biologically active in vivo. J Clin Invest 1991; 87: 2253–2257.
24. Hansson G. Immune and inflammatory mechanisms in the development of atherosclerosis. Br Heart J 1993; 69: S38–S41.
25. Faruqi R, DiCorleto P. Mechanisms of monocyte recruitment and accumulation. Br Heart J 1993; 69: S19–S29.
26. Poston R, Haskard D, Coucher J, Gall N, Johnson-Tidey R. Expression of intercellular adhesion molecule-1 in atherosclerotic plaques. Am J Pathol 1992; 140: 665–673.
27. Stemme S, Rymo L, Hansson G. Polyclonal origin of T lymphocytes in human atherosclerotic plaques. Lab Invest 1991; 65: 654–660.

28. Raines E, Ross R. Smooth muscle cells and the pathogenesis of the lesions of atherosclerosis. Br Heart J 1993; 69: S30–S37.
29. Ross R. The pathogenesis of atherosclerosis – a perspective for the 1990s. Nature 1993; 362: 801–809.
30. Ferns G, Raines E, Sprugel K, Motani A, Reidy M, Ross R. Inhibition of neointimal smooth muscle accumulation after angioplasty by an antibody to PDGF. Science 1991; 253: 1129–1132.
31. Bini A, Fenoglio J, Mesa-Tejada R, Kudryk B, Kaplan K. Identification and distribution of fibrinogen, fibrin and fibrin(ogen) degradation products in atherosclerosis. Use of monoclonal antibodies. Arteriosclerosis 1989; 9: 109–121.
32. Glagov S, Weisenberd E, Zarins C, Stankunavicius R, Kolettis G. Compensatory enlargement of human atherosclerotic coronary arteries. N Engl J Med 1987; 316: 1371–1375.
33. De Feyter P, Serruys P, Davies M, Richardson P, Lubsen J, Oliver M. Quantitative coronary angiography to measure progression and regression of coronary atherosclerosis. Value, limitations, and implications for clinical trials. Circulation 1991; 84: 412–423.
34. Ernst C. Abdominal aortic aneurysm. New Engl J Med 1993; 328: 1167–1172.
35. Lichtlen P, Nikutta P, Jost S et al. Anatomical progression of coronary artery disease in humans as seen by prospective, repeated, quantitated coronary angiography. Relation to clinical events and risk factors. Circulation 1992; 86: 828–838.
36. Davies M. A macroscopic and microscopic view of coronary thrombi. Circulation 1990; 82: 1138–1146.
37. Constantinides P. Plaque fissures in human coronary thrombosis. J Atheroscl Res 1966; 6: 1–17.
38. Tracy R, Devaney K, Kissling G. Characteristics of the plaque under a coronary thrombus. Virchows Arch Pathol Anat 1985; 405: 411–427.
39. Richardson P, Davies M, Born G. Influence of plaque configuration and stress distribution on fissuring of coronary atherosclerotic plaques. Lancet 1989; ii: 941–944.
40. Lendon C, Davies M, Born G, Richardson P. Atherosclerotic plaque caps are locally weakened when macrophage density is increased. Atherosclerosis 1991; 87: 87–90.
41. Davies M, Richardson P, Woolf N, Katz D, Mann J. Risk of thrombosis in human atherosclerotic plaques: role of extracellular lipid, macrophage, and smooth muscle cell content. Br Heart J 1993; 69: 377–381.
42. Mizuno K, Miyamoto A, Satomura K, et al. Angiographic coronary macromorphology in patients with acute coronary disorders. Lancet 1991; 337: 809–812.
43. Nissen S, Gurley J, Booth D et al. Differences in ultravascular plaque morphology in stable and unstable patients. Circulation 1991; 84: 436–437.
44. Davies M, Woolf N, Rowles P, Pepper J. Morphology of the endothelium over atherosclerotic plaques in human coronary arteries. Br Heart J 1988; 60: 459–464.
45. Burrig K. The endothelium of advanced arteriosclerotic plaques in humans. Arteriosclerosis Thrombosis 1991; 11: 1678–1689.
46. Davies M, Bland J, Hangartner J, Angelini A, Thomas A. Factors influencing the presence or absence of acute coronary artery thrombi in sudden ischaemic death. Eur Heart J 1989; 10: 203–208.
47. Tofler G, Stone P, Maclure M et al. Analysis of possible triggers of acute myocardial infarction (the MILIS study). Am J Cardiol 1990; 66: 22–27.

3

The pathology of ischaemic heart disease

INTRODUCTION

The clinical expression of coronary atheroma falls into a number of well defined entities. At different times individual patients may have each of these. Stable angina refers to cardiac pain initiated by exercise in which the threshold of work which initiates symptoms remains constant for years. Rest pain is not present. A proportion of patients with stable angina develop episodes of pain or ischaemia detected by continual ECG monitoring in the absence of pain (silent ischaemia) at rest.

In unstable angina episodes of pain at rest occur which often increase in severity over several days (crescendo angina). ECGs recorded during these episodes record transient myocardial ischaemia but not infarction. Acute myocardial infarction has the sudden onset of persistent pain with ECG signs of myocardial muscle death. Sudden death can occur with or without prodromal pain in subjects with or without a known history of previous heart disease. The essence of the clinical picture of coronary atheroma is therefore of a chronic disease on to which acute episodes are superimposed.

THE PATHOLOGY OF ANGINA

Stable angina

Angiographic studies in vivo have shown that patients whose pain is predictable and provoked by a constant level of cardiac work have segments of more than 50% diameter (75% cross-sectional area) stenosis in one or more epicardial coronary arteries. The evidence for regarding this degree of stenosis as significant is derived from the practical clinical experience of symptomatic, as compared with asymptomatic patients, and the theory of flow in tubes. At a standard perfusion pressure, flow begins to fall sharply when the lumen is narrowed by 75% in cross-sectional area and causes a significant drop of pressure across the stenosis. Such in vitro work also suggests that the length of the stenotic segment and the number of stenotic segments existing in series also influence flow by progressively increasing turbulence.

An atheromatous plaque causing this degree of obstruction has converted a low-resistance conduction vessel into one with significant resistance to flow. To some extent, this can be offset by a compensatory fall in resistance within the distal intramyocardial vascular bed. However, there will be a point at which this vasodilatory capacity within the myocardium is exhausted and the stenosis due to atheroma in the epicardial arteries becomes flow-limiting, usually on exercise.

Autopsy studies on patients who had stable exertional angina in life have confirmed the presence of multiple segments of stenosis, usually in more than one major coronary artery. When compared with clinical angiographic studies, pathological studies show a far higher proportion of main left coronary artery stenosis and of involvement of all three coronary arteries. This reflects the inevitable bias of studying subjects who have died of coronary atherosclerosis; clinical series will contain more patients with single-vessel disease.

At autopsy, the appearances of coronary stenosis are best appreciated by examining arteries which have been distended at physiological pressure during fixation. In such arteries, the lumen is seen to be approximately circular in shape, suggesting that the slit- and star-shaped lumens often illustrated in the literature are to a large extent artefacts of examining collapsed arteries.

Stenosis can be classified[1] by their possession of certain basic characteristics; atheromatous plaques may be concentric (Fig. 3.1) or eccentric (Figs 3.2, 3.3) with regard to the residual lumen and may be fibrous or contain, in addition, a variable amount of lipid (Figs 3.3, 3.4). Plaques that are situated eccentrically with respect to the residual lumen allow the retention of an arc of normal medial muscle on the opposite wall of the vessel. The greater the arc of normal vessel wall that surrounds the residual lumen, the greater will be the capacity for variation in muscle tone to produce significant alterations in resistance

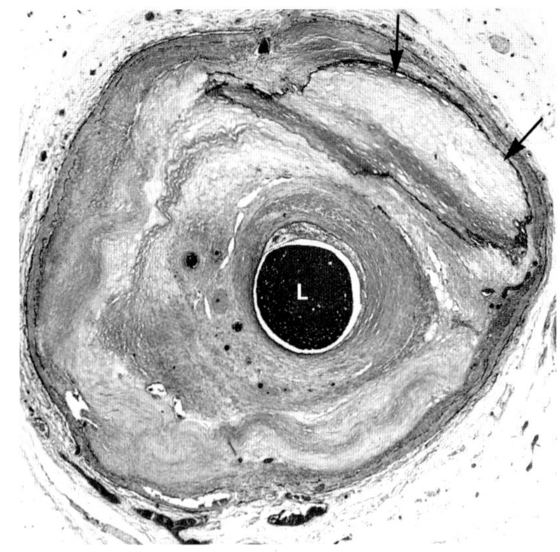

Fig. 3.1 Concentric atherosclerotic plaque. The lumen (L) contains angiographic medium. The lumen is central with high-grade stenosis due to concentric intimal fibrosis. There is no lipid core present but calcification (arrows) has occurred.
Haematoxylin–eosin × 15

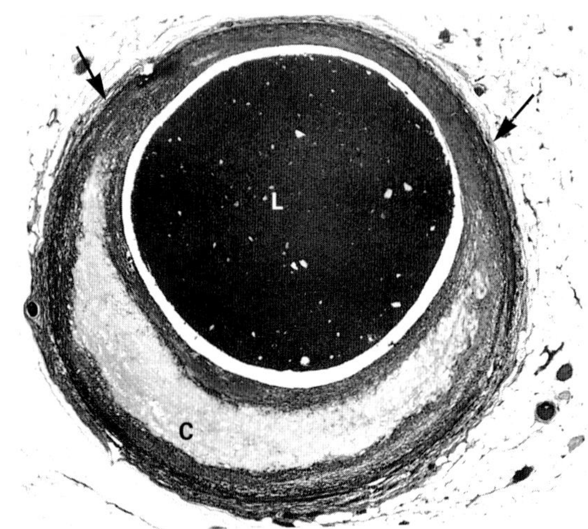

Fig. 3.2 Eccentric atherosclerotic plaque. The lumen (L) is eccentric with retention of an arc of normal vessel wall (arrows). The plaque contains a large lipid core (C). The degree of stenosis is mild.
Haematoxylin–eosin × 15

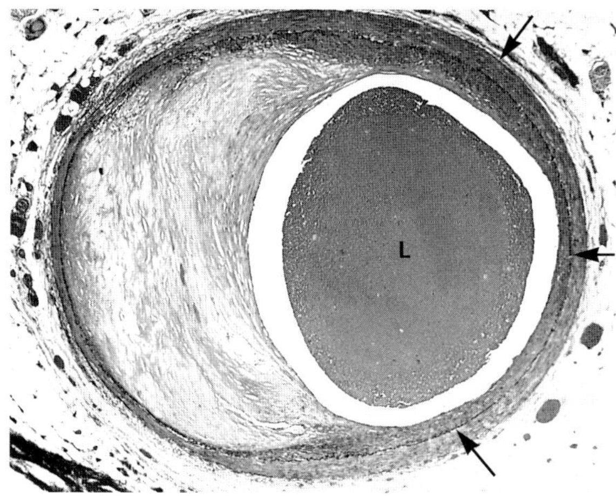

Fig. 3.3 Eccentric atherosclerotic plaque. The lumen (L) is eccentric with retention of an arc of normal vessel wall (arrows). The plaque is solid and fibrous. The degree of stenosis is mild to moderate.
Haematoxylin–eosin × 14

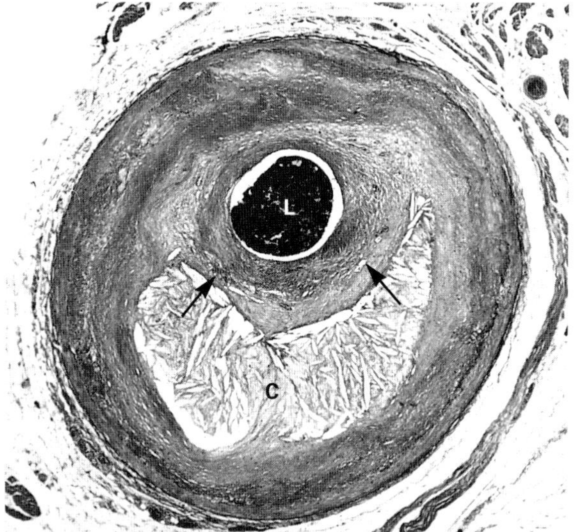

Fig. 3.4 Lipid-rich plaque — high-grade stenosis. The lumen (L) is eccentric but there is no arc of normal vessel wall. The plaque contains a lipid core (C) and has a thick fibrous cap (arrow).
Haematoxylin–eosin × 15

across the stenosis. It has been calculated that with plaques causing >75% cross-sectional area stenosis, if the arc of normal vessel wall occupies >16% of the circumference of the residual lumen of the artery, normal variation in smooth muscle tone could significantly reduce blood flow.[2]

Beneath atheromatous plaques, the media undergoes striking atrophy[3] and the internal elastic lamina is often disrupted. In concentric stenosis, the majority of the medial muscle is lost and this, associated with the thickened and rigid intima, precludes any significant variation in lumen cross-sectional area. Clinical angiographic studies confirm that a high proportion of eccentric stenosis can be varied in degree by drugs, such as ergonovine and nifedipine, but concentric stenosis remain unaltered.

Patients with coronary atheroma can therefore have stenotic segments that are fixed in the degree of stenosis and those that have the potential for undergoing some degree of alteration. The proportion of the two types of stenosis, fixed or variable, has been reported in several pathological series with divergent results. In some series, variable stenosis has been found to be predominant,[4] in other series more rare.[1] There is however considerable individual variation from patient to patient, and group data are biased by the selection of different types of patient and clinical presentation. However, it is certain that a proportion of patients with stable angina will have some segments of variable high-grade stenosis whereas others will have stenosis that is all fixed. In a pathological study confined to patients with stable angina and excluding those with diabetes, it was found that 56% of patients had at least one segment of eccentric high-grade stenosis with the potential for variation. In a small subset of patients, all the high-grade lesions were eccentric in type.[1]

Plaques may also be purely fibrous or contain a pool of extracellular lipid encapsulated within the intima. In addition to stenosis formed by different permutations of the basic characteristics of eccentric or concentric and fibrous or lipid, the majority of patients with stable exertional angina also have arterial segments in which the lumen is occluded by connective tissue within which there is more than one new vascular channel (Fig. 3.5). This appearance is regarded as indicative of recanalisation of an originally occlusive thrombus.[5] Segments in which the lumen is totally occluded by fibrous tissue but within which new vessel formation has not occurred are also thought to indicate old occlusive thrombi. Collaterals frequently develop within the adventitia of

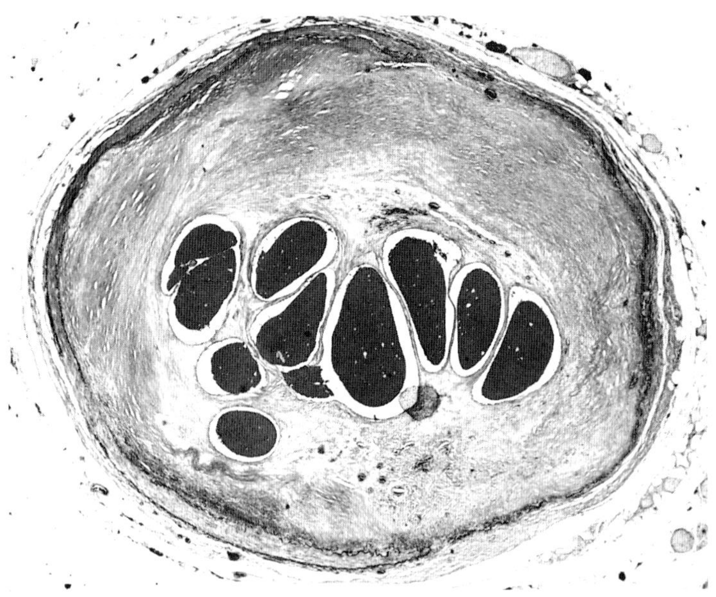

Fig. 3.5 Coronary artery recanalisation. There are 10 separate luminal channels within dense intimal fibrosis.
Haematoxylin–eosin × 16

chronically occluded vessels bridging the proximal and distal segments of artery. The presence of such recanalised or chronically occluded arterial segments at autopsy is not confined to patients who have had previous myocardial infarction; in one pathological study[1] of patients with stable angina, 85% of patients with healed infarcts were found to have such recanalised stenosis, but 65% of such patients without healed infarcts had similar arterial lesions.

Other morphological features of stenotic segments of possible functional significance include vascularisation of the intima, calcification and inflammatory cell infiltration in the adventitia. Thickening of the intima, whether focal, as in the formation of atheromatous plaques, or more diffuse leads inevitably to the appearances of new capillary vessels within the vessel wall itself. In normal human coronary arteries, the intima and media are avascular structures but beneath atheromatous plaques new capillaries extend into the media from the adventitia, breach the internal elastic lamina and reach the intima. This enhanced network of small vessels in the adventitia adjacent to coronary plaques can be easily identified in angiograms, during life and at autopsy.[6]

The stimulus for the ingrowth of capillaries to the intima is probably hypoxia of the deeper layers of the intima that would normally derive oxygen from the arterial lumen. Rupture of these small capillaries which enter the base of the plaque leads to some extravasation of red cells into the plaque. It has been postulated that this bleeding may expand the plaque from within and potentially cause thrombosis.[7] Two factors militate against the validity of this concept, which has been contested. The capillaries would be subject to an external transmitted force from the arterial lumen, which would limit bleeding. Those pathological studies which have reconstructed plaques which have a large intraplaque thrombus find that inevitably an entry point into the lipid core from the arterial lumen via a cap tear can be found. Large intraplaque thrombi also contain a large amount of fibrin and platelets rather than just extravasated red cells. It can be concluded that plaque haemorrhage from transmedial capillaries is a common but inconsequential complication of atheroma.

A heavy adventitial chronic inflammatory response is common in atherosclerotic coronary arteries. The response is largely lymphocytic (both T and B) and plasma cell in type, sometimes with the formation of lymphoid follicles. Some cases have an associated increase in mast cells in the adventitia. In part the inflammatory response is due to an immune reaction to oxidised LDL.

Unstable angina

Several clinical conditions are associated with episodes of transient myocardial ischaemia with pain at rest for which the major precipitating factor appears to be a reduction in myocardial blood flow. The ischaemia is not of sufficient duration to result in structural damage to the myocardium. Transient episodes may be silent and not associated with pain. The clinical conditions range from the crescendo type of unstable angina through variant angina of the Prinzmetal type to episodes of silent ischaemia at rest detected by Holter monitoring in patients whose clinical picture is otherwise that of stable exertional angina. The prognosis of these conditions is very diverse and it seems unlikely that a single pathophysiological mechanism can be responsible. Two basic mechanisms are thought to exist, an abnormality of vasomotor tonal responses and thrombosis, but in any individual patient it may be difficult to ascertain which is predominant.

Thrombosis and unstable angina

Patients with the crescendo form of unstable angina in whom the pain is unpredictable, comes on at rest and increases in severity or frequency are known to have a substantial risk of developing acute myocardial infarction. In the majority of cases the symptoms ultimately settle and patients may be left with exertional angina or recover completely. Early angiographic studies in such patients showed that the extent and severity of atheroma was no different to that in patients with stable angina. Unstable angina, however, is characterised by the possession of an eccentric stenotic lesion with irregular or concave outlines,[8,9] over which an intraluminal filling defect, thought to represent thrombus, is common. These angiographic appearances have been designated as type II in contrast to the smooth outlines of type I angiographic lesions found in stable angina. Post-mortem studies (Figs 3.6–3.8)[10,11] and angioscopy[12] have shown that these appearances indicate a disrupted plaque with overlying mural thrombus. The attacks of pain are mediated by combinations of intermittent complete occlusion with spontaneous lysis restoring antegrade flow within a few minutes, by superimposed local vascular spasm and by distal platelet emboli.

There is pathological evidence of intramyocardial platelet emboli in up to 40% of fatal cases of crescendo unstable angina.[13,14] Such emboli are specific for segments of myocardium downstream of arteries containing disrupted

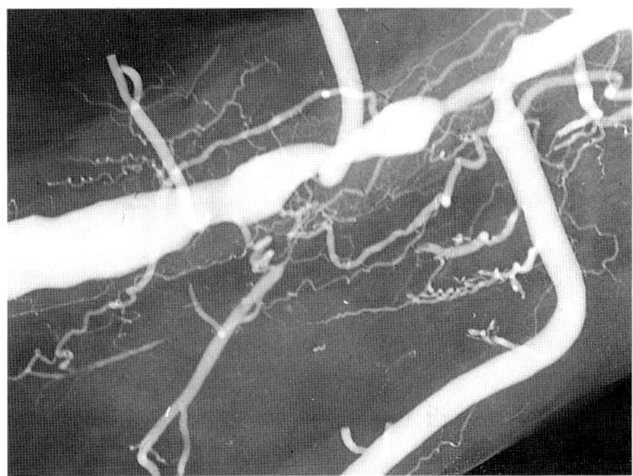

a)

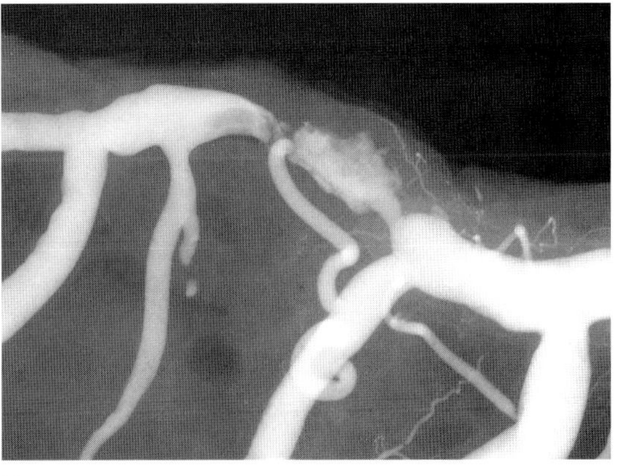

b)

Fig. 3.6 a,b Angiographic appearances of angina. In (**a**) with stable angina there are smooth indentations of the wall into the vascular lumen. In (**b**) with unstable angina there is a segment of high-grade stenosis with an irregular outline and a filling defect in the lumen.

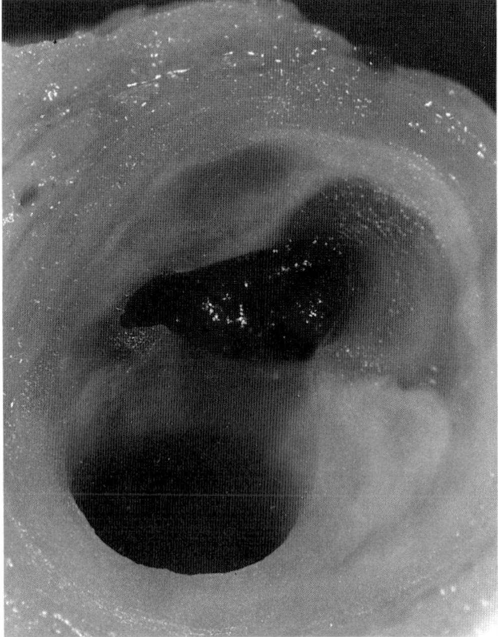

Fig. 3.7 Plaque disruption with mural thrombus. In this perfused fixed coronary artery a mass of thrombus projects into the lumen from a disrupted plaque.

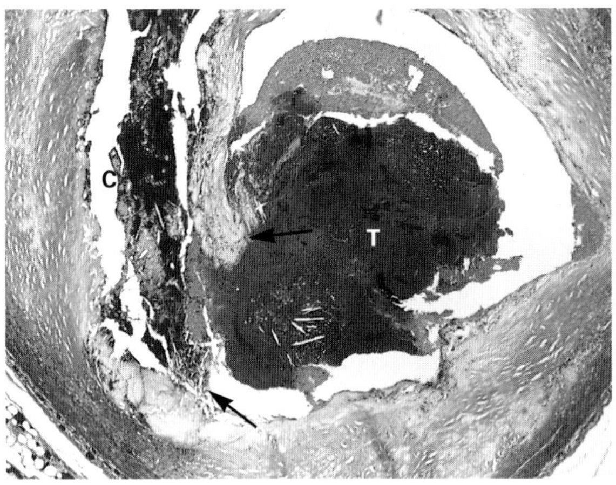

Fig. 3.8 Plaque disruption with mural thrombus. A plaque with a large lipid core (C) has undergone a cap tear (arrows) and thrombus (T) projects from the plaque into the lumen. The thrombus contains some cholesterol extruded from the plaque.
Haematoxylin–eosin × 38

plaques, confirming the embolic nature of platelet masses in the myocardium (Fig. 3.9). Peak excretion of metabolites of thromboxane[15] coincide with episodes of pain, suggesting that thrombosis and platelet activation have a role in precipitating

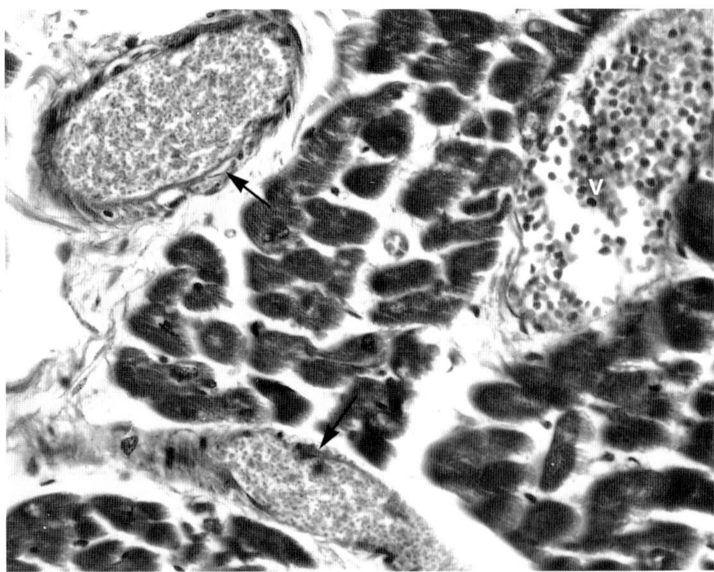

Fig. 3.9 Unstable angina — platelet emboli. Intramyocardial arteries (arrows) are plugged by a mass of platelets recognisable as small dot-like bodies which are much smaller than the red cells in an adjacent venule (V). There was a disrupted plaque with mural thrombus upstream.
Picro–Mallory trichrome stain × 160

ischaemic attacks. Circulating levels of fibrinopeptide A are significantly higher in patients with unstable angina than in those with stable angina, which suggests that thrombin generation is occurring. While the clinical concept of unstable angina is that of preservation of myocardial integrity without ECG evidence of structural damage, more sensitive tests such as plasma elevations of myocardial enzyme isoforms do show that some myocardial necrosis is present.[16]

Comparisons have been made of the tissue removed by atherectomy in cases of unstable and stable angina.[17] Overall there is an association of unstable angina with evidence of thrombus in the atherectomy material but many cases have florid smooth muscle proliferation alone, and conversely a small proportion of samples removed from subjects with stable angina contain recent thrombus.

Angina due to variations in vasomotor tone

Spasm of focal segments of the coronary artery tree is well established as the cause of attacks of rest pain and ST-segment elevation typical of the Prinzmetal type of variant angina. Many of the patients have coexistent atheroma, either with an irregular outline to the lumen or focal stenosis on angiography; pathological studies have not reported normal vessels free from atheroma in Prinzmetal's angina.[18] The segmental nature of the arterial spasm in most cases suggests that there must be a local reason for enhanced medial tone; there is some tenuous evidence of a more generalised smooth muscle abnormality in an association with oesophageal spasm, migraine and Raynaud's phenomenon.

Undoubted cases of rest pain due to spasm, superimposed on a high-grade stenosis due to an eccentric plaque, are described. In one case, the arterial lesion responsible was excised at the time of inserting vein grafts thereby establishing its nature beyond doubt.[19] Such work indicates that, for unknown reasons, a particular atheromatous lesion has acquired a hypersensitivity to vasoconstrictor stimuli. One possibility is that the endothelium at this site is deficient in the production of endothelium-derived relaxing factor. Experimental atherosclerosis, in which endothelial damage is known to occur, increases the arterial sensitivity to vasoconstrictor stimulation and in human coronary atherosclerosis the normal vasodilator action of intracoronary acetylcholine is paradoxically converted to vasoconstriction.[20] Alternative explanations for focal vascular hypersensitivity include infiltration of the adventitia by chronic inflammatory cells, which interfere with the neural release of mediators, or the release, from mast cells in the adventitia, of histamine[21] and leucotrienes which act directly on medial smooth muscle.[22] These hypotheses concerning the role of adventitial chronic inflammatory cells are based on autopsies of single cases; it is not clear why the many stenoses that have such an adventitial infiltrate do not show similar abnormalities of tonal responses.

THE PATHOLOGY OF ACUTE MYOCARDIAL INFARCTION

An understanding of myocardial infarction has to be based on the fact that the anatomy of the coronary arteries is regional, i.e. each segment of myocardium has its own blood supply with little cross-over with adjacent segments.

Anatomy of the coronary arteries

The great majority of individuals possess two coronary arteries opening from the right and left aortic sinuses respectively. The level at which the arteries arise, in relation to the junction between the aortic sinuses and the root of the aorta (supra-aortic ridge), varies. Most ostia are a few millimetres above this ridge but an origin a centimetre or more into the aorta or from the sinus itself is not unusual. The main left coronary artery varies considerably in length, from being at one extreme over a centimetre in length to, at the other extreme, being absent; in this latter case, the left anterior descending and left circumflex arteries open from the left aortic sinus by separate orifices.

The branches of the left anterior descending artery supply the anterior two-thirds of the interventricular septum and the anterior wall of the left ventricle, comprising at least 50% of the overall mass of the left ventricular myocardium. The first septal perforating branch running backward into the interventricular septum is constant in position but the epicardial branches of the left anterior descending artery vary in pattern; there may be a division into two relatively large arteries immediately after the first septal branch or a single artery may pass to the apex of the ventricle.

The left circumflex artery passes laterally in the left atrioventricular groove, and branches supply the lateral wall of the left ventricle, including the antero-lateral papillary muscle.

The right coronary artery runs in the atrioventricular groove around the right ventricle to reach the posterior wall of the left ventricle, supplying the postero-medial papillary muscle in most cases. The right ventricular myocardium is supplied by branches of the right coronary artery, the first of which, the conus branch, in approximately 30% of hearts has a small separate orifice in the right aortic sinus.

The right and the left circumflex arteries are inversely related in size (Fig. 3.10), and therefore in the proportion of the posterior wall of the left ventricle that each supplies. The term dominance is used to express this relation. In right dominant individuals (70% approximately), the posterior descending artery is derived from the right coronary artery; in left dominant individuals it is derived from the left circumflex artery. The posterior descending coronary artery supplies the posterior third of the ventricular septum by perforating branches which meet the corresponding branches of the left anterior descending coronary artery. At the apex of the left ventricle, the anterior and posterior descending arteries meet. In many hearts, the anterior descending artery is longer than the posterior descending artery and turns the apex to supply a portion of the posterior wall of the left

a)

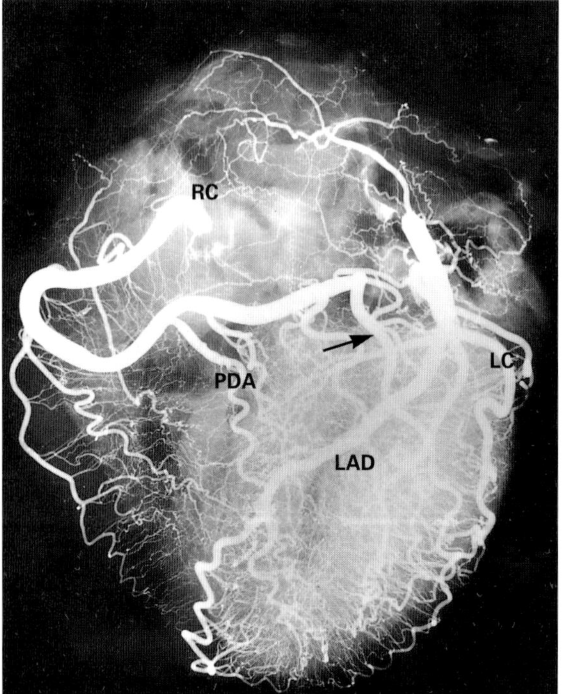

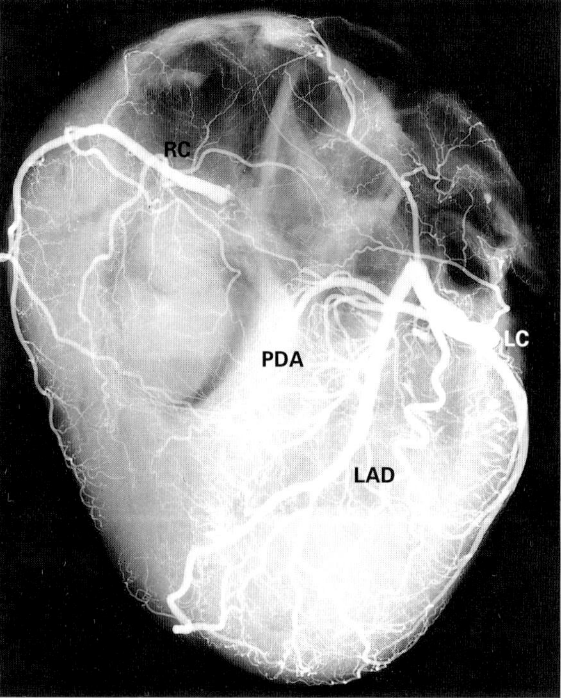

b)

Fig. 3.10 a,b Variations in normal coronary anatomy. In these post-mortem angiograms of normal hearts the rich vascular supply of the left ventricle is obvious. In (**a**) the right coronary artery is large (RC), supplies the posterior wall of the right and left ventricles, including the posterior descending artery (PDA), and extends on to the posterior wall of the left ventricle (arrow). The left circumflex artery is small (LC). In (**b**) the right coronary (RC) artery is small and the posterior descending (PDA) coronary artery arises from the left circumflex. In both hearts the left anterior descending coronary artery (LAD) supplies a very large proportion of the left ventricular muscle.

ventricle. Dominance, as defined so far, is absolute and can be determined at a glance from angiograms or by dissection of the coronary arteries. However, the blood supply to the posterior wall of the left ventricle is also important and here dominance can be used in a relative rather than an absolute sense. The right coronary artery, after giving origin to the posterior descending branch, may extend across on to the posterior wall of the left ventricle. If it does, branches supply the left ventricular myocardium until the point at which the termination of the left circumflex artery is met. In extreme cases, the left circumflex artery is absent and the right coronary continues to supply the whole lateral wall of the left ventricle. At the other extreme, the left circumflex artery crosses the posterior crux of the heart to reach and supply the right ventricle, the right coronary artery being represented only by the conus branch opening directly from the aorta.

The posterior medial papillary muscle is supplied by whichever artery, right or, more rarely, left circumflex, has reached the posterior aspect of the left ventricle. The most representative situation is for the left anterior descending artery to supply over 50% of the left ventricular mass, comprising the anterior two-thirds of the interventricular septum and about half the posterior wall, including the papillary muscle, which represent 20–30% of the left ventricular mass, and for the left circumflex artery to supply the lateral wall, including the anterolateral papillary muscle, making up 10–20% of the left ventricular mass.

Intramyocardial vasculature

The epicardial arteries throughout their courses send penetrating branches into the myocardium. The distribution of these intramyocardial vessels has been studied by microinjection with radio-opaque media by conventional anatomical techniques.[23]

The intramyocardial arteries which supply the arteriolar bed fall into two distinct groups. One has straight, non-tapering vessels of approximately 200 μm external diameter with a well developed media. These extend to the endocardial surface before breaking up into a plexus of smaller arteries. This system also supplies a straight artery running up the centre of the heads of each papillary muscle. The second system forms branches throughout the full thickness of the ventricular wall; its branches taper down rapidly to arteries of an external diameter of approximately 50 μm and these form the great bulk of intramyocardial vessels with a defined medial muscle coat. Accompanying these vessels are veins which also have well developed medial muscle although a thinner wall and larger external diameter. In normal hearts there is little communication either between the two arterial systems or between arteries and veins. In diseased hearts with stenosing coronary disease very rich cross-flow is established between both arterial systems and also by the arteriovenous connections. Such cross flow is particularly developed within the inner third of the myocardium by enlargement of vessels in the subendocardial plexus. Such intramyocardial collateral flow must be distinguished from the opening of communications between epicardial arteries which are visible angiographically. The exact site and size of the human intramyocardial vessels, which either determine the major component of resistance or are responsible for variations in flow to different regions of the myocardium, is not certain.

Collateral flow

Stenosis or occlusion of a coronary artery creates a pressure differential between the distal vessel and adjacent normal coronary vessels. Such pressure differences invoke collateral flow between the normal vessel and the distal segment of the diseased vessel.

While the epicardial coronary arteries are rightly regarded as end vessels, implying that sudden occlusion leads to ischaemic damage, this concept is physiological rather than anatomical. In a normal heart if a low viscosity fluid is injected into one coronary artery orifice it emerges from the other. Collateral flow in diseased hearts is therefore probably established by the remodelling of existing vessels rather than by neogenesis.

It is not possible to demonstrate collaterals at autopsy other than by injection techniques.

Such techniques show three levels of collateral flow. Short segments of complete occlusion may be followed by the enlarging of adventitial vessels in the immediate region and at least by post-mortem angiography can fill the distal vessel readily. The connections between adjacent coronary arteries are often small epicardial arteries or the atrial arteries. Collateral flow leads to enlargement of the artery with a characteristic corkscrew appearance on angiography. Finally, anastomoses develop within the myocardium itself with the opening of a rich subendocardial plexus of vessels which have a large lumen and thin wall. Arterio-venous communications are established, allowing good cross-flow between adjacent vascular beds.

Acute myocardial infarction — definitions

The term myocardial infarction, used correctly, means necrosis of myocytes due to a reduction or cessation in their blood supply. Providing that the subject, whether an experimental animal or a human, survives a period of 8–12 hours after the inception of necrosis the resulting pattern of necrosis can be recognised morphologically as a loss of enzyme activity in the non-viable myocardium. It must be emphasised that most morphological methods of recognising irreversible necrosis depend on survival for a sufficient period for structural changes to develop; in experimental studies, in which conditions of tissue preparation can be made optimal, a minimum of 4–6 h is required.

Any infarct can be categorised as regional, i.e. encompassed within the territory of myocardium supplied by one major coronary artery, or diffuse (Fig. 3.11). Any infarct can also be categorised as subendocardial or transmural. In addition to areas of infarction that are visible macroscopically, there are microscopic foci of necrosis which can

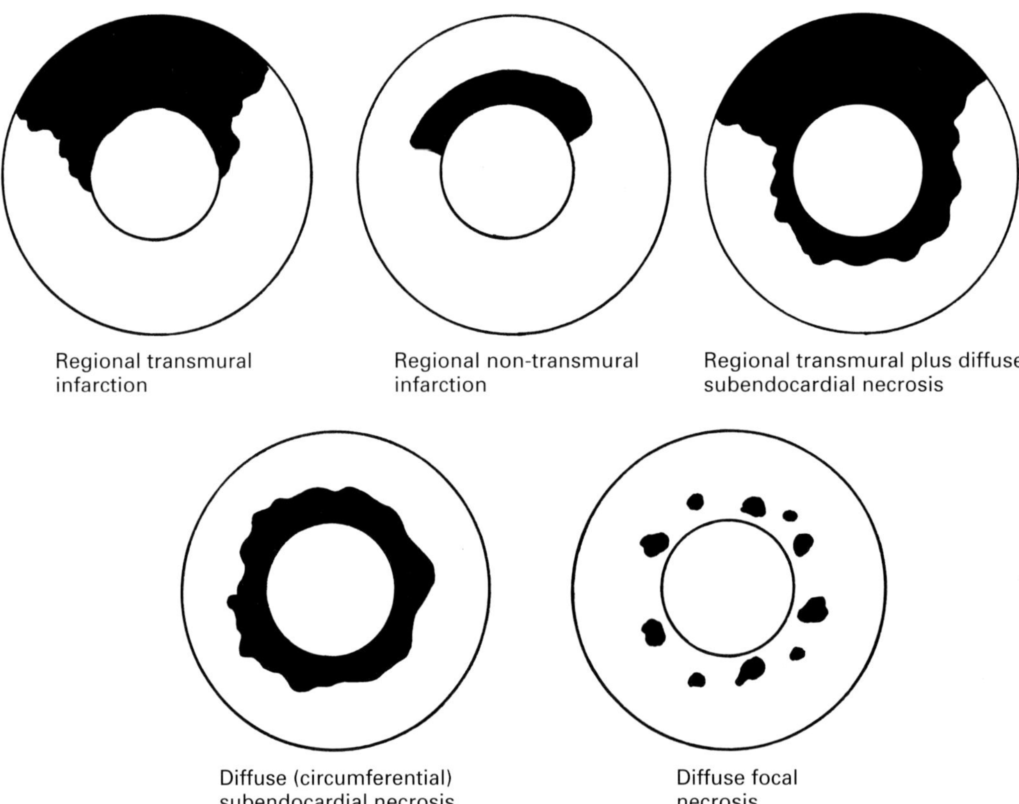

Fig. 3.11 Patterns of human myocardial infarction (necrosis).

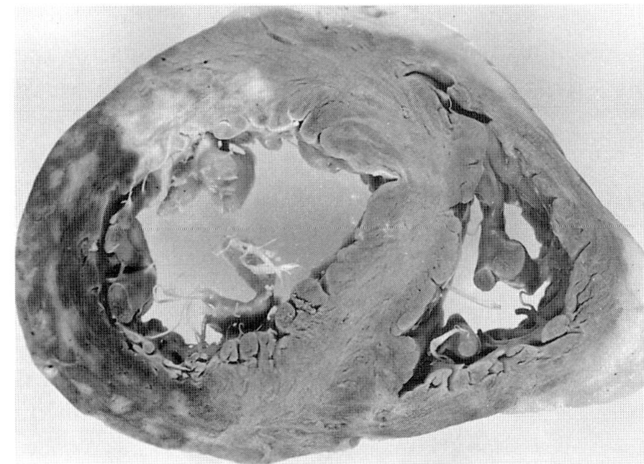

also be categorised as regional or diffuse in distribution. There is clinical and experimental evidence that there are separate pathogenetic mechanisms for these different forms of necrosis, the majority of which can be categorised as regional transmural (RTM) (Figs 3.12, 3.13), regional subendocardial (RSE), diffuse subendocardial (DSE) or focal microscopic.

Fig. 3.12 Regional myocardial infarction. By 3–4 days infarcts are easily recognised by a yellow central area with a rim of deep red tissue in fresh macroscopic specimens. This infarct is full-thickness and in the lateral wall, corresponding to an acute occlusion of the left circumflex artery.

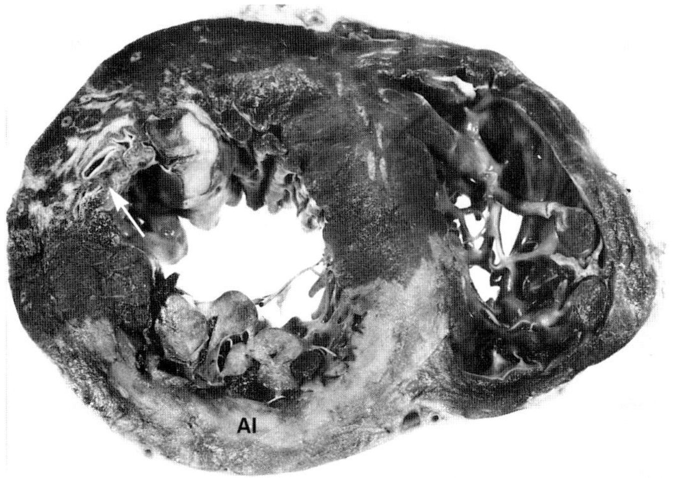

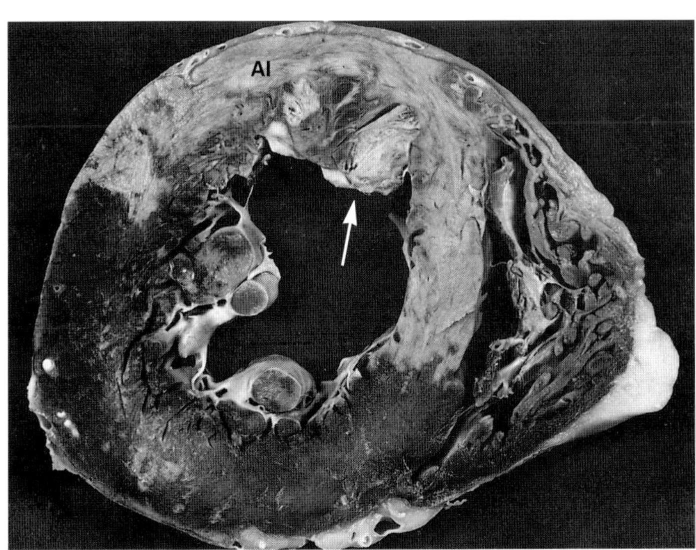

Fig. 3.13 a,b Regional transmural infarction. (**a**) A transverse slice of ventricular muscle has been stained to show succinic dehydrogenase activity. There is a transmural zone of enzyme loss indicating acute infarction (AI) involving the posterior wall of the left ventricle, the posterior third of the interventricular septum and the posteromedial papillary muscles. The area of infarction corresponds to the zone supplied by the right coronary artery. On the anterolateral wall of the left ventricle there is a non-transmural fibrous scar (arrow) indicating previous infarction. (**b**) In a transverse short axis slice of the ventricles stained for succinic dehydrogenase activity there is a transmural region of acute infarction with enzyme loss (AI) in the anterolateral and septal walls of the left ventricle. This corresponds to the area of distribution of the left anterior descending coronary artery. Mural thrombus is forming over the infarct (arrow).

Electrocardiographic changes are accurate in determining the regional distribution of necrosis but, although emphasis is often placed on the distinction between Q and non-Q wave infarction, implying that it distinguishes transmural from non-transmural infarction, pathological studies[24] show this assumption to be only partially true. Microscopic foci of necrosis probably occur in patients with ST-segment changes, but how long such elevation or depression must persist to indicate that at least some myocytes have undergone necrosis is not known. ST-segment elevation is thought to indicate subepicardial ischaemia, ST-segment depression subendocardial ischaemia; the formal proof of this is tenuous.

Pathogenesis of infarction in man

Clinical angiographic studies of Q wave regional infarction show that within the first hour the subtending artery is totally occluded in over 90% of cases, but subsequently re-opens spontaneously in up to 30% of cases.[25] Fibrinolytic therapy will restore antegrade flow in a far higher proportion of cases and during this re-opening phase angiography shows filling defects within the lumen which are thought to represent thrombus. In the re-opened vessel, a stenosis with a type II configuration is frequently present, suggesting an underlying fissured plaque. The efficacy of thrombolytic therapy in restoring flow suggests that thrombosis is the major element in the occlusion, although coexistent spasm may be present.

Pathological studies of regional transmural infarctions (Figs 3.12, 3.13)[26] have revealed that the supplying artery is totally occluded in over 90% of cases, suggesting that persistent occlusion is related to greater risk of a fatal outcome,[27] possibly because of large infarct size. Reconstruction of the microanatomy of these occlusive thrombi[11,28,29] confirms that there is an underlying disrupted plaque in approximately three quarters of cases (Figs 3.14, 3.15). At the proximal end of the occlusion within the intima there is a mass of predominantly platelet thrombus which is contiguous through a fissure in the cap with the main mass of thrombus within the lumen. Adjacent to the plaque fissure the thrombus has a high platelet content but more distally there is a higher fibrin and red blood cell content. The

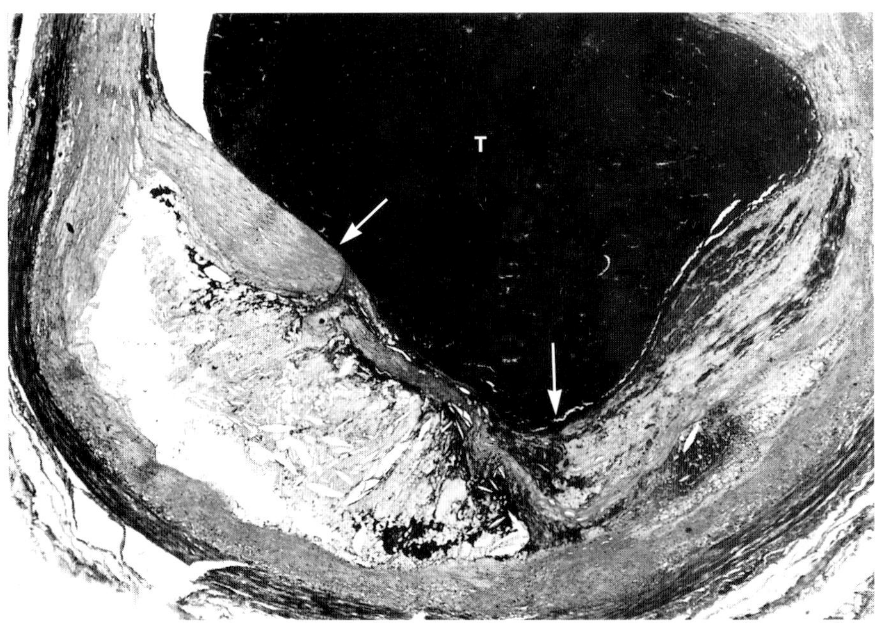

Fig. 3.14 Occlusive coronary thrombosis. A large lipid rich plaque has undergone disruption with a tear in the plaque cap (arrows). There is thrombus (T) occluding the vessel lumen. The plaque did not appear to cause high-grade stenosis prior to the disruption.
Picro–Mallory trichrome stain × 74

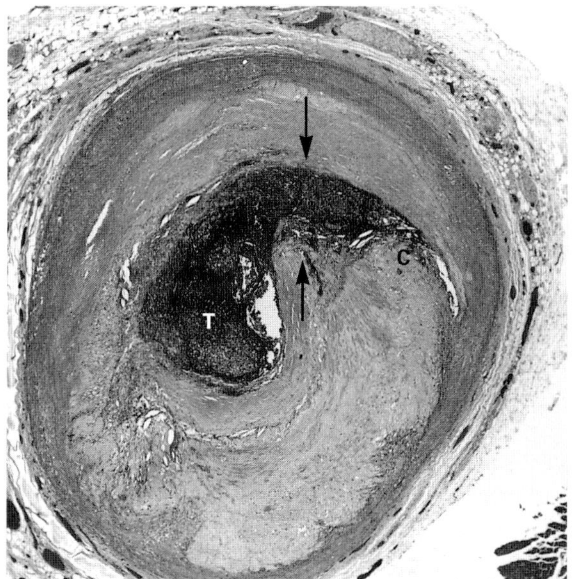

Fig. 3.15 Occlusive coronary thrombus. A plaque causing high-grade stenosis has undergone disruption (arrows) producing a typical comma shaped thrombus (T) with its tail in the plaque (C) and the head occluding the lumen.

microstructure of the thrombus is consistent with a phasic progression and the distal propagation is of a 'stasis' type, suggesting that thrombus growth continued after the vessel was occluded. Clinical evidence from radiolabelled fibrinogen supports this view. Radiolabelled fibrinogen and platelets given after the onset of infarction can be shown to localise to the occluded artery. Post-mortem studies, however, show that it is the distal tail rather than the proximal head of the thrombus which is labelled.[30]

The magnitude of the fissure varies: at one extreme the amount of intraintimal thrombosis and size of the fissure is small, needing reconstruction from serial histological sections for its detection, while at the other extreme the plaque cap is lost over a centimetre and fragments of intima and extruded lipid are mixed with thrombus occluding the lumen.

A minority (c. 25%) of occlusive thrombi associated with regional infarcts in man are not related to deep plaque injury and are due to more superficial injury. In smaller vessels such as the left marginal and posterior descending arteries, thrombosis develops at points of high-grade stenosis over intact plaques without deep intimal injury. In some of these, infiltration of the endothelium and intima by lipid macrophages is present, a phenomenon known to be associated with thrombus in experimental atheroma. This form of thrombosis may represent loss of the endothelial layer and superficial damage to the intima, exposing collagen to platelets. Only in small arteries or at points of high-grade stenosis is the stimulus for thrombosis sufficient to produce occlusion.

Autopsy studies show that regional subendocardial (non-transmural) infarction (Fig. 3.16) in man is not uncommon, particularly in association with unstable angina or in sudden ischaemic death. Pathological studies confirm that, in common with transmural infarction, there is recent plaque disruption in the supplying artery. In contrast to transmural infarction, there is a far lower incidence of total arterial occlusion[31] and a correspondingly higher incidence of the distal segment of the artery being patent and filling either by antegrade flow over mural thrombus or more rarely by well-developed collateral flow. Distal propagation of thrombus is virtually never found in non-transmural infarction. This pathological distinction is very similar to that found on clinical angiography between Q-wave and non-Q-wave infarction, where rich collateral development is common in the latter situation.[32] This is also in accord with the view that in non-transmural infarction there remains viable myocardium at risk should another acute thrombotic episode develop in the same artery. There are also differences in the histological structure of transmural and non-transmural infarct; the latter is far more frequently made up of coalescence of focal areas of necrosis of different ages.

Diffuse (non-regional) subendocardial necrosis (Fig. 3.17) may occur in man in the absence of any structural coronary artery obstruction and reflects an overall fall in myocardial perfusion accentuated in its effect on the subendocardial zone. The vulnerability of the subendocardial zone to ischaemic damage can be confirmed, and in part explained, by studies in animal models. Subendocardial muscle, as compared with subpericardial muscle, has a 20% higher oxygen

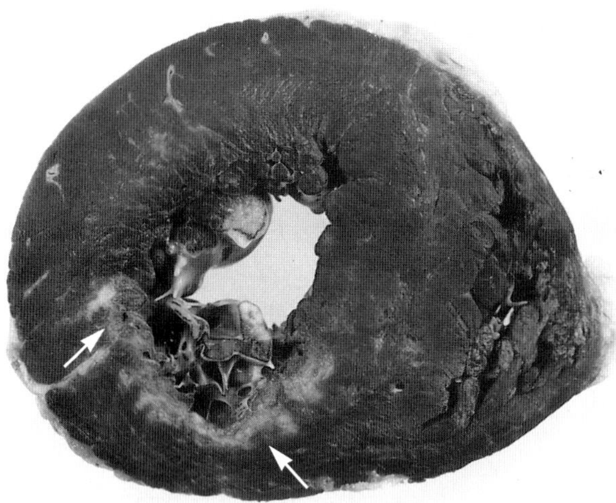

Fig. 3.16 Non-transmural regional infarction. In a short axis transection of the ventricles stained for enzyme activity there is a regional area of enzyme loss (arrows) but this is confined to the subendocardial zone.

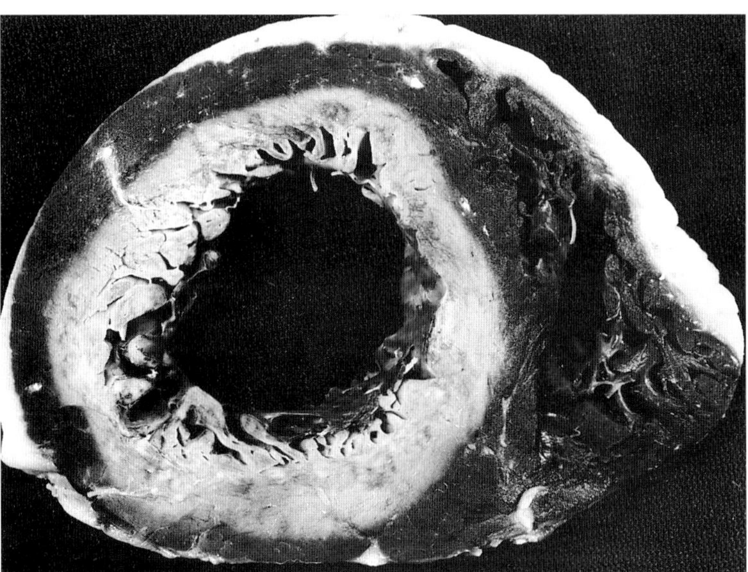

Fig. 3.17 Diffuse subendocardial infarction. In this transverse section of the ventricles stained for enzyme activity there is a circumferential subendocardial zone of enzyme loss. The outline is smooth and typical of myocardial hypoperfusion in the context of normal coronary arteries.

utilisation per gram of tissue, produces lactate readily, undergoes necrosis first under ischaemic conditions and, in conscious animals, has a higher resting blood flow.[33] Significant decreases in aortic diastolic pressure, reduction in diastolic duration and increase in left ventricular diastolic pressure all produce a decrease in the proportion of total flow entering the subendocardial muscle. The physiological basis of subendocardial underperfusion has been shown to result from the

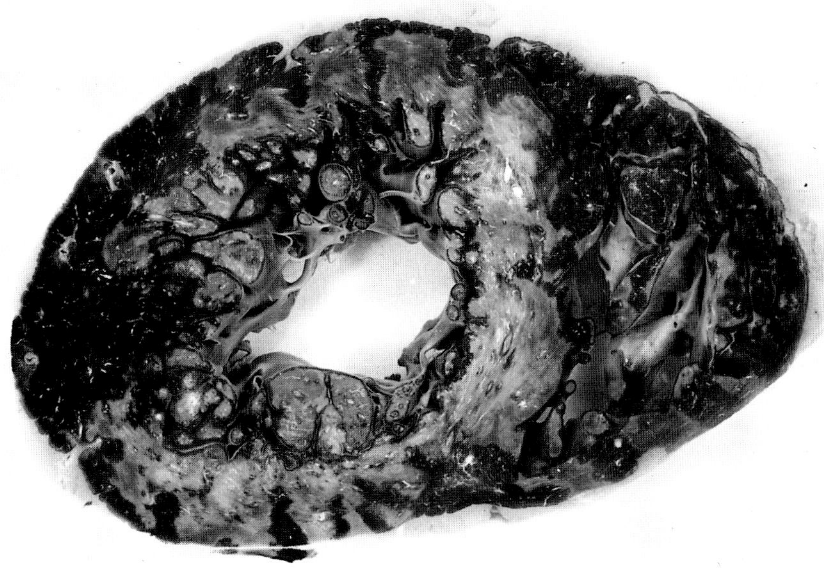

Fig. 3.18 Myocardial infarction and diffuse necrosis in cardiogenic shock. In this transverse slice of ventricular muscle stained for enzyme activity there is a regional area of enzyme loss involving the whole thickness of the septum. In addition there is diffuse subendocardial necrosis involving the papillary muscles. The diffuse necrosis has an irregular outline which contrasts with the smoother outline in Figure 3.17. Irregular necrosis is most typical of general hypoperfusion superimposed on diffuse coronary disease.

higher pressure generated in the subendocardial zone in systole; as a result, the intramyocardial vessels of this zone are empty and offer greater impedance to reflow in diastole. Subendocardial necrosis may also occur in carbon monoxide poisoning and prolonged hypoglycaemia. Diffuse subendocardial necrosis is common in human end-stage triple-vessel disease, particularly when small vessels are involved as in diabetes mellitus and hypercholesterolaemia. Diffuse subendocardial necrosis may develop when regional infarction is complicated by cardiogenic shock (Fig. 3.18). The central zones of the papillary muscle are the most vulnerable component of the subendocardial tissues and undergo necrosis first. At autopsy, many patients with a large regional infarct can be observed to have recent necrosis of the centre of the contralateral papillary muscle.

Multifocal microscopic foci of necrosis (Fig. 3.19) are of very diverse origin. In the subendocardial zone they appear to represent an early stage of more confluent necrosis and are almost ubiquitous at the margins of larger areas

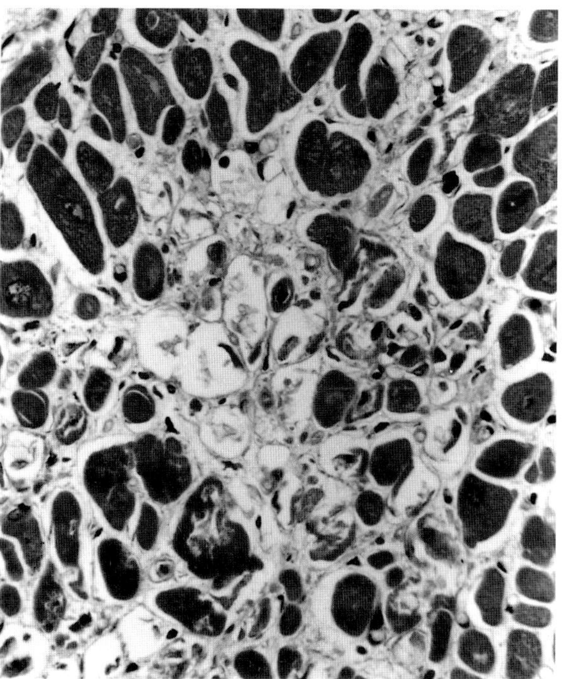

Fig. 3.19 Focal microscopic myocardial necrosis. There is a focus of myocyte loss without destruction of the stroma. Within the focus of damage there is a mixed inflammatory cell infiltrate where macrophages predominate. Such foci heal to leave small focal stellate scars.

of infarction. In the subpericardial zone microscopic foci of necrosis are related to the occurrence of intramyocardial platelet emboli.[13,14] Any patient dying after prolonged hypoxia or hypotension will have these microscopic foci of necrosis as a preliminary stage of diffuse non-regional ischaemic damage. In severe left ventricular hypertrophy such microscopic foci of necrosis are common without obvious impairment of coronary blood flow or hypoxia. High catecholamine levels, both iatrogenic or natural, as in raised intracranial pressure, are also causes of these small foci of myocardial necrosis. Modern treatment with very high doses of inotropic agents to sustain cardiac output leads to such foci of necrosis. The 'myocarditis' reported to occur in patients with phaeochromocytomas reflects the inflammatory response to small foci of necrosis due to high levels of catecholamines.

METABOLIC AND STRUCTURAL CONSEQUENCES OF EXPERIMENTAL CORONARY ARTERY OCCLUSION

Animal models provide insight into the structural and metabolic events that occur in human infarction.[34] A limitation of these models is that they represent an abrupt cessation of flow rather than the intermittent obstruction which precedes the final occlusion in many episodes of human infarction. Nevertheless, the structural changes bear a very close similarity to those seen in human infarction.

The experimental model used most frequently is ligation of the left circumflex coronary artery in the anaesthetised dog. Within 1–2 min of ligation a portion of the lateral wall of the left ventricle ceases to contract. A majority of the dogs survive but a minority develop increasing numbers of ventricular ectopic beats which culminate in the sudden onset of ventricular fibrillation. In those that survive a minimum of 8–12 h, autopsy reveals an area of infarcted muscle in the lateral wall of the left ventricle. The size of the infarct varies depending on the degree of collateral formation which existed previously and on the basic coronary artery anatomy.

Functional changes

Myocardial ischaemia can be defined as a level of ATP consumption above that which can be provided by a particular coronary blood flow.[35] The characteristics of myocardial metabolism mean that such ischaemia is translated into structural damage within a relatively short time. Within 20 s following complete coronary occlusion systolic contraction diminishes and ceases by 1–2 min. The electrocardiogram changes by 30 s. If flow is re-established within 20–40 min, necrosis can be totally prevented; if flow is not re-established, some myocyte necrosis is inevitable.

Biochemical changes

Seconds after coronary arterial occlusion tissue oxygen levels fall in the affected segment of myocardium and mitochondrial aerobic glycolysis ceases.[35] Anaerobic glycolysis becomes the only source of new high-energy phosphates using glycogen as a substrate. Creatinine phosphate levels fall to virtually zero within 2–3 min and are the first back-up system to regenerate ATP from adenosine diphosphate (ADP) by donation of a high energy phosphate group. ATP levels within the cell begin to fall significantly only after 2–3 min and cannot therefore be the immediate cause of cessation of contraction which begins to decline within 20 beats of the induction of ischaemia. Intracellular acidosis appears within this time-span and may directly affect contractile protein reaction with calcium; intracellular acidosis, in part, reflects lactate production from glycogen stores; the depletion of stainable glycogen granules is the first morphological evidence of ischaemia. Phosphate also accumulates within the myocyte very rapidly following the breakdown of creatinine phosphate.

Within seconds of ischaemia, there is also evidence of a membrane functional abnormality with loss of intracellular potassium ions probably responsible for the rapid development of alterations in the configuration of the action potential. The intracellular sodium levels do not change initially. Brief periods of ischaemia can be reversed without leading to tissue necrosis. The best indication of irreversible cell damage is disruption of the cell membrane; such changes can be detected by electron microscopy after 40 min of ischaemia.[36] The biochemical events leading to the transition from reversible to irreversible ischaemia are not entirely clear. It is tempting to postulate that membrane integrity is energy-dependent and that irreversible damage is the result of the loss of control of intracellular ionic and osmolar homoeostasis. However, the degree of necrosis does not directly correlate with levels of ATP and, although restoration of ATP production is a necessary prerequisite for survival, it is not the key factor. The increasing acidosis and calcium accumulation within the myocyte activates phospholipases in the cell membrane but such changes are probably very late and associated with the development of structural changes. The rise in intracellular calcium is due to an increased influx; an excess of intracellular calcium is known to inhibit mitochondrial ATP production and to destabilise membranes.

Structural changes following experimental infarction

Ultrastructural changes can be observed within the reversible phase of ischaemia, including mitochondrial swelling and glycogen depletion. Within 40 min of total occlusion the changes are more severe, including disruption of cristae within swollen mitochondria, sarcoplasmic swelling, clumping of chromatin within the nuclei and total loss of glycogen; irreversible change has occurred once granular electron-dense deposits of calcium appear within mitochondria and there are breaks in the cell membrane.

Although ultrastructural changes occur within 40 min of occlusion, changes visible on light microscopy cannot be recognised before at least 4–8 h have elapsed. The first recognisable histological feature is an accumulation of polymorphs within the interstitial tissues which may start as early as 4 h and last for up to 3 days. Beyond this time, macrophages are the dominant cells. Individual muscle cells become hyper-eosinophilic (coagulative necrosis) with nuclear pyknosis followed by loss of cross-striations and by 4–5 days they have disintegrated, to be phagocytosed by macrophages. Perfusion within the central zone of an infarct is absent, because of persistent occlusion of the major artery and destruction of the capillary bed by the necrotic process. Thus, within this central zone, the changes described above are retarded or absent. Repair of these infarcts is dependent on a rim of granulation tissue at the junction with viable tissue which contains intact perfused capillaries. Fibroblasts extend inward into the infarct from about 7–10 days; the whole process takes up to 8 weeks to produce a solid mass of fibrous tissue.

Evolution of acute infarction and reperfusion injury

Experimental models provide an opportunity to study the evolution of infarction by removing the arterial clip and re-establishing flow at varying times; sacrifice 4 days later allows the extent of necrosis to be identified on light microscopy. Such work reveals that infarction is not an instantaneous process in which all the myocardial cells at risk undergo death at the same moment. Infarcts reperfused after intervals longer than 6 h are no different morphologically to those that have not been reperfused. The infarct is transmural and extends from endocardium to pericardium. Comparison of non-perfused and reperfused infarcts at time-intervals up to a maximum of 6 h after occlusion shows that re-establishing blood flow reduces the infarct size by a factor related to time. This reduction in size is in the depth to which infarction extends through the wall of the subendocardial zone and not in the centrifugal extent of the infarct.[37] Limitation of infarction by reperfusion within the period from 40 min to 4–6 h is therefore due to sparing of the sub-pericardial zone; this has given rise to the concept that infarction spreads as a wavefront through the ventricular wall from endocardium to pericardium over 6 h. Although there has been much clinical interest in the concept of reduction in infarct size in man by reperfusion, the failure of reperfusion of experimentally induced infarction to limit spread in a lateral direction strongly suggests that a similar state will exist in man. The therapeutic hope must be to reduce the number of infarcts that progress to become transmural.

A comparison of infarcted areas that have been reperfused with those in which flow was not re-established reveals significant functional and structural differences. Within minutes of reperfusion, the myocardial cells undergo explosive swelling due to water entering the cell. Calcium ions also pour into the cell, invoking focal shunting together of sarcomeres forming 'contraction bands' within the cell, recognisable on light microscopy. This tonic contracture often disrupts the cell, leading to extrusion of mitochondria into the interstitial spaces. Contraction band necrosis is recognisable histologically within 20 min of the onset of infarction in contrast to the traditional form of 'coagulative' necrosis which requires survival for at least 4–6 h before it is recognisable.

Reactive free radicals toxic to cell membranes and organelles are known to develop in ischaemic myocardium. Further production of such radicals occurs on reperfusion. Potential sources include the myocytes, polymorphs and endothelial cells. Myocyte damage releases complement activation factors[38] leading to adhesion of polymorphs to capillary endothelium and their passage into the interstitial tissues. This accumulation of polymorphs in the tissue is the first morphological feature of necrosis recognisable on light microscopy, in both human and experimental infarction. Polymorphs within the tissues release cytotoxic factors including free radicals, such as oxygen, and enzymes such as elastase. Reperfusion is also associated with evidence of microvascular damage which may result in a progressive decrease in blood flow (no-flow phenomenon) in areas of ischaemic damage following reperfusion.[39] At a structural level, this is associated with the obliteration of the capillary lumen by endothelial swelling and the formation of plugs of polymorphs and red blood cells. Interstitial haemorrhage and oedema are present, reflecting capillary damage. In man and in animals, a characteristic macroscopic appearance of haemorrhagic infarction is produced. The mechanism of endothelial damage may involve interactions with neutrophils and also production of free radicals within the endothelium itself; in animal experiments a range of scavengers or inhibitors of free radical production will reduce the degree of vascular damage, as judged by endothelial swelling and the number of polymorph plugs, as well as reducing infarct size. The concordance of these two effects makes it difficult to determine if the protective effect is primarily on the myocyte or on the vasculature.

MORPHOLOGICAL CHANGES IN HUMAN MYOCARDIAL INFARCTION

The microscopic appearances of human myocardial infarcts are complex. Some regional infarcts are a single area of necrosis, which is apparently identical in structure although there is always an irregular lateral border with focal areas of viable myocardium mixed with necrotic areas. A surviving subendocardial band of muscle up to 10 cells in thickness is also almost universal. The central zone of such infarcts comprises totally necrotic myocytes with no vascular perfusion. In contrast, other infarcts appear to represent the confluence of multifocal areas of necrosis of different ages. Such appearances suggest that in some cases arterial obstruction is complete and sudden, whereas in others it is staccato in origin with repeated episodes of occlusion and reperfusion. Although there are complicated descriptions of the microscopic changes designed to date exactly the onset of infarct they can provide a rough approximation only because the process of necrosis does not involve every myocardial cell at risk at the same moment and the reparative process does not proceed at an identical rate throughout the infarcted area.

Coagulation necrosis is the typical appearance of myocardial muscle cells seen in well-established regional transmural infarction following complete cessation of blood flow to the area. The muscle cells become hypereosinophilic but otherwise appear little affected until 24 h, following which the cross-striations vanish and the myofibrils begin to coalesce as granular debris (Fig. 3.20). The earliest histologically recognisable changes at 12–24 h is the accumulation of polymorphs within the interstitial tissue (Fig. 3.21).

In contraction band necrosis (Fig. 3.22), dense eosinophilic transverse bands are present within the muscle cell. These represent telescoped sarcomeres and the cell is often greatly shortened

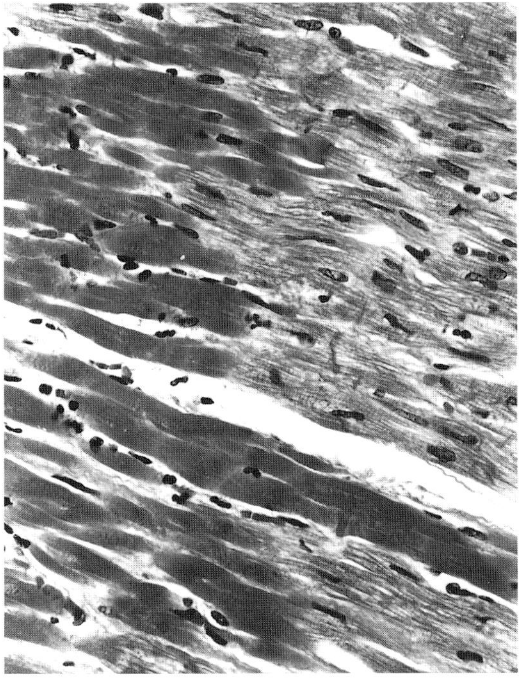
a)

in length. Such cells are often contiguous at the intercalated disc with an apparently normal cell. This form of necrosis is more common in situations in which flow is known to have been restored; in man, as in the experimental model, the morphological changes probably represent a reperfusion phenomenon.

In any area of necrosis, a distinction has to be made between those instances in which the whole tissue is dead, including the stroma and vascular component and those in which only the muscle cells have died. The former is often known as colliquative necrosis and usually found in the centre of regional transmural infarcts. The reparative process takes place only at the margins where the infarct abuts on to tissue with viable stroma and vessels. Amorphous hyaline muscle fibres, which have undergone little change other than total loss of striations, and nuclei may persist for many weeks or months incarcerated in the centre of such infarcts. From 3–5 days, macrophages, fibroblasts and capillaries begin to

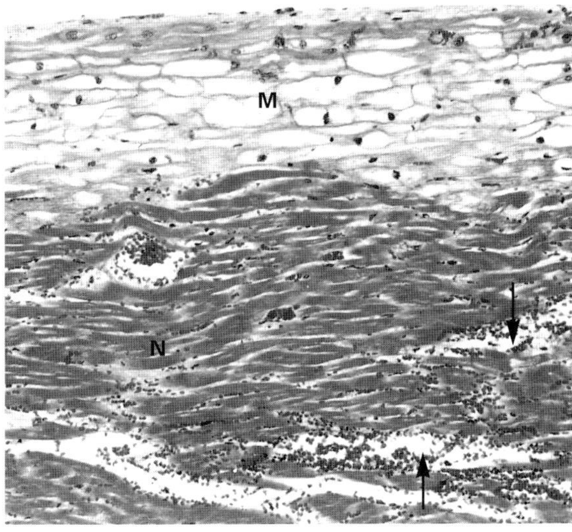

b)

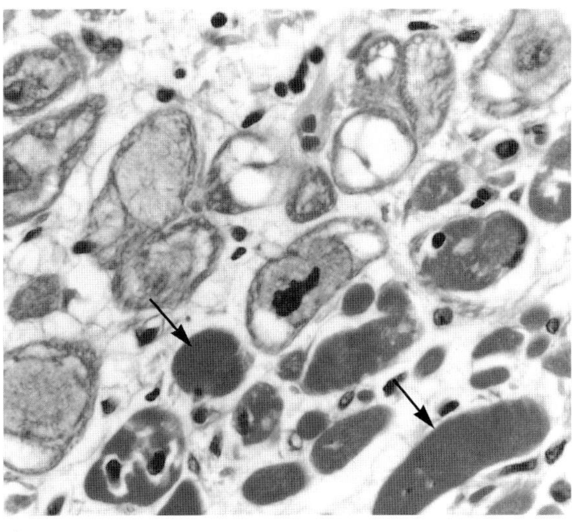
c)

Fig. 3.20 a,b,c Microscopic changes in infarction. (**a**) The myocytes undergoing necrosis have become deeply eosinophilic but no pronounced polymorph response has developed. The surviving myocytes are mixed with the dead myocytes at the margin of this infarct which was approximately 18 hours in duration by clinical data. (**b**) There is a zone of necrosis in which the myocytes are hypereosinophilic and undergoing coagulative necrosis (N). All nuclear detail has gone. Some red cell extravasation (arrow) has occurred into the interstitial tissue, suggesting that reperfusion may have occurred. Adjacent to the dead myocytes is a zone (M) in which the cells are empty and vacuolated (myocytolysis) but nuclei are still present. Such myocytes are thought to be viable but inert (hibernating). Infarction was 3 days in duration by history. (**c**) At the margins of an area of infarction myocytes often appear vacuolated with large vesicular nuclei. These are thought to be viable and undergoing a repair or hypertrophic process. Adjacent myocytes which are shrunken and eosinophilic (arrow) are not viable.
(**a**) Haematoxylin–eosin × 105
(**b**) Haematoxylin–eosin × 60
(**c**) Haematoxylin–eosin × 175

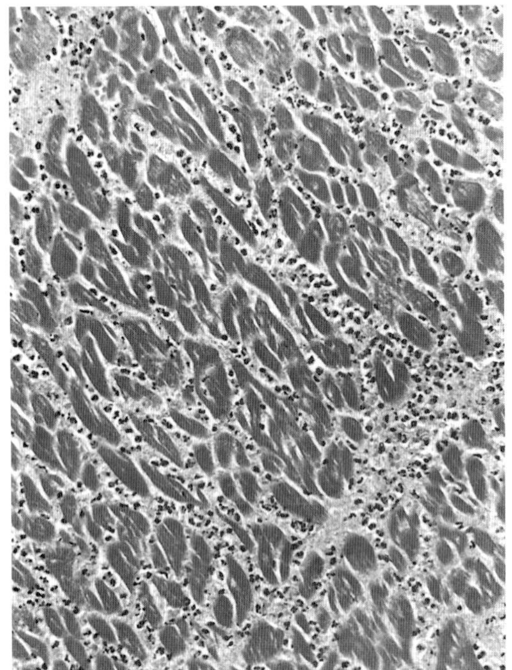

Fig. 3.21 Microscopic changes in infarction. The earliest sign of necrosis is that some myocytes appear hypereosinophilic and a little shrunken in association with infiltration of the interstitial tissue by polymorphs. 24 hours by history. Haematoxylin–eosin × 60

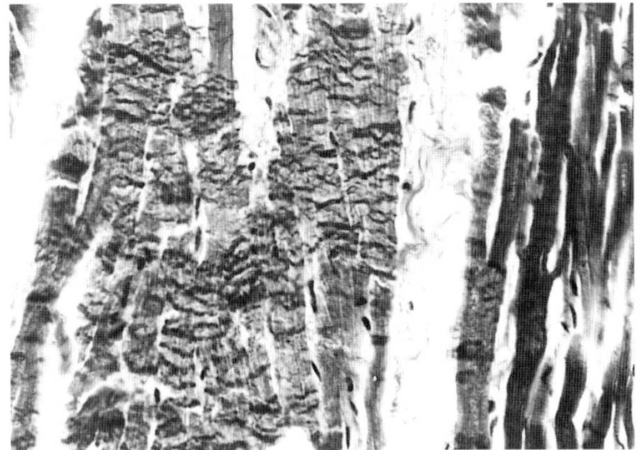

Fig. 3.22 Microscopic changes in infarction. The myocytes show brightly eosinophilic cross banding. Such appearances of contraction bands suggest reperfusion has occurred and can be seen as early as 6 hours but only occur with reperfusion and are therefore often absent. Haematoxylin–eosin × 95

extend into the infarct from the periphery (Fig. 3.23). Collagen deposition begins by 7–10 days and may take many weeks to transform the infarct into a fibrous scar. The ingrowth of capillaries into the area of infarction is mediated by release, within the infarct, of a myocardial angiogenesis factor closely related in structure to angiogenesis factors elaborated by tumour cells.

In areas of infarction in which the stroma has not undergone necrosis, the reparative process is far more rapid. In part, this may be due to the smaller size of the foci of necrosis but it is also due to the presence of viable stromal cells within the area. In such areas, the myofibrillary structure of the muscle is lost, leading to the formation of hyaline masses after which macrophages appear within the sheath of the original muscle cells. The stroma collapses and coalesces to allow some proliferation of collagen to leave ultimately a small focal scar, often containing some residual lipofuscin. Microscopic focal areas of acute necrosis in which the stroma has survived are common in ischaemic heart disease, particularly at the margins of large areas of necrosis. They are also characteristic of microembolic myocardial damage. Such foci are also found in severe cardiac hypertrophy irrespective of the presence or absence of significant coronary atheroma; a range of factors, including excess catecholamine levels, thyrotoxicosis and potassium deficiency, can lead to similar foci.

Myocytolysis is a further expression of ischaemic damage to myocardial cells (Fig. 3.20). The cells become large and vacuolated, often to the point at which virtually no myofibrils remain. At the same time, the nuclei persist and mitochondrial enzyme activity remains. The appearance is often seen immediately beneath the endocardium or around blood vessels within areas which otherwise show conventional coagulative necrosis. The change is thought to indicate muscle cells which have lost the ability to maintain normal ionic gradients with the interstitial fluid and are only just viable. There is some evidence, based on biopsies taken at the time of aortocoronary bypass grafting, that myocytes showing moderate degrees of myocytolysis can revert to normal over a prolonged period; this finding forms a potential morphological basis for a chronic stunned or hibernating myocardium in which function returns after revascularisation.[40]

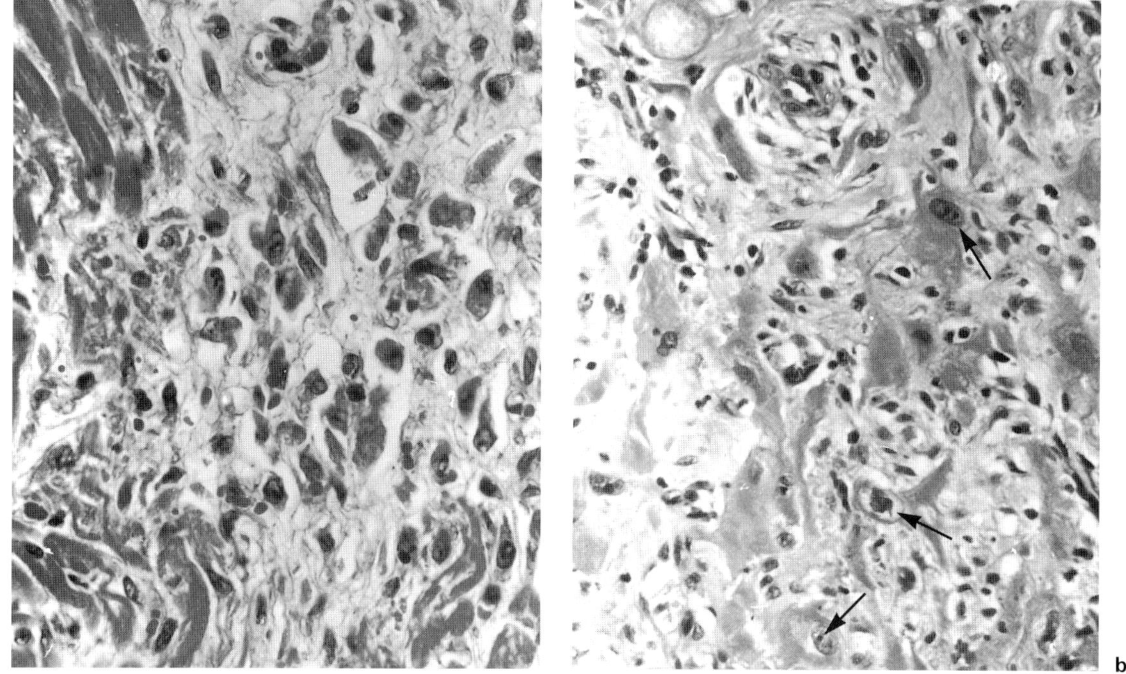

Fig. 3.23 a,b Microscopic changes in infarction. (**a**) At the margin of an area of infarction there is intense macrophage accumulation and proliferation of fibroblasts and vascular ingrowth is occurring. (**b**) At the margin of this area of infarction fibroblast proliferation is surrounding isolated surviving myocytes (arrows) which may develop considerable nuclear enlargement. Such fibrosis leads to irregularly arranged islands of myocardial tissue embedded in scars.
(**a**) Haematoxylin–eosin × 160
(**b**) Haematoxylin–eosin × 160

FACTORS INFLUENCING INFARCT SIZE

Thrombotic occlusion of a coronary artery leads to a segment of myocardium being 'at risk'. The actual mass of muscle that has undergone infarction by 6–12 h, however, may be significantly less than the mass at risk. In man, blood flow may be restored in an antegrade manner by spontaneous or therapeutic lysis of the occluding thrombus; this mechanism may be a major factor in the production of non-transmural rather than transmural infarction. Infarct size is also influenced by the degree of collateral flow. There are considerable interspecies differences in the degree to which collateral flow exists between adjacent arteries in the epicardium of normal hearts. The importance of collaterals can be judged by the relation of time to the proportion of the area of myocardium at risk that has undergone necrosis when a major coronary artery is ligated. In the guinea pig, collateral flow is so rich that no infarction develops. In the pig, the area at risk is virtually all irreversibly damaged by 1 h; in the dog, 6 h are needed for an equivalent degree of necrosis to occur. Man lies somewhere between these two extremes. Collaterals develop following the creation of a pressure gradient between two vascular beds. In the pig such collaterals develop in the subendocardial zone of the myocardium; in the dog they are epicardial. In man, collateral development is more likely to occur in patients who have stenosis that predates the development of thrombosis. Collateral flow may completely prevent infarction following complete occlusion of a major coronary artery. In man, collateral development takes place on the epicardial surface, where enlarged, rather tortuous vessels develop linking of separate regional territories, and by a vascular plexus in the subendocardial zone of the left ventricle. However, despite the presence of well-developed collateral vessels, minimal resistance is considerably higher than in a normal vascular bed. Canine collateral vessels develop a new medial muscle coat with vasoconstrictor responses; however, nothing is known about the responses of human collaterals. In man, when antegrade flow is re-established by organisation of thrombi in segments of artery occluded for some time, or occurs in collateral vessels in the adventitia, flow probably develops far too slowly to influence infarct size. Such means of re-establishing flow, however, may influence whether postinfarct angina develops. Collateral flow can be reliably demonstrated at post-mortem only by angiography; consequently it is not widely studied by pathologists.

FACTORS INFLUENCING PROGNOSIS AFTER REGIONAL TRANSMURAL INFARCTION

Intensive care in the first 48 h of acute myocardial infarction is orientated to the recognition of ventricular fibrillation followed by resuscitation by defibrillation; in effect, sudden deaths are avoided. Even small infarcts can cause sudden ventricular fibrillation.[41] By 48 h, the risk of ventricular arrhythmias is virtually over, providing no further ischaemic myocardial necrosis occurs. Infarct size, i.e. the proportion of the total left ventricular muscle mass which has been lost, is directly related to the subsequent mortality. Cardiogenic shock is a major cause of mortality and occurs in patients whose infarcts involve >40% of the total left ventricular muscle mass.[42] It is these patients who enter a vicious cycle of hypoperfusion and progressive subendocardial infarction.

ATRIAL ARRHYTHMIAS IN ACUTE MYOCARDIAL INFARCTION

Acute sinus node dysfunction is commonly seen in the acute stages of infarction and reflects a multifactorial problem which resolves in the majority of cases. The range of putative mechanisms are well reviewed by James.[43] They include occlusion either proximal to or within the nodal artery. Although such instances have been described, they are rare. Infarction of the node and surrounding atrial muscle is also described. The node is immediately adjacent to the pericardium and will be involved 'pari passu' in any pericarditic process. The reversibility of sinus node dysfunction in most cases of acute infarction suggests that factors such as local hypoxia, acidosis and hyperkalaemia are responsible rather than permanent structural damage. Atrial fibrillation has similar associations but is significantly more common if atrial infarction is present.

CONDUCTION DEFECTS IN ACUTE INFARCTION

The pathogenesis, pathology and prognosis of atrioventricular block complicating postero-inferior infarction differ from those of anterior infarction.

In posterior infarction, the clinical features suggest that the phenomenon is one of reversible nodal dysfunction. Pathological studies show that there is an occlusion due to thrombosis in the artery giving rise to the nodal supply.[44] The thrombus, however, very rarely extends into the nodal artery itself and, in most instances, the node does not have histological evidence of gross ischaemic damage; indeed, the majority of patients who survive revert to sinus rhythm. The mechanism of the nodal inhibition has been postulated to be due to temporary hypoxia or to excess potassium ions released from adjacent necrotic myocardium. This necrotic myocardium could lie within the adjacent atrial muscle[45] or the upper interventricular septum, whose venous drainage passes back across the central fibrous body and through the nodal area. The rare cases of permanent nodal damage following posterior infarction are associated with occlusion of the nodal artery itself probably by emboli from more proximal thrombi. The size of a posterior-inferior infarct does not seem to be important in the pathogenesis of atrioventricular block.

In contrast, anterior infarction causes atrioventricular block by involving both bundle branches, either in potentially reversible hypoxic damage including myocytolysis or frank necrosis. As the infarcts must be far larger to affect both

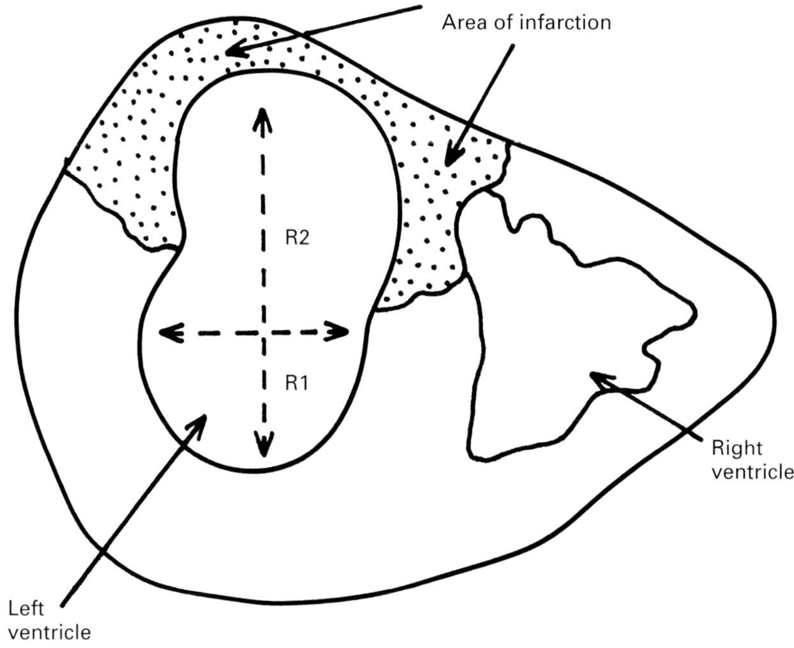

Fig. 3.24 Infarct expansion. In infarct expansion the area of infarction does not increase in area but stretches and thins bulging outward. This leads to the ventricular cavity being increased in diameter in one plane but not another (R1 <R2).

branches, they carry a worse prognosis. The high incidence of necrosis of the bundle branches is associated with a significant risk of residual conduction defects in those who do survive.

PATHOLOGICAL COMPLICATIONS OF ACUTE INFARCTION

Infarct extension and expansion

Stretching and thinning of the infarcted tissue (Figs 3.24–3.27)[46] within the first few days is associated with a high mortality and may progress to cardiac rupture. Such expansion is a feature of anterior transmural infarcts that involve >10% of the total left ventricular mass; infarct expansion carries an increased risk of developing mural thrombus. The enlargement of the infarct is due to combinations of simple stretching and tearing or sliding of muscle bundles relative to each other. The importance of such expansion is that a

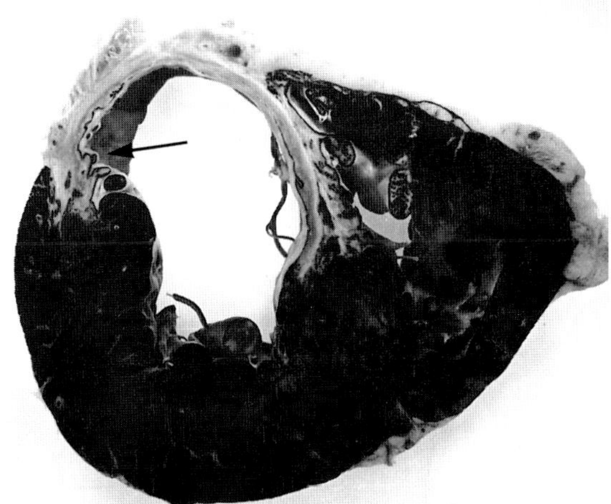

Fig. 3.25 Infarct expansion and ventricular remodelling. An anterior infarct has undergone expansion and thinning. Healing by fibrosis has fixed the shape of the expanded infarct and the free wall of the rest of the ventricle has undergone wall thickening due to hypertrophy. At one margin of the infarct (arrow) there are loops of surviving subendocardial muscle in the scar.

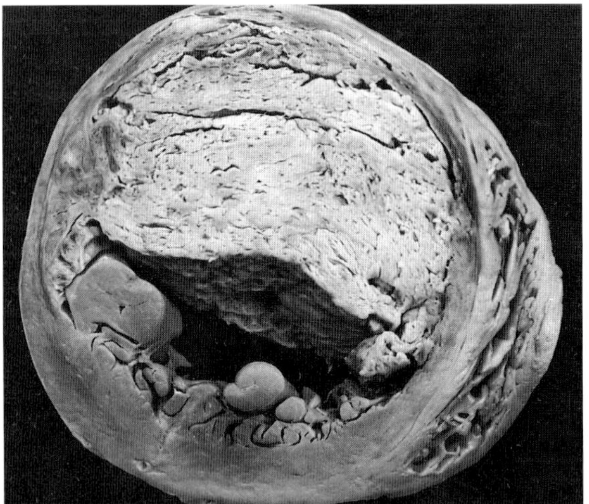

Fig. 3.26 Infarct expansion and mural thrombosis. An acute anterior infarct has undergone expansion to form an aneurysmal bulge which has filled with mural thrombosis.

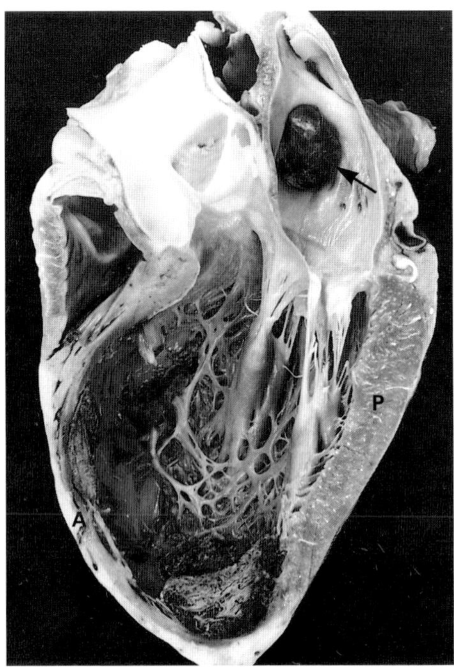

Fig. 3.27 Infarct expansion. In this long axis view there is expansion of an antero-septal infarction which has led to mural thrombus formation. The anterior wall (A) is thinner than the posterior wall (P) of the ventricle. There is also mural thrombus in the left atrial appendage (arrow).

permanent globular dilatation of the ventricle may result in detrimental effects on both left ventricular contraction and mitral valve function.[47] Expansion is less likely if there is pre-existing left ventricular hypertrophy. Expansion must be clearly separated conceptually from extension; in the latter further necrosis occurs; in expansion the volume of dead myocardium does not increase.

External cardiac rupture

Pericardial tamponade resulting from external cardiac rupture is responsible for 10–20% of the mortality of myocardial infarction and is the most common cause of death after ventricular arrhythmias and cardiogenic shock. Rupture is a complication of transmural infarction but there is no direct relation between infarct size and cardiac rupture, which is relatively more common in older women.[48]

The mechanism of myocardial rupture[49] is not clear but there are at least two variants. In some there is a slit-like tear between viable and non-viable muscle in an infarct that has not undergone expansion. Such ruptures occur within the first 2 days. In infarcts that have undergone expansion, the endocardium is torn with extravasation of blood between the muscle bundles; this form of rupture occurs typically from the fifth to the tenth day (Fig. 3.27). One report links accumulation of eosinophils within the infarct with an increased risk of rupture.[50]

Ventricular septal defects

Transmural infarcts of the interventricular septum may rupture, leading to the sudden acquisition of a left-to-right shunt at ventricular level. Septal rupture is a complication of both antero-septal and postero-septal infarction.[51] In the former case, the arterial occlusion is characteristically in the left anterior descending coronary artery above the first septal branch, in a patient who has not had previous symptoms of angina and in whom collateral flow is minimal. The resulting infarct is large. This, in association with the haemodynamic burden of a shunt, causes a high mortality. The shunt takes place initially through a ragged hole ranging from 1–3 cm^2 in size. It is rare for patients to survive; it is usually those with smaller defects who will develop a smooth-edged hole as the infarct heals. In antero-septal infarction, the defect is in the anterior or apical portion of the ventricular septum on the left side (Fig. 3.28) and opens into the right ventricular outflow or apex of the right ventricle. In posterior-septal infarction, ventricular septal defects occur behind the posterior medial papillary muscle on the left side and open into the right ventricle close to the septal cusp of the tricuspid valve. These defects have a strong association with aneurysms of the posterior wall of the left ventricle and with right ventricular infarction. Subsequent external rupture of the same posterior infarct that induced a septal shunt a day or two before is well recognised. It is difficult to assess the true relative frequency of anterior and posterior septal defects because in autopsy studies approximately equal numbers

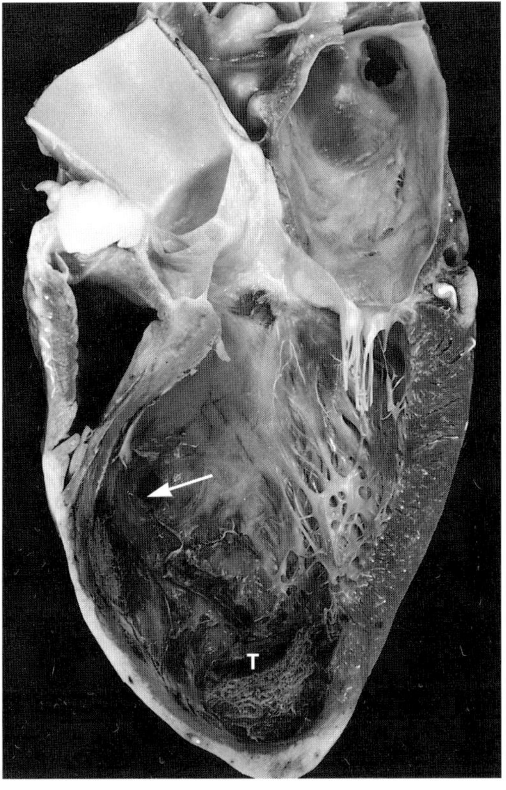

a)

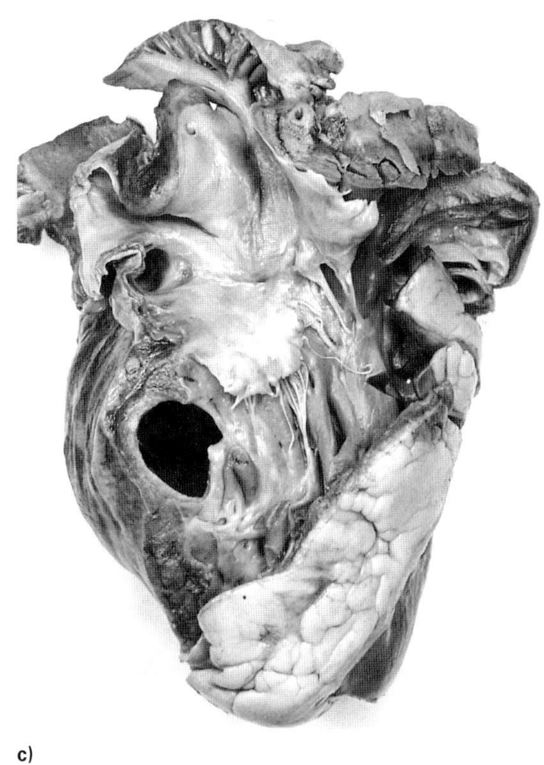

c)

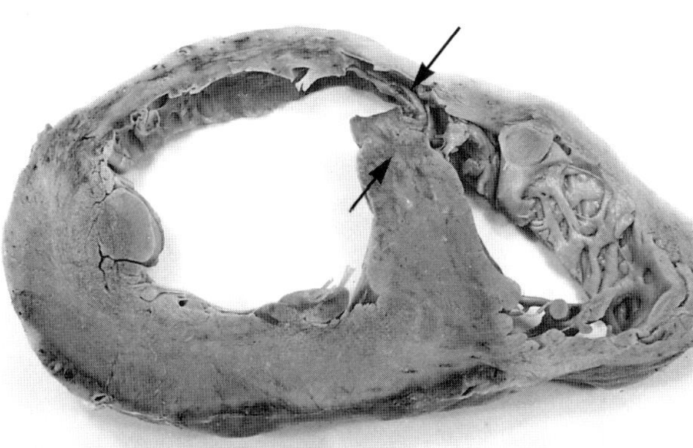

b)

Fig. 3.28 a,b,c Infarction and ventricular septal defect. (**a**) In this long axis view there is expansion and thinning of an apical anterior acute infarct. Thrombosis (T) is occurring over the endocardium at the apex. There is an acquired ventricular septal defect (arrow). (**b**) A ventricular septal defect (arrows) here complicates an antero-septal infarction which has not undergone marked expansion. (**c**) If the patient survives an acute ventricular septal defect due to infarction with healing, a smooth-edged round hole is produced in the septum.

have been reported whereas in clinical series the preponderance of anterior septal defects has been stressed. This difference may reflect the greater ease with which the anterior septal defect can be clinically diagnosed and surgically repaired.

Papillary muscle infarction

Necrosis of the papillary muscles is very common during acute infarction, being present to some degree in 15–30% of anterior and up to 50% of posterior infarctions. The greater frequency of posterior medial papillary muscle infarction reflects the blood supply from the right coronary artery whereas the antero-lateral group of papillary muscles is predominantly supplied by the left circumflex artery, a less common site of thrombosis. Papillary muscle infarction complicates both regional subendocardial and transmural infarction and is responsible for transient mitral regurgitation in the acute phase. In a tiny minority, < 1% of all fatal infarcts, a portion or all of a papillary muscle avulses. In the most severe form, the whole papillary muscle ruptures and the stump attached to the chorda passes in a flail-like motion across the mitral valve orifice, associated with torrential mitral regurgitation. Rupture of a subhead of a papillary muscle, to which only one or two chordae are attached, is less catastrophic and leads to prolapse of a portion of the cusp only (Fig. 3.29). Partial tears may heal to leave an elongated papillary muscle with a central fibrous isthmus. Rupture of the posterior papillary muscle is four to seven times more frequent than rupture of the antero-lateral papillary muscle, but in neither case is the infarct necessarily large or transmural.[52–54] There is a distinctive syndrome of rupture of the antero-lateral papillary muscle causing death from rapid onset of torrential mitral regurgitation due to a very small localised infarct resulting from thrombosis of the marginal branch of the left circumflex coronary artery.

Right ventricular infarction

In isolation, right ventricular infarction is very rare, but it may occur in patients with ischaemic heart disease who have pre-existing severe right ventricular hypertrophy. Between 20% and 50% of patients with postero-inferior infarcts of the

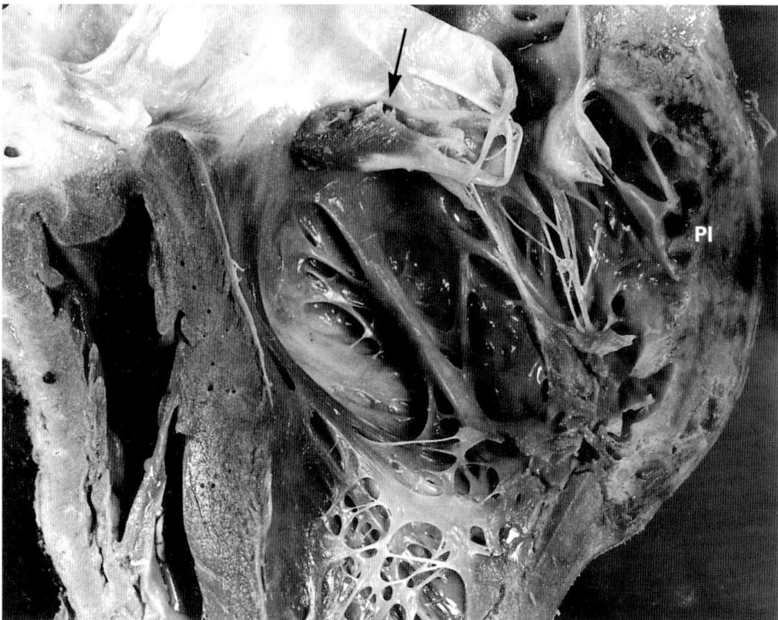

Fig. 3.29 Infarct expansion with papillary muscle rupture. In this long axis view there is an expanded and thinned acute posterior infarction (PI). One head of the posteromedial papillary muscle has ruptured (arrow).

left ventricle have some concomitant right ventricular necrosis. The incidence of right ventricular infarction in association with anterior infarction is far lower and many series contain no such cases. The right ventricular myocardium is supplied by the right coronary artery and the more proximal and the more complete the occlusion due to thrombosis the more likely it is for infarction to occur in the right ventricle. The effect of concomitant right ventricular infarction on clinical management has been of considerable interest:[55] it leads to severe heart failure and an enlarged liver without evidence of left-sided failure in the form of pulmonary oedema. Right ventricular infarction is an independent predictor of prognosis increasing the risk of death and major complications.

Ventricular aneurysms

The term aneurysm is used inconsistently in clinical cardiology, but a working morphological definition of it is a convex protrusion of the ventricular wall composed of collagenous replacement of the myocardium throughout its full thickness.[55] Such ischaemic aneurysms can result only from transmural infarction. There is a wide spectrum from, on the one hand, aneurysms with very diffuse bulges with a wide base (Fig. 3.30) to, on the other hand, very localised saccular bulges with a narrow neck (Fig. 3.31). Aneurysms present clinically with persistent ventricular arrhythmias, cardiac failure and systemic emboli from mural thrombosis within the aneurysm. All of these complications can be corrected by resection of the aneurysm. Late cardiac rupture is rare. The presence of mural thrombus is not a constant feature; aneurysms apparently identical in shape and size may be full of thrombus, obliterating the sac, contain some mural thrombus (Fig. 3.32) or have no thrombus. The wall of ventricular aneurysms is composed predominantly of collagen but calcification may occur,[57] particularly where the sac is lined by a thin coat of old thrombus.

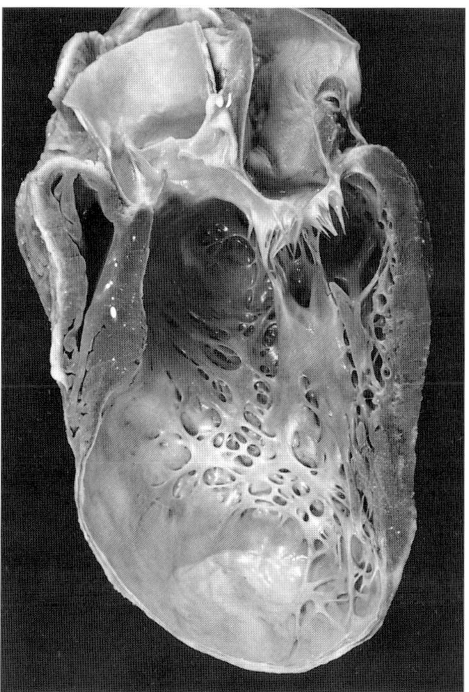

Fig. 3.30 Diffuse ventricular aneurysm. In a long axis view there is a chronic apical aneurysm with a wide base without mural thrombus. It developed following expansion of an acute infarct.

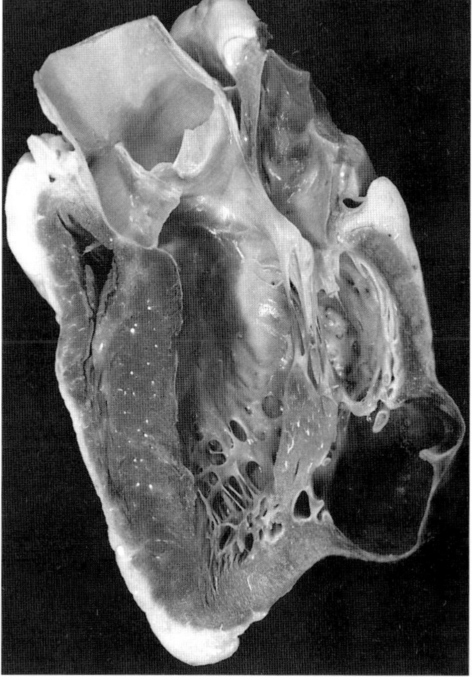

Fig. 3.31 Localised ventricular aneurysm. The posterior wall of the left ventricle shows a chronic aneurysm with a relatively narrow neck without mural thrombus formation.

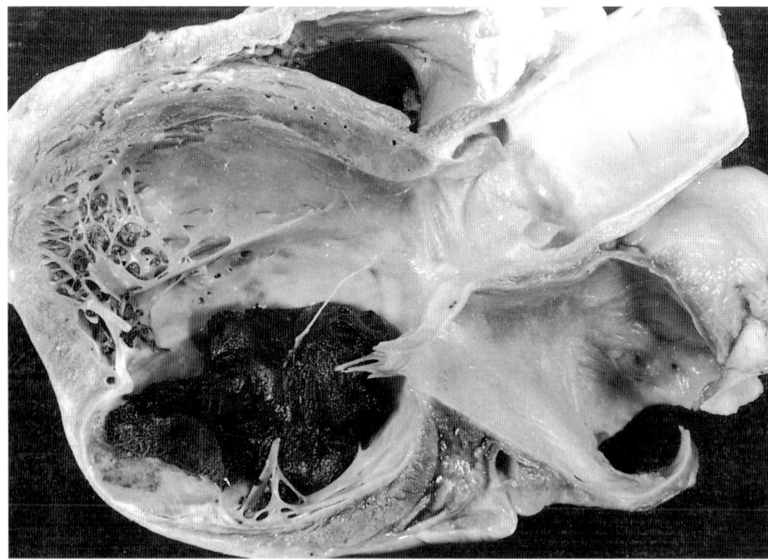

Fig. 3.32 Localised ventricular aneurysm with mural thrombus. The posterior wall of the left ventricle shows a chronic aneurysm in which there is a large mass of mural thrombus.

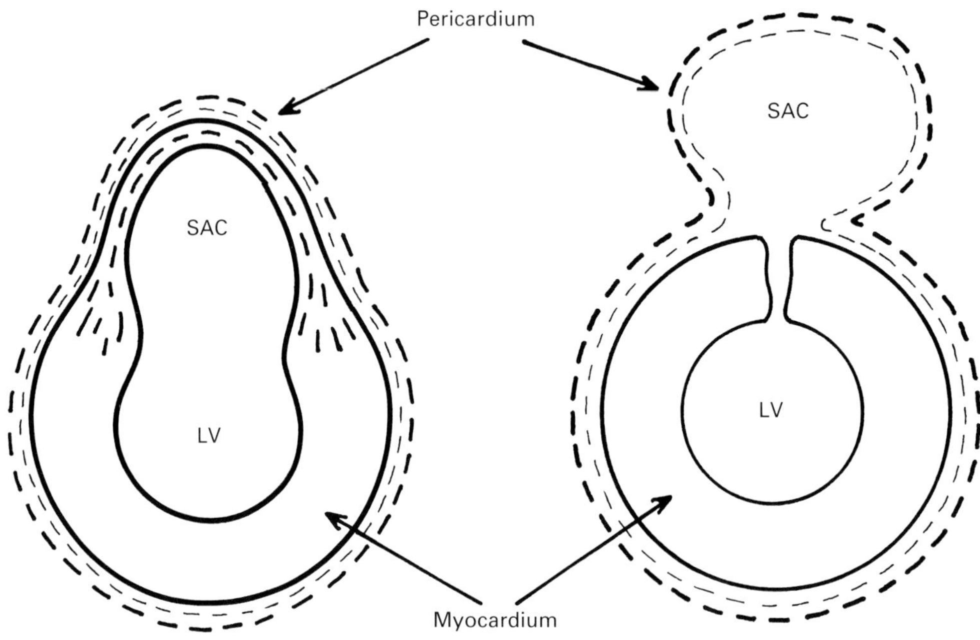

Fig. 3.33 True versus false ventricular aneurysm. In true aneurysms the wall of the sac is derived from the myocardium; in false aneurysms it is derived from the pericardium. The distinction is more theoretical than real.

The pathogenesis of aneurysm formation has been regarded either as expansion of the necrotic myocardium in the acute phase, with subsequent replacement fibrosis stabilising the new expanded shape, or the later expansion of an infarct which had already undergone fibrous replacement. A clinical study using serial two-dimensional echocardiography found that aneurysms developed in 35 of 158 patients (22%) with infarction, but the reported incidence varies widely. Early aneurysms developed within the period in intensive care in 15 patients and all were anterior and apical. Aneurysms developed within 3 months in a further 14 patients, including some on the posterior inferior wall.[58]

A different pathogenesis has been proposed for aneurysms which have a narrow neck opening into a large fibrous sac (Fig. 3.33). This form of aneurysm results from a ventricular tear which has led to a subpericardial haematoma, stopping just short of rupture into the pericardium in the acute stage. Organisation of the haematoma results in an aneurysmal sac to which the name pseudoventricular aneurysm has been applied[59] because the wall did not derive originally from ventricular myocardium. The distinction between true and pseudoaneurysms is more of theoretical than practical importance and localised saccular aneurysms intermediate in appearance between the two forms also occur. Aneurysms with a narrow neck and large external sac are also found in patients without coronary artery disease and must be presumed to be congenital in this case. Penetrating trauma such as knife wounds also leads to aneurysms with a similar shape.

Ischaemic cardiomyopathy

Cardiomyopathy is strictly indicative of a disease of the myocardium itself; hence the term ischaemic cardiomyopathy is a misnomer. The term is usually applied to chronic heart failure without anginal pain and a dilated left ventricle with generalised hypokinesia simulating the clinical picture of an idiopathic dilated cardiomyopathy. The pathology is usually of a dilated left ventricle with no increase in wall thickness, in which there is no evidence of a previous large regional infarct. There is widespread myocardial fibrosis with scarring throughout the subendocardial zone and papillary muscles. The characteristic coronary arterial pathology is of widespread stenosis in all the epicardial arteries and extreme development of intramyocardial collateral flow.

MYOCARDIAL INFARCTION WITH NORMAL CORONARY ARTERIES

The prevalence of patients who develop myocardial infarction and in whom subsequent angiography shows normal coronary arteries is between 1% and 3%. Clinical parameters include young age, a high proportion of women and the absence of classic risk factors of atheroma with the exception of smoking habit. As the number of pathological studies of this entity is very small, it is possible to list only potential mechanisms of action. In some cases, the development of thrombosis is out of proportion with the degree of underlying atheroma so that lysis restores a vessel outline which, at worse, is slightly irregular. In others thrombosis appears to have occurred in arteries which have

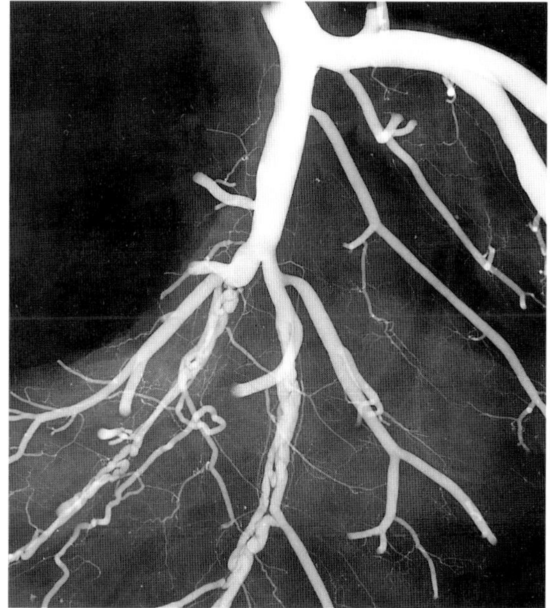

Fig. 3.34 Non-atherosclerotic coronary thrombosis. Post-mortem angiography showing recanalisation channels in branches of the left anterior descending coronary artery. Histology showed resolving thrombi but no lipid deposition or evidence of preceding atherosclerosis.

no morphological evidence of prior atherosclerosis (Fig. 3.34). The absence of classic risk factors for atheroma would suggest that enhancement of thrombosis is the major factor. Other possible precipitating mechanisms are emboli from minor abnormality of the aortic or mitral valve and unrecognised coronary artery dissection stopping at the point of subadventitial haematoma without an intimal tear. The majority of cases, however, probably represent spasm and can be regarded as forms of variant angina.[60] Spasm is not a phenomenon that can be recognised at autopsy and must be a presumptive diagnosis when there is an infarct supplied by a morphologically normal artery. Cocaine is a potent coronary vasoconstrictor and should always be considered in such cases.

VARIANTS OF ATHEROMATOUS CORONARY ARTERY DISEASE

Coronary artery lesions in hyperlipidaemia

The pattern of aortic and coronary atheroma differs in the five types of genetically determined hyperlipoproteinaemia.[61] Type I hyperlipoproteinaemia is not associated with enhanced atheroma. In homozygous type II hyperlipoproteinaemia there is severe diffuse involvement of the ascending aorta, often with heavy calcification superimposed on atheroma. Supra-aortic stenosis, valvular calcification and ostial stenosis may all result. The coronary arteries show widespread stenosis, often with diffuse intimal thickening containing numerous foam cells (Fig. 3.35) and there is a high incidence of left main disease. Heterozygous type II hyperlipoproteinaemia is closer to 'conventional' coronary atheroma but with a tendency to diffuse intimal disease, often with extension into small arteries. In type III and IV hyperlipoproteinaemia there is an increased risk of ischaemic heart disease but little evidence that the atheroma has features different from the usual form. In secondary hyperlipoproteinaemia, such as found in diabetes mellitus or myxoedema, there is usually even intimal involvement with abundant lipid-containing foam cells. Distal extension to small vessels such as the posterior

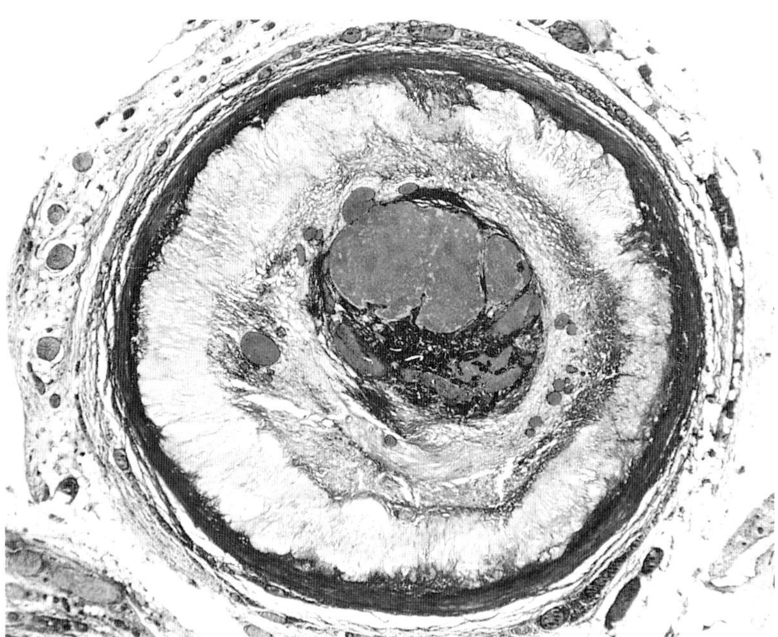

Fig. 3.35 Coronary disease in familial hyperlipidaemia. The coronary artery shows concentric diffuse intimal thickening infiltrated by numerous lipid containing foam cells. There is no formation of discrete plaques or lipid cores. The lumen is occluded by thrombosis due to superficial intimal injury and endothelial denudation. Haematoxylin–eosin × 38

descending or marginal arteries, and even to intramyocardial arteries, may occur.

Coronary ostial stenosis

Angiographic studies in vivo emphasise the rarity of ostial stenosis and that the majority of cases are found in association with widespread coronary stenosis. Thompson[62] found 27 examples in 2105 angiograms (1.2%) and Miller[63] found 35 in 4000 angiograms (0.8%). In only 10 of these 62 cases was the ostial stenosis isolated; all were relatively young women who had a low incidence of atheroma-related risk factors. These findings lead to speculation that isolated ostial stenosis might be due to aortic root dysplasia, intimal hyperplasia or a sphincter-like ring of smooth muscle in the ostium and not to atheroma. The results of the few pathological studies suggest an unusual distribution of atheroma rather than a different pathogenesis for ostial stenosis.[64] In some pathological series a very high incidence of ostial stenosis has been recorded[65] using casts of the aortic root but the functional significance of these findings is in doubt.

Sudden ischaemic cardiac death

Ambulatory monitoring and out-of-hospital resuscitation of sudden death victims in ischaemic heart disease shows that the onset of ventricular fibrillation is the common precipitating event for death. Study of resuscitated victims has also revealed that only a proportion of them, between 25% and 50%, will develop a clinically demonstrable infarct.[66] Sudden death, therefore, is not synonymous with death from early myocardial infarction. Detailed pathological studies of sudden ischaemic death suggest that victims fall into two basic groups. In the first, there is an acute arterial lesion, usually a disrupted plaque, over which either mural or occlusive thrombus has formed.[67,68] Recent myocardial necrosis may be demonstrable histologically. In this group, the onset of ventricular fibrillation reflects an acute ischaemic myocardium and the pathological process present in the subjects with acute coronary thrombi is essentially identical to that found in patients with unstable angina and acute infarction. In these patients, prodromal symptoms, albeit not recognised as indicating heart disease by the patient before the final attack, are not uncommon. In the second group, advanced coronary stenosis is present in association with myocardial scarring; often significant left ventricular hypertrophy is also present and frequently acute coronary thrombi are absent.[69] Re-entrant arrhythmias in a scarred, poorly functioning left ventricle are likely precipitating events for ventricular fibrillation in this latter group.

Divergent opinions exist on the relative frequency of the two basic groups. Recent pathological series[67,68] highlight the pre-eminence of the thrombotic group in sudden ischaemic death over all. Other series[69] in which the majority of patients are known to have ischaemic disease or old infarction and die without any prodromal warning will contain a high proportion of patients with widespread arterial stenosis and no acute coronary thrombi. Thus, patient selection predetermines the type of vascular pathology found in sudden ischaemic death.

THE PATHOLOGY OF CORONARY INTERVENTIONS

Angioplasty, in which a balloon is passed down a coronary artery over a guide wire until it passes through the section of stenosis and is then inflated to several atmospheres, has become an established treatment for discrete coronary stenosis. In another form of angioplasty laser energy is directed at the wall of the stenotic artery from an intracoronary catheter. Plaque tissue is burnt or vaporised. Various means of mechanical destruction or removal of coronary plaque tissue are also in use. In atherectomy a portion of the plaque is sucked into a hollow intracoronary catheter and then sliced off. The fragment is retrieved from the catheter, after which other cuts can be made into the plaque. In another system (Rotablator) a rapidly spinning disc disintegrates the plaque into microfragments which pass distally as flow is restored.

Mechanisms

Two mechanisms are responsible for an increase in arterial lumen size following balloon angioplasty.[70,71] In the first there is a simple mechanical stretching of the tissue, in particular the segment of normal vessel wall opposite an eccentric plaque. Recoil may occur within a short time and is one mechanism of restenosis. In extreme cases the segment of normal vessel wall may undergo medial necrosis with an inflammatory adventitial response, and repair by smooth muscle proliferation occurs. The second and more common mechanism of successful angioplasty is the creation of intimal and medial tears. The hoped for result is that the repair response of smooth muscle proliferation will smooth out the newly created irregular torn intima, leaving a larger lumen.[72]

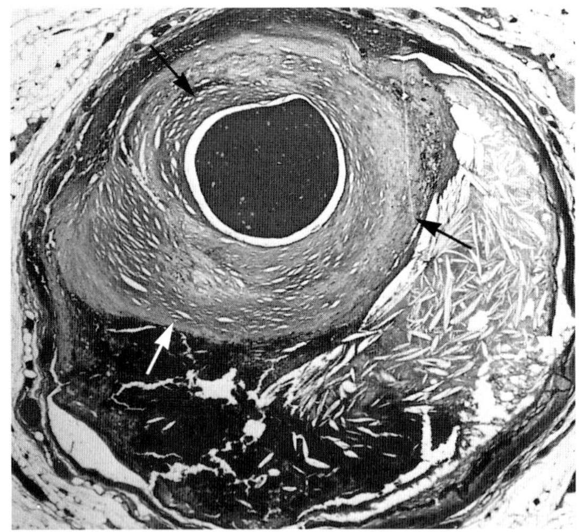

Fig. 3.36 Restenosis. Stenosis has reoccurred due to concentric intimal fibromuscular hyperplasia (arrows) superimposed on the underlying damaged plaque.

Repair responses

Angioplasty is nothing more than an intense injury to the vessel wall and invokes smooth muscle proliferation. Inevitably in angioplasty a very irregular surface is created in which a large amount of collagen is exposed and platelet adhesion occurs. The twin factors of controlling thrombosis with aspirin/heparin and creating high local blood flow prevent major thrombus formation but some platelet adhesion at the site is inevitable.

Restenosis

Restenosis is due largely to excessive smooth muscle proliferation (Fig. 3.36). The therapeutic problem is one of stopping this repair process exactly at the point at which the lumen is the desired size. The process cannot be prevented totally; a new intima with a smooth outline and non-thrombogenic surface must be created. To date a wide range of therapeutic agents, including aspirin and calcium antagonists, has not reduced the approximately 30% rate of restenosis observed clinically.

Mechanisms of smooth muscle proliferation

The problem can be simply stated. In angioplasty a stimulus is created; this causes the release of growth factors for which smooth muscle cells have receptors. Following the specific binding of growth factor to receptor there is a proliferative response involving activation of oncogenes.

The stimulus is mechanical trauma, exposure of collagen with platelet adhesion, release of tissue factor and damage to viable smooth muscle cells. This stimulus varies in magnitude and there is some evidence that the greater the extent of intimal and medial tearing the greater the likelihood of restenosis. It is not yet clear which growth factors are important in human restenosis. In animal models antibodies both to acidic growth factor released from damaged smooth muscle cells and to PDGF have been successful in reducing the smooth muscle response. An alternative approach is to apply at the site antisense oligonucleotides to oncogenes, thus preventing the final stage of proliferation.[73] There is evidence that some smooth muscle cells possibly derived from the media have a far greater capacity for persistent proliferation than those already within the intima in man.[74] Deeper tears may therefore have a greater risk of restenosis.

Restoration of the endothelial surface over the damaged intima in animal models is associated with the cessation of smooth muscle proliferation within the underlying intima. Little is known about the rate of re-endothelialisation at human angioplasty sites although there is a potential mechanism for seeding the site with autologous endothelial cells.

COMPLICATIONS OF ANGIOPLASTY

As discussed above, the borderline between an acceptable degree of smooth muscle proliferation and an excessive degree leading to restenosis is not clear-cut. Virtually all angioplasties create intimal tears and many enter the media. The exact proportion which enter the media is not known because angiographic appearances are not capable of defining the depth of tearing. Ultrasound and pathology studies, however, show the great majority of tears to enter the media. Once tears enter the media there is the potential for dissection either in the intimal/medial or medial/adventitial phase. Dissection in either of these planes can extend distally and even re-enter, leading to a double lumen. Dissection into the subadventitial plane is associated with a striking periadventitial inflammatory response. Plaques which contain a large lipid pool are subject either to extrusion of cholesterol-rich debris into the distal microvascular bed (Fig. 3.37) or out into the periadventitial tissue. In both cases a florid foreign body giant cell response may occur. Significant loss of the distal microvascular bed may occur.

Atherectomy and laser angioplasty

Both of these procedures also produce a florid smooth muscle proliferative response and can be followed by restenosis. The only essential difference in relation to complications is that plaque tissue is actually removed or destroyed. A surprisingly high proportion of atherectomy specimens contain medial tissue and some even have adventitia. There is therefore the risk of perforations or late localised aneurysms at the site of

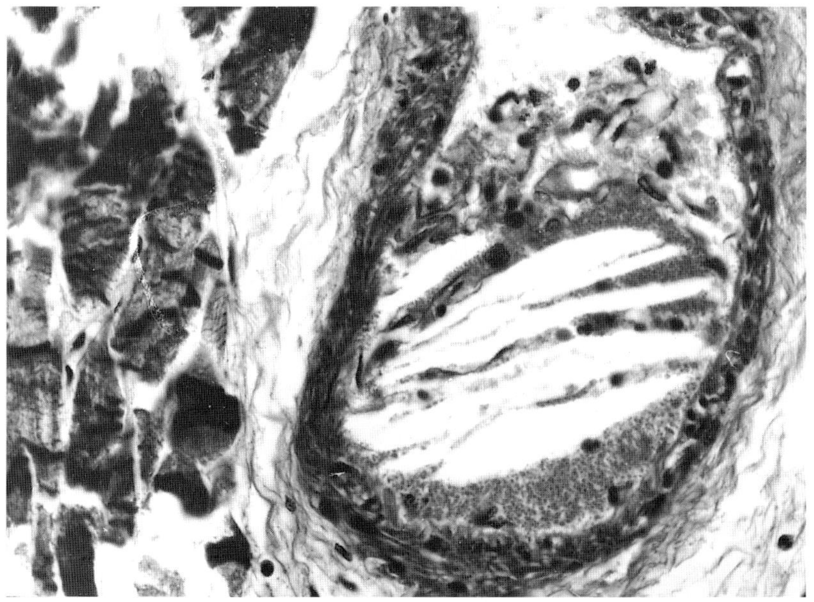

Fig. 3.37 Cholesterol embolisation. Following any manipulation of lipid-rich plaques in coronary arteries whether by angioplasty, endarterectomy or insertion of grafts, cholesterol-rich core material may embolise into the distal vascular bed. The artery is occluded by a mass of platelets surrounding crystals of cholesterol. The adjacent myocytes show contraction band necrosis.
Haematoxylin–eosin × 18

atherectomy. Pathological studies show that atherectomy often removes part of the normal vessel wall and leaves a great deal of residual plaque behind.[75]

PATHOLOGY OF CORONARY ARTERY BYPASS GRAFTS

Vascular grafts used to bypass stenotic segments of coronary arteries may be arterial or venous. Venous grafts are taken from leg veins, their side branches ligated and inserted into the aorta, being anastomosed to the coronary artery distal to the stenosis. The internal mammary arteries are dissected on pedicles and the distal end is anastomosed to the coronary artery.

All coronary vein grafts in which flow is established develop a new intimal layer due to fibromuscular proliferation.[76] This process appears to be inevitable and may be the result of a degree of endothelial damage and resultant platelet adhesion releasing mitogenic factors for smooth muscle cells, or the result of exposing a vein to arterial pressure. The process can be minimised in animals by antiplatelet drugs but, as similar intimal changes develop in arteriovenous shunts created for dialysis, it may also be a response of the venous intima to high flow and pressure. Intimal fibromuscular proliferation begins within 3 days of insertion of the graft and in most patients reaches a steady state by 1 month. A few patients show an exuberant intimal proliferation which may lead to occlusion, particularly at anastomotic sites. The degree to which the original media of the vein survives varies widely, both within different segments of the same vein and among patients. Where marked medial loss with replacement fibrosis has occurred, chronic dilatation of the graft often develops. Medial loss probably represents damage to the graft at insertion and examination of patent grafts in patients who have died within the first week often shows frank necrosis of the graft media.

The early fibromuscular proliferation that occurs within vein grafts has no direct link to graft atheroma, which is a time-related phenomenon that becomes manifest some years after insertion. Foam cells begin to accumulate diffusely within the most superficial layer of the neointima (Fig. 3.38). Discrete plaques do form and may relate to ligature sites of side branches. With

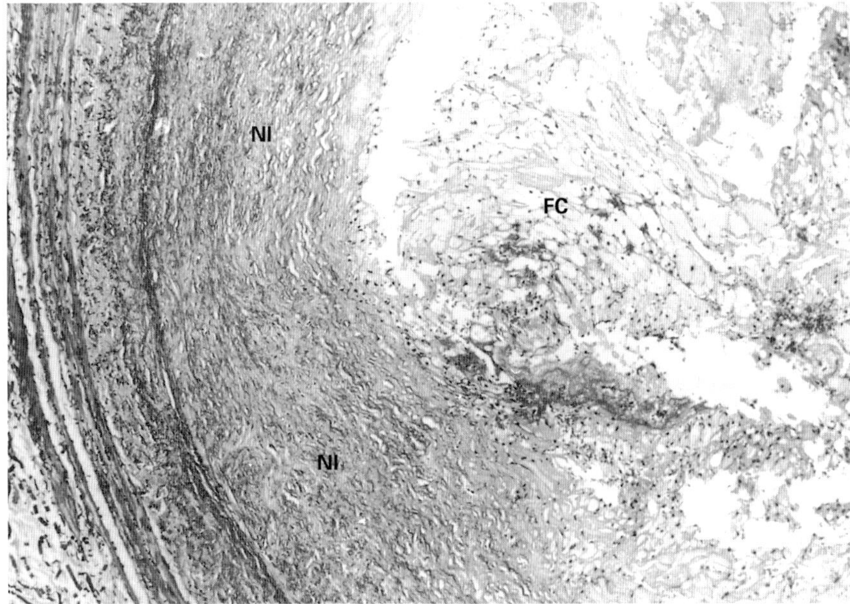

Fig. 3.38 Vein graft atheroma. The graft had developed a neointima (NI), indicating that long-term flow had been present. A zone of foam cell infiltration (FC) mixed with fragments of connective tissue and with thrombus formation has developed on the luminal aspect of the new intima.
Haematoxylin–eosin × 18

time, there is superficial breakdown of the neo-intima and the graft becomes lined by a mixture of foam cells, endothelial cells and strands of fine collagen over which friable thrombus forms. The final stage is graft occlusion by a mixture of cholesterol and thrombus.[77] There is some clinical evidence that graft atheroma is accelerated by hyperlipidaemia and reduced in patients with normal levels of high-density lipoprotein.[78]

In striking contrast to vein grafts internal mammary arteries are largely resistant to the development of atherosclerosis. Internal mammary artery grafts are small immediately after insertion but enlarge and dilate over some months. This long term function and survival is far better than venous grafts and most patients are given both forms of graft. The limitation of the internal mammary grafts is the difficulty in reaching the lateral and posterior walls of the left ventricle.

NON-ATHEROMATOUS CORONARY ARTERY DISEASE

Congenital anomalies

A vast number of variations in the origins of the coronary arteries from the aorta are described, many as case reports. Some variants cause no physiological abnormality, others are dangerous (Fig. 3.39).

The origin of both arteries from one aortic sinus or a single coronary orifice has no functional significance except when the artery passes between the aorta and pulmonary trunk.[79] In this case progressive intimal proliferation may occlude the artery, possibly due to intermittent external pressure. The artery may be the right coronary originating from the left aortic sinus, or the left anterior descending and circumflex artery arising from the right sinus. Arteries crossing from right to left, or vice versa, behind the aorta have a far lower incidence of intimal proliferation and the only danger of crossing anteriorly to the pulmonary trunk is inadvertent damage at cardiac surgery. The one coronary orifice in the pulmonary trunk has far more serious sequelae.[80] In patients who survive infancy (Fig. 3.40) a significant left-to-right shunt develops and the artery opening into the pulmonary trunk becomes aneurysmally dilated. Subendothelial fibrosis and calcification develop in infancy making early heart failure a common presentation. Late sudden death as the presenting symptom in adult life is also common. Aneurysmal dilatation of a coronary artery which opens as a congenital fistula into atria, ventricles or coronary sinus (Fig. 3.41) also occurs. Mural thrombosis may develop at the shunt sites leading to a risk of bacterial endocarditis.

When such a single dilated coronary artery is encountered at autopsy it must always be checked carefully for the exit point. Exit in the main pulmonary artery or coronary sinus is easily identified but entry between trabeculae of the left ventricle requires persistent gentle probing to identify the exit point.

In infants sudden death may be associated with atresia of a segment of coronary artery but the ostia are normal. The commonest pattern is for the first portion of the left anterior descending coronary artery to be a thread-like structure with a tiny lumen and a disorganised thick intima and media. The distal vessel is often fed by large collateral vessels crossing the outflow tract of the right ventricle from the right coronary. The condition is usually associated with marked papillary muscle fibrosis and calcification, which prompts a detailed examination of the arteries.

Spontaneous dissection of coronary arteries

Dissecting aneurysms of the ascending aorta may extend into the coronary arteries themselves, a complication that develops more frequently in relation to the right coronary artery. Dissection confined to the coronary artery may develop as a complication of procedures such as endarterectomy, insertion of vein grafts, cardiac catheterisation and angioplasty, as well as developing spontaneously. Spontaneous coronary artery dissection has several important differences from aortic dissection. In isolated coronary dissection, unlike aortic dissection, it is far less common to find an intimal tear. The process in the coronary arteries is at least initially a subadventitial haematoma and

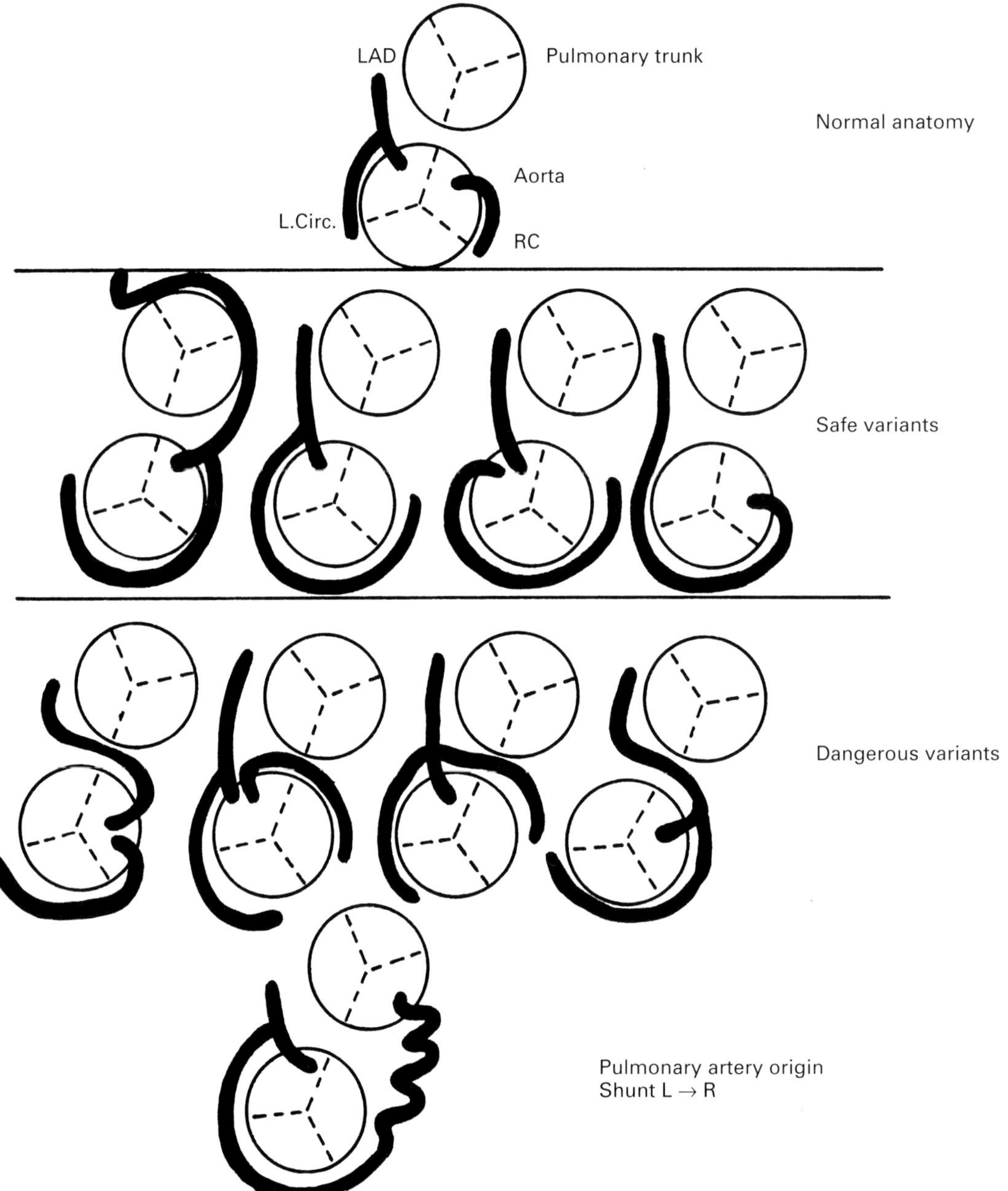

Fig. 3.39 Variants in coronary ostial origins. Some variants are physiologically safe apart from the danger of atherosclerosis and thrombosis jeopardising more myocardium if all the coronary arteries take origin from one common trunk. Variants in which a segment of coronary artery passes left to right (or vice versa) between the aorta and main pulmonary artery are dangerous because that segment of artery undergoes slow obliteration of the lumen. One orifice being in the pulmonary trunk and one in the aorta leads to high left to right flow and a tortuous dilated artery. Sudden death is a high risk.

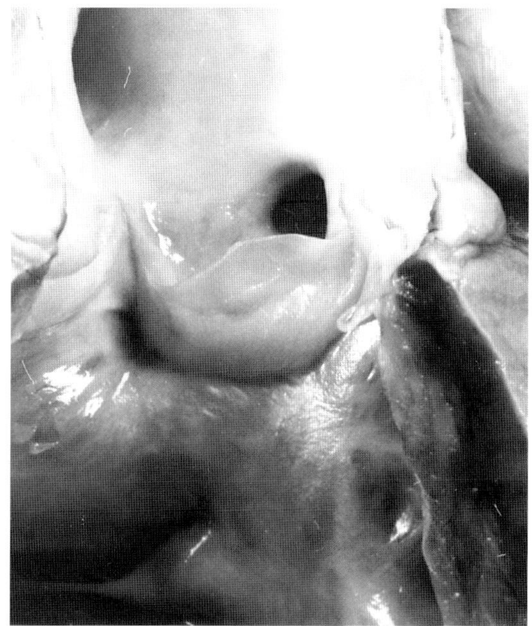

Fig. 3.40 Anomalous coronary artery. The pulmonary trunk shows the origin of the right coronary artery. The orifice is large because a high-flow shunt from aorta to pulmonary artery develops through the coronary bed. The left coronary origin was normally sited. Sudden death at 24 with normal exercise tolerance.

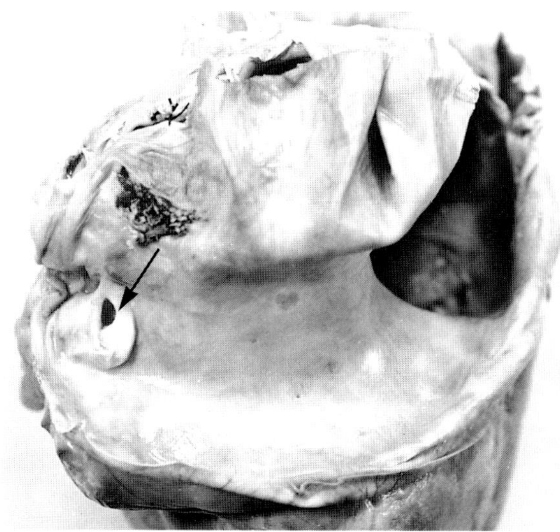

Fig. 3.41 Coronary artery fistula. The coronary sinus has been opened to show a fistula (arrow) into the left circumflex coronary artery. Both the artery and the sinus were widely dilated as a result of high blood flow.

the plane in which dissection develops is between the media and adventitia rather than within the media (Fig. 3.42). A review of the cases of spontaneous coronary dissection in the literature, most of which are case-reports, indicates characteristic features of the process.[81–83] There is a preponderance of women; 40% of cases occur in the puerperium. Presentation is with acute infarction, sudden death or unstable angina, with the left anterior descending artery being affected more commonly than the right, by a ratio of 4:1. Post-mortem studies, however, show that multiple dissections are common, suggesting that the basis lies in a generalised abnormality of the coronary arteries. Pathological studies also suggest the process begins as a subadventitial haematoma due to bleeding from vessels crossing into the most superficial layer of the media. Such haematomas may compress the arterial lumen, leading to ischaemic myocardial damage, or may invoke local arterial spasm. Resolution and organisation of the haematoma at this stage can lead to a return to normal angiographic appearances. In other cases, the haematoma leads to the development of an intimal tear and more major arterial disruption. Intimal tears can be invoked easily by apparently uneventful angiography in patients who have subadventitial haematomas.

Medial cystic change analogous to the changes seen in the aortic media with dissection are described inconsistently; an infiltrate of the adventitia with chronic inflammatory cells including eosinophils is frequently described. The basic structure of the media of the coronary arteries is very different from that of the aorta and an association of coronary artery dissection with diseases that produce cystic medial necrosis in the aorta, such as Marfan's syndrome, is not established. In one case, as yet unconfirmed, fibroblasts in the skin of a patient with spontaneous dissection of a coronary artery in the puerperium had impaired collagen synthesis.[83] No association with coronary atheroma is described. It is not known whether the tendency to coronary dissection is intermittent or persistent. Patients who develop

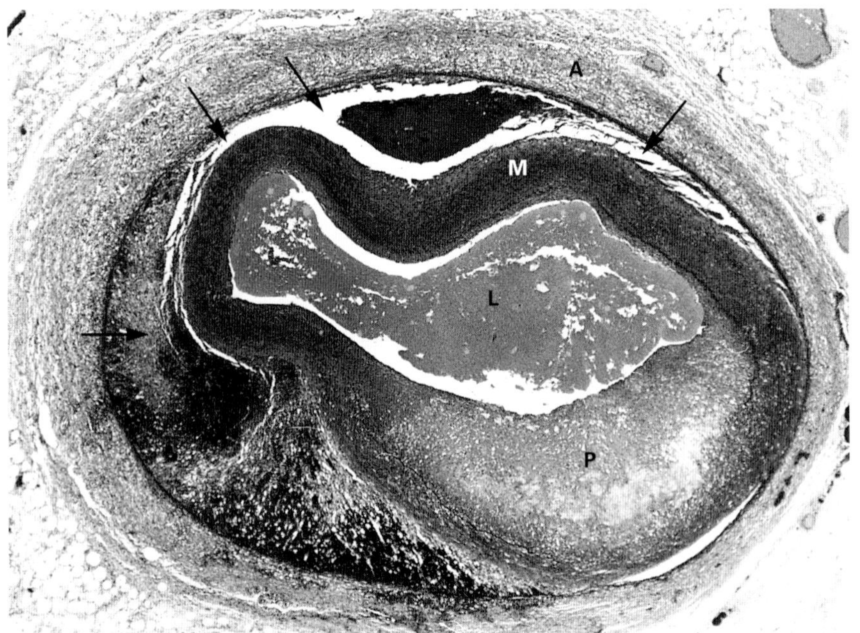

Fig. 3.42 Spontaneous coronary artery dissection. There is a dissection plane (arrows) containing red cells and fibrin between the media (M) and the adventitia (A). There is an atheromatous plaque (P) which is unrelated to the dissection. The lumen (L) contains post-mortem angiographic medium.
Haematoxylin–eosin × 18

dissection in the puerperium suggest that the tendency is intermittent, whereas in patients who develop dissection after apparently routine angiography the tendency may be persistent. On the other hand long-term survivors who have no further events are reported. A further possibility is that subadventitial haematomas develop after prolonged spasm.

Arterial bridging

At certain points, the epicardial arteries are covered by a layer of subepicardial myocardium. The phenomenon occurs in varying degrees in up to 50% of normal hearts. Reports suggest that external compression of the artery during systole can be detected angiographically, can be responsible for temporary occlusion or for myocardial infarction,[84] has been described to cause sudden death[85] and can play a part in inducing angina in hypertrophied ventricles, including hypertrophic cardiomyopathy. However, it must be emphasised that bridging is common in normal hearts[86] from subjects without any history of cardiac symptoms. Bridged arterial segments appear to be protected from atheromatous disease, but just proximal and distal to the bridge plaques do develop.

Coronary aneurysms

The terms coronary aneurysm, aneurysmal dilatation and coronary ectasia are all used to describe parts of a spectrum running from localised bulges in an otherwise angiographically normal artery through localised areas of dilatation in an artery with areas of stenosis to diffuse dilation of the whole artery. There is considerable overlap and inconsistency in the use of these terms by different authors but agreement exists that about 1.5% of coronary arteriograms in adults show appearances falling within this spectrum.[87–88] In all cases, the basic pathological process is one of medial loss. The commonest form is dilated ectatic segments of artery alternating with stenotic segments, suggesting that atheroma is responsible. Diffuse atheroma does lead to marked medial atrophy but the reason why stenosis should occur in some areas and dilatation in others is not known. Although diffuse ectasia without stenosis is associated with diffuse loss of medial muscle, often with some intimal calcification and minor lipid deposition, it is debatable whether that is sufficient evidence to regard the whole process as a variant of atheroma. Diffuse dilation of one artery in young individuals may represent a high-flow shunt into the pulmonary artery, atria or ventricles.

Localised saccular coronary aneurysms represent destruction or loss of the media in part of the circumference of the artery. A minority are due to congenital defects in the media but most represent the end-stage of an inflammatory process. Classic polyarteritis nodosa affects the coronary arteries as part of a systemic involvement of muscular arteries but in Kawasaki's disease (Fig. 3.43) the coronary arteries are almost exclusively involved. Kawasaki's disease, first described as endemic in Japan, presents as an acute febrile illness in children, associated with a skin rash, oral ulceration and cervical lymphadenopathy. Cardiac involvement may develop after a short latent period and is characterised by coronary aneurysms leading to thrombosis and myocardial infarction as the principal cause of death. Epidemics of the disease are characteristic worldwide and in Japan, and a viral aetiology is likely.[89] The coronary arterial involvement may be very widespread, leading to early death, or less severe, leaving a residual aneurysm which may be detected by angiography or thrombose to induce infarction in later adult life.[90–93]

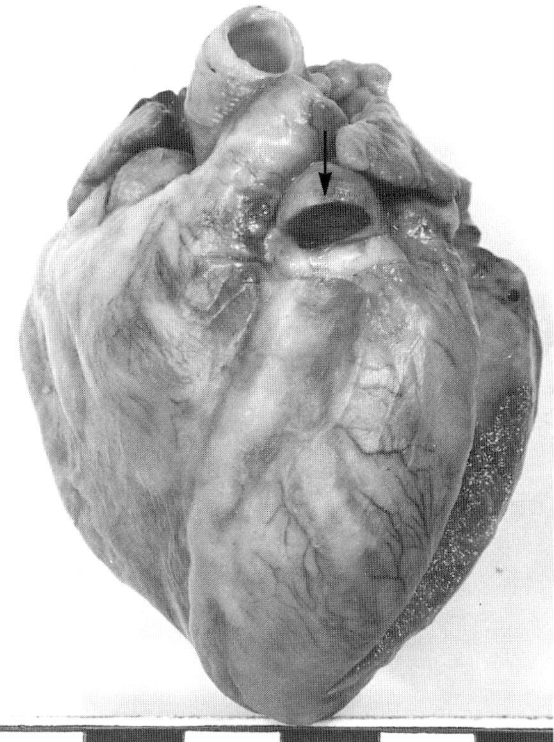

Fig. 3.43 Kawasaki disease. The heart from a case of sudden death in a child shows an aneurysm of the left anterior descending coronary artery associated with occlusive thrombosis (arrow).

REFERENCES

1. Hangartner J, Charleston A, Davies M, Thomas A. Morphological characteristics of clinically significant coronary artery stenosis in stable angina. Br Heart J 1986; 56: 501–508.
2. Brown B, Bolson E, Dodge H. Dynamic mechanisms in human coronary stenosis. Circulation 1984; 70: 917–922.
3. Isner J, Donaldson R, Fortin A, Tischler A, Clarke R. Attenuation of media of coronary arteries in advanced atherosclerosis. Am J Cardiol 1986; 58: 937–939.
4. Saner H, Gobel F, Salomonowitz E, Erlien D, Edwards J. The disease free wall in coronary atherosclerosis: its relation to degree of obstruction. J Am Coll Cardiol 1985; 6: 1096–1099.
5. Roberts W, Virmani R. Formation of new coronary arteries within a previously obstructed epicardial coronary artery (intra-arterial arteries). A mechanism for occurrence of angiographically normal coronary arteries after healing of acute myocardial infarction. Am J Cardiol 1984; 54: 1361–1362.
6. Barger A, Beeuwkes RI, Lainey L, Silverman K. Hypothesis: Vasa vasorum and neovascularization of human coronary arteries. A possible role in the pathophysiology of atherosclerosis. N Engl J Med 1983; 310: 175–177.
7. Barger A, Beeuwkes RI. Rupture of coronary vasa vasorum as a trigger of acute myocardial infarction. Am J Cardiol 1990; 66: 41G–43G.
8. Constantinides P. Causes of thrombosis in human atherosclerotic arteries. Am J Cardiol 1990; 70: 203–208.
9. Ambrose J, Winters S, Arora R. Angiographic evolution of coronary artery morphology in unstable angina. J Am Coll Cardiol 1986; 7: 472–478.

10. Levin D, Fallon J. Significance of the angiographic morphology of localized coronary stenosis: histopathologic correlations. Circulation 1982; 66: 316–320.
11. Davies M, Thomas A. Plaque fissuring — the cause of acute myocardial infarction, sudden ischaemic death and crescendo angina. Br Heart J 1985; 53: 363–373.
12. Sherman C, Litvack F, Grundfest W. Coronary angioscopy in patients with unstable pectoris. N Engl J Med 1986; 315: 913–919.
13. Falk E. Unstable angina with fatal outcome: dynamic coronary thrombosis leading to infarction and/or sudden death. Circulation 1985; 71: 699–708.
14. Davies M, Thomas A, Knapman P, Hangartner R. Intramyocardial platelet aggregation in patients with unstable angina suffering sudden ischaemic cardiac death. Circulation 1986; 73: 418–427.
15. Fitzgerald D, Roy L, Catella F, Fitzgerald A. Platelet activation in unstable coronary disease. N Engl J Med 1986; 315: 983–989.
16. Bitker H, Ravkilde J, Sigaard P, Jirgensen P, Hirder M, Thygesen K. Gradation of unstable angina based on a sensitive immunoassay for serum creatine kinase MB. Br Heart J 1991; 65: 72–76.
17. Garratt K, Edwards W, Kaufmann U, Vlietstra R, Holmes DJ. Differential histopathology of primary atherosclerotic and restenotic lesions in coronary arteries and saphenous vein bypass grafts: analysis of tissue obtained from 73 patients by directional atherectomy. J Am Coll Cardiol 1991; 17: 442–448.
18. Roberts W, Curry R, Isner J. Sudden death in Prinzmetal's angina with coronary spasm documented by arteriography: analysis of three necropsy cases. Am J Cardiol 1982; 50: 203–210.
19. Brown B. Observations linking the clinical spectrum of ischaemic heart disease to the dynamic pathology of coronary atherosclerosis. Arch Intern Med 1981; 141: 716–722.
20. Nabel EG, Selwyn AP, Ganz P. Large coronary arteries in humans are responsive to changing blood flow: an endothelium-dependent mechanism that fails in patients with atherosclerosis. J Am Coll Cardiol 1990; 16: 349–356.
21. Kohchi K, Takebayashi S, Hiroki T, Nobuyoshi M. Significance of adventitial inflammation of the coronary artery in patients with unstable angina: results at autopsy. Circulation 1985; 71: 709–716.
22. Forman M, Oates J, Robertson D. Increased adventitial mast cells in a patient with coronary spasm. N Engl J Med 1985; 313: 1138–1141.
23. Farrer-Brown G. Normal and diseased vascular pattern of myocardium of human heart. Br Heart J 1968; 30: 527–536.
24. Levine H. Subendocardial infarction in retrospect: pathologic, cardiographic and ancillary features. Circulation 1985; 72: 790–800.
25. Stadius M, Maynard C, Fritz J. Coronary anatomy and left ventricular function in the first 12 hours of acute myocardial infarction: the Western Washington randomized intracoronary streptokinase trial. Circulation 1985; 72: 292–301.
26. Davies M, Woolf N, Robertson W. Pathology of acute myocardial infarction with particular reference to occlusive coronary thrombi. Br Heart J 1976; 38: 659–664.
27. Kim CB, Braunwald E. Potential benefits of late reperfusion of infarcted myocardium. The open artery hypothesis. Circulation 1993; 88: 2426–2436.
28. Falk E. Plaque rupture with severe pre-existing stenosis precipitating coronary thrombosis. Characteristics of coronary atherosclerotic plaque underlying fatal occlusive thrombi. Br Heart J 1983; 50: 127–131.
29. Horie T, Sekiguchi M, Hirosawa K. Coronary thrombosis in pathogenesis of acute myocardial infarction. Histopathological study of coronary arteries in 108 necropsied cases using serial section. Br Heart J 1978; 40: 153–161.
30. Fulton W. Pathological concepts in acute coronary thrombosis: relevance to treatment. Br Heart J 1993; 70: 403–408.
31. DeWood M, Spores J, Notske R. Non-transmural (subendocardial) myocardial infarction in man; the prevalence of total coronary occlusion. Am J Cardiol 1981; 47: 459–464.
32. Piek JJ, Becker AE. Collateral blood supply to the myocardium at risk in human myocardial infarction. A quantitative post mortem assessment. J Am Coll Cardiol 1988; 11: 1290–1296.
33. Hoffman J. Coronary physiology and pathophysiology. In: Fox K, ed. Ischaemic heart disease. Lancaster: MTP Press, 1987: 69.
34. Reimer K, Jennings R, Cobb F. Animal models for protecting myocardium — results of the NHLBI co-operative study. Circ Res 1985; 56: 651–665.
35. Poole-Wilson P. Haemodynamic and metabolic consequences of angina and myocardial infarction. In: Fox K, ed. Ischaemic heart disease. Lancaster: MTP Press, 1987: 123–148.
36. Jennings R, Reimer K. Lethal myocardial ischaemic injury. Am J Pathol 1981; 102: 241–255.
37. Reimer K, Jennings R. The wave front phenomenon of myocardial ischemic cell death. II. Transmural progression of necrosis within the framework of ischemic bed size and collateral flow (myocardium at risk). Lab Invest 1979; 40: 633–644.
38. Rosen R, Swain J, Michael L. Selective accumulation of the first component of complement and leukocytes in ischaemic canine heart muscle. A possible initiator of an extramyocardial mechanism of ischaemic injury. Circ Res 1985; 57: 119–130.
39. Kloner R, Ganote C, Jennings R. The 'no-reflow' phenomenon after temporary coronary occlusion in the dog. J Clin Invest 1974; 54: 1496–1508.
40. Flameng W, Wouters L, Sergeant P. Multivariate analysis of angiographic, histological and electrocardiographic data in patients with coronary heart disease. Circulation 1984; 70: 7–17.
41. Grande P, Pederseb A. Myocardial infarct size: correlation with cardiac arrhythmias and sudden death. Eur Heart J 1984; 5: 622–628.
42. Alonso D, Scheidr S, Post M, Killip T. Pathophysiology of cardiogenic shock, quantifications of myocardial necrosis, clinical pathologic and electrocardiographic correlation. Circulation 1973; 48: 588–596.
43. James T. The coronary circulation and conduction system in acute myocardial infarction. Prog Cardiovasc Dis 1968; 10: 410–449.
44. Becker A. Atrioventricular conduction disturbances in acute myocardial infarction. In: Davies M, Anderson R, Becker A, ed. The conduction system of the heart. London: Butterworths, 1983: p. 161.
45. Bilbao F, Fabalza I, Vilanova J, Froufe J. AV block in

posterior acute myocardial infarction: a clinicopathological correlation. Circulation 1987; 75: 733–736.
46. Pirolo S, Hutchins GM, Moore W. Infarct expansion: pathologic analysis of 204 patients with a single myocardial infarct. J Am Coll Cardiol 1986; 7: 349–354.
47. Gaudron P, Eilles C, Kugler I, Ertl G. Progressive left ventricular dysfunction and remodelling after myocardial infarction. Circulation 1993; 87: 755–763.
48. Dellborg M, Held P, Swedberg K, Vedin O. Rupture of the myocardium: occurrence and risk factors. Br Heart J 1985; 54: 11–17.
49. Becker A, van Mantgem J. Cardiac tamponade: a study of 50 hearts. Eur J Cardiol 1975; 3: 349–358.
50. Atkinson J, Robinowitz M, McCallister H, Virmani R. Association of eosinophils with cardiac rupture. Human Pathol 1985; 16: 562–568.
51. Mann JM, Roberts WC. Acquired ventricular septal defect during acute myocardial infarction: analysis of 38 unoperated necropsy patients and comparison with 50 unoperated necropsy patients without rupture. Am J Cardiol 1988; 62: 8–19.
52. Nashimura R, Schaff H, Shub C, Gersh B, Edwards W, Tajik A. Papillary muscle rupture complicating acute myocardial infarction — analysis of 17 patients. Am J Cardiol 1983; 51: 373–377.
53. Wei J, Hutchins G, Bulkley B. Papillary muscle rupture of fatal acute myocardial infarction: a potentially treatable form of cardiogenic shock. Ann Intern Med 1979; 90: 149–153.
54. Barbour D, Roberts W. Rupture of a left ventricular papillary muscle during acute myocardial infarction. Analysis of 22 necropsy patients. J Am Coll Cardiol 1986; 8: 548–565.
55. Isner J, Roberts W. Right ventricular infarction complicating left ventricular infarction secondary to coronary artery disease: frequency, location, associated findings and significance from analysis of 236 necropsy patients with acute or healed myocardial infarction. Am J Cardiol 1978; 42: 885–894.
56. Tibbutt D. Pure left ventricular aneurysm. Br Med J 1984; 289: 450–451.
57. Roberts W, Kaufman R. Calcification of healed myocardial infarcts. Am J Cardiol 1987; 60: 28–32.
58. Visser C, Kan G, Meltzer G, Koolan J, Dunning A. Incidence, timing and prognostic value of left ventricular aneurysm formation after infarction. Am J Cardiol 1986; 57: 729–732.
59. Van Tassel R, Edwards J. Rupture of the heart complicating myocardial infarction. Analysis of 40 cases including nine examples of left ventricular false aneurysm. Chest 1972; 61: 104–106.
60. Legrand V, Deliege M, Henrard L, Boland J, Kulbertus H. Patients with myocardial infarction and normal coronary arteriogram. Chest 1982; 82: 678–685.
61. Roberts W, Ferrans V, Levy R, Fredrickson D. Cardiovascular pathology in hyperlipoproteinaemia: anatomic observations in 42 patients. Am J Cardiol 1973; 31: 557–570.
62. Thompson R. Isolated coronary ostial stenosis in women. J Am Coll Cardiol 1986; 7: 997–1003.
63. Miller A, Honey M, El Sayed H. Isolated coronary stenosis. Cathet Cardiovasc Diag 1986; 12: 30–34.
64. Stewart J, Ward D, Davies M, Pepper J. Isolated coronary ostial stenosis: observations on the pathology. Eur Heart J 1987; 8: 917–920.
65. Rissanen V. Occurrence of coronary ostial stenosis in necropsy series of myocardial infarction, sudden death and violent death. Br Heart J 1975; 37: 182–191.
66. Cobb L, Werner J, Trobaugh G. Sudden cardiac death. A decade's experience with out-of-hospital resuscitation. II. Outcome of resuscitation, management and future directions. Mod Conc Cardiovasc Dis 1980; 49: 31–42.
67. Davies M. Anatomic features in victims of sudden coronary death. Circulation 1992; 85: 1-19–1-24.
68. Van Dantzig J, Becker A. Sudden cardiac death and acute pathology of coronary arteries. Eur Heart J 1986; 7: 987–991.
69. Warnes C, Roberts W. Comparison at necropsy by age group of amount and distribution of narrowing by atherosclerotic plaque in 2995 five mm long segments of 240 major coronary arteries in 60 men aged 31–70 years with sudden coronary death. Am Heart J 1984; 108: 431–435.
70. Block P. Mechanism of transluminal angioplasty. Am J Cardiol 1984; 53: 69C–71C.
71. Colavita P, Ideker R, Reimer K, Hackel D, Stack R. The spectrum of pathology associated with percutaneous transluminal coronary angioplasty during acute myocardial infarction. J Am Coll Cardiol 1986; 8: 855–860.
72. Ueda M, Becker A, Fukimoto T. Pathological changes induced by percutaneous transluminal coronary angioplasty. Br Heart J 1987; 58: 635–643.
73. Simons M, Edelman ER, DeKeyser J-L, Langer R, Rosenberg RD. Antisense c-*myc* oligonucleotides inhibit intimal arterial smooth muscle cell accumulation in vivo. Nature 1992; 359: 67–70.
74. Chan P, Patel M, Betteridge L, Munro E, Schachter M, Wolfe J, Sever P. Abnormal growth regulation of vascular smooth muscle cells by heparin in patients with restenosis. Lancet 1993; 341: 341–342.
75. Umans V, Haine E, Renkin J, de Feyter P, Wijnst W, Serruys P. The mechanism of directional coronary atherectomy. Eur Heart J 1993; 14: 505–510.
76. Bourassa M, Campeau L, Lesperance J, Solymoss B. Atherosclerosis after coronary artery bypass surgery: results of recent studies and recommendations regarding prevention. Cardiology 1986; 73: 259–268.
77. Bulkley B, Hutchins G. Accelerated 'atherosclerosis': a morphological study of 91 saphenous vein coronary artery bypass grafts. Am J Cardiol 1976; 37: 124.
78. Neitzel G, Barboriak J, Pintar K, Qureshi I, Clement J. Atherosclerosis in aortocoronary bypass grafts. Morphologic study and risk factor analysis 6 to 12 years after surgery. Arteriosclerosis 1986; 6: 594–600.
79. Roberts WC. Major anomalies of coronary arterial origin seen in adulthood. Am Heart J 1986; 111: 941–962.
80. Taylor AJ, Rogan KM, Virmani R. Sudden cardiac death associated with isolated congenital coronary artery anomalies. J Am Coll Cardiol 1992; 20: 640–647.
81. Mathieu D, Larde D, Vasile N. Primary dissecting aneurysm of the coronary arteries: case report and literature review. Cardiovasc Intervent Radiol 1984; 7: 71–74.
82. Baker P, Keyhani-Rofagha S, Graham R, Sharma H. Dissecting hematoma (aneurysm) of coronary artery dissection: case report and evidence for a defect in collagen metabolism. Am J Med 1986; 80: 317–319.
83. Bonnet J, Aumailley M, Thomas D, Grosgogeat Y, Broustet J, Bricaud H. Spontaneous coronary artery dissection: case report and evidence for a defect in collagen metabolism. Eur Heart J 1986; 7: 904–909.

84. Felman A, Baughman K. Myocardial infarction: association with a myocardial bridge. Am Heart J 1986; 111: 784–788
85. Corrado D, Thiene G, Cocco P, Frescura C. Non-atherosclerotic coronary artery disease and sudden death in the young. Br Heart J 1992; 68: 601–607.
86. Ishall T, Hosoda Y, Osaka T, et al. The significance of myocardial bridge upon atherosclerosis in the left anterior descending coronary artery. J Pathol 1986; 148: 279–292.
87. Daoud A, Pankin D, Tulgan H, Florentin R. Aneurysms of the coronary artery: Report of 10 cases and review of the literature. Am J Cardiol 1963; 11: 228–237.
88. Swanton R, Lea-Thomas M, Coltart D, Jenkins B, Webb-Peploe M, Williams B. Coronary artery ectasia — a variant of occlusive coronary arteriosclerosis. Br Heart J 1978; 40: 393–400.
89. Seiguchi M, Takao A, Endo M, Asai T, Kawasaki I. On the mucocutaneous lymph node syndrome or Kawasaki disease. In: Yu P, Goodwin J, ed. Progress in cardiology. Philadelphia: 1985: p. 97.
90. Yanagawa H, Nakamura Y, Kawasaki T, Shigematsu I. Nationwide epidemic of Kawasaki disease in Japan during the winter of 1985–1986. Lancet 1986; ii: 1138–1139.
91. Shulman S, Rowley A. Kawasaki disease has a retroviral aetiology. Lancet 1986; ii: 545–546.
92. Kato H, Ichinose E, Yoshicka F, et al. Fate of coronary aneurysm in Kawasaki disease, serial coronary angiography and long-term follow-up study. Am J Cardiol 1982; 49: 1758–1766.
93. Brecker S, Gray H, Oldershaw P. Coronary artery aneurysm and myocardial infarction; adult sequelae of Kawasaki disease? Br Heart J 1987; 59: 509–512.

4

Diseases of the aorta and arteries

INTRODUCTION

Inflammatory disease involves the aorta and arteries of different sizes. Some of the named categories of aortitis and arteritis affect a particular size of artery; some have concomitant venous involvement, others do not. In general, aortic involvement leads to dilatation and aneurysm formation rather than obstruction but Takayasu's disease is an exception. Arteritis in medium and small arteries leads to obstruction and ischaemic organ damage. The clinical symptoms depend on the organ involved. This chapter considers those inflammatory disorders which affect arteries of an order of size down to 250 μm in external diameter. For a discussion of arteritis in the smaller arteries and arterioles the reader is referred to the books in this series on skin, renal and gastrointestinal pathology.

Non-inflammatory disorders of medium and small arteries, including the effect of hypertension, are described in the companion volume of this book. Non-inflammatory medial disease of the aorta leads to aneurysms, dissection and aortic root dilatation and is described here. Atherosclerosis in the aorta and major arteries such as the carotid and femoral is subtly different from that in the coronary arteries and is also described here.

INFLAMMATORY DISEASES OF BLOOD VESSELS

A wide range of inflammatory processes can lead to vascular damage all of which are brought together under the generic term vasculitis. There is little logic in the published classifications, which largely consist of cataloguing and correlating the size and type of vessel involved with the clinical features to produce a series of named entities which almost certainly overlap (Table 4.1). A comprehensive recent classification is that of Lie.[1]

A common theme of immune-mediated vascular damage runs through the vasculitides. At least four putative mechanisms have been described in animal models and human disease. Any particular vasculitic disease may have more than one mechanism.[2]

1. Circulating immune complexes

Deposition of immune complexes in the vessel wall will invoke a florid inflammatory response. The complexes vary in size, in their ability to activate complement, the degree to which the complexes penetrate the vessel wall, the class of immunoglobulin present and the proportions of antigen and antibody in the complex. IgG activates complement via the classic pathway, IgA and IgE via the alternative pathway. Variations in the properties of the immune complexes found at the site of vascular damage militate for the wide range of human vasculitic diseases. Immune-complex-mediated vasculitis includes polyarteritis nodosa due to deposition of complexes containing the surface antigen of hepatitis B virus, drug hypersensitivity vasculitis, the vasculitis seen in association with various malignancies, serum sickness and Henoch–Schönlein purpura. Immediate hypersensitivity due to IgE in immune complexes has been suggested in both polyarteritis nodosa and Churg–Strauss syndrome.

Table 4.1

Infective			Syphilis
			Tuberculosis
			Rickettsial
			Bacterial-fungal
Non-infective			
	Large arteries/aorta		
			Takayasu's disease
			Giant cell aortitis/arteritis
			Rheumatoid
			Ankylosing spondylitis
	Medium arteries		
			Polyarteritis nodosa
			Kawasaki's disease
		With granulomas	
			Wegener's granulomatosis
			Churg–Strauss syndrome
		With collogen disease	
			Rheumatoid
			Systemic lupus
			Dermatomyositis
	Small arteries		
			Serum sickness
			Henoch–Schönlein purpura
			Drug-induced angiitis
			Malignancy associated vasulitis,
			Cryoglobulinaemia
			Good pasture's syndrome

2. Antibody-mediated

Cytotoxic or complement fixed antibodies with a specificity targeted to the endothelial cell have been found in Goodpasture's syndrome, systemic lupus and Kawasaki's disease.[3]

3. Antineutrophil cytoplasmic autoantibodies

Antibodies to either a serine protease contained in the azurophilic lysosomal granules of polymorphs and monocytes or to leucocyte myeloperoxidase are a feature of Wegener's granulomatosis, some microscopic forms of polyarteritis and the Churg–Strauss syndrome. While possession of the autoantibody does not necessarily mean that the subject has the disease, in those with clinically expressed disease there is a good correlation of activity and antibody levels. It is thought that either the antibodies cause neutrophil activation in situ, releasing free radicals, or the enzymes are bound to components of the vessel wall such as the basement membrane, following which T-cell-mediated immune reactions are triggered at the site.[4]

4. Direct infection of endothelial cells

Herpes virus, mycoplasma, rickettsiae and the HTLV-1 virus are all capable of directly infecting the endothelial cell, either altering its expression of receptors for complement and adhesion molecules or causing direct cytotoxicity.

It should however be emphasised that in most of the named clinical entities of vasculitis either nothing is known of the pathogenesis or there is more than one putative mechanism. Only serum-sickness-related vasculitis is simple and easy to understand in terms of pathogenesis.

Infective causes of vasculitis

Syphilis

Of the chronic granulomatous infections, including tuberculosis, leprosy and syphilis, it is the last that has a particular predilection for causing cardiovascular disease. After the initial infection untreated cases pass through primary, secondary and tertiary stages as resistance to the organism increases. Cardiovascular manifestations are a complication of the third stage and represent tissue responses in a highly resistant state, yet for some unknown reason there is a local breakdown in this immunity after a latent period of years. About one-third of untreated patients with primary syphilis will develop the tertiary complications. Of these as many as 80% will have cardiovascular lesions.[5] A third of these will be the coincidental finding at autopsy of a segment of syphilitic aortitis without clinical effect. Syphilitic aortitis has a particular predilection for the

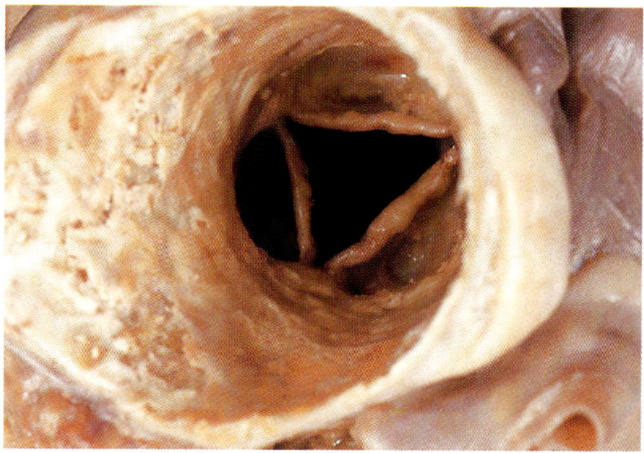

Fig. 4.1 Syphilitic aortitis. The intimal surface of the root of the aorta is dilated with the intima pitted and wrinkled. All three commissures of the aortic valve are separated. The edge of the cusps is rolled and thickened but this is a consequence of regurgitation and not part of the syphilitic process.

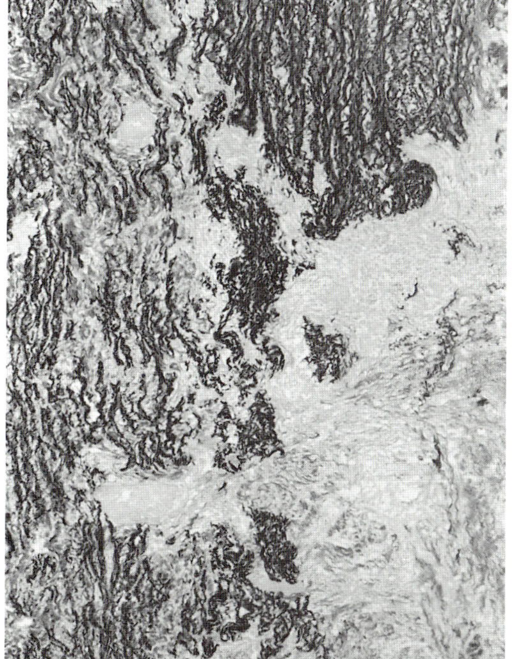

a)

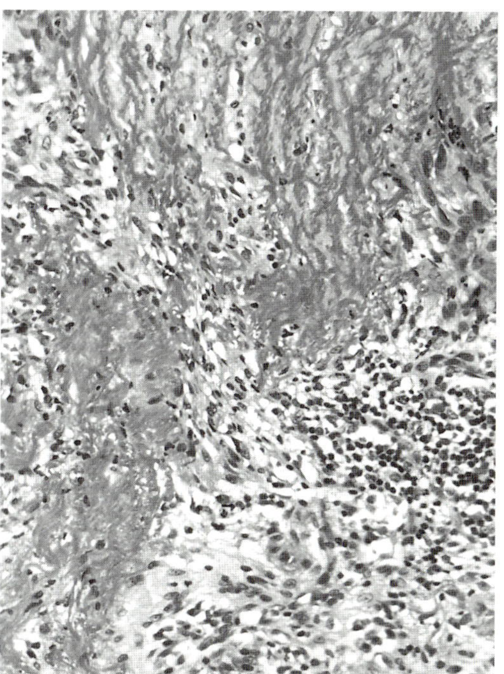

b)

Fig. 4.2a, b Syphilitic aortitis. (**a**) Stains to demonstrate the elastic tissue in the aortic media show irregular focal areas of total destruction alongside areas where the elastic pattern is more normal. (**b**) In the areas of destruction there is necrosis of the tissue with a florid inflammatory cell infiltrate consisting largely of plasma cells. Fibroblastic proliferation and endothelial swelling is also prominent.
(**a**) Elastica/Van Gieson × 95
(**b**) Haematoxylin–eosin × 95

ascending aorta, often occurring as a discrete band just above the aortic valve. It may, however, involve the whole of the ascending aorta or any segment of the thoracic and abdominal aorta. The involved segment may simply dilate, this being typical of the form confined to the proximal ascending aorta, or give rise to fusiform or saccular aneurysms. The intimal surface viewed en face shows a wrinkled and pitted appearance (tree bark scarring) on to which diffuse atherosclerosis is superimposed (Fig. 4.1). As discussed in Chapter 6, tree bark scarring is an indication of focal medial destruction and can occur in any form of aortitis as well as in non-inflammatory medial destruction.

When the proximal ascending aorta is involved the commissures of the aortic valve cusps separate; in conjunction with root dilation this leads to aortic regurgitation (Fig. 4.1). The bases of the aortic cusps are not involved but the free edges often develop nodular thickening as a secondary result of regurgitation. A diffuse sheet of calcification in the aortic wall (egg-shell calcification) is often a striking feature and is confined to the affected segment of aorta. Scarring of the intima around the coronary orifices leads to ostial stenosis and angina. The best method of judging ostial stenosis is to see if probes or catheters of known dimensions can be passed. If a probe of more than 1 mm diameter cannot be passed there is significant stenosis at the ostia.

The histology of the aorta in syphilis shows focal areas of destruction of the media with an infiltrate of lymphocytes and plasma cells (Fig. 4.2). The inflammatory cells are seen both within the areas of medial destruction and generally throughout the adventitia. There is some fibrous thickening of the adventitia but the overall thickness of the aortic wall is reduced. Small focal areas of destruction in the media are located around the vasa vasorum which show endothelial proliferation and obliteration of the lumen. Very occasionally organisms can be found.[6] In part the medial destruction may be ischaemic in origin, due to vascular damage in the vasa vasorum possibly relating to the production of a mucopolysaccharidase by the spirochaete which damages endothelial connections, but it is also caused by cell-based immune-mediated tissue damage to the media itself. Small foci of necrosis with adjacent giant cells (microgummata) are found in more acute cases.

Saccular aneurysms occur (Fig. 4.3) in 10–40% of patients with aortitis.[5] They are not associated with a risk of dissection but can expand to erode or press on adjacent tissues and rupture is a definite risk. Most aneurysms occur in the aortic arch where compression or erosion into the right bronchus, the superior vena cava or the right pulmonary artery occur. Descending thoracic aneurysms may compress the oesophagus, trachea or recurrent laryngeal nerve. Abdominal aneurysms are rare; in John Hunter's time syphilitic aneurysms of the popliteal artery were described. The histology of syphilitic aneurysms is identical to that of syphilitic aortitis but with more advanced medial destruction.

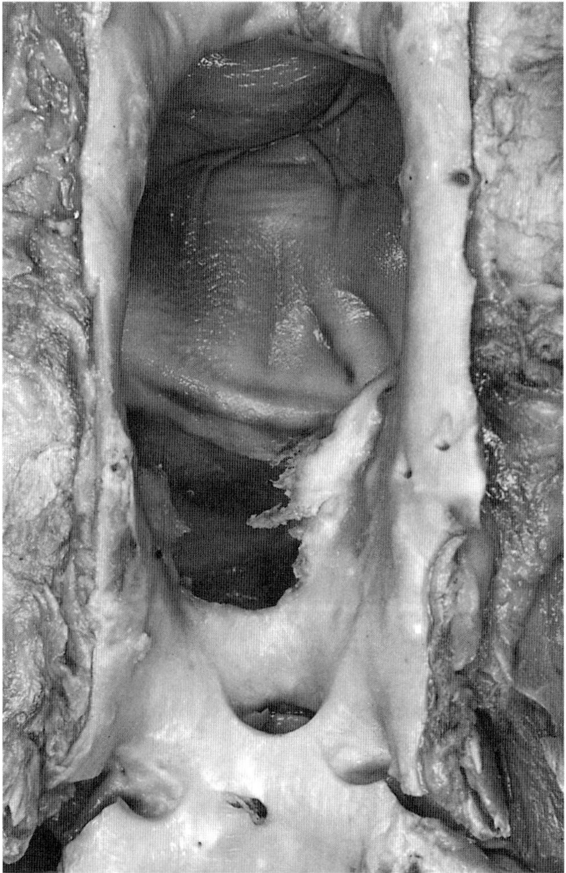

Fig. 4.3 Syphilitic aneurysm of aorta. There is a saccular, well-defined aneurysm in the lower thoracic aorta. Concomitant aortic regurgitation due to involvement of the ascending aorta was also present.

Syphilitic gummas are now the rarest manifestation of cardiovascular involvement. The gumma forms a grey expanded mass (Fig. 4.4) with areas of necrosis but without caseation. While any segment of the ventricular myocardium can be involved the upper interventricular septum is the site of predilection. The mass of tissue replaces the muscular interventricular septum at the base, along with the membranous septum, and then extends into the atrial septum destroying the A-V node. The gumma also surrounds the aortic valve and fills the sinuses, distorting and thickening the cusps. The histology is of dense fibrosis with ghost remnants of the original tissue. Fibrinoid necrosis of structured tissue is present. There is a pleomorphic infiltrate in which plasma cells predominate with marked endarteritis obliterans of small arteries. The cardiac gumma is often clinically misdiagnosed as a tumour due to its expanded form. A-V block and aortic regurgitation are common both to syphilitic aortitis and gumma formation.

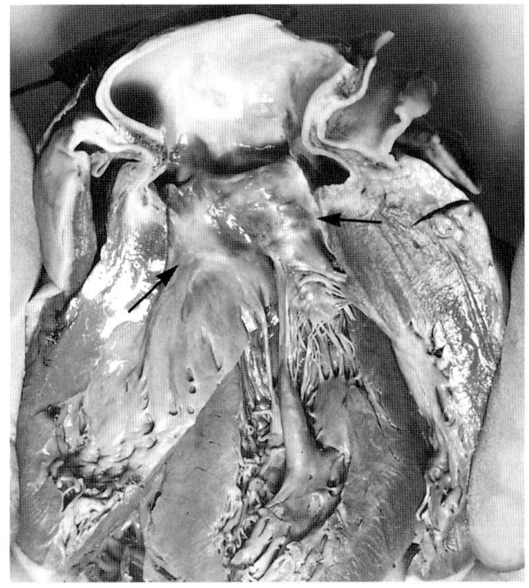

a)

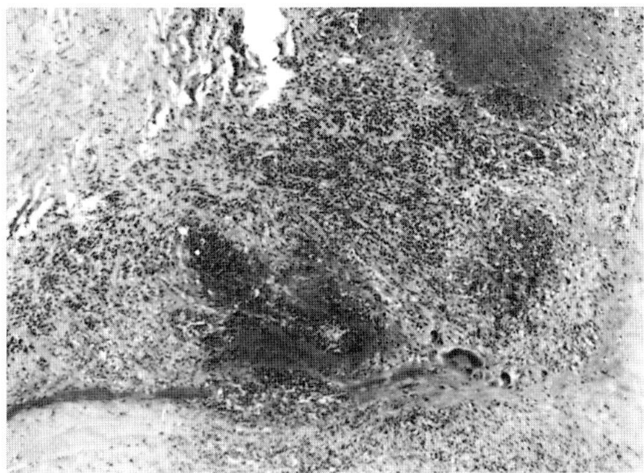

b)

Fig. 4.4 a,b Syphilitic gumma. (**a**) There is an ill defined mass (arrows) at the base of the aorta behind one aortic cusp. The mass extends into the membranous septum. (**b**) The histology shows fibrinoid necrosis of connective tissue with a surrounding chronic inflammatory infiltrate including giant cells.

Tuberculous aortitis

Even in the heyday of tuberculosis only 100 cases of involvement of the aorta were published by 1960.[7] Most cases are extension from tuberculous lesions in the vertebrae directly into the aorta to produce a local aneurysm. Direct deposition of organisms via miliary spread into the aortic media without adjacent periaortic disease is also described.[8] Vessels which enter a cavitating pulmonary tuberculous lesion may be eroded and bleed into the cavity. Concomitant tuberculosis elsewhere is a putative factor in the immunological damage to the aorta in Takayasu's disease.[9]

Fungal and bacterial aneurysms

The term mycotic aneurysm is ill defined. The term is usually applied to aneurysms of the aorta and smaller arteries such as the cerebral or coronary vessels that arise in subjects who have or have had recent bacterial or fungal endocarditis. In the aorta sharply defined saccular aneurysms develop (Fig. 4.5) with a high risk of rupture. In the cerebral arteries small aneurysms not unlike those seen in polyarteritis nodosa develop and carry a high risk of intracerebral or subarachnoid haemorrhage. Several possible mechanisms exist for the formation of mycotic aneurysms. An embolus containing organisms may impact in small and medium-sized arteries. A local inflammatory response to the viable organism itself may destroy the vessel wall locally. This mechanism seems most likely in acute staphylococcal endocarditis. The local inflammatory response may be immune in response but to bacterial antigens without viable

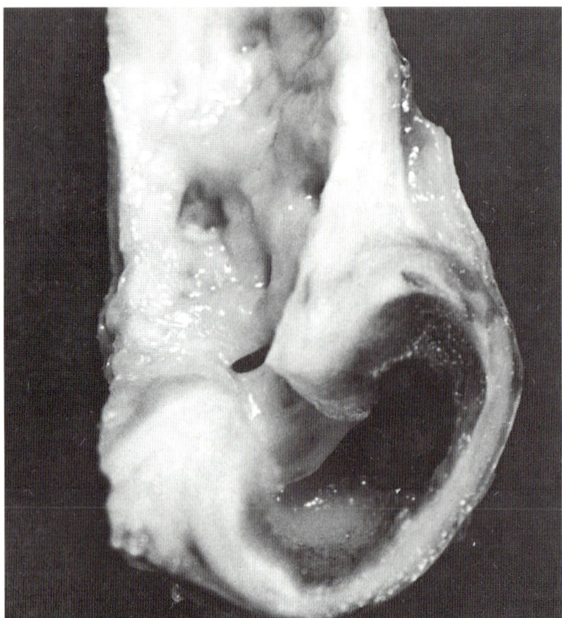

Fig. 4.5 Bacterial aneurysm of aorta. There is a sharply defined saccular aneurysm with a narrow neck in the thoracic aorta. Bacterial endocarditis of the aortic valve had been treated some weeks earlier. Detected as a mass attached to the aortic wall on chest X-ray and CT scan.

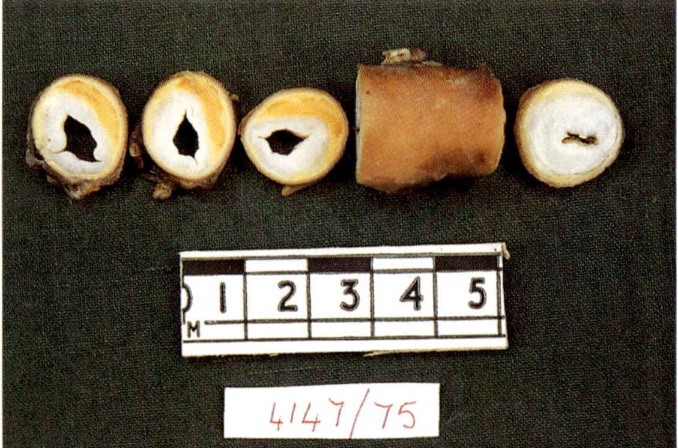

Fig. 4.6 Aorta in Takayasu's disease. The segment of aorta with extreme thickening of the wall significantly reducing the lumen was excised from a woman of 29 with stenosis of the thoracic aorta. The striking feature is concentric intimal fibrosis. Some lipid is present but the appearances are totally unlike atheroma in the aorta.

organisms being present. Both these mechanisms occur associated with emboli occluding the artery and, particularly in the brain, haemorrhage is compounded by infarction. A different mechanism must be present in mycotic aneurysms of the aorta. The lesion appears to be a localised destruction of the media, possibly due to deposition of organisms or immune complexes in the aortic wall via the vasa vasorum.

Takayasu's aortitis

The striking feature of this form of aortitis is the conversion of segments of the aorta and its major branches, or very rarely the pulmonary artery, into narrowed, rigid segments (Fig. 4.6). In essence it is a focal stenosing aortic disease.[10,11] Histologically the striking feature is intimal fibromuscular proliferation, often with some superimposed thrombosis which becomes organised into the thickened intima. Throughout the vessel wall there is a diffuse pleomorphic infiltrate of inflammatory cells, including plasma cells. The media may atrophy and focal destruction of the elastic tissue occurs. Small giant cells may occur but fibrinoid necrosis is not a feature.

The disease is markedly more common in the Far East, although sporadic cases occur worldwide, including Europe. Its pathogenesis is largely unknown, although there are some interesting associations with rheumatoid disease and HLA B5. Up to half of the patients are said to have concurrent tuberculosis elsewhere.[9] The clinical presentation is extremely variable because of the many different segments of aorta which can be involved and to the varying degree of collateral development. In the early stages there is evidence of an acute phase response with elevated C reactive protein and α-2-globulin. The chronic stage, in which most patients present, is dominated by obstruction of segments of the aorta or its major branches to the arms and neck. Angiographic classifications exist which delineate the pattern of disease[12] (Table 4.2).

Table 4.2 Classification of the distribution of Takayasu's disease based on angiographic demonstration of lesions in the aorta

Ia	Arch of aorta and branches
Ib	Aortic root
IIa	Thoracic
IIb	Abdominal
III	Multiple lesions combining I and II

Because there is no specific test or feature of the disease it is difficult to exactly delineate its limits. Some cases do develop dilated segments of aorta proximal and distal to the narrow segments. A small number of cases develop ascending aortic aneurysms and aortic regurgitation in addition to narrow distal segments of aorta. The definition should, however, stop short of giving the name Takayasu aortitis to aneurysms without any associated narrowed segments simply because they occur in patients from the Middle East.

Giant cell aortitis and arteritis

Giant cell aortitis and arteritis has a characteristic histological appearance in which there is fragmented elastic tissue associated with a striking giant cell response in addition to a diffuse infiltration of the wall with chronic inflammatory cells.[13] Fibromuscular intimal proliferation may become prominent as the lesions heal. There is clear evidence of a systemic upset and the onset is usually acute in elderly subjects. There is a raised ESR and a characteristic rapid response to steroids. There is a clear clinical association with polymyalgia rheumatica but the pathogenesis is entirely unknown. There is also a relation to HLA-DR4.

The symptoms depend on which arterial bed is involved. The most common form involves the extracranial arteries, including the temporal arteries.[14] Presentation is with headache, pain and tenderness on the scalp, muscle pain in the jaw and general malaise. Segments of the temporal artery may be swollen, tender and pulseless. Biopsy of the temporal artery has become a standard method of obtaining a cast iron diagnosis but it has its problems and false negatives are common.[15] The difficulties are due to several factors.

1. Sampling errors — the lesions characteristically are very focal and may be missed
2. The inflammatory process responds very rapidly to steroids which are often given early to minimise pain and the risk of ophthalmic nerve artery involvement — the percentage of positive biopsies falls to 20% within a week of steroids
3. Even without therapy the lesions are focal and at different stages of evolution.

A reporting scheme is described in which three histological categories are included; any of these is consistent with the diagnosis of giant cell temporal arteritis. In the classic fully developed acute stage of the disease there is a segmental inflammation not involving the whole circumference of the artery. Biopsies taken in this acute stage will however often show circumferential involvement. The media is predominantly involved with an infiltrate of lymphocytes, plasma cells and macrophages. In florid cases necrosis of tissue occurs (Fig. 4.7). Giant cells cluster around the ends of fragments of the internal elastic lamina in areas of necrosis. This giant cell response is not necessarily part of the basic process and can occur in any situation where elastic destruction occurs. In the absence of giant cells the lesions are often described as atypical non-granulomatous arteritis but this does not imply that the pathogenesis or course of the disease, if the clinical picture is otherwise typical, is different. In the healing phase of temporal arteritis fibrosis replaces the damaged media and extends between breaks in the elastic laminae into fibromuscular intimal proliferation. It is this healed phase that gives rise to most difficulty in diagnosis. Breaks in the elastic lamina and some intimal fibromuscular hyperplasia are common age-related changes in subjects without a clinical diagnosis of previous temporal arteritis. It is best to report the features and conclude that they are consistent with a clinical diagnosis of temporal arteritis.

Studies are reported in which a search has been made at autopsy for other arteries involved in cases of the polymyalgia rheumatica syndrome. About 15% show aortic lesions[16] and sporadic lesions are found in renal, mesenteric and splenic arteries. Giant cell aortitis (Fig. 4.8) is probably related to temporal arteritis in that the age distribution is identical and similar systemic manifestations occur. The presentation may be with aortic regurgitation due to root dilation, or aortic rupture and localised aneurysm formation. In the aorta the histology is characteristic and there are plates of necrotic elastic laminae at the margins of which giant cells form.

Another variant of giant cell arteritis involves

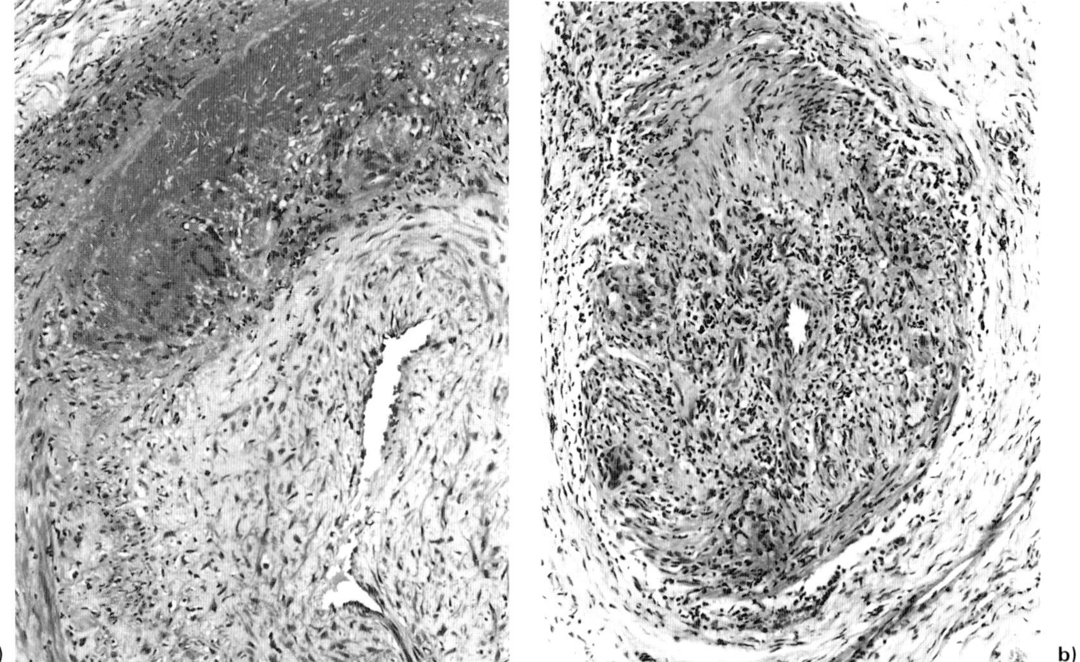

Fig. 4.7 a,b Temporal arteritis. (**a**) There is marked necrosis of medial tissue associated with a local giant cell response to fragmented elastic. The intima shows florid fibromuscular hyperplasia. This would be reported as active temporal giant cell arteritis. (**b**) There is florid fibromuscular intimal proliferation with a diffuse inflammatory infiltrate throughout the vessel wall. Giant cells are not a feature. This would be reported as atypical non-granulomatous arteritis. The clinical history and response to steroids was, however, typical of temporal arteritis.
(**a**) Haematoxylin–eosin × 165
(**b**) Haematoxylin–eosin × 42

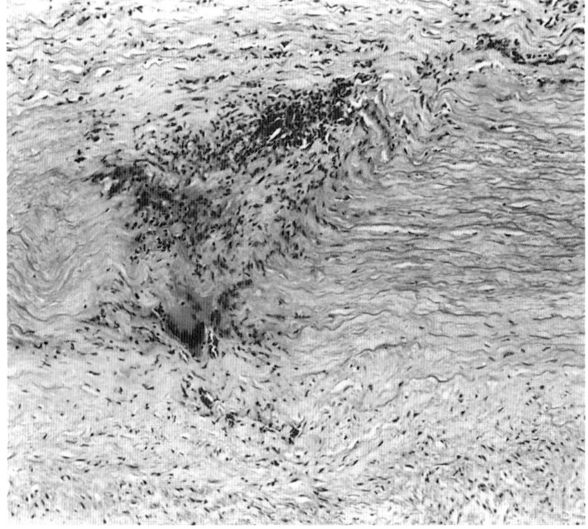

Fig. 4.8 Giant cell aortitis. There are areas of acellular media in which smooth muscle cells have been lost but the elastic laminae remain. At the margins of these necrotic plates of media there is an inflammatory infiltrate with giant cells related to fragmented elastic laminae.
Haematoxylin–eosin × 16

visceral arteries alone without cranial or aortic lesions.[1] Yet another possible variant exists in which granulomatous lesions occur only in the intracranial arteries and the classic systemic symptoms of polymyalgia rheumatica are absent. This form is related to malignant lymphomas and may be virally induced.[17]

It is questionable whether there is a unifying pathogenetic mechanism in all these forms of giant cell aortitis and arteritis. The association of giant cells and elastic laminae has suggested that some form of elastolysis followed by an immune reaction is the basic mechanism. Against this is the fact that induction of giant cells by fragmented elastic may occur in any destructive arteritis. Search for immune complexes has produced contradictory results.

Polyarteritis and its variants

Polyarteritis nodosa is a potentially lethal vasculitis with a 50% mortality within 3 months. In common with many of the vasculitides there is a systemic disorder with fever, weight loss and myalgia grafted on to symptoms related to the particular vascular bed involved.[18] In adults the disease is twice as common in men as in women and occurs in middle life. An infantile form also occurs with no specific pathological features to distinguish it from the adult form.

The histological appearances are the key to diagnosis. In the acute phase there is focal necrosis of the full thickness of the arterial wall. This necrosis is localised to short segments of the artery and in these segments is often eccentric, being confined to one segment of the circumference. The necrotic areas are brightly eosinophilic ('fibrinoid necrosis') due to insudation of fibrinogen being converted to fibrin in the acute inflammatory process that develops. Immunoglobulins and immune complexes are present in some cases. The localised nature of the inflammatory process coupled with the transmural destruction of the vessel wall leads to small, pea-sized aneurysms (Fig. 4.9), hence the term nodosa.

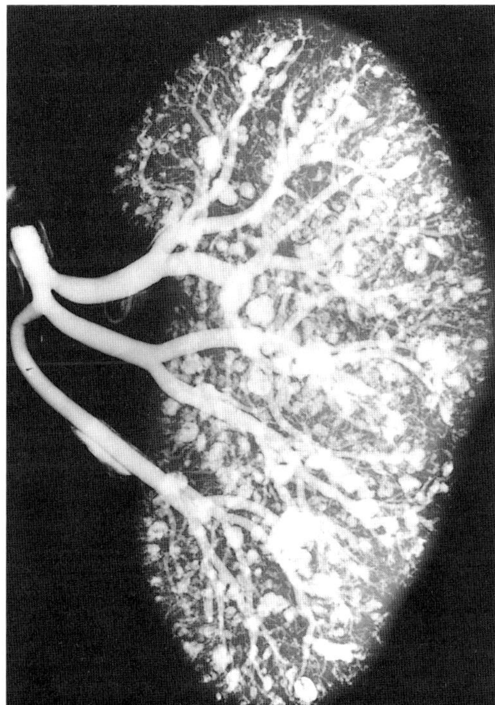

Fig. 4.9 Polyarteritis nodosa. Renal post-mortem angiogram showing multiple small aneurysms up to 0.5 cm in diameter. Similar aneurysms were present in coronary and cerebral arteries.

In the acute phase of the arteritis (Fig. 4.10) the cell response is predominantly neutrophilic, being rapidly followed by a more pleomorphic infiltrate including eosinophils, lymphocytes and macrophages. Subsequently intense fibroblastic proliferation develops which converts the affected arterial segment into scar tissue, usually with obliteration of the lumen by fibromuscular intimal proliferation.

Polyarteritis is divided into two forms, the classic form affecting medium-sized arteries and that affecting arterioles (microscopic polyarteritis). The latter is predominantly a renal glomerular disease.[19] The classic form of polyarteritis may affect the arteries in the heart, kidney, gastrointestinal tract, brain and skin. Pulmonary involvement is rare. In affected arteries small aneurysm formation can be identified by angiography and symptoms result from both bleeding due to rupture of aneurysms and occlusion of arteries. In the myocardium widespread small focal infarcts

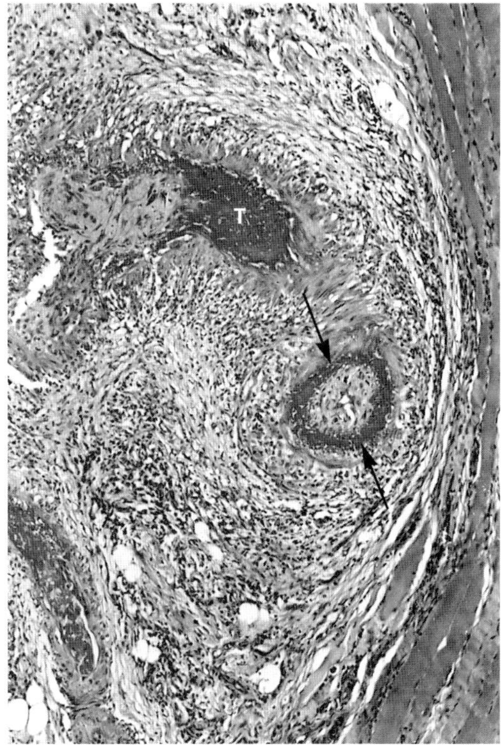

Fig. 4.10 Polyarteritis nodosa. A skeletal muscle artery showing a ring of fibrinoid necrosis (arrows). Another segment of the artery shows thrombosis (T) and intimal proliferation. There is a diffuse inflammatory infiltrate through the vessel wall.
Haematoxylin–eosin × 65

are produced. Biopsy of skin and muscle is a means of obtaining a tissue diagnosis but is positive in only 30% of cases. Cardiac biopsies usually show the effects of ischaemia rather than the actual vascular lesions responsible for it because the arteries which are affected are subepicardial and not obtained.

The pathogenesis of polyarteritis is heterogeneous. Immune complex deposition is common and is thought to result from hepatitis, tumour antigens and drugs. Drug-related polyarteritis is often associated with a higher proportion of eosinophils in the vascular lesions. A wide range of drugs have been implicated including phenylbutazone, D-penicillamine and chlorpropamide.[20] There is also a strong association with hairy cell leukaemia.

In the microscopic form of polyarteritis the renal glomeruli are the primary target with the production of segmental necrotising glomerular lesions. The pathogenesis is rather different from macroscopic polyarteritis, immune complexes being absent and antineutrophil cytoplasmic autoantibodies levels in the plasma often high.

Kawasaki's disease

In its fully expressed form this is an acute febrile illness in children below the age of 5 who develop conjunctivitis, inflammation of the oral mucosa and tongue, cervical lymphadenopathy and an erythematous skin rash. The rash is accentuated over the palms and soles, which become bright red and then desquamate. The clinical picture is characteristic when fully developed but many milder cases are probably misdiagnosed as rubella. The name mucocutaneous lymph node syndrome is sometimes used.[21] A proportion of cases, including those in whom the systemic symptoms were mild, develop coronary arteritis. The exact proportion who develop this complication is unclear but studies by angiography and echocardiography suggest cardiac complications may develop in up to 40% of cases (Chapter 3). In contrast to polyarteritis nodosa, in Kawasaki's disease the main epicardial coronary arteries are selectively involved (Fig. 4.11). The arteries show transmural inflammation with fibrinoid necrosis and characteristically the arteries dilate over long segments. Focal aneurysms develop within 2–4

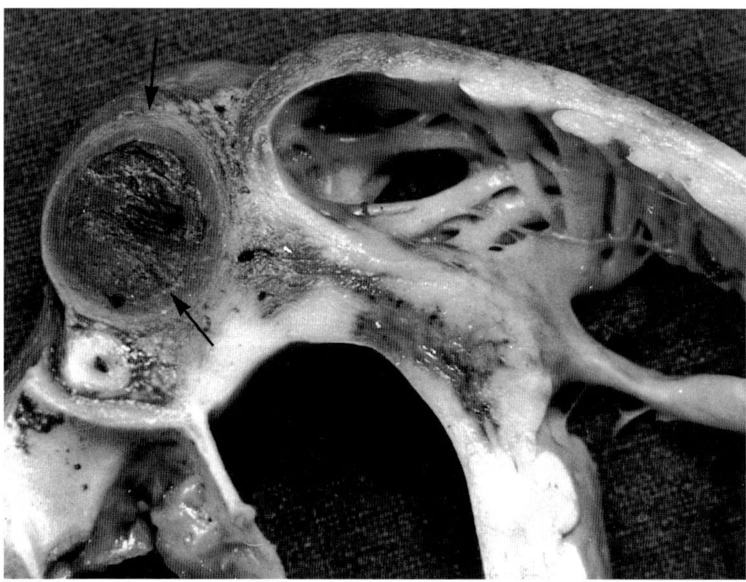

Fig. 4.11 Kawasaki's disease. Transverse section of both ventricles in a child of 6 who died suddenly 14 days after a febrile illness with a skin rash. The left anterior descending aorta (arrows) is greatly dilated and filled with thrombus. The myocardium shows areas of pale necrosis.

weeks of the onset of symptoms. It is estimated that 3–5% of cases develop sufficient arteritis that thrombosis of a major vessel occurs, leading to sudden death or acute myocardial infarction. The degree to which generalised dilatation occurs has some prognostic value; diameters of over 4 mm in a major epicardial artery imply that regression will not occur. Those cases which do not resolve develop aneurysms and a tendency to coronary thrombosis long after the acute phase illness is over.

Fatal cases are unmistakable by naked-eye examination. There is massive diffuse dilation of several segments of the epicardial arteries which are occluded by thrombosis. The left ventricle is dilated and shows various stages of infarction. The myocardium and valves often show a concomitant infiltrate with lymphocytes, suggesting that a pancarditis is present, but this is difficult to assess in the face of ischaemic myocardial damage. If arteritis is present in organs outside the heart, the case is probably best regarded as infantile polyarteritis nodosa. This potential overlap of Kawasaki's disease and infantile polyarteritis highlights the tendency of all the vasculitic entities to merge into each other.

Wegener's granulomatosis

This condition is an entity characterised by the concordance of granulomatous necrotising lesions of the upper and lower respiratory tract with a systemic vasculitis involving many organs including the kidney where a proliferative glomerulonephritis is a common cause of death. It occurs at any age and in either sex but is more common in association with the HLA-DR2 and B8 antigens. Untreated, most patients die within 2 years but immunosuppression is usually effective in prolonging life. The lungs, nasal sinuses and kidneys

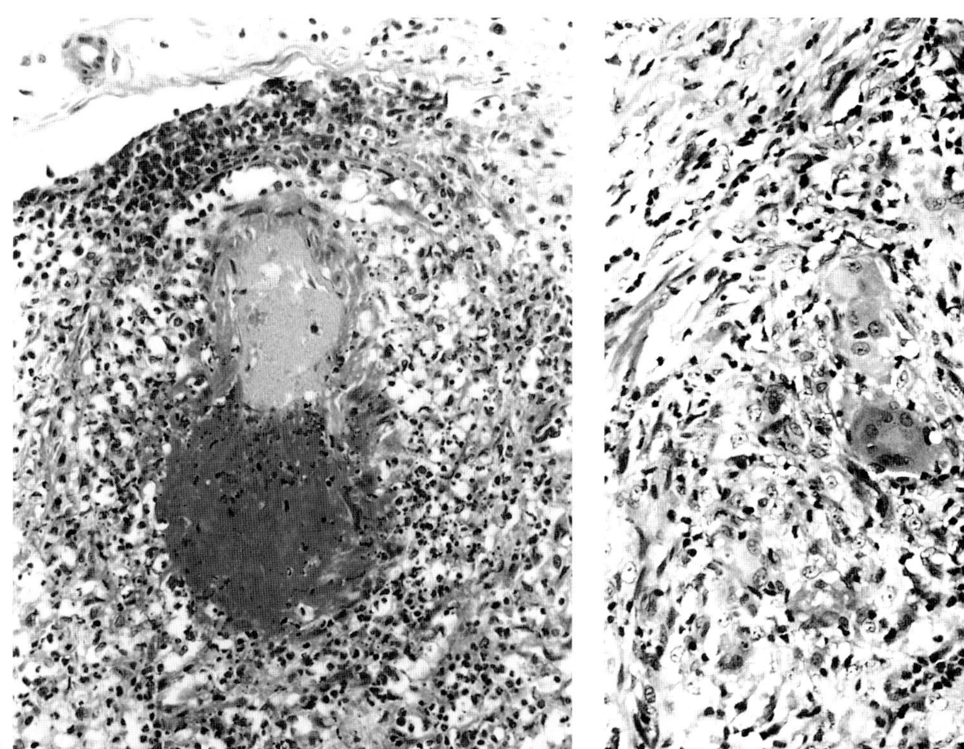

Fig. 4.12 a,b Wegener's granulomatosis. (**a**) A small coronary artery shows eccentric fibrinoid necrosis and infiltration of the wall by inflammatory cells including polymorphs. (**b**) Adjacent to the artery in (**a**) there is a loosely arranged granuloma with giant cells.
(**a**) Haematoxylin–eosin × 65
(**b**) Haematoxylin–eosin × 175

are conjointly involved in over 90% of cases, joints, eyes, ears conjointly in 60–70%, skin in 45%, the CNS in 22% and the heart only in 12% of cases.[22] The initial complaints of most patients are sinusitis and nasal obstruction or ulceration. These are followed by cough, dyspnoea and haemoptysis as lung involvement develops and haematuria followed by renal failure when the kidneys become involved.

The pulmonary lesions in Wegener's granulomatosis are those most easily recognised. Pulmonary X-rays show solid opaque lesions up to 5 cm across within the lungs. Macroscopically the lesions are solid and grey. Histological examination shows central areas of coagulative necrosis in which the outlines of the tissue, particularly blood vessels, are retained. Granulation tissue is prominent. Vasculitic lesions in adjacent arteries may or may not be present. Extrapulmonary lesions are dominated by a vasculitis with involvement of a wide range of vessel sizes. In the heart both epicardial and intramyocardial vessels are involved. The arteritis is histologically similar to polyarteritis nodosa (Fig. 4.12) with the addition that giant cells are present either adjacent to the artery wall or in areas of tissue necrosis. Veins also are involved. A myocarditis with giant cells in the absence of vascular lesions is also reported.[23]

The pathogenesis of the condition is not clear; antineutrophil autoantibodies are present in most cases. Titres of more than 1/40 seem constantly related to tissue lesions.

The Churg–Strauss syndrome

The Churg–Strauss syndrome has affinities, at least in morphological terms, with the macroscopic form of polyarteritis nodosa. In the pulmonary and systemic arteries a necrotising vasculitis occurs. The features which separate the Churg–Strauss syndrome are a history of severe asthma which precedes the vasculitis, often by some years, and a circulating hypereosinophilia of more than 5×10^9 l. In the vasculitic phase plasma IgE levels are very high and there is a systemic illness with fever, a high ESR and weight loss. Up to 70% of cases develop widespread pulmonary infiltrates.

The histological appearances are those of an eosinophilic vasculitis in association with extravascular granulomas. The vascular lesions involve a considerable spectrum of vessel size down to

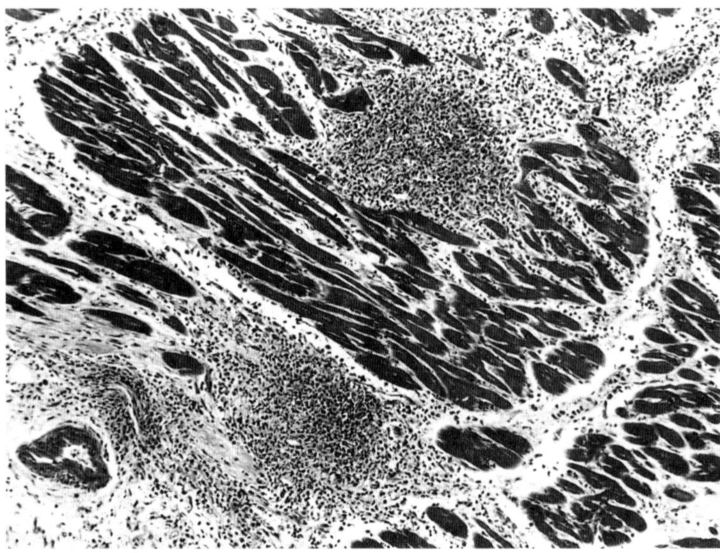

Fig. 4.13 Myocardium in Churg–Strauss syndrome. The myocardium shows nodular aggregates of lymphoid cells with large numbers of eosinophils centred on small arteries and veins although many larger arteries in the myocardium are not involved.
Haematoxylin–eosin × 19

arteriolar level and may also involve veins (Fig. 4.13). There is focal transmural necrosis of vessels, with an inflammatory infiltrate in which eosinophils predominate over lymphocytes and macrophages. The extravascular granulomas have poorly formed centres with some small giant cells and macrophages arranged in a palisaded manner more reminiscent of a rheumatoid nodule than sarcoidosis. Eosinophils are present in large numbers. Vasculitic lesions occur in the gastrointestinal tract, spleen and heart but such involvement is less common than in Wegener's granulomatosis. Death is usually from right ventricular failure secondary to lung disease. The persistent hypereosinophilia can evoke endomyocardial fibrosis (Chapter 6) and this is a more common form of cardiac involvement than coronary arteritis in the Churg–Strauss syndrome.

The exact relation of the Churg–Strauss syndrome and polyarteritis nodosa is not known and they may form part of a spectrum. Asthma is said to be absent in classic polyarteritis nodosa, this being predetermined by the fact that if asthma is present the disease is classified as Churg–Strauss syndrome. One view is that the conditions overlap and the pattern of the disease is determined by the route by which the unknown antigens enter the body — if via the respiratory tract pulmonary lesions develop, if via the intestine they do not.[19]

Thromboangiitis obliterans (Buerger's disease)

This disease may or may not exist as a distinct clinical and pathological entity.[24] The diagnosis depends on inclusion and exclusion criteria which, if strictly used, do seem to define an entity, albeit a rare one. The clinical features are lower limb ischaemia progressing to gangrene occurring in males below the age of 45 who smoke. A migratory thrombophlebitis precedes the limb gangrene and both arteries and veins are found to be occluded in amputation specimens. An important negative aspect is that atherosclerosis is absent. This exclusion is usually made by an absence of risk factors such as hyperlipidaemia, including hypertriglyceridaemia, and by vascular ultrasound demonstrating a normal aorta and iliac arteries. From this definition it is clear that the diagnosis over the age of 50 is difficult due to the inevitable presence of concomitant atherosclerosis. In its pure, strictly defined form there is an excess of cases in subjects who are HLA A9- and B5-positive and the link with cigarette smoking is very strong. Antibodies to collagen are present in around 80% of cases.[25]

The pathological features of necessity are described from amputation specimens and most are late in the disease. In end stage both arteries and veins are solid fibrous chords bound together in dense periadventitial fibrous tissue. In the minority of cases in which an earlier stage of the active disease is still present both arteries and veins contain thrombi with a high polymorph content. There is transmural inflammation but without necrosis, elastic fragmentation or giant cells. Episodic thrombosis and recanalisation occur. An important negative point is the absence of cholesterol emboli in small arteries.

Vasculitis in collagen–vascular disease

Many of the connective tissue disorders are associated with aortitis and arteritis. In severe rheumatoid arthritis vasculitis is common in the small arteries and veins surrounding the nodules or within highly inflamed periarticular tissues. Rarely a disseminated vasculitis of the polyarteritic type develops.[26] In systemic lupus a necrotising arteritis of medium-sized arteries (cerebral, coronary, renal) and down to arteriolar level in the skin and renal glomeruli occurs. Immunoglobulins are present in the vascular lesions. A wide range of symptoms including purpura, skin gangrene, cerebral and myocardial infarction and renal failure occur. Local aneurysm formation similar to polyarteritis also occurs. The advent of arteritis in systemic lupus is a poor prognostic sign. In rheumatoid arthritis an aortitis may involve the ascending aorta in a manner identical to ankylosing spondylitis but is less severe. An identical aortitis develops in Reiter's syndrome. All of these inflammatory lesions in the aorta have almost identical histological appearances and detailed clinical data; HLA status and serology are needed to separate them. All produce aortic incompetence (Chapter 6).

NON-INFLAMMATORY AORTIC DISEASE

With age the aorta, particularly the thoracic portion, dilates and becomes less elastic. This change is associated with a change in compliance; the aorta becomes a rigid tube leading to a more rapid rise in systolic pressure and a widened pulse pressure. These physiological changes are due to structural changes in the media the degree of which is sufficient to blur the distinction between normality and pathological change.

At birth there are about 35 elastic laminae arranged in parallel in the aortic media; this number rises to 55 or above in the adult.[27] Between the elastic laminae are packed smooth muscle cells surrounded by fine collagen and a considerable amount of glycosaminoglycan. Vessels from the adventitia penetrate the outer fifth of the media and form an arcade at this level. The inner four-fifths of the normal media is avascular.

In what is called 'physiological arteriosclerosis' the intima thickens and by the age of 20 develops fine elastic laminae that blur the structural distinction between intima and media. The elastic laminae in the media thicken and often reduplicate, making counts of the laminae in a transect very difficult. By late middle age some fragmentation of elastic laminae is common (Fig. 4.14). Smooth muscle cells diminish in density and the elastic laminae lie closer together. In other aortas smooth muscle proliferation in the inner third of the media appears to occur, widening the gap between the elastic laminae. With age the amount of stainable glycosaminoglycan rises and may even form small cystic spaces. Finally, in

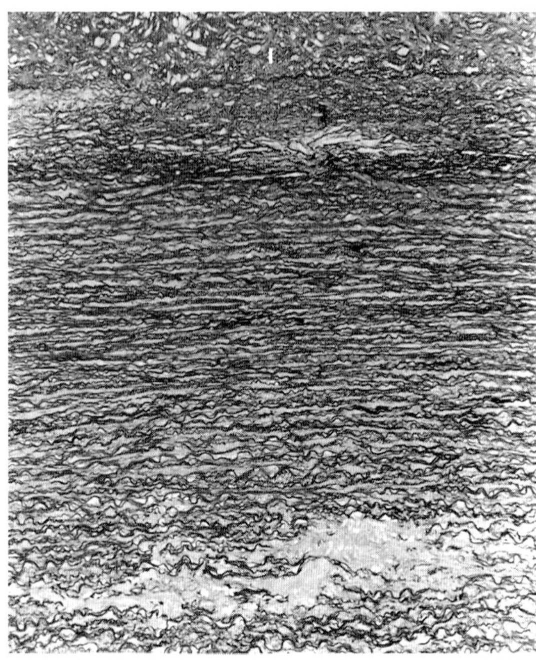

Fig. 4.14 Age change in aortic media. The intima (I) is thickened. The elastic laminae in the inner third of the media are straighter and closer together than normal. In the outer third of the media the laminae are wavy but there is focal disruption with cystic change.
Elastica/Van Gieson × 16

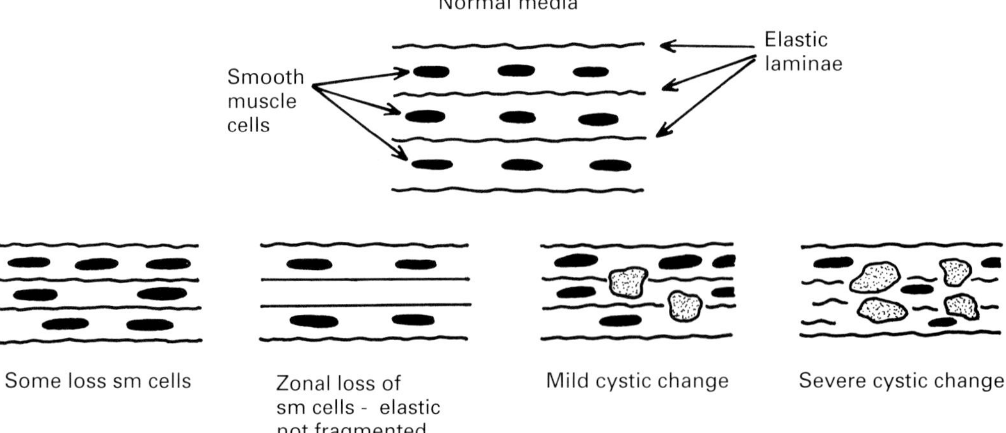

Fig. 4.15 Spectrum of non-inflammatory medial disease

many aortas from subjects over the age of 70 large areas of media become virtually acellular, in other words smooth muscle cell death has occurred.

These complex changes (Fig. 4.15), which can be summarised as any permutation of 1) elastic fragmentation, 2) smooth muscle loss, 3) cystic change and 4) fibrosis, make the concept of normality in an aorta from an elderly person well nigh impossible. All that can be said is that an assessment must be made of the degree of change in relation to age. Given that this spectrum of change occurs in ageing alone it has been regarded as 'non-specific'.[28] This concept should not obscure the fact that a more severe degree of these changes does occur in certain genetic disorders of connective tissue synthesis such as Marfan's disease (Figs 4.16, 4.17). The medial changes of age are accelerated by hypertension. The changes are in the broadest sense a progressive failure of the medial smooth muscle cell to maintain the connective tissue matrix of the media and in particular the elastic laminae. It is perhaps not surprising that genetic defects in the synthesis of key components of the connective tissue enhance and accelerate the morphological changes that occur with age.

The aorta in inherited connective tissue disorders

Effects of medial non-inflammatory disorders

The simplest result of medial damage is dilation of the aorta, which is an almost inevitable

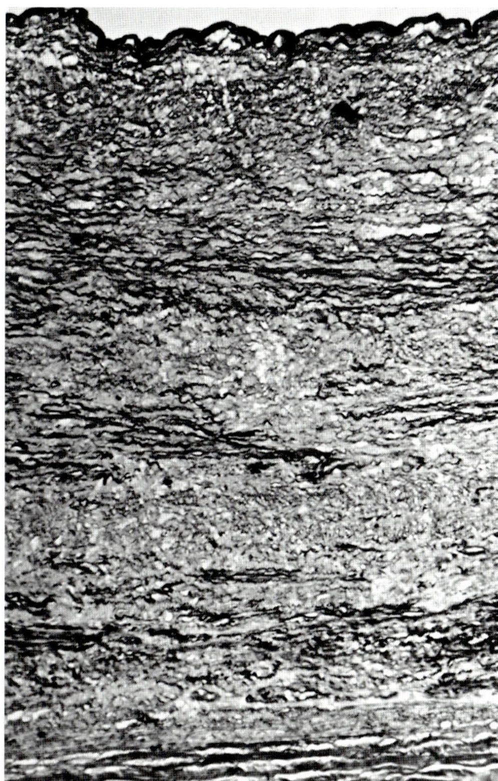

Fig. 4.16 Non-inflammatory aortic medial change. Throughout the media there are large areas in which the elastic laminae are destroyed but cystic change is minimal. Elastica/Van Gieson × 16

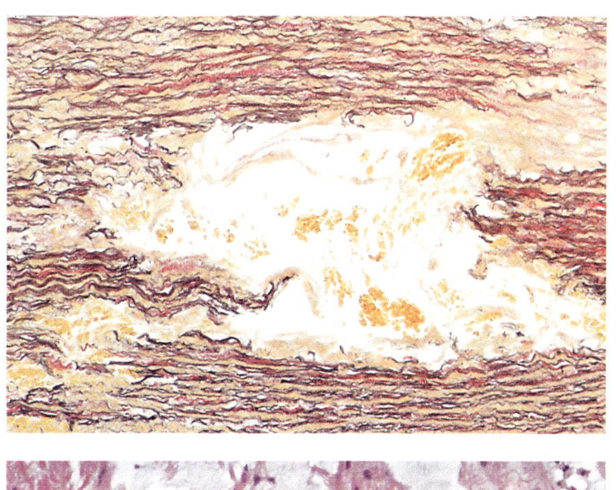

a)

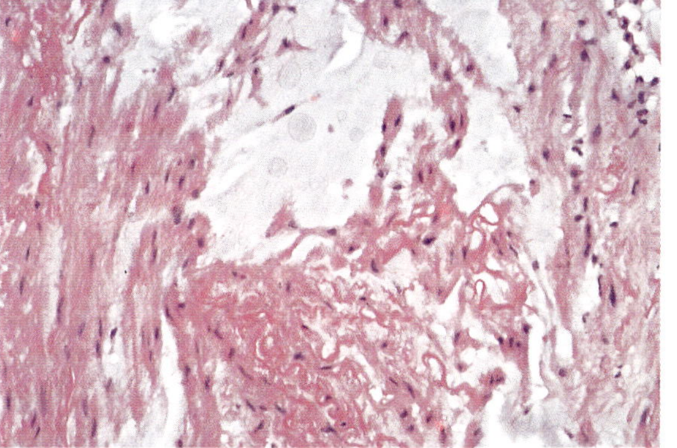

b)

Fig. 4.17 a,b Marfan's disease — aortic media. The classic histological hallmark of Marfan's disease is disruption of laminae leaving an open space in sections stained with elastica/Van Gieson. In haematoxylin and eosin stains these spaces contain blue connective tissue mucin.
(**a**) Elastica/Van Gieson × 65
(**b**) Haematoxylin–eosin × 65

consequence of getting old. Simple dilatation is of consequence only when there is sufficient change in the ascending aorta to induce aortic regurgitation. Trivial degrees of aortic regurgitation are now recognised by Doppler flow studies to be common in both hypertension and old age. A more serious consequence is the formation of aneurysms. Clear distinction must be made between saccular or fusiform aortic aneurysms and aortic dissection. In the former the wall of the aneurysm is derived from the full thickness of the media. In the latter there is an intimal tear from which blood tracks along the media in a plane well out towards the adventitia. This dissection tract ruptures outward, usually at a point somewhere distal or proximal to the intimal tear. In general, inflammatory destruction of the media causes saccular or fusiform aneurysms and not dissection. Both aneurysms and dissection complicate non-inflammatory medial disease.

Marfan's syndrome

Marfan's syndrome is an autosomal dominant hereditary disease characterised by cutaneous, ophthalmic and cardiovascular involvement. The disease was first described in a 5-year-old girl by Marfan in 1896. Since then other clinical manifestations have been added to the original description and significant progress has been made regarding the pathogenesis of the disease.

The diagnostic criteria for Marfan's syndrome have been recently reviewed[29] and include:

1. Family history of Marfan's syndrome
2. Musculoskeletal abnormalities such as tall stature, increased ratio of upper to lower body segment over two standard deviations above the mean value for age, thoracic deformities such as pectus excavatum or scoliosis, cutaneous stretch marks (striae atrophicae), arachnodactyly and high-arched palate
3. Ophthalmic abnormalities such as subluxation of the lens and myopia
4. Cardiovascular abnormalities such as dilatation of the aortic root, aortic dissection, mitral and/or aortic valve prolapse and/or regurgitation.

The cardiovascular manifestations are important in that approximately 90% of Marfan patients ultimately die of cardiovascular causes, the average age at death being 32 years.[30]

Marfan's syndrome can be associated with congenital heart defects such as tetralogy of Fallot, atrial septal defect and bicuspid aortic valve. The frequency of these congenital heart defects in Marfan's is higher than in the general population.[31]

Marfan's syndrome affecting the heart in infants has somewhat different clinical manifestations[32] from the syndrome in adults; the mean age at death is only 16 months. The main cause of death is congestive heart failure secondary to both mitral and tricuspid regurgitation. The frequency of mitral regurgitation is significantly higher than in the adult with Marfan's disease (89% vs 13%). Infants with Marfan's disease also have an extremely high frequency of tricuspid regurgitation, which is virtually unknown in adults. The frequency of a positive family history is much lower than in the adult group. Pathology reports of patients with the infantile form describe myxomatous changes in the atrioventricular valves, with thickened and elongated chordae tendineae and redundant pulmonary valve cusps. Histologically, there is disruption of elastic fibres both in the ascending aorta and the main pulmonary artery, as well as fragmentation of collagen in the valves.

In Marfan's syndrome in adults the cardiovascular findings include dilatation of the aortic

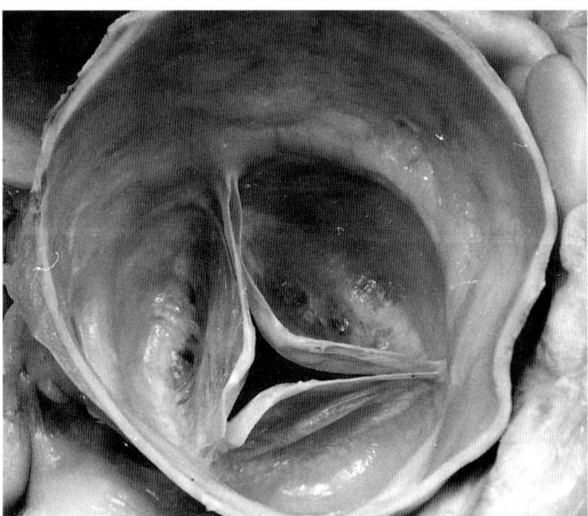

Fig. 4.18 Aortic root in Marfan's syndrome. Viewed from above the aortic root is dilated and the aortic cusps fail to meet allowing regurgitation to occur.

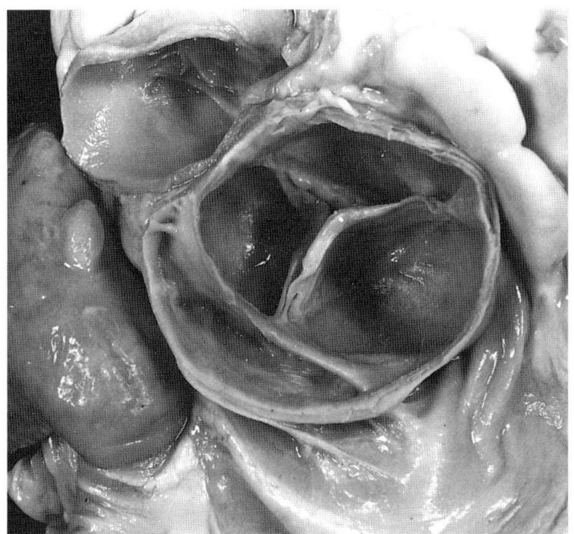

Fig. 4.19 Aortic root in Marfan's syndrome. Viewed from above there is a healed dissection tear in the aorta just above one commissure.

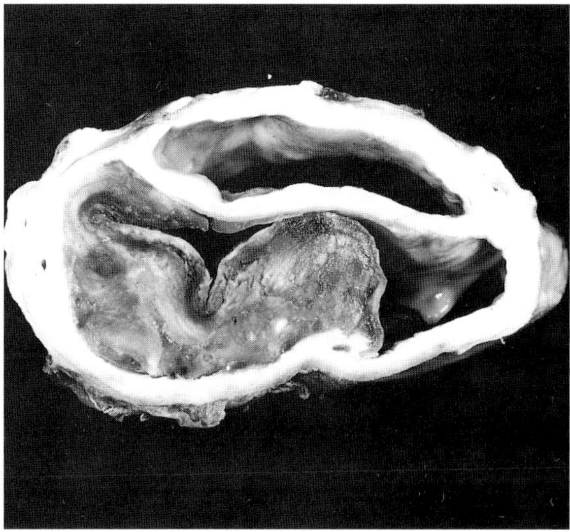

Fig. 4.20 Chronic dissection of aorta in Marfan's syndrome. Segments of thoracic aorta in which there was a chronic dissection tract filled with thrombus have been resected.

root (Fig. 4.18), with or without aortic dissection (Fig. 4.19), and aortic regurgitation. The dilatation of the aortic root generally starts above the level of the coronary ostia; the aortic valve cusps become thinner and stretched and are not able to coapt, leading to aortic regurgitation. Aortic dissection is the main cause of death in patients with Marfan's syndrome. The dissection usually involves the root of the aorta and the ascending aorta and tends to rupture into the pericardial sac, resulting in cardiac tamponade and death. One or more chronic dissection tracts may however occur (Fig. 4.20). Established risk factors for aortic dissection are a family history of dissection, and a dilated aortic root. However, some patients with Marfan's syndrome develop aortic dissection with a non-dilated aorta. Clinically, aortic dissection can be quite easily diagnosed by trans-oesophageal echocardiography; this has become the best available tool for patients' follow-up and to detect any changes in the size of the aortic root, i.e. progressive dilatation, which should lead to surgical treatment. The cut-off point regarding diameter of the aortic root has been defined as 5.5 cm. Beyond that point the patient should be recommended to have surgical treatment, even if he or she is asymptomatic and there is no evidence of dissection.[33] Serial echocardiographic follow-up of patients with Marfan's syndrome suggests that dilatation of the aortic root is a prognostic sign regarding dissection.

Recent surgical reviews of surgical treatment of aortic root dilatation, aortic dissection and other cardiovascular complications in patients with Marfan's syndrome[34] show that the early surgical mortality rate varies between 0 and 7.7%, whereas the late mortality rate can reach 27%. The mean follow-up was 7 years.

Long-term follow-up studies[35] have shown that at least 70% of Marfan patients will show an increase in the aortic root measurements at 3 years, with an 'overall rate' of dilatation of 2 mm per year. The importance of carrying out serial echocardiograms in order to measure the aortic root cannot be overemphasised.

In adults with Marfan's disease aortic regurgitation is the result of root dilatation; mitral regurgitation is also common and is due to a combination of ring dilatation, cusp expansion and dilatation of the left ventricle. In some patients ventricular dilatation is out of proportion with the degree of aortic and mitral regurgitation. This suggests that defects of the intramyocardial connective tissue are also present. Arrhythmias and sudden death may occur in such patients.

The genetic defect of Marfan's syndrome has recently been identified. Previous studies searching for defects in collagen types I and III did not show any positive results but abnormalities of the fibrillin gene have now been identified. Fibrillin is one of the microfibrillary elements of the extracellular matrix and is found in many tissues, including periosteum, corneal stroma, glomeruli, bronchioles, the suspensory ligament and the aortic media. Fibrillin is a glycoprotein with a molecular weight of 350 000 kDa, and a high content of cystein residues.[36] Its structure contains an epidermal-growth-factor-like motif, as well as a tissue-growth-factor-β motif. It has been suggested that fibrillin is associated with other components of the extracellular matrix such as fibronectin, elastin and amyloid substance P. Studies using monoclonal antibodies to fibrillin showed abnormal staining patterns in the aortas of a majority of patients with Marfan's syndrome. Later, by means of linkage analysis, the fibrillin gene (FBN1) was localised in chromosome 15q15-q21.[37] A second gene (FBN2) is on chromosome 5 and is particularly associated with arachnodactyly and lens problems.[38]

The gene defect in Marfan's disease may express itself in structural changes in the media. These in their fully developed form include elastic fragmentation with the formation of cystic spaces filled with connective tissue mucins (Fig. 4.15). These changes are, however, often focal and other areas of the media look structurally normal.

Other genetic defects of connective tissue synthesis

Ehlers–Danlos syndrome

The 10 described clinical variants of the Ehlers–Danlos syndrome have a variable cardiovascular component; the dominant features are however hyperelastic skin, poor wound healing, joint hypermobility, intestinal rupture and hernias.[39] Cardiovascular manifestations include aortic dissection (EDS I, II), aortic dilatation, aortic regurgitation and aortic rupture (EDS I, II, IV, VI, XI), mitral valve prolapse and regurgitation (I, II, III, V, VI, VIII, X) and spontaneous rupture and arteriovenous fistulae in peripheral arteries (IV). The arterial disease in type IV is often a significant part of the clinical picture, responsible for haemorrhage and fistulae. The arterial wall appears thin with fragmentation of the internal elastic lamina. In dermal vessels evidence of periadventitial haemorrhage in the form of haemosiderin deposition is often present. In the mitral valve the changes consist of replacement of the fibrosa by loosely arranged myxomatous tissue differing from idiopathic mitral prolapse only by its greater degree. The aortic medial changes are similarly rather non-specific, with thinning of the media, some elastic disruption and formation of small cystic spaces.

Cutis laxa

In cutis laxa the skin is deeply folded and emphysema is the dominant clinical feature. Dilation of the aorta and major arteries is prominent, with a histological appearance identical to that in Marfan's syndrome. Mitral valve prolapse is common but the disease is too rare to estimate the risk of aortic dissection and rupture.

Osteogenesis imperfecta

The principal symptoms relate to bone fragility. In all four genetic types aortic dilatation, aortic regurgitation and mitral valve prolapse can occur. The aortic medial changes are very similar to Marfan's syndrome but medial calcification may occur as an additional feature.

DISSECTION OF THE AORTA AND ARTERIES

Dissection of the aorta is a different entity from dissection of smaller arteries such as the coronary, mesenteric or renal vessels.

In the aorta an intimal tear is almost inevitably present. Three patterns have been recognised. The classification (Fig. 4.21) is largely aimed as a guide to surgical management.[40]

Type 1. The dissection tear is in the ascending aorta within 2–3 cm of the aortic valve (Figs 4.22, 4.23). The tear is clean-cut and straight, almost looking like a cut. It may be in the long axis or the

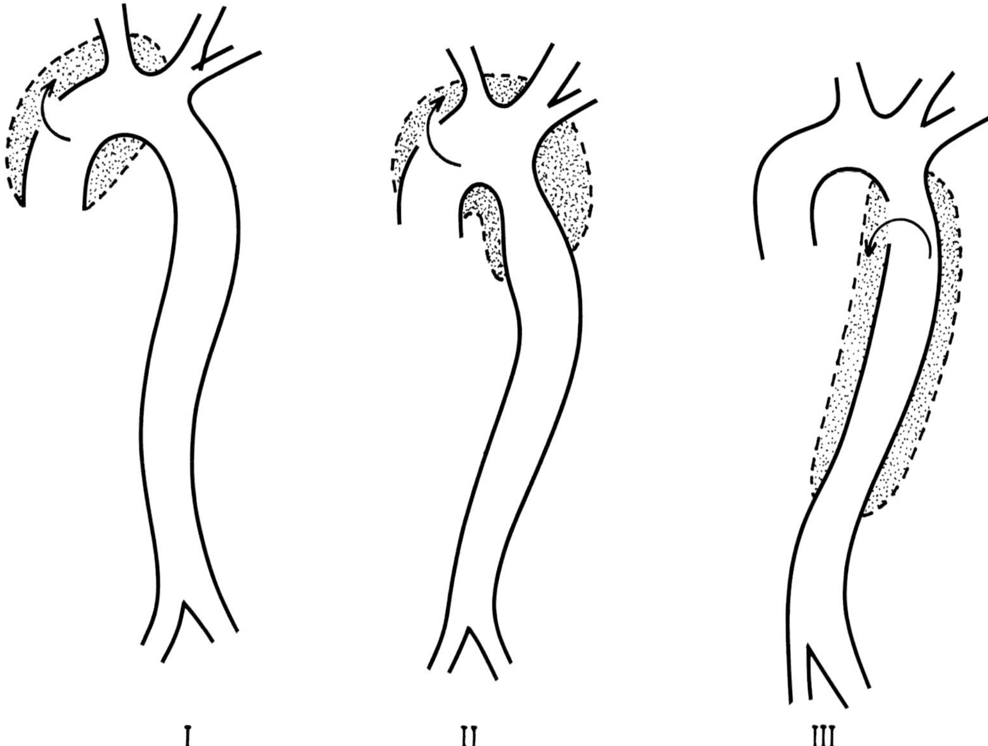

Fig. 4.21 Classification of aortic dissection

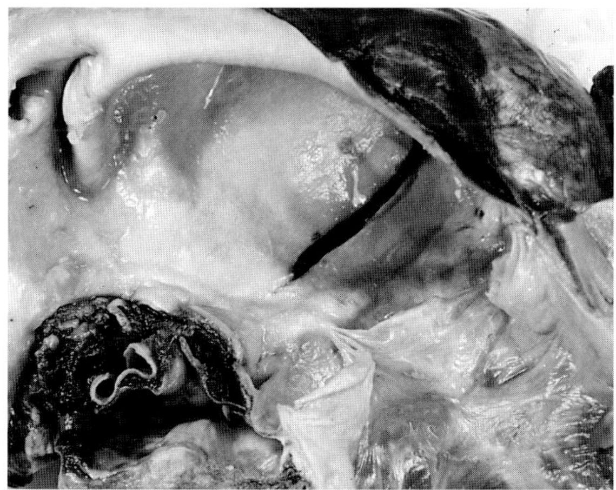

Fig. 4.22 Type I aortic dissection. There is a transverse intimal tear 2 cm above the aortic valve. Dissection was confined to the ascending aorta.

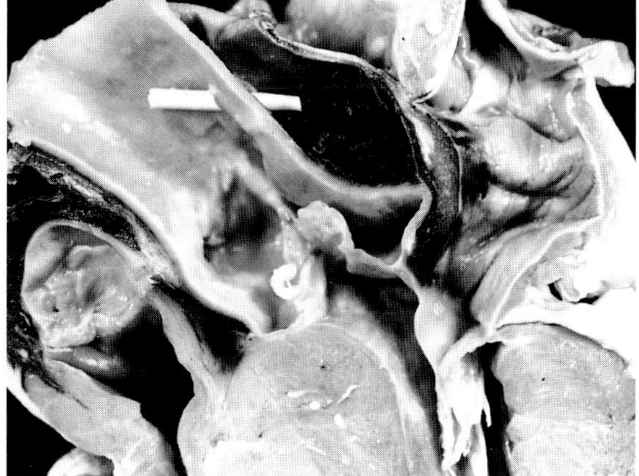

Fig. 4.23 Type I aortic dissection. There is a vertical tear in the ascending aorta which leads to a dissection tract in the media. This tract dissects downward to the aortic valve.

transverse axis of the aorta or T-shaped. Transverse tears may be circumferential. The dissection plane is in the outer quarter of the media and extends distally around the arch to the left subclavian artery. Dissection may extend into the carotid, brachial or right coronary artery. Blood in the lumen of the dissection tract may occlude the lumen of these arteries by external pressure. External rupture may occur at any point but haemopericardium or right haemothorax is the most common final event. Survival without surgical intervention is rare.

Type 2. The tear is as in type 1 but dissection is not confined to the ascending aorta (Fig. 4.24). The sites of external rupture are identical.

Type 3. The intimal tear is distal to the left subclavian origin and dissection passes distally (Fig. 4.25). Rupture is into the left pleural cavity or the peritoneum.

It must be emphasised that the classification is arbitrary and many Type 1 dissections may extend throughout the whole aorta. Involvement of renal, mesenteric and intercostal arteries is common with dissection tracts below the diaphragm. The commonest site of the intimal tear (>60%) is in the ascending thoracic aorta, with a steadily diminishing frequency distally. Tears in the abdominal aorta are the rarest.

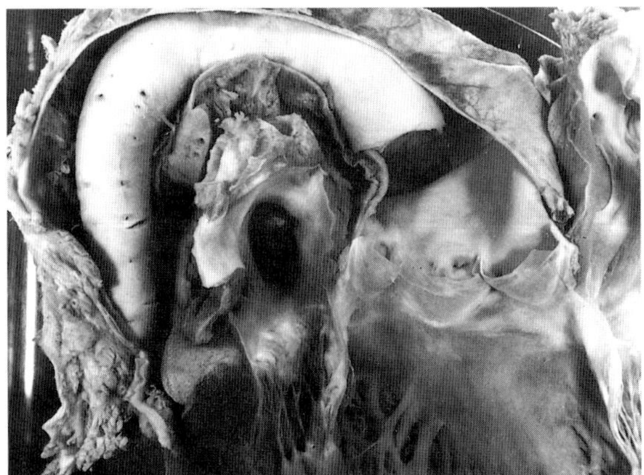

Fig. 4.24 Type II aortic dissection. There is a complete circumferential intimal tear and a dissection tract which extends round the arch and down the descending aorta. Intercostal arteries have been torn away in the dissection process.

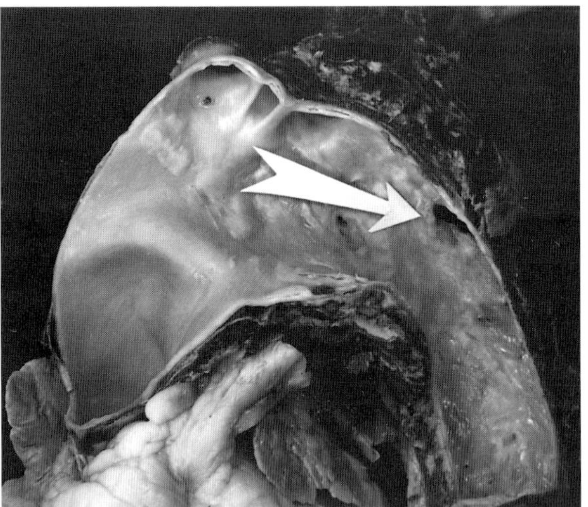

Fig. 4.25 Type III aortic dissection. There is a vertical intimal tear just distal to the left subclavian artery.

Natural history and progression of aortic dissection

The presenting feature is severe chest and back pain. Other symptoms depend on the site of the dissection. Ascending aortic dissection may extend proximally to just above the aortic valve. One or more cusps attached to a flap of aortic wall prolapse, leading to acute aortic incompetence. Extension of dissection into major aortic branches may occlude the right coronary artery leading to myocardial infarction, the carotid artery leading to strokes, the brachial arteries leading to loss of radial pulse, the mesenteric arteries leading to intestinal ischaemia, the renal arteries leading to renal failure and the intercostal arteries leading to spinal cord ischaemia. The external wall of the dissection tract is weak and blood often exudes outward, causing pericarditis, pleurisy or peritonitis, before a final fatal rupture. Untreated, the condition probably has a mortality of above 95% from external rupture. Surgical repair of the dissection by inserting a Teflon graft and obliterating the track is possible and better results are obtained with more localised dissections. A small percentage of dissections do resolve and the patient survives without surgical intervention. Resolution is either by a second distal intimal tear, reducing pressure in the dissection tract and creating a double lumen, or by the thrombus in the tract organising to ultimately create a thick-walled external sac communicating with the aortic lumen by a single orifice with smooth, white edges.

Pathogenesis of aortic dissection

The normal aorta is exposed to considerable circumferential and longitudinal stress in systole which its structure seems adapted to accommodate. Dissection tears are sudden events in which the sharp edge suggests an abrupt mechanical tear. Hypertension is a risk factor for dissection but clearly an aortic wall abnormality is also required. This abnormality of the media may be expressed in abnormal morphology. There is an increased frequency of a wide range of medial abnormalities in aortas which have undergone dissection, including elastic fragmentation, smooth muscle loss and cystic changes frequently described together as 'cystic medial necrosis'. A proportion of cases show laminar medial necrosis of smooth muscle cells but it is always difficult to know if this is secondary to dissection rather than its cause. The frequency of significant medial changes is highest in aortas which are dilated before dissection developed and in those from patients with Marfan's syndrome. These circumstances are also those in which evidence of previous episodes of localised dissections are more common. A very significant (at least 40%) proportion of healed dissections, however, occur in aortas which are not dilated and in which the media is morphologically normal.

In examining surgical resections of dissection as many possible areas of media remote from the tract itself should be examined. The tract contains a layer of organising thrombus and occurs in the outer part of the media in the plane in which the vasa vasorum run. A number of strands of evidence suggest that biochemical abnormalities of the connective tissue in the media underlie dissection. In Marfan's syndrome the abnormal fibrillin leads in some way to weakness in the adhesion of elastin and other connective tissue components. Dissection of the aorta may be familial and unassociated with any other stigmata of Marfan's disease. While often regarded as a *forme fruste* of Marfan's, i.e. a defect in the fibrillin gene but with phenotypic expression confined to the aorta, this supposition is as yet unsubstantiated. In experimental animals' lathyrism, the feeding of beta-amino propionitrile compounds and copper deficiency lead to dissection.

Another alternative view of dissection is that the primary event is bleeding from the vasa vasorum forming an intramedial haematoma which then ruptures into the lumen through the intima. The theory is based heavily on the reported cases of aortic dissection without an intimal tear. The proportion is reported to be as high as 15%.[41] We personally have never seen such a case.

Extra-aortic dissection

Dissection of smaller arteries contrasts sharply to aortic dissection in having a genuine very low incidence of an intimal tear. The lesions are more like subadventitial haematomas and compress the lumen from outside, causing organ ischaemia. The condition is rare but occurs in coronary arteries (Chapter 3), renal arteries and mesenteric arteries. In renal and hepatic arteries fibromuscular dysplasia is a concomitant feature.

Traumatic dissection with an intimal tear in the plane between adventitia and media is a complication of any procedure which penetrates any size of artery with needles, catheters or pressure lines, as well as all forms of angioplasty.

AORTIC, CAROTID, ILIAC AND FEMORAL ATHEROSCLEROSIS

All stages of plaque development can be observed in the aorta. In a similar manner to coronary atherosclerosis the percentage of the intimal surface of the aorta covered by plaques relates to risk factors such as hyperlipidaemia and hypertension. The number of aortic plaques on a population basis can also be related to the overall risk of atherosclerosis-related cause of death. While in statistical terms in large numbers of subjects the amount of carotid, femoral, aortic and coronary atherosclerosis at autopsy is related, many individuals have lesions in one site alone. This is particularly true of lower limb ischaemia and suggests that there may be subtle differences in risk factors for coronary and peripheral arterial atherosclerosis.

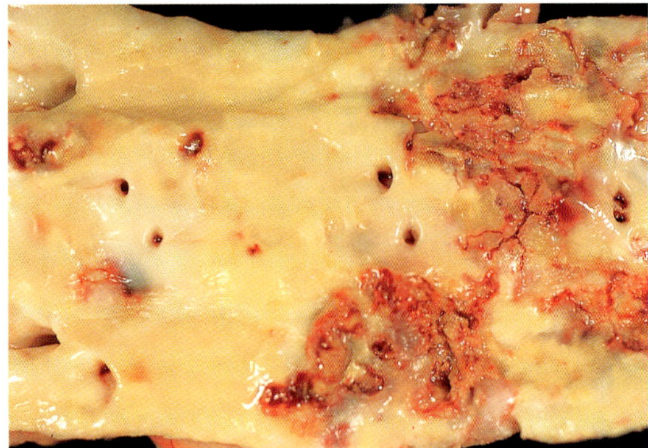

Fig. 4.26 Aortic atherosclerosis. Below the renal artery much of the intimal surface is covered by thrombus due to ulcerated plaques.

In the aorta the number of plaques increases from the ascending to the abdominal aorta and is maximal below the renal arteries. In the aorta it is common to find ulcerated plaques covered by thrombus exposed to the blood flow (Fig. 4.26). Plaques which ulcerate have a large lipid core the exposure of which initiates thrombosis. Distal embolisation to the lower limbs of a mixture of platelet-rich thrombus mixed with lipid, including cholesterol crystals, is a complication of ulcerated aortic plaques.

Hypercholesterolaemic angiitis

A rare acute clinical syndrome consisting of combinations of fever, muscle pain, lower limb ischaemia (purple toes), livido reticularis on the skin of the trunk, renal failure and transient cerebral or intestinal symptoms may develop following widespread embolisation of cholesterol from aortic plaques. What has been called hypercholesterolaemic angiitis[42] is often misdiagnosed as a systemic polyarteritis. Biopsy of muscle or kidney shows occlusion of arteries in the size range 100–300 μm external diameter by needle-shaped cholesterol crystals. Local inflammatory cell infiltration also occurs. The symptoms are most striking in the lower half of the body, reflecting the extent of abdominal atherosclerosis but also occur with striking cerebral signs after any surgical operation in which the ascending aorta is cross-clamped, from squashing plaques. The initiation of anticoagulation in a patient who has clinically silent large areas of aortic ulceration can also precipitate the syndrome. Intra-aortic balloon pumps are another precipitating factor.

Lower limb ischaemia

The great majority of lower limb ischaemia is due to proximal atherosclerosis in the aorta, iliac and femoral arteries. Two syndromes exist: intermittent claudication, i.e. muscular pain in the legs on exercise, and gangrene of the toes or feet. Stenosis and chronic occlusions in the iliac, femoral and popliteal arteries arise by the same mechanisms as described for the coronary arteries (Chapter 2), i.e. primary atherogenesis with superimposed thrombosis. Local collateral flow is often well developed. Bypass operations using vascular grafts and endarterectomy, either at open operation or via atherectomy catheters, are used in a manner identical to the techniques used in the coronary arteries.

Gangrene of the toes or feet may be superimposed on the clinical picture of intermittent claudication. Pathological examination of amputated specimens suggests that a major factor in acute ischaemia is occlusion of the smaller distal arteries. The lumen may be occluded by recent thrombus, with or without cholesterol crystals, or may be occluded by smooth muscle proliferation. In the latter case several new vascular channels may be present in the original lumen. The arterial wall does not show the changes of atherosclerosis and these occlusions of small arteries are most likely to be the result of emboli.

Carotid and cerebral atherosclerosis

Plaque formation is enhanced at the bifurcation of the internal and external carotid from the common carotid artery. Such plaques may grow to cause stenosis at the origin of the internal carotid artery but the effects are often minimised by collateral flow established with branches of the external carotid artery on the same side or via anastomoses in the circle of Willis with the vertebral system or the other internal carotid artery.

A major factor in symptoms is the superimposition of thrombosis on the carotid lesion. Some plaques ulcerate, leaving a shallow crater covered by platelet-rich thrombus. Intermittent embolisation of small fragments of predominantly platelet thrombus leads to transient ischaemic attacks lasting minutes or hours but resolving clinically within 24 hours. Small platelet aggregates forming 'white bodies' within retinal arteries can be seen in life. The number of episodes can be reduced by aspirin therapy. Subjects with such ulcerated plaques who are having transient ischaemia are at considerable risk of developing more major thrombosis at the site. Where the carotid plaque is not in itself causing high-grade local stenosis, a chronic ulcer containing thrombosis may persist for periods of months. High-grade stenosis predisposes to larger occlusive thrombi in the carotid artery. Endarterectomy at open surgery is used to relieve both plaques acting as a nidus for emboli and those causing stenosis.

It is not the purpose of this book to consider stroke in detail. Sufficient to say that cerebral infarction can result from any of the following processes:

1. Occlusive thrombus in the carotid arteries
2. Embolic thrombosis in the circle of Willis
3. Primary thrombosis in relation to atherosclerosis in the circle of Willis

Primary thrombosis in the intracerebral arteries of the circle of Willis is probably the least common. In the intracerebral arteries atherosclerosis may cause high-grade stenosis. The plaques are rich in lipid-filled foam cells and lipid cores are far less common than in the coronary arteries. The mechanism of thrombosis is usually superficial intimal injury rather than deep plaque disruption.

ANEURYSMS OF THE AORTA

Clear distinction must be made between saccular or fusiform aneurysms, in which the wall of the lesion is derived from the whole thickness of the aortic wall, and dissection of the aorta. In dissection there is an intimal tear leading to a tract in the media. The dissection tract contains blood clot and thrombus which may compress the original lumen. Because the outer wall of the tract consists largely of adventitia, external rupture is common.

Diffuse or saccular aneurysms

Aneurysms are defined as permanent localised dilatations of an artery or the aorta and are pulsatile in life. Aneurysms contrast to ectasia in which the dilatation is far more diffuse and also to the dilatation of arteries which results from high flow. In true aortic aneurysms the wall of the sac is derived from all the constituents of the aortic wall. In so called false aneurysms the wall is not composed of all the wall components but is due to organisation of an extravascular haematoma following traumatic perforation of the aorta. While the distinction between 'true' and 'false' is made a great deal of in the literature in reality both lesions pulsate and carry a high risk of external rupture. The pathogenesis of aortic aneurysms differs depending on the site in the aorta, the clinical symptoms and the geographic origin of the patient.

Abdominal aortic aneurysms

Aneurysms of the abdominal aorta are most common below the renal arteries and above the aortic bifurcation. The majority are probably due to atherosclerosis. Ultrasound examination of the abdominal aorta in life shows that small clinically silent aneurysms are common. This confirms a number of autopsy studies in which the frequency of incidental aneurysms is around 5%.[43] The frequency of aneurysms discovered on routine ultrasound in life depends on the definition of an aneurysm. Some use a figure of 5 cm in width, others 7 cm. Leaving definitions aside, however, it is clear that there is increasing awareness of how common abdominal aneurysms are in Western populations which have a high frequency of atherosclerosis. In contrast, aneurysms of the thoracic aorta are becoming very rare. Atherosclerotic aortic aneurysms are up to nine times more common in men than in women, are related to smoking, develop over the age of 50 and may be familial on account of genetic factors distinct from the lipid abnormalities leading to atherosclerosis itself.

Atherosclerotic abdominal aortic aneurysms are usually fusiform and involve the whole circumference of the aorta. It is, however, common for the aneurysmal bulge to be more pronounced on one side, left or right. The wall consists of dense hyaline fibrosis varying in thickness with laminated old and recent thrombus adherent to the inner surface of the aneurysm sac. The diameter ranges from 5–30 cm. Diffuse atherosclerosis is present in the aorta above the aneurysm. Abdominal ultrasound provides an opportunity to follow the natural history of these aneurysms. The natural progression is by expansion, leading ultimately to rupture into the retroperitoneal tissues and peritoneal cavity. The rate of increase in diameter increases as the aneurysm enlarges and rates above 0.5 cm per annum or an overall diameter of more than 7 cm are probable indicators of the need for surgical intervention to forestall rupture. Nevertheless, the time of surgical intervention for asymptomatic aneurysms is a complex decision.

Histological examination usually shows very little evidence of residual medial structures and the wall of the aneurysms is hyaline fibrous tissue. The aneurysm is lined by a complex mixture of thrombus of all ages mixed with cholesterol.

Pathogenesis of aortic atherosclerotic aneurysms

The essential cause of any aneurysm is medial destruction and there is a paradox in the concept that atherosclerosis, an intimal disease, causes aneurysms. The reasons why these abdominal aneurysms are regarded as atherosclerosis are the concordance of the site of the aneurysm with the site of maximum plaque formation, the presence of cholesterol in the aneurysm wall, the age distribution and the concordance of many of the conventional risk factors for atherosclerosis with those of abdominal aneurysm. Intimal atherosclerosis does lead to widespread medial loss in many arteries yet only in the abdominal aorta is aneurysm formation common. The mechanism of medial loss may be direct pressure atrophy, hypoxia or an inflammatory-mediated damage. An adventitial chronic inflammatory response is common in atherosclerosis in general and large numbers of lymphocytes, macrophages and plasma cells are often present in the wall of atherosclerotic aneurysms. A slightly different view is held about aneurysms of the abdominal aorta in which there is dense periadventitial fibrosis extending into the retroperitoneal tissues associated with a florid chronic inflammatory response, including lymphoid follicles.[44] Fibrosis surrounds nerves and endarteritis obliterans is prominent. The fibrosis may extend to encroach on the ureters or the vena cava. Ultrasound investigation in life identifies the aneurysm wall to be unusually thick.

These so-called 'periaortitic' or inflammatory atherosclerotic aneurysms are thought to be part of the overall spectrum of atherosclerotic disease in which an autoimmune response to altered LDL is involved. The periaortitis type of atherosclerotic aneurysm comprises up to 10% of all lower abdominal aortic aneurysms and, apart from a slightly reduced risk of rupture and an increased risk of ureteric involvement, the clinical correlates are little different from the more usual atherosclerotic aneurysms.

Non-atherosclerotic saccular aortic aneurysms

Aneurysms which are not due to atherosclerosis are due either to inflammatory aortitis or non-inflammatory medial degeneration. In order to elucidate the pathogenesis all the data that can be gathered about the clinical state of the patient (ESR, serology for syphilis, HLA status, presence or absence of rheumatoid factor), the presence of other aortic lesions (stenotic segments) and histological evidence from the media at the margins of the aneurysm must be considered together. It is usually possible to distinguish inflammatory from non-inflammatory causes. The former have focal medial destruction associated with chronic inflammatory cells, the latter elastic fragmentation, smooth muscle loss and cystic change without inflammation. Once the distinction is made further diagnosis depends on clinical rather than histological data. Personal experience suggests that the aetiology of the larger proportion of either group remains unexplained.

Post-traumatic saccular aneurysms

Sudden deceleration causes shear forces to be exerted on the aorta at the junction of mobile and more fixed areas, producing tears. Most such tears transect the aortic wall and are rapidly fatal. A small proportion tear the intima and media, stopping short at the adventitia. Healing occurs, leaving a linear smooth area in which the media is discontinuous. Over time localised saccular aneurysms may develop and may be seen on a chest X-ray years after a road traffic accident. The aneurysm sac has a highly characteristic histological appearance with a sharp-edged defect in an otherwise normal media. Typical sites are just

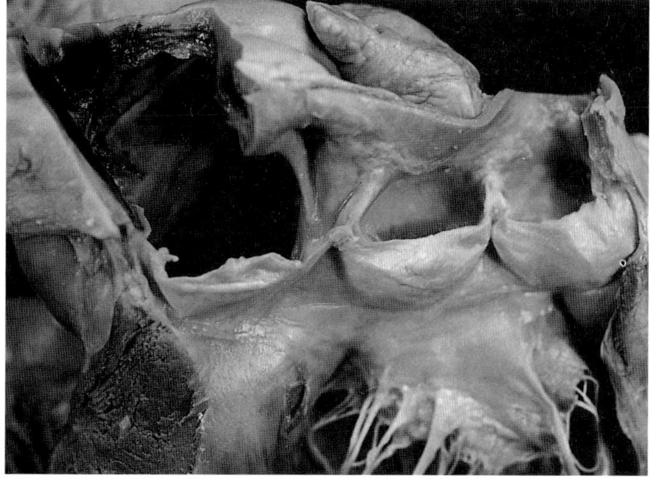

Fig. 4.27 Aneurysm of the sinus of Valsalva. There is saccular dilatation of the right coronary sinus in a patient with Marfan's syndrome.

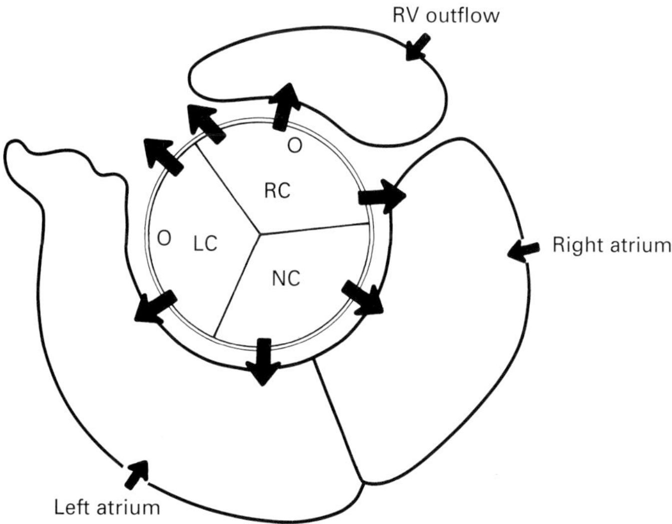

Fig. 4.28 Potential sites of rupture of aneurysms of the sinus of Valsalva.

above the aortic valve and just distal to the left subclavian artery. Late rupture is a complication and if identified in life these aneurysms are usually surgically removed.

Aneurysms of the sinus of Valsalva

Aneurysms may develop in any of the three sinuses (Fig. 4.27) or rarely in all three. Such aneurysms may be isolated abnormalities which develop in adult life, may complicate genetic defects of connective tissue synthesis such as Marfan's disease or may be part of a congenital defect which includes a small ventricular septal defect. The last particularly involves the right coronary sinus. The pathogenesis may be partial defects in the fusion of the aortic root with the heart or a general weakness of the connective tissue of the valve sleeve tissue. The danger associated with such aneurysms is of rupture into an adjacent chamber with formation of a shunt (Fig. 4.28).

REFERENCES

1. Lie J. Coronary vasculitis. A review of the current scheme of classification of vasculitis. Arch Pathol Lab Med 1987; 111: 224–233.
2. Kazatchkine M, Seifert P, Nydegger U. Immunological processes in the vascular wall. In: Camilleri J-P, Berry C, Fiessinger J-N, Bariety J, ed. Diseases of the arterial wall. London: Springer-Verlag, 1989: 391–419.
3. Leung D. Immunoglobulin antibodies present in the acute phase of Kawasaki syndrome lyse cultured vascular endothelial cells stimulated by gamma interferon. J Clin Immunol 1986; 77: 1428–1435.
4. Kallenberg C. Autoimmunity to lysosomal enzymes: new clues to vasculitis and glomerulonephritis. Immunol Today 1991; 12: 61–64.
5. Jackman J, Radolf J. Cardiovascular syphilis. Am J Med 1989; 87: 425–433.
6. Virmani R, McAllister HJ. Pathology of the aorta and major arteries. In: Lande A, Berkmen Y, McAllister H, ed. Aortitis: clinical, pathologic and radiologic aspects. New York: Raven Press, 1986: 7–53.
7. Silbergleit A, Arbulu A, Defever B, Nedwicki E. Tuberculous aortitis – surgical resection of ruptured abdominal false aneurysm. JAMA 1965; 193: 333–335.
8. Felson B, Akers P, Hall G. Mycotic tuberculous aneurysm of the thoracic aorta. JAMA 1977; 237: 1104–1108.
9. Gajaraj A, Victor S. Tuberculous aortoarteritis. Clin Radiol 1981; 32: 461–466.
10. Nakao K, Ikeda M, Kimata S. Takayasu's arteritis. Clinical report of eighty-four cases and immunological studies of seven cases. Circulation 1967; 35: 1141–1155.
11. Hall S, Barr W, Lie J. Takayasu arteritis. A study of 32 North American patients. Medicine 1985; 64: 89–99.
12. Lupi-Herrera E. Takayasu's arteritis. Clinical study of 107 cases. Am Heart J 1977; 93: 94–103.
13. Lie J. Disseminated visceral giant cell arteritis: Histopathologic description and differentiation from other granulomatous vasculitides. Am J Clin Pathol 1978; 69: 229–305.
14. Wilkinson I, Russel R. Arteries of the head and neck in giant cell arteritis. A pathological study to show the pattern of arterial involvement. Arch Neurol 1972; 27: 378–391.
15. Klein R, Campbell R, Hunder G. Skip lesions in temporal arteritis. Mayo Clin Proc 1976; 51: 504–510.
16. Klein R, Hunder G, Stanson A. Large artery involvement in giant cell (temporal) arteritis. Ann Intern Med 1975; 83: 806–812.
17. Cupps T. Isolated angiitis of the nervous system: prospective diagnostic and therapeutic experience. Am J Med 1983; 74: 97–105.
18. Frohnert P, Sheps S. Long-term follow up study of periarteritis nodosa. Am J Med 1967; 43: 8–14.
19. Fauci A, Haynes B, Katz P. The spectrum of vasculitis: clinical, pathological and therapeutic considerations. Ann Intern Med 1978; 89: 660–676.
20. Mullick F, McAllister HJ, Wagner B. Drug-related vasculitis: clinicopathologic correlations in 30 patients. Hum Pathol 1979; 10: 313–325.
21. Dajani AS, Taubert KA, Gerber MA et al. Diagnosis and therapy of Kawasaki disease in children. Circulation 1993; 87: 1776–1780
22. Fauci A. Wegener's granulomatosis: a prospective clinical and therapeutic experience with 85 patients for 21 years. Ann Intern Med 1983; 98: 76–85.
23. Weidhase A, Grone H, Unterberg C, Schuff-Werner P, Wiegand V. Severe granulomatous giant cell myocarditis in Wegener's granulomatosis. Klin Wochenschr 1990; 68: 880–885.
24. McKusick V, Harris W, Ottesen O. Buerger's disease. A distinct clinical and pathologic entity. JAMA 1962; 181: 93–100.
25. Adar R. Cellular sensitivity to collagen in thromboangiitis obliterans. N Engl J Med 1983; 308: 1113–1116.
26. Lakhanpal S, Conn D, Lie J. Clinical and prognostic significance of vasculitis as an early manifestation of connective tissue disease syndrome. Ann Intern Med 1984; 101: 743–748.
27. Bouissou H, Pieraggi M, Julian M. Age-related morphological changes of the arterial wall. In: Camilleri J-P, Berry C, Fiessinger J-N, Bariety J, ed. Diseases of the arterial wall. London: Springer-Verlag, 1989: 71–78.
28. Schlatmann T, Becker A. Pathogenesis of dissecting aneurysms of aorta. Comparative histopathologic study of significance of medial changes. Am J Cardiol 1977; 39: 21–26.
29. Pyeritz R. The Marfan syndrome. Am Fam Physician 1986; 34: 83–94.
30. Stasiecki P, Arnold G. Das Marfan-Syndrome. Med Klinik 1989; 84: 590–594.

31. El Habbal M. Cardiovascular manifestations of Marfan's syndrome in the young. Am Heart J 1992; 123: 752–757.
32. Geva T, Sanders S, Diogenes M, Rockenmacher S, Van Praagh R. Two-dimensional and Doppler echocardiographic and pathologic characteristics of the infantile Marfan syndrome. Am J Cardiol 1990; 65: 1230–1237.
33. Treasure T. Elective replacement of the aortic root in Marfan's syndrome. Br Heart J 1993; 69: 101–103.
34. Pasic M, von Segesser L, Carrel T, Laske A, Bauer E, Turina M. Surgical treatment of cardiovascular complications in Marfan syndrome: a 27 year experience. Eur J Cardiothorac Surg 1992; 6: 149–155.
35. Hwa J, Richards J, Huang G et al. The natural history of aortic root dilatation in Marfan syndrome. Med J Aust 1993; 158: 558–562.
36. Dietz H. Molecular biology of Marfan syndrome. J Vasc Surg 1992; 15: 927–928.
37. Francke U, Furthmayr H. Genes and gene products involved in Marfan syndrome. Sem Thorac Cardiovasc Surg 1993; 5: 3–10.
38. Tsipouras P, Del Mastro R, Sarfarazi M et al. Genetic linkage of the Marfan syndrome, ectopia lentis, and congenital contractural arachnodactyly to the fibrillin genes on chromosomes 5 and 15. N Engl J Med 1992; 326: 905–909.
39. Depairon M, Lapiere C. Cardiovascular alterations in inherited connective tissue disorders. In: Camilleri J-P, Berry C, Fiessinger J-N, Bariety J, ed. Diseases of the arterial wall. London: Springer-Verlag, 1989: 513–527
40. De Bakey M, Walter S, Cooley D. Dissecting aneurysms of aorta. J Thorac Surg 1965; 49: 130–149.
41. Wilson S, Hutchins G. Aortic dissecting aneurysms: causative factors in 204 subjects. Arch Pathol Lab Med 1982; 106: 175–180.
42. Smith M, Ghose M, Henry A. The clinical spectrum of renal cholesterol embolization. Am J Med 1981; 71: 174–180.
43. Auerbach O, Garfinkel L. Atherosclerosis and aneurysms of aorta in relation to smoking habits and age. Chest 1980; 78: 805–809.
44. Parums D. The spectrum of chronic periaortitis. Histopathology 1990; 8: 589–600.

5

Myocardial disease

CARDIAC HYPERTROPHY

Hypertrophy is the increase in individual myocyte size, and thus ventricular muscle mass, which follows an increase in cardiac workload. Hypertrophy may involve the whole of either the right or left ventricle. Examples of generalised right or left ventricular hypertrophy are seen in pulmonary or systemic hypertension and in aortic or pulmonary stenosis. The work that the ventricle experiences can be divided into pressure, where the ventricle ejects against an increased aortic or pulmonary pressure (afterload), or volume, where the ventricle is overfilled in diastole prior to contraction (preload). The two processes produce very different ventricular shapes (Figs 5.1, 5.2) and may have a different effect on the shape of individual myocytes. Both volume and pressure load increases initiate a hypertrophic response which is largely restricted to the ventricle experiencing the stimulus. This must imply that whatever the trigger mechanism it operates locally within the myocardium.

Hypertrophy may also be regional or focal rather than an overall response within the myocardium. Following a regional infarct the remaining viable myocardium undergoes hypertrophy (remodelling). Adjacent to a microscopic focal scar myocytes increase in size while those more distant remain normal.

A further consideration is that the workload carried by the heart varies with overall physical activity. An increase in physical activity, for example by trained athletes, is accompanied by an increase in total heart size. This is usually regarded as a physiological adaptation rather than hypertrophy but the borderline between what is physiological, i.e. reversible, and pathological, i.e. fixed and irreversible, is not clear-cut.

All of these definitions and factors must be born in mind when using the term cardiac hypertrophy. Cardiac hypertrophy is perhaps the most loosely used word adopted in autopsy reports, often qualified as mild, moderate or severe. The limitations of such a terminology are not always appreciated by clinicians who may be using the

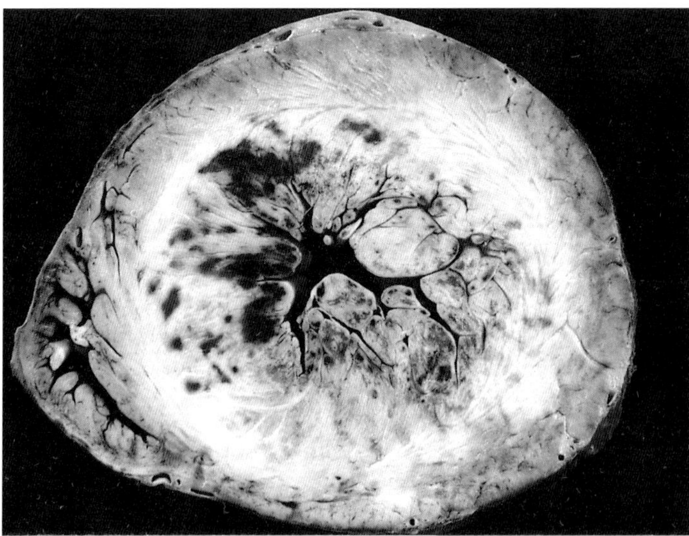

Fig. 5.1 LV hypertrophy due to aortic valve stenosis. The left ventricle is thick walled with a small cavity. In such hearts the myocytes have a markedly increased width. Death after cardiac surgery reperfusion injury produced myocardial haemorrhage.

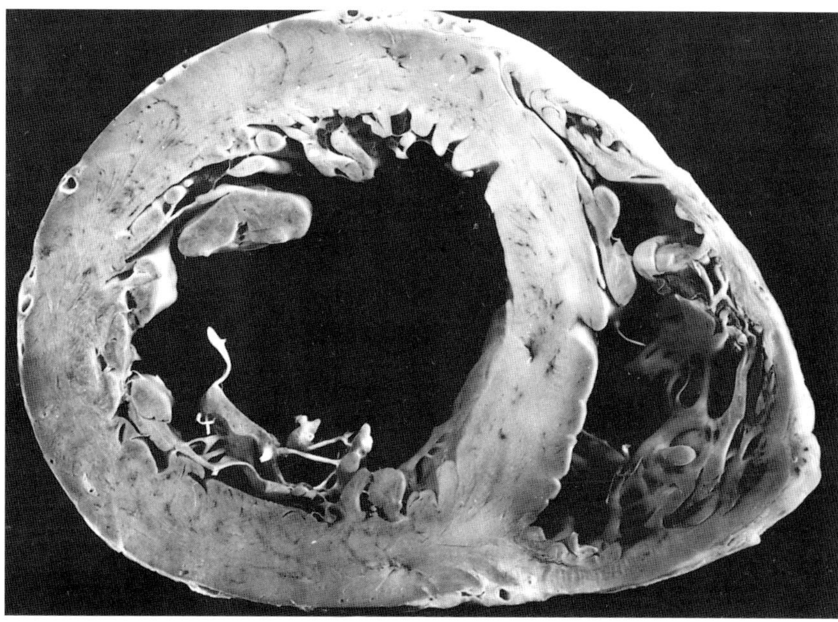

Fig. 5.2 LV hypertrophy due to aortic valve regurgitation. When compared with Figure 5.1, although the isolated left ventricular mass was virtually identical the wall thickness is not markedly abnormal and the cavity diameter is increased. Myocyte width in such volume-loaded ventricles may not be increased.

word hypertrophy to signify something quite different in an equally unquantified manner. The ways in which cardiac hypertrophy can be measured at autopsy are discussed in Chapter 12.

MORPHOLOGICAL CHANGES IN HYPERTROPHY

MYOCYTE ADAPTATION

In hypertrophy the overall volume of any particular myocyte increases. The increase in size may be predominantly in diameter or in length, but in most circumstances both increase. Increase in size is associated with an increase in both mitochondrial and myofibrillary protein content and the formation of additional sarcomeres. An increase in nuclear size is often striking, with an increase in total nuclear DNA content occurring as the cells become polyploid.[1] Myocyte nuclear ploidy increases with age irrespective of the presence or absence of hypertrophy; in adult hearts 4N and 8N myocytes make up approximately 25% of the population. In hypertrophy this proportion increases and myocytes occur which are up to 32N. As far as is currently known the number of myocyte nuclei does not increase. Mitosis has never been unequivocally shown in adult human myocytes. There are however hints[2] that some form of amitotic splitting may occur; certainly in hypertrophy the number of myocytes with more than one nucleus rises.[3] Use of PCNA staining confirms that under the stimulus to hypertrophy DNA synthesis in the myocyte occurs.[4] Nuclear changes of hypertrophy, i.e. an increase in nuclear volume, area and DNA content, are often very striking in the myocytes adjacent to focal areas of necrosis and focal scars.

The increase in myocyte diameter is most striking in pressure load hypertrophy such as follows aortic valve stenosis. In volume overloaded ventricles myocyte diameter increases to a lesser degree although the nuclear changes of hypertrophy do develop.

In addition to morphological adaptation in hypertrophy myocytes undergo phenotypic modulation. In the process of hypertrophy fetal-type cardiac proteins are re-expressed by the myocyte.

In rodent models of hypertrophy there is a re-expression of the beta-myosin heavy chain form rather than the usual alpha-myosin heavy chain found in the normal ventricle. In human ventricular myocardium, however, the beta form of the heavy chain is normally retained into adult life. Atrial natriuretic factor is however re-expressed in hypertrophic ventricular muscle in man.[5] The re-expression of genes controlling fetal-type proteins in hypertrophy is difficult to explain in terms of benefit. One view[6] is that it is entirely fortuitous and that in hypertrophy a master gene is triggered which initiates a whole series of gene expressions. Some of these, such as DNA synthesis, are beneficial but others are just coincidental. In skeletal muscle such a master gene (myo-D) is known but does not appear to be present in the myocardium.

MECHANISMS OF HYPERTROPHY INDUCTION

In addition to volume and pressure load, adrenergic stimulation and thyroid and growth hormone excess are well known clinical causes of cardiac hypertrophy. There are now compelling reasons based on the ability of inhibitors to prevent hypertrophy that both angiotensin II and endothelin are involved.

The exact nature of the system recognising the need for hypertrophy is, however, not clear. Thyroxine and growth hormone excess are exogenous factors affecting the whole myocardium. The very restricted response to volume and pressure overload suggests an internal recognition/triggering system. In isolated myocytes stretching alone will induce increased mRNA levels and upregulation of the c-*myc* and c-*fos* oncogenes.[7] Adrenergic receptor density rises and thus the cell is more sensitive to the effect of adrenergic compounds in increasing myocyte protein synthesis. In part therefore the stimulus is mechanical, acting on the myocyte. In hypertrophied myocardium an increase in TGF-β as well as acidic and fibroblast growth factors also occurs. This may be originating in interstitial cells or myocytes. All of these growth factors initiate some of the changes observed in hypertrophy when added to myocytes in culture.[6]

INTERSTITIAL TISSUE ADAPTATION IN HYPERTROPHY

In hypertrophy the total DNA content of the myocardium rises. This is due in part to the increase in ploidy of the myocyte nuclei but in equal measure to hyperplasia of interstitial connective tissue cells. The total content and concentration of collagen in the myocardium rises as ventricular hypertrophy develops.[8] In this regard pressure and volume overload have different effects. In volume overload the increase in collagen occurs after some years; in contrast, in pressure overload collagen synthesis begins to outstrip the adaptive response of the myocyte much earlier. This replacement of myocytes by interstitial fibrosis is particularly striking in the subendocardial zone. Increasing interstitial fibrosis is important in altering ventricular compliance, hindering diastolic relaxation and therefore ventricular filling. It is also important because fibrosis once initiated is less likely to be reversible. The adaptation of the microvascular system in hypertrophy is a contentious subject. If myocytes increased in size and the number of capillaries remained the same the capillary density would fall. Many studies suggest that capillary density does not fall, implying that formation of new capillaries has occurred. Whatever the capillary density, an increase in the diameter of myocytes will increase the distance between the capillary lumen and the interior of the myocyte, with a resulting effect on oxygen diffusion. The subendocardial fibrosis so characteristic of pressure load hypertrophy probably implies that some myocyte death is the stimulus to interstitial fibroblastic cells. Equally, interstitial connective tissue cells can be stimulated to produce growth factors as the result of altered mechanical stresses, or may be stimulated by release of growth factors by myocytes themselves stimulated by different mechanical stress patterns.[9]

VENTRICULAR SHAPE ADAPTATION

Pressure load hypertrophy is characterised by a symmetric increase in wall thickness with retention of a normal cavity size demonstrated by echocardiography in life. At autopsy the left ventricular cavity may be reduced in size or virtually obliterated (Fig. 5.1). This probably reflects a tendency for the heart to arrest in systole, or be in rigor. The ventricular wall thickening is usually symmetric although left ventricular pressure load hypertrophy from any cause will accentuate the septal width relative to the posterior wall. Ratios of septal to posterior wall thickness in the range of 1.3–1.5 must not be taken in isolation to indicate hypertrophic cardiomyopathy. In volume overload the left ventricular cavity is increased in size while the wall thickness remains normal (Fig. 5.2) or is reduced. When viewed in a longitudinal section the interventricular septum is sigmoid in shape in all hearts. In pressure overload the subaortic bulge of the septum may be accentuated and protrude beneath the aortic valve. Again, in isolation this must not be taken as indicating hypertrophic cardiomyopathy. In rare cases this septal hypertrophy causes some obstruction to the outflow of blood from the left ventricle and may be resected surgically at the time of aortic valve replacement. The phenomenon of reactive hypertrophy causing ventricular outflow obstruction is however far more common in the right ventricle.

The mechanisms involved in the adaptation to volume overload are not entirely clear. One view is that myocyte shape changes occur with the formation of elongated thinner individual cells.[10] Another view denies this and sees ventricular wall thinning as due to slippage of myocytes relative to each other.[11] This process involves alterations of myocyte arrangement so that a transect of the ventricular wall passes through fewer layers of myocytes. Whatever the processes involved, once established ventricular dilatation has occurred it persists even after a defective valve is replaced and the volume overload removed.

CARDIAC FAILURE

This is probably the most difficult term to define in clinical cardiology. At one level it may be used to imply that myocardial contractility is diminished in an apparently asymptomatic individual; at the other extreme the term is applied to a distinct clinical entity in which cardiac function has failed to provide sufficient blood flow to certain key organs, invoking a set of neurohumoral responses which retain fluid and raise blood pressure (Fig. 5.3). All these processes throw further load on an already failing heart.

Traditionally, cardiac failure is divided into acute (e.g. following myocardial infarction) and

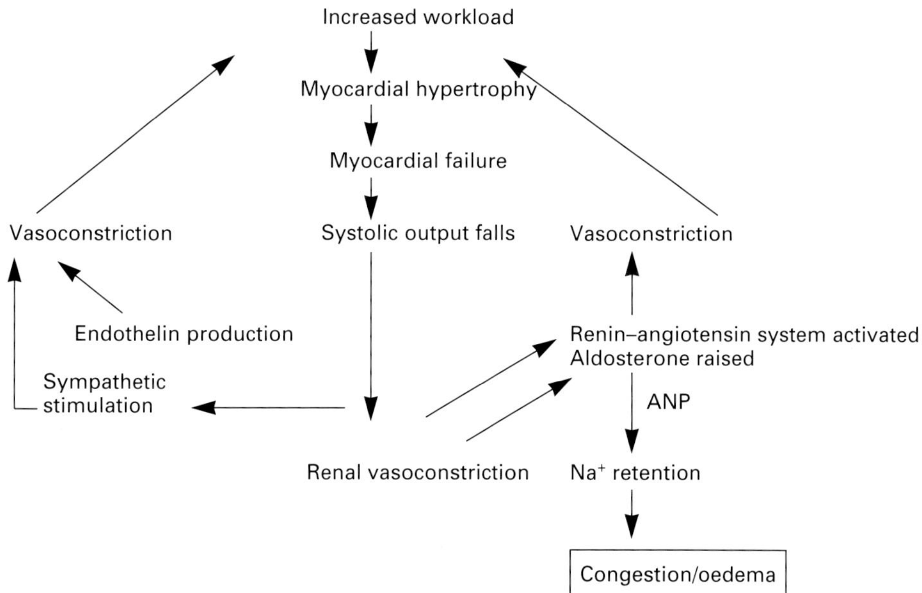

Fig. 5.3 Mechanism of cardiac failure.

chronic (e.g. mitral stenosis). It has been traditional to consider left and right ventricular failure as separate entities although once secondary physiological responses have occurred strain is increased on both ventricles. Increased left-sided pressures inevitably lead to pulmonary venous hypertension followed by pulmonary arterial hypertension, throwing an increased load on the right ventricle.

MORPHOLOGICAL CORRELATES OF CARDIAC FAILURE

It is not easy, or indeed possible in many cases, to confirm the presence of cardiac failure at autopsy. The initial myocardial response to increased workload is hypertrophy. There is no sharp dividing line between the hypertrophic response and cardiac failure and no specific histological, biochemical or function change in the myocyte which indicates cardiac failure. Quantification at electronmicroscopic level of the relative proportions of the myocyte occupied by myofibrils, mitochondria and sarcoplasm does show changes that can be related to left ventricular function. As the ejection fraction (that proportion of the diastolic volume of blood ejected at each systolic beat) falls, the number of myofibrils falls and that of sarcoplasma devoid of organelles rises.[12] This phenomenon occurs in a wide range of diseases, including ischaemia, cardiomyopathies and hypertrophy, but it only becomes striking when cardiac dysfunction is already far advanced. It is thus a late secondary morphological change precipitating a further decline in function rather than a primary factor in causing heart failure.

While usually measured by quantitative electronmicroscopy, the loss of myofibrils can be appreciated by light microscopy as viable but empty vacuolated myocytes. This change has been called myocytolysis but the name is confusing because it is also used for myocyte necrosis in ischaemia and for myocyte damage in cardiac rejection. While there is no structural abnormality which can be correlated with failure in the hypertrophic myocardium it has long been felt that there is a functional abnormality. So far no primary deficit has been demonstrated in coronary flow, O_2 extraction or energy utilisation. Uptake of glucose and fatty acids is normal. ATPase activity of myosin is reduced but this may be a secondary rather than a primary event. Beta-adrenergic receptor density is reduced in the failing myocardium, which becomes functionally denervated and has a poor response to sympathetic stimulation. The whole complex question of whether there is a primary defect within the myocyte which precipitates failure after the development of hypertrophy is well reviewed by Schlant and Sonnenblick.[13]

PRIMARY MYOCARDIAL DISEASE

MYOCARDITIS

In morphological terms acute non-specific myocarditis means the presence of inflammatory cells in the interstitial tissues of the myocardium. The acute inflammatory cell infiltration of myocardial infarction is excluded from this definition.

In acute non-specific myocarditis the inflammatory infiltrate is a mixture of T lymphocytes and macrophages, associated with morphological evidence of myocyte damage and necrosis. Particularly in children interstitial cells with the central bar of nuclear chromatin characteristic of Anitschow cells may be found. These must not be taken in the absence of Aschoff bodies to indicate acute rheumatic disease. A few eosinophils may occur in non-specific myocarditis, but large numbers of eosinophils and giant cell formation are typical of granulomatous myocarditis. Many cases of acute myocarditis have a short clinical course, often of days only, with severe cardiac failure and arrhythmias. The pathology of cases dying this rapidly usually presents no difficulty, virtually every block of myocardial tissue showing a profuse interstitial inflammatory infiltrate. The infiltrate both surrounds individual myocytes and occurs as aggregates around blood vessels. Either subepicardial or subendocardial accentuation of the infiltrate can occur. Macroscopically the heart is dilated but not increased in weight and mural thrombi may be present in either ventricle. The myocardium may appear mottled with alternating pale and haemorrhagic areas or may be normal in colour. Acute myocarditis may be associated with a concomitant pericarditis.

There would be little difficulty with the term acute non-specific myocarditis if all cases conformed histologically to the pattern described so far. Unfortunately, many do not. The problem can best be appreciated from the clinical viewpoint. The clinical diagnosis of acute myocarditis is made when a previously fit patient presents with the sudden onset of fever, flu-like symptoms, rapidly progressive heart failure and arrhythmias in the absence of any other disease such as pneumonia. Such patients may recover completely, die in the acute phase or after an initial improvement slowly deteriorate over some years. Because of the histological similarity of acute non-specific myocarditis to cardiac transplant rejection it was felt that immunosuppression and/or steroid therapy might improve the prognosis in patients with a clinical diagnosis of acute myocarditis. A controlled trial was needed. This trial necessitated a firm tissue diagnosis to be made and cardiac biopsies were widely used for this purpose. It rapidly became apparent that the correlation between the clinical and pathological diagnosis of acute myocarditis was imperfect. In 28 reported series comprising 2636 patients with acute myocarditis on clinical grounds, the percentage found to have a positive cardiac biopsy ranged from 0–63% with an average of 16%.[14] In part this wide range was due to variation in the morphological criteria for myocarditis being used.

BIOPSY DIAGNOSIS OF ACUTE NON-SPECIFIC MYOCARDITIS — DALLAS NOMENCLATURE

To co-ordinate and rationalise trials of therapy in acute myocarditis an international panel of

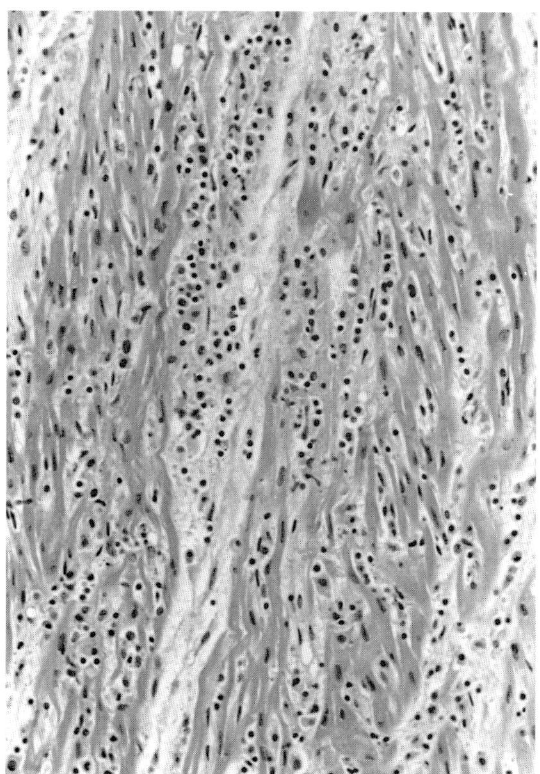

Fig. 5.4 Acute myocarditis. The myocardium from a subject of 13 who died suddenly after a febrile illness. There is a diffuse interstitial infiltrate of mononuclear cells which are largely lymphocytes.
Haematoxylin–eosin × 65

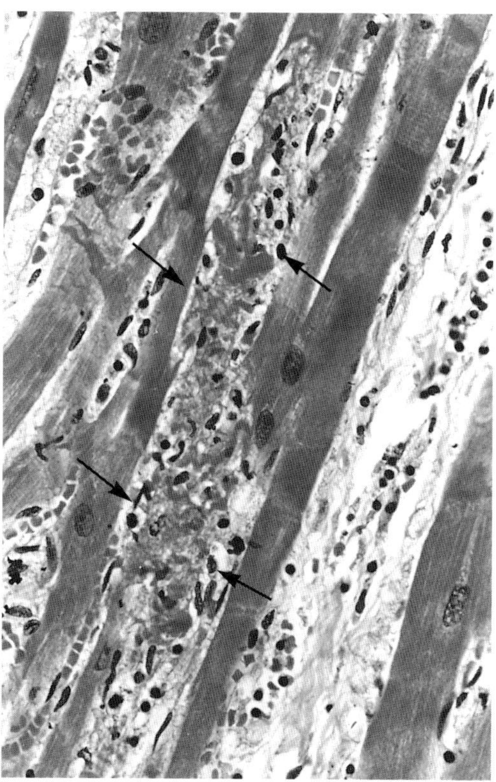

Fig. 5.5 Acute myocarditis. The diagnosis of acute myocarditis requires evidence of active myocyte loss. A necrotic myocyte is shown (arrows) associated with lymphocytic infiltration of the interstitial tissues.
Haematoxylin–eosin × 260

pathologists met and laid down the criteria for the diagnosis.[15]

The first essential was that acute non-specific myocarditis must only be used as a morphological diagnosis when there is concordance of T cell infiltration and myocyte damage in the absence of fibrosis (Figs 5.4, 5.5) and myocyte hypertrophy. This ensures that more chronic conditions such as a dilated cardiomyopathy are excluded. Secondly, terms such as resolving or healed myocarditis, previously used when biopsies showed some fibrosis, were to be confined to cases where a previous biopsy had shown acute myocarditis. Certain facts follow from these definitions — the most important being that positive identification of interstitial mononuclear cells as T lymphocytes by immunohistochemistry (Fig. 5.6) is mandatory. It is all too easy in routine haematoxylin–eosin-stained sections to overinterpret endothelial nuclei as lymphocytes. It is, however, unresolved how many T lymphocytes are needed for the diagnosis. Figures such as more than 5 per high-power field are suggested but this begs the question of how many such high-power fields should contain lymphocytes. In part the problem is also one of the focal nature of myocarditis in living subjects. To exclude acute myocarditis at least five good (>2 mm) biopsies are required.

Distinction between active acute myocarditis in which myocyte damage is occurring and chronic myocarditis in which there is a lymphocytic infiltration alone is also regarded as important, but it is not always easy to make under the microscope, depending as it does on the recognition of acute myocyte loss.

The Dallas criteria have proved invaluable in unifying the reporting of biopsies but have led to a marked reduction in the frequency of biopsy-positive cases of myocarditis. When the biopsy findings of patients presenting with a clinical diagnosis of myocarditis are reported under strict Dallas criteria three groups emerge. First there are morphologically confirmed cases of acute myocarditis, but this group proves to be small: usually not more than 10% of cases overall. A second group shows fibrosis and myocyte hypertrophy suggesting that, despite a short clinical history, the disease is of long standing. Patients with an incipient dilated cardiomyopathy appear to be precipitated into becoming symptomatic by viral infections such as influenza without this being due to a direct viral effect on the heart. A final group shows no evidence of myocarditis or of a dilated cardiomyopathy and the reason for acute myocardial dysfunction is totally unexplained by the biopsy. There is as yet no clear evidence that immunosuppression improves the diagnosis in any of the three groups, although several uncontrolled trials are published.[14]

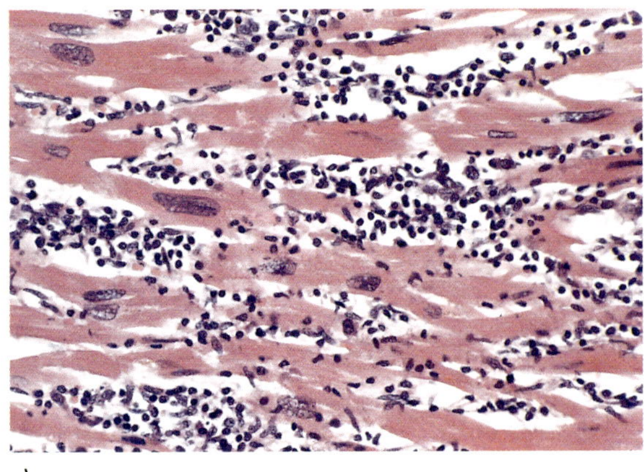

a)

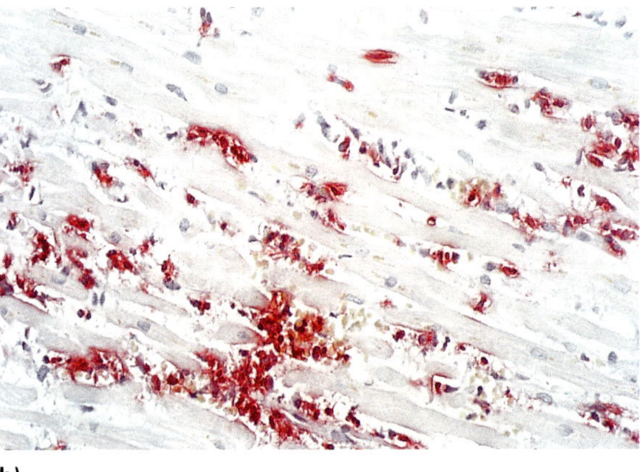

b)

Fig. 5.6 a,b Acute myocarditis. (**a**) Diffuse infiltration of the interstitial tissues with mononuclear cells. (**b**) Immunohistochemical staining with a pan T cell antibody shows most of the interstitial cells to be T lymphocytes. (**a**) Haematoxylin–eosin × 540

PATHOGENESIS OF HUMAN ACUTE NON-SPECIFIC MYOCARDITIS

The current view is that the great majority of cases of non-specific myocarditis that occur in subjects who were previously well, not immunocompromised and not taking drugs known to produce hypersensitivity are infective, due predominantly to the intracellular growth within myocytes of viruses but occasionally by protozoa.

VIRAL AETIOLOGY

A wide range of viruses (Table 5.1) can be cardiotoxic.[16] Some infect the myocardium as part of a generalised viral disease. Myocarditis in such cases is only one aspect of the disease albeit potentially fatal if severe. Studies of common childhood viral diseases, such as mumps, in the acute stage show that abnormalities of the electrocardiogram occur frequently. This is taken to indicate subclinical myocarditis. Myocarditis confirmed at autopsy is an occasional cause of mortality in all common childhood virus infections and is reported in the literature as isolated case reports. The enteroviruses, and in particular group B Coxsackie virus, are more cardiotropic and may produce myocarditis as the sole clinical feature.

Table 5.1 Viruses causing human myocarditis

	Viruses causing myocarditis in isolation or as dominant clinical feature	Viruses causing myocarditis as one feature of a systemic disease
Picornavirus	Coxsackie A Coxsackie B Echovirus ? Adenovirus	Poliovirus Hepatitis A
Orthomyxovirus		Influenza A Influenza B
Paramyxovirus		Mumps — Measles Respiratory syncytial virus
Rubivirus		Rubella
Arbovirus		Yellow fever — Dengue
Poxvirus		Vaccinia
Herpes virus		Varizella zoster CMV Epstein–Barr virus Herpes simplex

While there are many facets to the mounting evidence that enteroviruses, and in particular Coxsackie B, are the main cause of human myocarditis and pericarditis, only isolated case reports exist in which the virus was isolated from myocardial biopsies or at autopsy. While it is usual to attempt viral isolation from myocardial tissue, it is very unlikely to be successful. The question is whether this fact exonerates a virus; many other facts suggest it does not. Both in situ hybridisation and PCR have been used to demonstrate enteroviral genomic material in human acute myocarditis. Even with such sophisticated techniques, however, the positive rate overall is variable, averaging 30%.

In situ hybridisation does not necessarily show the viral genomic material to be at the sites of maximum myocardial injury. The main data implicating viral infection is serological. One problem is that enteroviruses are endemic in the population and serological evidence of previous infection in the form of IgG antibodies is very common in control populations. Serological proof of recent infection in a patient with myocarditis is best made by the presence of viral-specific IgM. The reported range of positive enteroviral serology in patients with clinical myocarditis and pericarditis is very wide, averaging 37% (range 3–78%).[17] The frequency with which the heart is involved is indicated by the 1965 European epidemic of Coxsackie B5 infection. In 1160 subjects 5.3% developed pericarditis and 5 (0.4%) myocarditis. There were two fatalities from myocarditis, indicating that the risk of death is high when myocarditis occurs. The WHO data for 1975–1985 give the rank order of cardioselectivity for typed enteroviruses as (highest to lowest) Coxsackie B2, B3, Echo 16, Coxsackie B6, B1, A4, B5, B4, Echo 22, 14, 11, Coxsackie A9, Echo 9, 30, Coxsackie A16 and Echo 4.[17] A feature of enteroviral myocarditis is the higher attack rates in infants, a frequent concomitant pericarditis and a tendency to develop after physiological stress such as pregnancy.

Pathogenesis of myocardial damage in viral myocarditis

One compelling piece of evidence linking enteroviral infection with human myocarditis is the affinity of Coxsackie B group viruses to cause the disease in rodents, particularly mice. Thus excellent models exist. One lesson from such models is that a viraemic phase is followed by a short phase in which the virus can be isolated from the heart. This is followed by a phase of intense myocardial damage with myocyte death; in this phase the virus has apparently vanished and cannot be isolated. Both from man and mouse it is apparent that many viruses can be cardioselective but among these only a proportion are cardiotoxic, i.e. cause myocyte death. Within one type of virus strains can be virulent or avirulent. On the host side physiological state, age and mouse strain are other variables in determining whether myocarditis occurs.

The sequence of events in infection of myocytes with picornaviruses (of which enteroviruses are part), both in vivo and in culture, has been extensively studied[18] in the mouse. Picornaviruses are small viruses containing a single RNA strand with positive sense, allowing genomic RNA to be directly translated. There is a capsid containing four structural proteins (VP1–VP4). The basic cycle of replication can be divided into stages.

Viral attachment. The viral capsid has affinity for certain receptors on the target cell. These include ICAM-1, MHC antigens and T cell receptor proteins. The exact human myocyte receptor targeted by the Coxsackie virus is unknown as yet.

Viral penetration. Receptor-mediated uptake of picornaviruses involves complexing of several receptor molecules with the virus and the transport across the cell wall into lysosomes.

Uncoating of viral genome. The protein capsid of the virus undergoes proteolytic degradation by host enzymes to release the viral genome.

Genomic translation. Poly (C) tracts at the non-coding region of the viral RNA attract entry of ribosomes. The viral RNA initially encodes a single protein, which is split to form the capsid proteins. A virally encoded polymerase now induces formation of more RNA. Negative sense complementary RNA is produced from the original infecting positive sense RNA. The negative sense RNA is subsequently converted into the positive form and used to continue replication or for incorporation in new infectious particles within the cytoplasm of the host cell. A striking feature is the rapid shutdown of host cell protein and RNA synthesis. The mechanism involves displacement of host RNA/ribosome complexes and their replacement by viral complexes. Alterations in the poly(C) portion of the virus can radically alter the viral capacity to damage host cells and probably accounts for the variation in virulence even with one strain of virus.

Assembly of virus. This occurs within the cytoplasm with the RNA being constituted and subsequently covered by the capsid.

Release of virus. Release of virus is achieved most easily by lysis of the infected cell. Such lysis is preceded by increased plasma membrane permeability. The dying cells, necessary for the histological diagnosis of myocarditis in man by the Dallas criteria, are the morphological correlate of viral release. The mechanism of cell death may be a simple shutdown of host protein synthesis or the more active degradation by a virally encoded protease.

Persistent enteroviral infection

A major advance in the possible understanding of enteroviral infection of the myocardium came from in situ hybridisation. Several studies[19–21] show viral genomic material within scattered, apparently viable myocytes in subjects with acute myocarditis or dilated cardiomyopathy without any other evidence of an infectious virus being present. This data raises questions over whether a cycle of cell infection, replication and cell death is the only process occurring in enteroviral myocarditis.

There is evidence that long-term chronically infected cells in culture may release Coxsackie

B3 in small amounts over years. This may reflect lysis of only a small number of cells at any particular point in time with division of the cells providing a steady supply of new hosts. An alternative explanation is that chronically infected cells may survive for long periods, releasing from time to time infective virus. Such cells may have a high content of negative strand RNA and be defective in producing infectious virus. Chronically infected cells may have diminished contractile function. Both these mechanisms have implications for the long-term outlook of those who survive an attack of acute viral myocarditis and run a risk of developing a dilated cardiomyopathy.

Immune mechanisms in myocyte death in myocarditis

The cycle of viral replication within the cell, followed by cell death, followed by release of new viral particles and infection of more cells is usually broken by viral-neutralising soluble antibodies. A subsidiary defence mechanism is the stimulation of interferon production in the inflammatory process invoked by cell death. Interferon enhances the resistance of the remaining myocytes to further viral infection. Ingestion of dying infected myocytes by macrophages leads to activation and presentation of viral antigens to lymphocytes. Viral-specific T cells may lyse infected cells before viral replication is complete. Activated macrophages may however invoke autoantibodies targeted to non-viral components of the myocyte. These may be due to antigens shared by the virus and the myocyte, to new antigens produced by complexes of viral and myocyte components or to normal cellular antigens exposed to macrophages as the cell dies. Several normal myocyte components, including cardiac myosin, mitochondrial components, adenosine nucleotide translocator protein (ATP/ADP carrier) and a ketoacid dehydrogenase, are highly antigenic and readily invoke autoantibody formation. Another major group of neoantigens to which autoantibodies form belong to the heart shock protein group. Autoimmune responses mediated either by cytotoxic T cells or through complement-mediated mechanisms can destroy non-infected myocytes. Experimental models in the mouse suggest that the bulk of myocytes destroyed are in fact not infected by virus. Injection of myosin with adjuvant into rodents induces a histological picture of myocarditis identical to that which follows viral infection.[22]

Myocarditis caused by other viruses

Of the other viruses listed in Table 5.1 evidence of cardiotoxicity is largely in the form of histological reports of myocyte damage and lymphocytic infiltrate in subjects dying of either systemic infections in which the myocarditis is only a part of the clinical picture (examples being rabies, yellow fever, dengue and polio) or the common less severe viral infections in which myocarditis is a sporadic serious complication (examples being mumps, measles and chicken pox). The histological picture in both groups is identical. Care has to be taken at autopsy to distinguish true myocarditis from hypoxic damage to the myocardium in terminally ill patients. Terminal vascular collapse will cause widespread focal myocyte necrosis and if patients survive a few days a macrophage response occurs. T lymphocytes are not present in large numbers. This problem in differential pathological diagnosis is particularly seen in patients dying of influenza or chicken pox pneumonitis who have profound terminal hypoxia. Positive confirmation of direct viral infection of the myocardium by isolation or immunological methods is the ultimate test for the diagnosis of viral myocarditis in such circumstances.

Cytomegaloviral infection of the myocardium has become much more common due to both cardiac transplantation[23] and deficits in immunity occurring in AIDS. Cytomegalovirus has been extensively studied in animal models and appears primarily to target endothelial cells. Some strains have selectivity for myocardial vascular endothelium. Only where immune responses are depressed does the virus achieve infection of adjacent myocytes (Fig. 5.7). Alterations in MHC and lymphocyte receptors on the surface of the myocyte may also play a role. Histologically the only distinguishing feature of cytomegaloviral infection is the characteristic intranuclear and intracytoplasmic inclusions which can occur in both endothelial cells and myocytes. Conventional light microscopy is the least sensitive

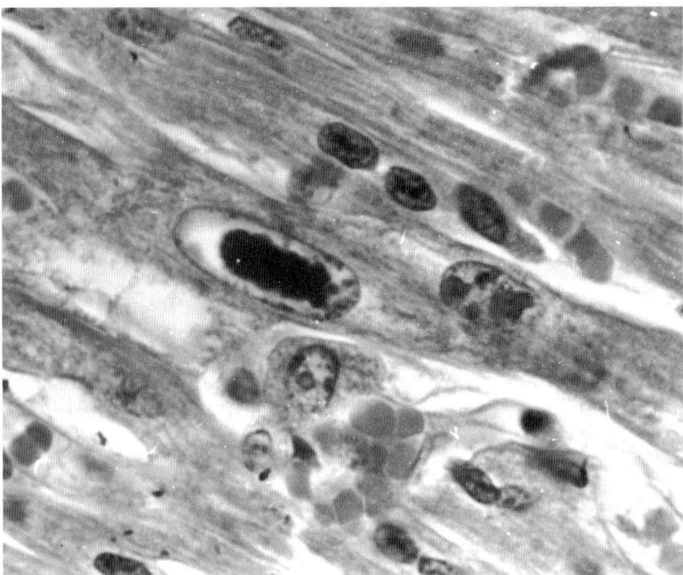

Fig. 5.7 Cytomegalovirus in the myocardium. There is a large intranuclear occlusion in a myocyte.
Haematoxylin–eosin × 280

means of detection, which can be greatly improved in biopsies by use of immunohistochemistry or in situ hybridisation. Excellent commercial antibodies are available for this task.

LYME DISEASE

The spirochaete *Borrelia bergdorferii*, injected by tick bites, causes both an acute and chronic febrile illness with myalgia, lymphadenopathy and mild arthritis.

A small proportion of cases develop an acute myocarditis often associated with atrioventricular or interventricular conduction blocks. Biopsy shows typical non-specific myocarditis and there are reports of the organism being identified by special histological stains.[24] Although isolated cases occur there is no serological evidence to suggest that the organism is a common cause of myocarditis or cardiomyopathy in general.

PROTOZOAL MYOCARDITIS

Two protozoa cause an acute non-specific myocarditis, these being *Trypanosoma cruzi* (Chagas disease) and *Toxoplasma gondii.*

Chagas disease

Chagas disease (South American trypanosomiasis) is a major cause of cardiac death and disability in areas of the world in which *T. cruzi* and its vector reduviid bug are endemic. The trypanosome multiplies in the intestine of the vector insect and is excreted in its faeces to infect the human host via skin abrasions, bites or mucous membranes. The vector is essential for passage of the trypanosome and the geographic distribution of the disease is determined by the distribution of the insect, from the Rio Grande (southern USA) to the south of Argentina. In man the disease is biphasic. An acute illness develops 1–3 months after infection and is characterised by a 10% mortality from acute myocarditis and/or meningoencephalitis. Histologically at this stage there is an acute non-specific myocarditis[25] with areas of myocyte necrosis. Organisms within myocytes (pseudocysts) are common. The chronic stage develops after a latent period of some years (up to 20), and may not be preceded by a clinically recognised acute phase. The heart in the chronic stage represents the end result of a chronic myocarditis in which inflammatory activity and myocyte loss have continued at a low level.

The heart is enlarged, with dilatation of both ventricles. The ventricular wall is thinned, often

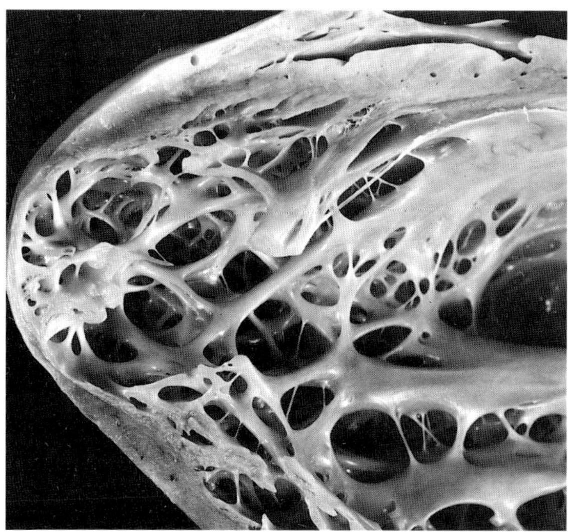

Fig. 5.8 Chronic Chagas disease — apical aneurysm. The apex of the left ventricle shows localised fibrosis with thinning of the wall.

with a marked regional accentuation to produce aneurysms. The most characteristic site is the apex of the left ventricle (Fig. 5.8) or on the posterior wall of the left ventricle just below the atrioventricular ring. Histological examination shows both focal and diffuse fibrosis with areas of inflammatory infiltration and myocyte loss.[26] Loss of myocytes, and a macrophage response at the margins of what appears to be an expanding scar are very typical. At this stage the organism is very rarely identifiable. A further striking feature of the disease is the accentuation of the inflammatory process around nerves and ganglia. A marked reduction of the number of ganglia in the heart is characteristic. The clinical picture of the chronic stage is that of cardiac failure with a particularly striking frequency of arrhythmias and conduction defects. Worldwide, Chagas disease is probably the commonest cause of chronic heart block.

The pathogenesis of the continuing myocyte loss in chronic Chagas disease is uncertain. On one hand it may be due to the repetitive re-infection by the organism of a small number of myocytes. Mitigating against this view is the rarity of the organism despite examining many tissue sections. It seems likely that the organism does persist in the tissue but that either it invokes a cellular and humoral immune response directed at normal components of myocytes and ganglia, or some product of the organism binds to the surface of cells, creating a new autoantigenic complex. Continuing damage is thus autoimmune rather than due to direct infection of the target cell.

Toxoplasmosis

Toxoplasmosis is due to infection with a

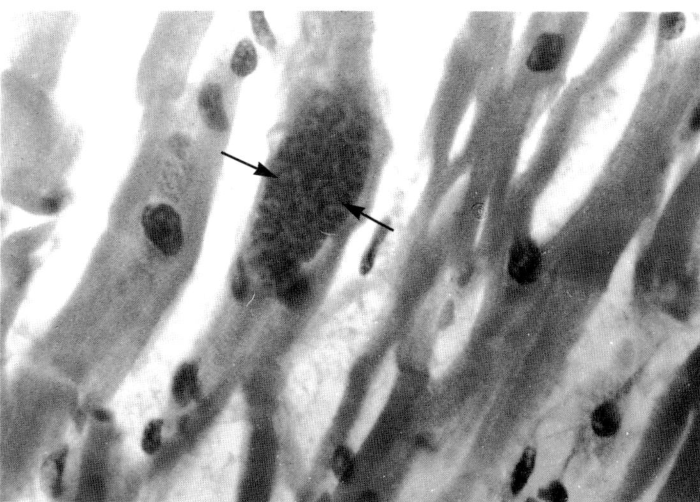

Fig. 5.9 Myocardial toxoplasmosis. A myocyte (arrows) is distended by the organisms to produce the so-called pseudocyst. The adjacent myocardium does not show an inflammatory infiltrate which is rather typical of the disease. The patient was immunosuppressed. Haematoxylin–eosin × 280

sporozoon protozoon, *Toxoplasma gondii*, which is endemic in cats. Oocytes are passed in the faeces, infect soil and thus pass to man. The parasite is distributed worldwide and is common, with prevalence rates between 20% and 100% in adults in all geographic populations studied by antibody screening. An acute phase follows infection, whether this is by transplacental congenital infection or acquired later in life. The acute phase is usually significant only in neonates and carries a high risk of fatal myocarditis or meningoencephalitis. In later life the acute phase often passes unnoticed and myocarditis is a problem only when infection is reactivated following immunosuppression in transplantation or AIDS infection. The histological picture is of an acute, non-specific myocarditis; the only distinguishing feature is if a myocyte filled with the organism is present.[27] These pseudocysts (Fig. 5.9) are usually easy to find in fatal cases but cardiac biopsy in living subjects is far less reliable due to the small amount of tissue that there is to examine. The infected myocytes are often remote from areas of inflammation and myocyte destruction, once again raising the possibility that much of the myocyte death may be related to an immune response rather than the direct effect of the organism per se.

DRUG-RELATED MYOCARDITIS

A wide range of drugs are known to invoke myocarditis, which has been divided into a toxic form in which the damage is cumulative and dose-related and a hypersensitivity type in which the response occurs soon after the drug is administered.[28]

Toxic myocarditis is due to agents causing myocyte death by their direct action on the cell. While usually given the name myocarditis, toxic damage to the myocardium differs from all the other myocarditis processes in that the cell response is largely a reaction to cell death rather than its cause. Myocyte death is usually focal, often involving one or two cells only, and occurs over a period of time, allowing the appearance of lesions of widely differing age ranging from recent cell death through a local inflammatory response to healing fibrotic focal scars. Death may occur rapidly, however, when very large numbers of myocytes are damaged before fibrosis appears. The inflammatory infiltrate is very pleomorphic and usually focal in relation to myocyte death. The macrophage is the predominant cell but occasional eosinophils may also appear. The presence of easily recognised myocyte death distinguishes toxic from hypersensitivity myocarditis. Damage to small arterioles and capillaries within the myocardium, taking the form of endothelial swelling, platelet aggregation and neutrophil plugging, may be a striking feature and is particularly found in cyclophosphamide toxicity.[29]

A wide range of drugs have been reported to cause toxic myocarditis, including antimony compounds, arsenic, emetine, fluorouracil, lithium and phenothiazines. The speed of onset and severity of symptoms depend on the total dose of drug given and the period of time over which it was given. There is a continual spectrum between, at one end, acute toxic myocarditis where large doses of drug are given rapidly, producing death of many myocytes, and, at the other extreme, drug-related cardiomyopathy. In drug-related cardiomyopathies small doses of drugs, usually antimetabolites used in treating malignancy, are given over long periods and produce slowly cumulative myocardial damage. The cardiomyopathy produced by these antimetabolite drugs is discussed later in this chapter. In hypersensitivity myocarditis the inflammatory infiltrate is often dominated by eosinophils and the picture suggests that the lesions are all of the same stage and age. Vasculitis is a concomitant feature and is associated with infiltration of the walls of intramyocardial arteries and veins by inflammatory cells; fibrinoid necrosis is rare.

In contrast to toxic myocarditis, hypersensitivity myocarditis resolves rapidly, often without residual fibrosis, when the offending drug is withdrawn. The first group of drugs to be identified to cause hypersensitivity myocarditis were sulphonamides but a far wider range has emerged including methyldopa, penicillin, phenylbutazone, streptomycin, sulphonylureas and tetracycline.[30] The pathogenesis of the phenomenon of hypersensitivity myocarditis may lie in combinations of drug metabolites with tissue constituents being antigenic and initiating an antibody response which in turn activates complement and stimulates cytokine expression in the tissues. No long-term sequelae follow resolution of the disease.

NON-DRUG RELATED TOXIC MYOCARDITIS

Toxic myocarditis, that is myocyte necrosis with a resultant inflammatory cell response, occurs following exposure to a number of substances which are not therapeutic agents. The prime example is diphtheria (Fig. 5.10). The organism at its primary site in the larynx and trachea produces a powerful cytotoxic exotoxin responsible for causing necrosis of the respiratory epithelial surface and the formation of a membrane of necrotic tissue. In severe cases exotoxin is absorbed systemically and will affect nerves and myocardial tissue. In fatal cases the striking feature is widespread myocyte cell death with hypereosinophilic amorphous intracellular coagulative necrosis. A florid macrophage and fibroblastic response occurs. The conduction system, including the AV node and proximal bundle branches, are particularly involved, leading to heart block which may persist permanently in survivors.

Focal myocyte death is also a feature of prolonged high levels of circulating catecholamines.

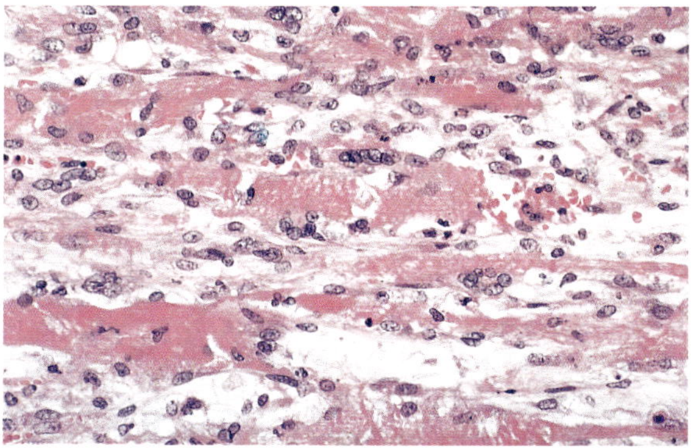

Fig. 5.10 Fatal diphtheric myocarditis. There is widespread myocyte necrosis which has invoked a florid interstitial inflammatory infiltrate. In contrast to viral myocarditis the infiltrate is very pleomorphic with macrophages as a major component.
Haematoxylin–eosin × 160

The phenomenon is best demonstrated by the myocardial changes which occur in patients with phaeochromocytomas of the adrenal gland. In such patients a combination of hypertension and focal myocardial damage ultimately leads to a hypertrophied heart to which the name cardiomyopathy is often applied. Considerable clinical resolution may follow removal of the adrenal tumour. The histology is very typical of a long-standing toxic effect with focal scars at all stages of development in association with foci of recent myocyte death with an inflammatory mononuclear response. The foci are usually small, involving two or three myocytes, and are maximal in the subendocardial region of the left ventricle. It is uncertain whether long-standing oral administration of sympathetic-stimulating drugs such as amphetamines can cause a similar degree of damage.

GRANULOMATOUS MYOCARDITIS

The formation of giant cells and granulomatous inflammation is characteristic of two diseases, sarcoidosis and idiopathic giant cell myocarditis.

Sarcoidosis

The frequency with which patients who have clinically diagnosed sarcoidosis are known to have cardiac involvement is less than 5% in life but is reported to vary widely from less than 15% to 58% in autopsy series.[31,32] This range probably reflects different definitions, i.e. whether there was a single microscopic focus discovered at autopsy or whether there was clinical evidence of cardiac involvement. Conversely, only approximately 50% of patients discovered at autopsy to have cardiac sarcoid were diagnosed in life. Up to 40% of patients with cardiac sarcoid do not have involvement of other organs.

Morphological forms of cardiac sarcoid

There is a wide range of morphological forms of myocardial sarcoid[33] matched by a similar range of clinical symptoms. A regional form of sarcoid occurs[34] in which initially there is a mass of enlarged pale tissue containing abundant giant cell granulomas. This mass may occupy the upper ventricular septum and extend into the atria, producing complete atrioventricular block. In other cases the mass is within the ventricular muscle and impairs contraction. At autopsy the mass is white and fibrous (Fig. 5.11) and is easily mistaken for other conditions such as a gumma or a fibrous tumour. Regional masses of sarcoid resolve ultimately by fibrosis and contraction leading to ventricular aneurysm formation (Fig. 5.12) in either ventricle. There is some evidence that treatment with steroids enhances the risk of aneurysm formation.[34] Regional ventricular involvement is strongly associated with recurrent ventricular tachycardia and may be cured by resection of the affected area. The high risk of ventricular arrhythmias in myocardial sarcoid means there is a high risk of sudden death.

More diffuse cardiac sarcoid leads to widespread fibrosis and the clinical picture of either a restrictive or dilated cardiomyopathy. Rarer patterns of cardiac sarcoid include involvement of the pericardium with effusions and ultimately constrictive pericarditis[35,36] and granulomas within cardiac valves. Valvular granulomas occur in up to 3% of cases but are usually coincidental findings.[34] Involvement of papillary muscles may cause mitral regurgitation.[37] Many patients with cardiac sarcoid experience chest pain, and the possibility that this is due to microvascular involvement is often raised. Pathological reports are limited but granulomas have been found in or around intramyocardial arteries.[31] Some of the widespread fibrosis in myocardial sarcoid may represent obliteration of small intramyocardial vessels. Myocardial biopsy, as would be anticipated from the focal nature of the disease, is rarely diagnostic.[38] Positive biopsies are however reported in up to 50% of cases with clinically proven myocardial sarcoid. Negative biopsies have no value in excluding the diagnosis. The histological picture of myocardial sarcoid is that of non-caseating focal granulomas identical to the disease in any other organ. Where there is a localised mass the centre may be amorphous collagen but it is usually possible to see discrete granulomas at the edge (Fig. 5.13). Neither myocyte necrosis nor eosinophilic infiltration is usually present.

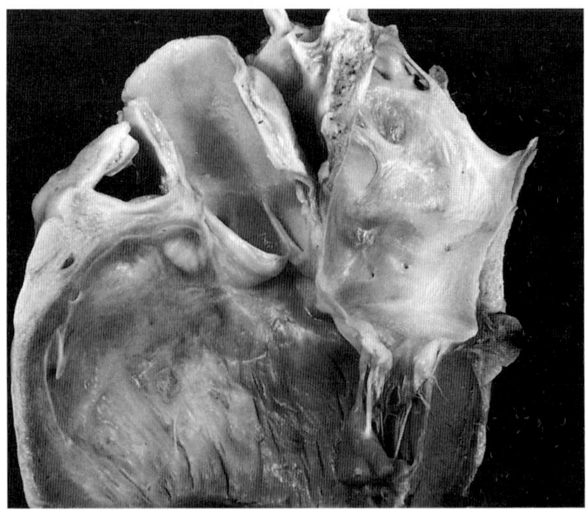

Fig. 5.12 Myocardial sarcoidosis. In this long axis view of the left ventricular outflow the anterior-septal wall is thinned and bulges outward. Systemic sarcoidosis present, treated with steroids for some years.

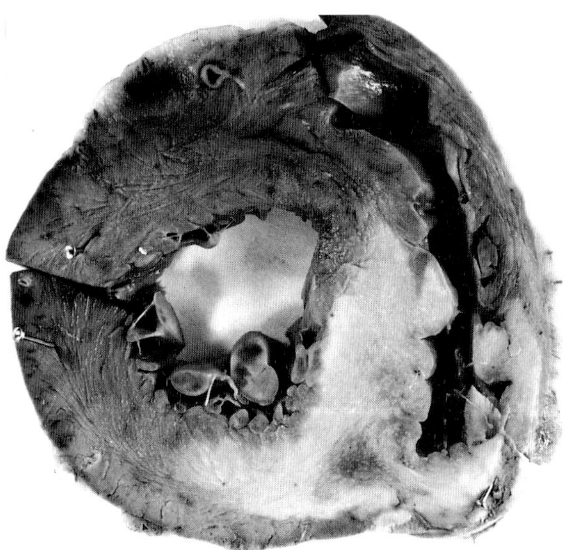

Fig. 5.11 Myocardial sarcoidosis. In this transverse short axis section of the ventricles there is a white mass in the posterior wall of the left ventricle, the interventricular septum and the posterior wall of the right ventricle. In this active stage of the disease the mass does not encroach on the ventricular chambers or extend into the pericardium. Such features in an echocardiogram or at autopsy are pointers against the mass being a tumour.

Idiopathic giant cell myocarditis

In its classic form (Figs 5.13, 5.14) this condition is readily recognised both macroscopically and microscopically.[39] A common presentation is a few days of fever, arrhythmias and heart failure followed by sudden death. At autopsy there are macroscopically visible serpiginous areas of myocardial necrosis throughout both ventricles. The irregular outline of the focal areas of necrosis scattered throughout the full thickness of the left ventricular wall contrasts with the diffuse sub-endocardial necrosis that follows prolonged hypoperfusion of the myocardium. Microscopic examination (Fig. 5.15) shows focal areas of frank myocyte necrosis with granulation tissue and early organisation at the margins of which there is a florid inflammatory response including eosinophils, macrophages and giant cells. The giant cells are multinucleated, occur at the margins of the necrotic areas and, when the myocytes are cut in cross-section, appear roughly round in shape. In areas in which the myocytes are seen in longitudinal section the giant cells are elongated and strap-shaped. The giant cells have been shown to be of macrophage origin[40] and the shape is determined by their being confined within the original sarcolemmal sheath of a dead myocyte.

The pathogenesis of this form of giant cell myocarditis is unknown. There must be some specific factor invoking the giant cell response since myocyte necrosis from infarction or viral myocarditis does not invoke this cell response. No virus has been implicated so far although measles might be hypothesised to be a candidate. There is an association with other autoimmune diseases and with thymomas.[41] Autoimmunity to myocyte antigens, such as myosin, that are common in human dilated cardiomyopathy are, however, not associated with giant cell formation. Immunisation of Lewis rats with myosin and an adjuvant will invoke a giant cell myocarditis;[42] in contrast, in mice giant cells are not a feature of autoimmune myocarditis.

The advent of diagnostic biopsies in patients suspected of suffering from acute myocarditis has

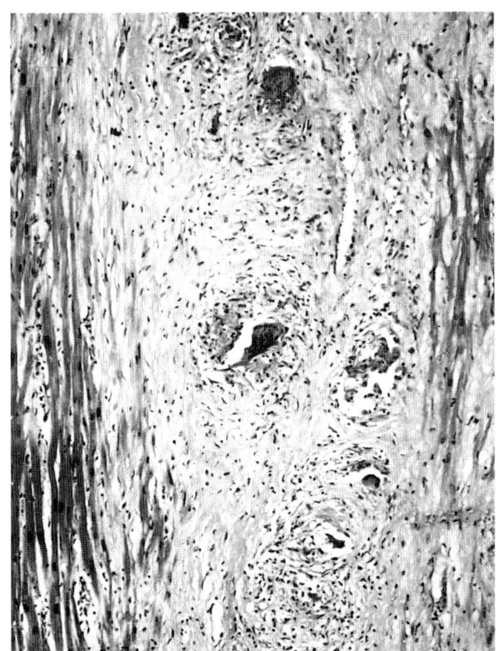

Fig. 5.13 Myocardial sarcoid — histology. In myocardial sarcoid there is retention of discrete follicular giant cell granulomas although these may coalesce to form larger areas. Inflammation in the tissue remote from the granulomas is minimal and the involvement is often very regional. Haematoxylin–eosin × 65

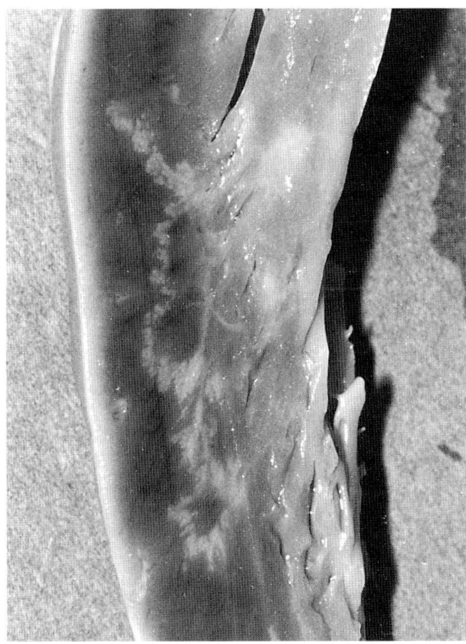

Fig. 5.14 Idiopathic acute giant cell myocarditis. The myocardium shows serpiginous areas of necrosis with a red centre and yellow rim.

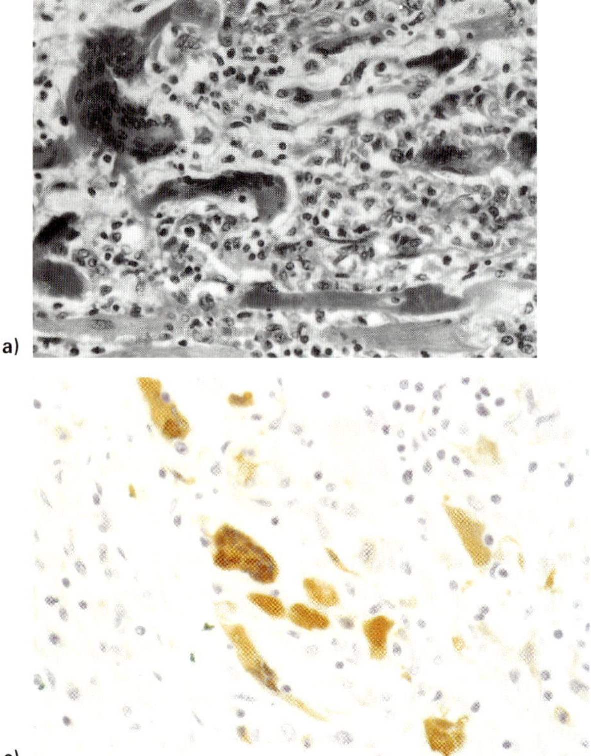

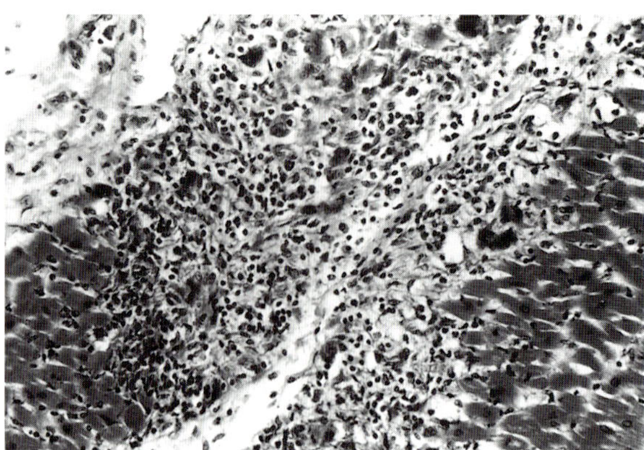

Fig. 5.15 a,b,c Idiopathic acute giant cell myocarditis. (**a**) The edges of the areas of necrosis show intense inflammatory infiltrate with eosinophils a major component. The giant cells, when seen in planes which show the myocytes in their long axis, are elongated and strap-shaped. (**b**) In tissue planes which show myocytes in cross-section the giant cells appear round in shape and packages of involvement have a follicular shape simulating sarcoid. The number of eosinophils and the absence of epithelioid cells are however helpful features. (**c**) The giant cells mark (brown) when antibodies against CD68 are used identifying them as being of macrophage origin.
(**a**) Haematoxylin–eosin × 200
(**b**) Haematoxylin–eosin × 125

shown some cases of giant cell myocarditis to have a less severe clinical course, and resolution with immunosuppression is reported. Some cases require emergency cardiac transplantation but recurrence in the transplanted heart is reported.[43]

Other forms of granulomatous (giant cell) myocarditis

Most cases of giant cell myocarditis can be characterised as either being sarcoidosis or idiopathic giant cell myocarditis (Table 5.2). Intermediate and overlapping forms occur, however, and will continue to cause considerable semantic difficulty until a classification based on aetiology becomes available.

In some patients with systemic sarcoidosis the cardiac involvement is very acute and indistinguishable from idiopathic giant cell myocarditis. It is therefore always necessary to search routinely for giant cell granulomas in other organs.

In Wegener's granulomatosis (Chapter 4) there is a fibrinoid necrosis/vasculitis in intramyocardial vessels associated with perivascular granulomas. Focal areas of myocardial necrosis occur but are not usually surrounded by giant cells. Cases are described, however, in which a diffuse giant cell myocarditis and vascular fibrinoid lesions coexist. In some cases of florid idiopathic giant cell myocarditis an occasional vessel showing transmural inflammation can be

Table 5.2 Contrasting features of different forms of giant cell myocarditis

	Idiopathic giant cell myocarditis	Cardiac sarcoid
Clinical onset	Rapid	Insidious
Macroscopic	Serpiginous necrosis right and left ventricle	White scarring as a) regional mass; b) diffuse
Microscopic	Necrosis with giant cells at periphery	Fibrosis with peripheral granulomas — no necrosis
	Eosinophils present	Eosinophils absent
Extracardiac lesions	Absent	May be present

found but their presence in large numbers is unusual.

These transitional forms of giant cell myocarditis have been used to suggest that idiopathic giant cell myocarditis is not a discrete entity but the common end point of a number of disease processes. Be that as it may, the majority of cases of florid giant cell myocarditis do not have evidence either of sarcoidosis or a general vasculitis.

There are two final forms of giant cell lesions encountered within the myocardium; neither however are likely to be confused with those types described so far. In acute rheumatic fever there are interstitial granulomas (Chapter 6) with a well-defined histological appearance. Small granulomas scattered through the interstitial tissue and unrelated directly to myocyte damage may occur in a number of conditions (Fig. 5.16).

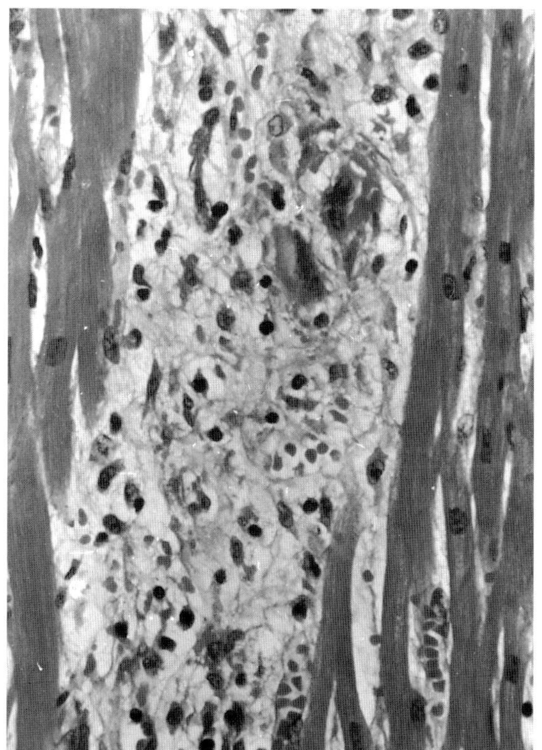

Fig. 5.16 Non-specific giant cell granulomas. The interstitial tissues contained small ill-defined granulomas without any other inflammation, vasculitis or necrosis. Incidental autopsy finding.
Haematoxylin–eosin × 160

These include drug reactions, myocarditis, rejection or incidental findings at autopsy.

In infants calcification of dead myocytes, whether because of myocarditis or from previous vascular hypoperfusion, is common. Such foci of calcification can invoke a florid foreign-body giant cell response.

CARDIOMYOPATHY

INTRODUCTION TO DEFINITIONS

The term cardiomyopathy is used to signify myocardial disease that is due neither to pressure and volume overload nor to ischaemic heart disease. Beyond this point the classification and terminology become complex; in part this is because the underlying tissue processes and pathogenesis of many of the conditions encompassed by the term cardiomyopathy remain unclear. A classification based on cellular mechanisms and aetiology is therefore impossible. The WHO[44] has highlighted this uncertainty by expressing the view that once the mechanism of myocardial dysfunction is known, the disease ceases to be called a cardiomyopathy and becomes a 'specific' heart muscle disorder. This usage, which excludes the term cardiomyopathy from being used at all once there is a known cause, has not achieved wide acceptance. The term cardiomyopathy continues to be used in the clinical context for myocardial dysfunction due to disease primarily of the myocardium itself.

The most widely used classification (Fig. 5.17) is based on the abnormalities in ventricular function that can be observed clinically.[45] In dilated cardiomyopathy (DCM) the abnormal function is predominantly expressed as a loss of systolic contractile power leading to a decreased LV ejection fraction. In functional terms the end systolic left ventricular volume is increased. The result is a dilated, thin-walled left ventricle with a large cavity. In hypertrophic cardiomyopathy (HCM) the left ventricular muscle is thickened and the left ventricular cavity small. Hypertrophic cardiomyopathy is associated with abnormalities in diastolic function and enhanced early systolic contraction. In restrictive cardiomyopathy (RCM) the left ventricle often appears

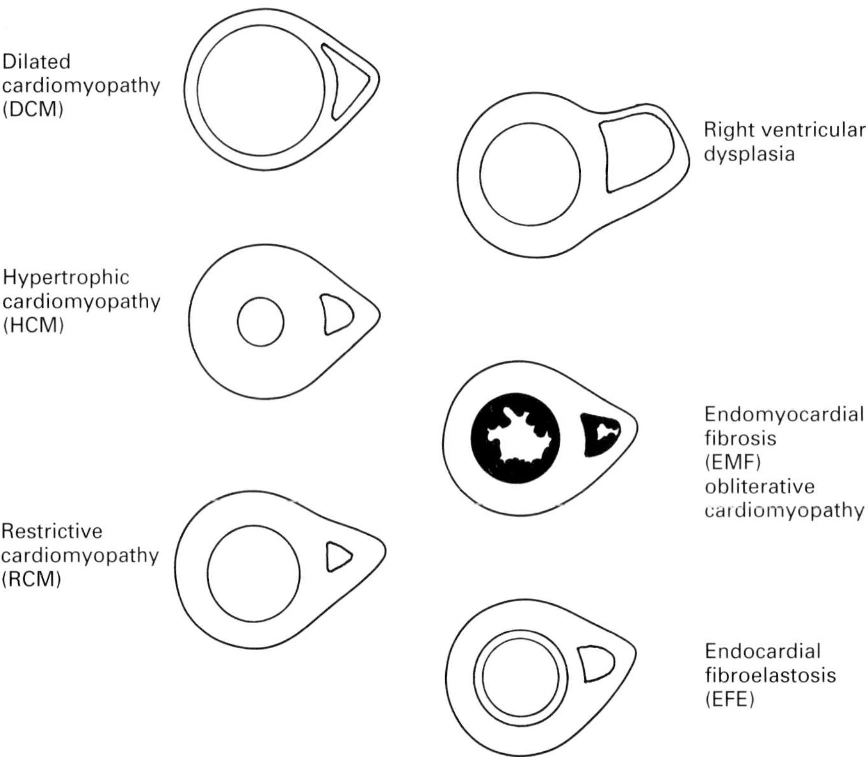

Fig. 5.17 Diagram of left and right ventricular morphology in cardiomyopathy

normal in size and volume but diastolic relaxation is impaired; the result is that the left ventricle can be filled only by increasing left atrial pressure with a resultant back pressure on the right side of the heart; severe right ventricular hypertrophy results. A subgroup of the restrictive cardiomyopathies is due to primary thickening of the endocardium rather than an abnormality of the heart muscle itself; an example is endocardial fibroelastosis (EFE). Yet another group of cardiomyopathies related to the restrictive group is where thrombosis forms on the endocardium of either the right or left ventricles and becomes incorporated and organised, both restricting ventricular relaxation and slowly obliterating the ventricular cavity (obliterative cardiomyopathy). An example is endomyocardial fibrosis (EMF), related to hypereosinophilia in temperate climates but also occurring as a tropical disease without a relation to hypereosinophilia.

Clinically many patients show functional abnormalities which transcend these divisions. For example, many subjects with a dilated cardiomyopathy have concomitant diastolic abnormalities and difficulty in left ventricular filling as well as a loss of systolic power. Despite this difficulty it is usually possible to fit most patients with a cardiomyopathy into the dilated, restrictive, hypertrophic or obliterative forms using the preponderant functional abnormality as shown by echocardiography in life. With the increasing use of cardiac biopsy and availability of explanted hearts it is realised that each functional group has a wide range of often overlapping pathology.

A further difficulty in clinical terminology arises over patients who present with rhythm and conduction problems rather than abnormalities of contractile function. Most cases of this arrhythmogenic type of cardiomyopathy lie closest to the dilated group and often have an enlarged left ventricular cavity although systolic function is preserved. Many such patients are labelled as ‘arrhythmias due to underlying cardiomyopathy’. One form of arrhythmogenic cardiomyopathy, right ventricular dysplasia (RVD), is unique in that it predominantly involves the right side, producing a dilated, thin-walled ventricle with extensive replacement of the myocardium by fat and adipose tissue.

A final difficulty lies in the use and definition of the term 'acute myocarditis'. On the clinical side there are patients who present with the sudden onset of cardiac failure in association with arrhythmias; on the pathological side an intense infiltration of lymphocytes and/or eosinophils and/or macrophages is found in the interstitial tissues of the myocardium in association with evidence of myocyte damage. When these two aspects, clinical and pathological, concur there is no difficulty about using the term acute myocarditis. It is, in effect, an acute form of a dilated cardiomyopathy. In clinical practice the term 'acute myocarditis' is often used without biopsy confirmation of the tissue finding and the supposition of the presence of interstitial inflammation is made based on the short clinical history, often in association with fever. The difficulties that these assumptions by the clinician make have been discussed earlier in this chapter.

All these semantic problems should not be allowed to assume too great a significance. In clinical practice, as well as in pathology, most patients can be fitted into the dilated, hypertrophic or restrictive cardiomyopathy group without undue difficulty. The word cardiomyopathy should be used, qualified by what is known about the functional and pathogenetic mechanisms. For example, alcoholic dilated cardiomyopathy, amyloid restrictive cardiomyopathy or familial hypertrophic cardiomyopathy are widely used and readily understood terms. It is to be hoped that the pathogenesis of the most common type of case, idiopathic dilated cardiomyopathy, will become better understood in the future.

HYPERTROPHIC CARDIOMYOPATHY

The major distinguishing morphological feature of this form of cardiomyopathy is the presence of ventricular hypertrophy without cavity dilatation. The ventricular hypertrophy is recognised clinically and pathologically both as an increase in ventricular mass and wall thickness. The ventricular hypertrophy may be symmetrical, i.e. involve the whole left ventricle, or asymmetrical, involving one segment only. When thickening is asymmetrical it most frequently involves the interventricular septum but can involve any segment of either ventricle. Symmetrical hypertrophy can only be assumed to be 'cardiomyopathic' when causes such as hypertension or valve disease have been rigorously excluded.

The archetypal form of hypertrophic cardiomyopathy (Fig. 5.18) is the familial type, associated with sudden death and originally described by Donald Teare.[46] It is now recognised that a significant proportion of such families have genetic abnormalities of beta heavy chain cardiac myosin (MHC). A wide range of missense mutations (currently 34 but increasing steadily) and deletions in the DNA coding the head and head/rod region of beta heavy chain myosin gene on chromosome 14 (designated CMH1 gene) have now been described.[47] Those mutations that produce the greatest change in the net charge in the molecule produce the more severe clinical manifestations, whereas some mutations appear relatively benign. Approximately 50% of cases of hypertrophic cardiomyopathy have now been shown to have abnormalities in the beta heavy chain of the cardiac myosin. Linkage studies in families with no abnormality of the myosin gene have identified at least four other genes that produce an identical disease. These are on the long arm of chromosome 1 (CMH 2 gene), the long arm of chromosome 15 (CMH 3 gene) and chromosome 11 (CMH 4 gene).

CMH 2 and 3 genes encode for troponin T and tropomyosin respectively; both are muscle sarcomere fibrillary proteins. It now seems clear that what is present is abnormal contractile filament formation with a loss of their normal spatial arrangement. This in turn leads to abnormal myocyte shape and the functional response of hypertrophy. The disease can therefore be regarded as a dysgenesis of myofibrillary contractile proteins. Both normal and mutant beta heavy chain myosin (MHC) are transcribed to some degree in circulating lymphocytes; this allows examination of MHC messenger RNA using a ribonuclease protection assay and identification of deletions, abnormal splicing and

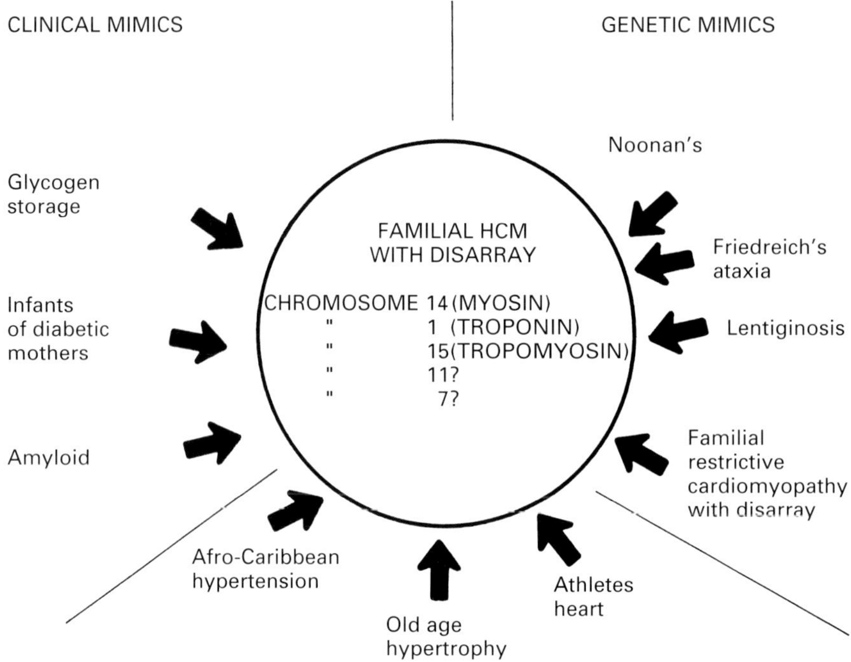

Fig. 5.18 Familial cardiomyopathy and possible related conditions — see diagram itself. The archetypal hypertrophic cardiomyopathy is the familial form. A number of conditions may mimic the morphology of the left ventricle but have no relation in pathogenetic terms. A number of other conditions have either inappropriate degrees of hypertrophy or disarray of myocytes but their genetic background remains unclear.

missense mutations in the gene on chromosome 14 from blood samples. One of the most striking features of hypertrophic cardiomyopathy is that of the wide phenotypical expression of the disease in the heart. This wide variation is found even within one family, i.e. among people who have the same mutation of the same gene. The variation is so wide that only formal genetic analysis will identify all the cases in a family. The variations have led to speculation that other genes also control the hypertrophic response. One candidate is polymorphism in the ACE gene. Of the three alleles of the gene (ID, DD, II), two are associated with higher levels of circulating angiotensin.

Clinical features of hypertrophic cardiomyopathy

The commonest presenting feature of families with hypertrophic cardiomyopathy is sudden death in one member following which echocardiographic screening of other members reveals more cases. Syncopal attacks, often on exercise, are common. Other presenting features include angina-type pain and dyspnoea. The risk of sudden death is maximal in adolescence and subsequently declines, although it never disappears. Proven cases of hypertrophic cardiomyopathy do however occur in subjects over 60 years of age,[48] sometimes as coincidental findings in autopsies, and the disease must not be considered necessarily lethal or disabling. A small proportion of patients finally develop congestive cardiac failure and the left ventricular cavity dilates.[49]

Echocardiography in life in patients with hypertrophic cardiomyopathy is very useful in demonstrating the small left ventricular cavity and asymmetric left ventricular wall thickening. It is very efficient in demonstrating the long axis of the left ventricular outflow tract. The most typical form of hypertrophic cardiomyopathy, originally recognised by Teare, involves the interventricular septum which bulges out to the left below the aortic valve. In systole the thickened septum and the anterior cusp of the mitral valve come together with great force, effectively obliterating the left ventricular outflow before systole is complete.[50] Very high pressures are generated in the left ventricle as a result. This process led to names such as idiopathic hypertrophic subaortic stenosis (IHSS), asymmetric septal hypertrophy (ASH) or obstructive cardiomyopathy being used in the past. These have now been largely superseded by the term hypertrophic cardiomyopathy (HCM). The high pressures across the outflow tract, although generated during systole, in fact occur after most of the blood has been ejected, and the concept of outflow obstruction is strictly incorrect.

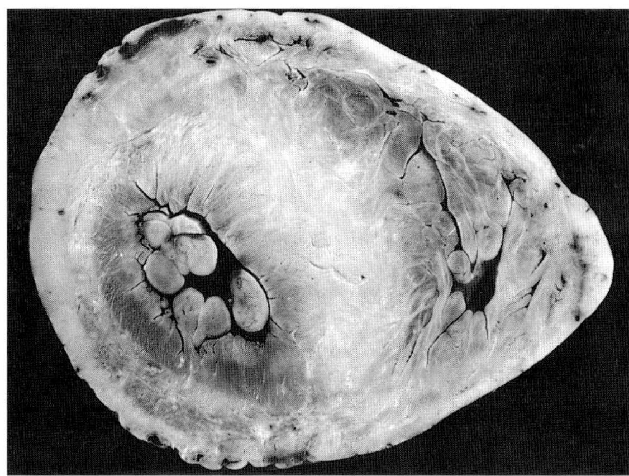

Fig. 5.19 Familial hypertrophic cardiomyopathy. Transverse section of both ventricles. The septum is disproportionally thick (4.1 cm) compared with the posterior wall of the left ventricle (1.9 cm). The cut surface of the septum is whorled, with areas of fibrosis. The right ventricular wall is uniformly thick and involved in the process. This specimen could not be anything other than familial hypertrophic cardiomyopathy.

Pathological features of hypertrophic cardiomyopathy

While the greater proportion of cases can be easily recognised macroscopically the very protean manifestations of hypertrophic cardiomyopathy must be appreciated. Overall the first impression for the examining pathologist is usually of a heart which appears unduly heavy for its volume. Once the heart is opened the reason for this impression is found to be a thick-walled left ventricle with a small cavity.

The standard methods by which many pathologists open the heart in the direction of blood flow in fact obscures the findings in hypertrophic cardiomyopathy. The disease is best appreciated either in transverse slices of the intact ventricles or in a long axis cut through the left ventricular outflow. The former approach allows the small cavity and thick walls of either ventricle to be well seen. Hypertrophic cardiomyopathy often produces asymmetric hypertrophy, i.e. one segment of the ventricle is much thicker than the rest (Fig. 5.19). The area most frequently involved is the interventricular septum, with extension on to either the anterior or posterior wall. The thickness of the septum can be compared to the thickness of the posterior wall of the

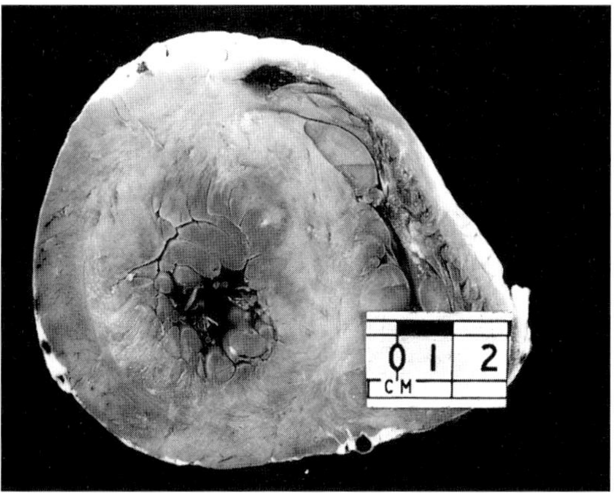

Fig. 5.20 Familial hypertrophic cardiomyopathy. Transverse section of both ventricles. The LV is concentrically thickened without any of the whorled fibrosis on the cut surface that is seen in Figure 5.19.

left ventricle and ratios above 2 are common in hypertrophic cardiomyopathy. The cut surface of the septum in such classical cases has a whorled appearance very like that of uterine fibroids.

This classic form of hypertrophic cardiomyopathy accounts for over 60% of cases. The next most common variant is for the left ventricular thickening to be virtually symmetric (Fig. 5.20). In part this is because the actual disease involves the whole ventricle, but in part it is due to a

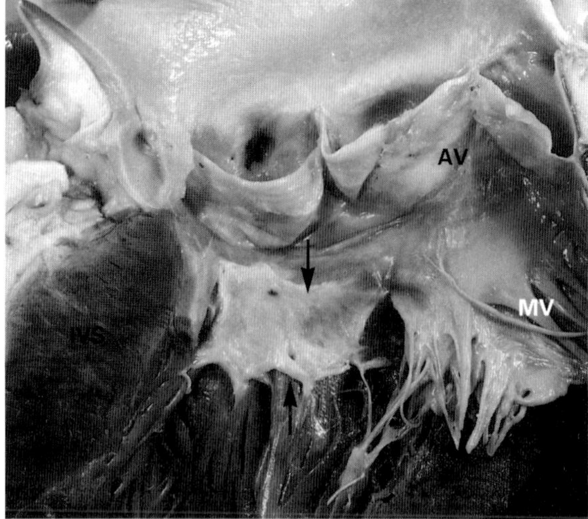

Fig. 5.21 Familial hypertrophic cardiomyopathy. The LV outflow is cut longitudinally. The interventricular septum (IVS) is disproportionately thick. On the endocardial surface of the septum (arrow) below the aortic valve (AV) there is a patch of white endocardial thickening. This patch has a very discrete sharp lower border which corresponds exactly to the lower edge of the mitral valve (MV). When it forms a mirror image of the anterior cusp and has a well-defined lower margin the lesion is pathognomonic of HCM.

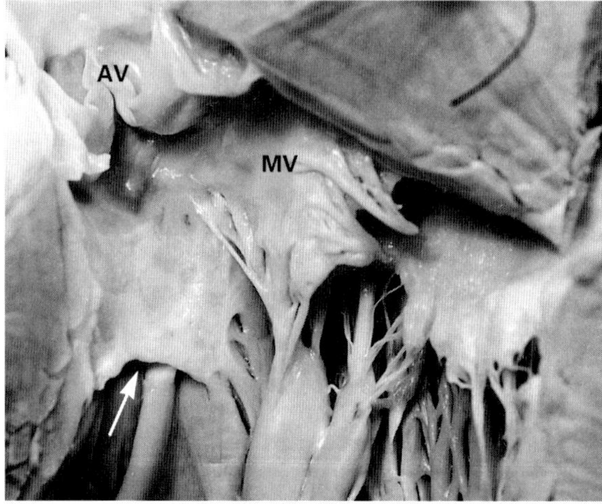

Fig. 5.22 Familial hypertrophic cardiomyopathy. Below the aortic valve (AV) there is a patch of endocardial thickening (arrow). As in Figure 5.21 this has a sharp lower border corresponding to the shape of the anterior cusp of the mitral valve. Mechanical damage causes the anterior cusp of the mitral valve (MV) to thicken and chordal rupture may occur, as it did in this case.

purely secondary hypertrophic response. Other variants include involvement of other segments of the left ventricle without septal involvement. In one particular variant only the apex of the left ventricle is involved in the hypertrophic response; this form appears to be more common in Japan, while the classic asymmetric septal form is most common in Europe and the USA.[51]

The right ventricle is also involved in many cases. The common pattern is for the anterior wall of the right ventricular outflow to be involved, together with the left ventricle. Rare cases of isolated right ventricular involvement are known.

In hypertrophic cardiomyopathy the left ventricular outflow has a very characteristic macroscopic appearance (Figs 5.21, 5.22). Below the aortic valve on the endocardium of the upper interventricular septum there is a discrete transverse band of endocardial thickening. This thickening may be several millimetres in depth. The lower border is sharply defined and corresponds exactly to the level of the lower edge of the anterior cusp of the mitral valve. A patch of endocardial thickening corresponding to the mitral valve chordae may also be present.

The endocardial thickening is due to direct trauma to the septum. When echocardiograms of the left ventricular outflow in hypertrophic cardiomyopathy are studied, the anterior cusp of the mitral valve can be seen to move forward in early systole (systolic anterior motion) to hit the septum, bounce off and then be forced back again on to the septum. The endocardial thickening microscopically contains smooth muscle proliferation, collagen and elastic fibrils. It is often vascularised but not inflamed. The anterior cusp of the mitral valve also suffers traumatic damage and becomes thickened by surface fibrosis. In extreme cases, chordae may rupture due to mechanical damage.

Cases of hypertrophic cardiomyopathy in which there is massive hypertrophy of the upper septum may be treated surgically to enlarge the LV outflow tract. The mitral valve may or may not be replaced at the same time (Figs 5.23, 5.24).

Some warnings must be given about the mitral valve impact lesion of hypertrophic cardiomyopathy. Firstly, it is not necessarily present and is, for example, absent in forms of the disease such as apical cardiomyopathy that do not involve the upper interventricular septum. Secondly, the more diffuse and mild endocardial thickening on the upper septum seen in any dilated left ventricle or

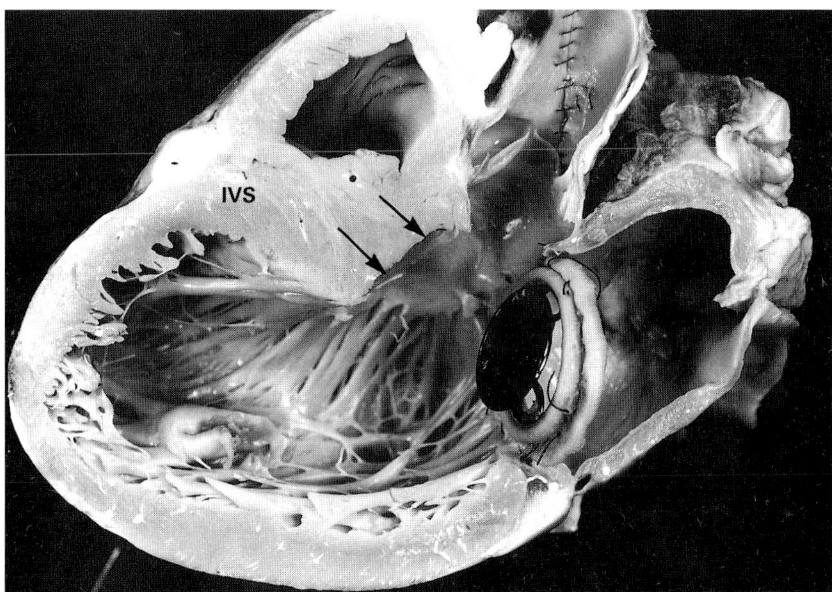

Fig. 5.23 Surgical treatment of hypertrophic cardiomyopathy. A case of familial HCM has been treated surgically to excise a segment of the interventricular septum (IVS). The surgical excision surface is straight (arrows) and has enlarged the LV outflow. Residual abnormally thick muscle remains in the upper septum but the rest of the ventricular wall is normal. The mitral valve has been replaced by a tilting disc prosthesis, further enlarging the LV cavity through the removal of the anterior cusp of the mitral valve and some papillary muscles.

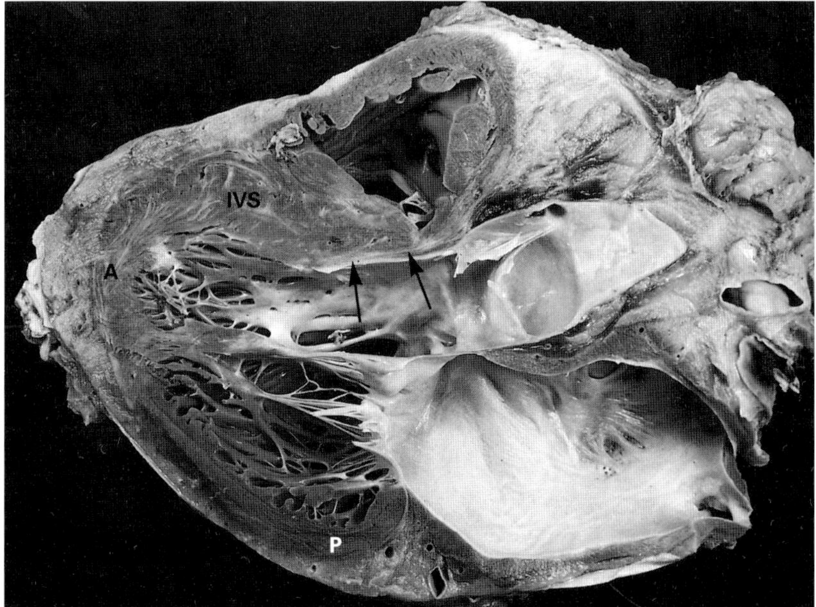

Fig. 5.24 Surgical treatment of familial hypertrophic cardiomyopathy. In this long axis plane abnormal whorled and thick muscle is present at the apex (A) and in the interventricular septum (IVS). The posterior wall of the LV (P) is normal. Muscle had been removed from the LV outflow some years before leaving a straight edge with endocardial thickening (arrows). Unlike in Figure 5.23 the mitral valve had not been replaced.

with age must not be overinterpreted. In hypertrophic cardiomyopathy the lower border of the endocardial fibrosis is very sharply defined and exactly matches the outline of the mitral anterior cusp.

A final problem with the macroscopic recognition of hypertrophic cardiomyopathy is that a small minority of cases in which the diagnosis is sound on genetic grounds express none of the macroscopic features described so far. Some cases enter a late phase in which the ventricle thins and dilates, simulating exactly a dilated cardiomyopathy. Others with a more than usual degree of restrictive-type physiology do not develop a thick-walled left ventricle at any stage. Thus, while it is often possible to give a positive macroscopic diagnosis, it is unwise to give dogmatic opinions on whether hypertrophic cardiomyopathy is absent before detailed histology. When giving firm macroscopic diagnosis of HCM it is also wise to remember that some totally unrelated conditions such as amyloid can produce massive septal enlargement and closely mimic hypertrophic cardiomyopathy.

Microscopic appearances

There is a very characteristic microscopic change reflecting the altered myocyte shape in the

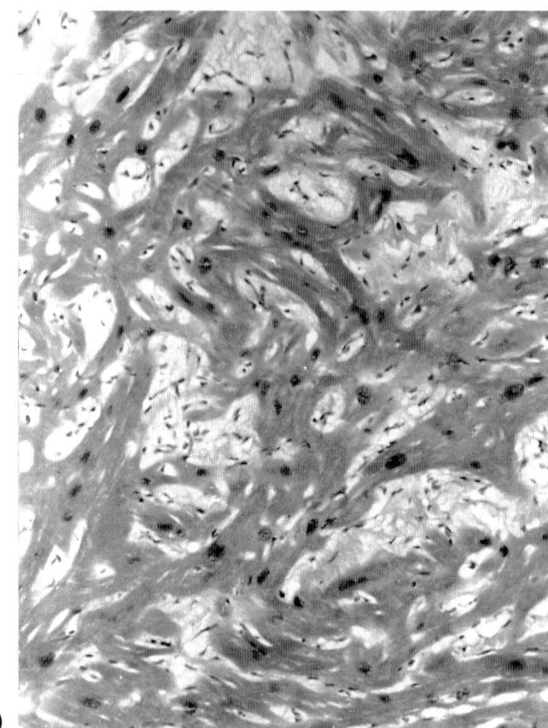
a)

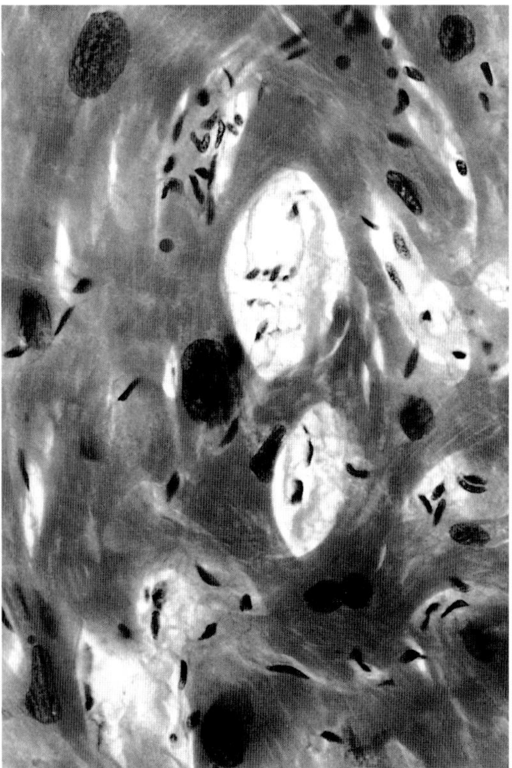
b)

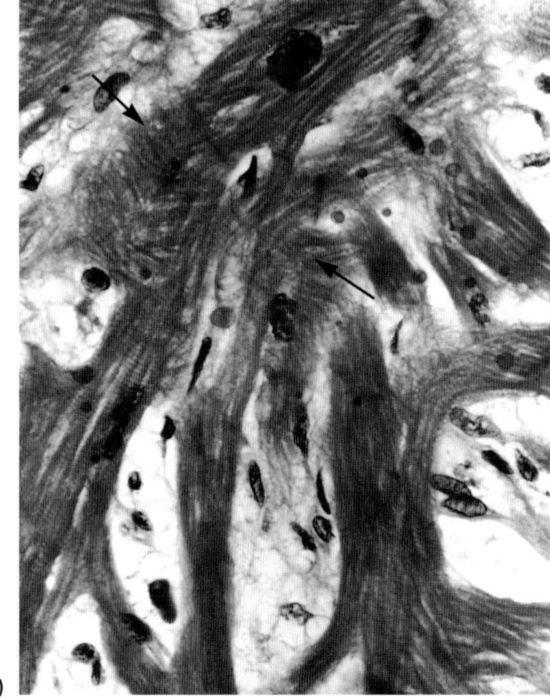
c)

disease.[52,53] Focal areas of the myocardium show bizarre myocytes in which there is extreme nuclear pleomorphism and the internal myofibrillary arrangement is disorganised (Fig. 5.25). These myocytes appear bizarre in shape, losing the rather oblong form of normal cells. Cell-to-cell adhesion appears to occur at many points, not just at the end of the long axis. These shape changes are reflected in myocytes being arranged in whorls, often around a central focus of collagen. These central foci often contain very pleomorphic fibroblasts, suggesting that considerable connective tissue proliferation is occurring. More macroscopic interweaving and whorling of large blocks of myocytes is also present, interspersed with thick bands of collagen.

This constellation of abnormal features has been given the overall name of myocardial disarray. It must be noted that this occurs at three levels. One is within the cell and is myofibrillary disorganisation. Another is at ordinary microscopic level, while another is semi-macroscopic. Ideally all levels of disarray are present. Intracellular myofibrillary disorganisation alone is of very low specificity.

The specificity of myocardial disarray for hypertrophic cardiomyopathy has been widely discussed and is a contentious subject. The first facet of this difficulty is that disarray is not evenly distributed throughout the ventricle. Its maximum presence coincides with the macroscopic areas of hypertrophy but disarray is also present in areas of the ventricle that look macroscopically normal. A feature of hypertrophic cardiomyopathy is that areas of myocardium that appear histologically normal, areas with ordinary hypertrophy and areas with disarray are often mixed and contiguous. A second difficulty is that small foci of apparent disarray can be found in normal hearts, particularly where the anterior wall of the right ventricle abuts on to the interventricular septum. While such focal areas in normal hearts have a passing resemblance to disarray they are more an interdigitating of myocytes and the whorling around foci of connective tissue is absent. A final difficulty is that a small number of cases that fit the clinical criteria of hypertrophic cardiomyopathy have no disarray. In part the difficulties have been solved by the development of a scoring system for disarray based on examining multiple areas of myocardium. It is then clear that, quantitatively, disarray is indicative of hypertrophic cardiomyopathy.[54]

In hypertrophic cardiomyopathy intramyocardial arteries in the range of 200–400 μm external diameter may show pronounced dysplastic changes with narrowing of the lumen due to disorganised smooth muscle proliferation in the intima and media (Fig. 5.26). These vascular changes have been linked to fibrous scarring in the myocardium and progression to a dilated left ventricle. The vascular changes are undoubtedly very

Fig. 5.25 a,b,c Disarray in hypertrophic cardiomyopathy. (**a**) Marked myocyte nuclear enlargement is present although some immediately adjacent myocytes have normal nuclei. Myocytes run in a circular fashion around foci of connective tissue. There is very marked myocyte nuclear pleomorphism. (**b**) The general orientation of myocytes in this field is at right angles to the short axis of the frame. Focal areas occur however in which myocytes run at right angles to this enclosing small areas of connective tissue. (**c**) In sections stained to enhance the myofibrillary architecture the disorientation within individual cells can be appreciated (arrows).
(**a**) Haematoxylin–eosin × 16
(**b**) Haematoxylin–eosin × 160
(**c**) PTAH × 160

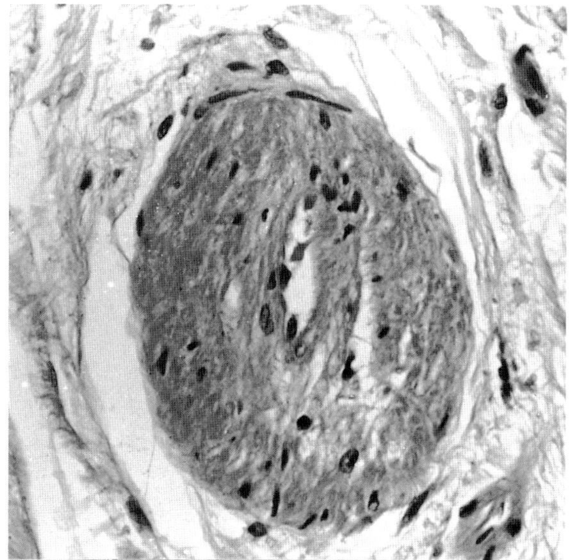

Fig. 5.26 Small-vessel change in hypertrophic cardiomyopathy. An intramyocardial artery shows extreme disorganisation of the smooth muscle within the media and loss of the distinction between the layers of the vessel wall. Relative to its external diameter the lumen is very small. The functional effect on flow is unknown although these changes have been related to the onset of myocardial fibrosis. Haematoxylin–eosin × 16

pronounced in some cases of hypertrophic cardiomyopathy but absent in others. Similar changes but involving smaller numbers of arteries may occur in old age and in severe hypertrophy from any cause.[55]

Phenotypic expression of hypertrophic cardiomyopathy

Both macroscopically and microscopically the disease is very variable both in the segment of the heart involved and in the degree of disarray. It is a feature of the disease that not every myocyte is involved. Clinical studies suggest that the hypertrophy first appears in the adolescent growth phase[56] and, although infant cases are described, symptoms or death are rare below about 12 years of age. Why the hypertrophy is regional is unknown. One view is that a stimulus for hypertrophy such as hypertension or unequal sympathetic innervation to the myocardium modulates the phenotypic expression. Studies of families known to have the same mutation of the beta heavy chain myosin gene show that within one family every phenotypic and clinical expression within the heart can occur.[49] Such phenotypic diversity is the rule rather than the exception.

Variations of hypertrophic cardiomyopathy

The disease described by Teare and having genetic abnormalities of myofibrillary proteins can be regarded as the archetypal form of hypertrophic cardiomyopathy.

Other hypertrophic conditions exist which may or may not have a similar basis in myofibrillary dysgenesis (Fig. 5.18). These include the following.

Neonatal diabetic cardiomyopathy. Infants born of mothers suffering from diabetes are unduly large and even allowing for large size have organomegaly. Disproportionate left ventricular hypertrophy can be demonstrated both by echocardiography in life and at autopsy. The septal thickness is often increased relative to the posterior wall. Disarray is notoriously difficult to assess in the immature heart and is probably not reliably identified. For what it is worth disarray is probably absent and the condition is due to excess growth-hormone-like substances. In infants who survive the hypertrophy ultimately resolves but may take up to 2 years.

Afro-Caribbean hypertensive cardiomegaly. Hypertension is common in Afro-Caribbean subjects and in some cases cardiac hypertrophy is disproportionately severe for the level of hypertension. Hearts in excess of 550 gms in weight with a thick LV wall and small cavity which simulate hypertrophic cardiomyopathy occur. Myocardial disarray is absent but sudden death can occur. Similiar hearts occur in renal hypertension in any race. The myocardial response is thought to be due to high levels of circulating angiotensin either renal in origin or due to polymorphisas of the ACE gene.

Disarray without hypertrophy and with restrictive physiology. Familial cases are encountered in which there are ECG abnormalities, evidence of restrictive cardiac physiology, no evidence of hypertrophy on echocardiography or autopsy and a risk of sudden death, and in which typical disarray is widely distributed in the myocardium on histology.[57] The genetic basis is as yet unknown.

Athlete's heart. Distinctive physiological adaptations occur in highly trained athletes and these, coupled with a considerable increase in left ventricular muscle mass, make the distinction of what is pathological and what lies in the range of adaptation to high physical demand very difficult. Athletes often have resting bradycardia between 40 and 60 beats a minute and cardiac stroke output is high. Sinus bradycardia, marked sinus arrhythmia and ectopic junctional rhythms are common due to high vagal tone. Athletes whose sport or progression involves isometric exercise (weight lifting, rowers) develop cardiomegaly with normal or decreased cavity dimensions and a thick ventricular wall. Those whose sport is isotonic (runners) have a ventricle retaining its normal relative dimensions. Asymmetry of greater than 1.3 in septal to posterior wall ratios is unusual and a wall thickness of 16 mm in the left ventricle defines the limit of normality. While all these guidelines are useful in screening live athletes, at autopsy there may be real problems in distinguishing the extreme of adaptation from hypertrophic cardiomyopathy, which accounts for about one quarter of sudden deaths in athletes. The problem is compounded by the use of steroids in some athletic categories. These even further accentuate heart mass and may be associated with sudden death in subjects without histological or genetic evidence of hypertrophic cardiomyopathy.

Noonan's syndrome. This syndrome is characterised by short stature, a webbed neck, mild mental deficiency and cardiac abnormalities including pulmonary stenosis and a hypertrophic cardiomyopathy which may involve either ventricle. The phenotype is variable and many cases are not clinically diagnosed. There is some disarray in the ventricular myocardium but this usually falls short of the degree seen in familial hypertrophic cardiomyopathies. The gene has not been located.

Friedreich's ataxia. This is due to an autosomal recessive gene on chromosome 9 but it is not known which protein is involved. Most cases present initially with ataxia in late childhood and adolescence while cardiac symptoms appear in adult life. The expression in the heart is very variable. At one extreme the heart may be macroscopically normal but show widespread disarray on microscopy, at the other extreme the macroscopic and microscopic features are identical to those of familial hypertrophic cardiomyopathy. In general, however, the hearts are macroscopically not strikingly abnormal and areas of fibrosis and disarray are present on microscopy.[58]

Conditions simulating hypertrophic cardiomyopathy

A number of conditions simulate hypertrophic cardiomyopathy because they produce asymmetric septal thickening detectable on echocardiography. The conditions are unlikely to be confused with true hypertrophic cardiomyopathy once microscopy is available but do create difficulties in clinical diagnosis. Examples are amyloid heart disease, sarcoidosis, acromegalic heart disease and glycogen storage disease. Two of the lysosomal storage enzyme deficits also mimic hypertrophic cardiomyopathy very closely.

Glycogen storage disease

In Pompe's disease (Type II glycogenosis) an autosomal recessive gene on chromosome 17 causes accumulation of glycogen because of a lack of the lysosomal enzyme alpha glycosidase. Glycogen can be made but not broken down. Massive deposition occurs in the myocardium leading to a grossly hypertrophied heart in infancy. The heart shows combinations of extreme wall thickening with either a small or enlarged cavity. Either a hypertrophic or restrictive physiological pattern occurs. The ventricular septum is often disproportionately thickened. Histological examination shows accumulation of large amounts of glycogen in enlarged, rather vacuolated myocytes (Fig. 5.27). Myofibrillary loss may become extreme. Diagnosis can be made in life by the absence of alpha glycosidase in skeletal muscle biopsies.[59] Most patients die before the age of two.

Fabry's disease

Fabry's disease is due to deficiency in a galactosidase A lysosomal enzyme that catabolises neutral glycophosphosphingolipids. The accumulation of glycophosphosphingolipid in tissues leads to angiokeratomas, corneal opacities, and peripheral and central CNS disorders. Cardiac

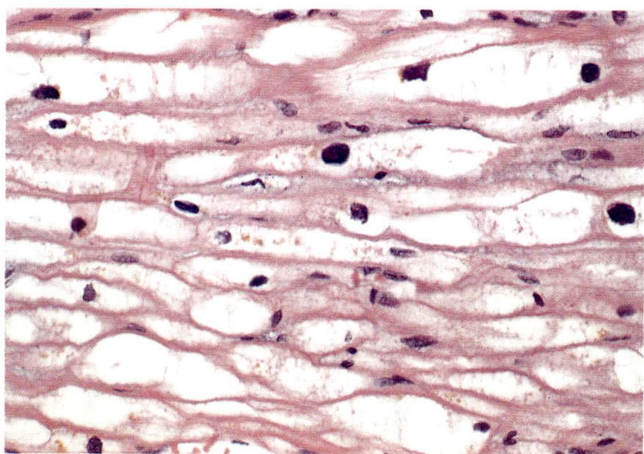

Fig. 5.27 Glycogen storage disease. Virtually all the myocytes appear vacuolated and are devoid of myofibrils. Haematoxylin–eosin × 41

involvement is common and consists of combinations of aortic and mitral regurgitation with very asymmetric ventricular hypertrophy. The posterior wall of the left ventricle or the septum is often disproportionately thick. When septal involvement is striking and the systemic manifestations minor, genuine clinical confusion with true familial hypertrophic cardiomyopathy can occur. The histology of the myocardium shows hypertrophied myocytes with vacuolisation of the cytoplasm and myofibrillary disorganisation. In biopsies on light microscopy the appearances can mimic familial hypertrophic cardiomyopathy. Electron microscopy, even on material which has been processed for light microscopy, will however show the very characteristic concentric lamellae inside myocytes.[60,61]

DILATED CARDIOMYOPATHY

The predominant functional abnormality in dilated cardiomyopathies is a reduction in systolic contractile function reflected by echocardiography and in pathology specimens as an increase in left ventricular cavity dimensions, with a reduction in wall thickness (Fig. 5.28). It is in aetiological

a)

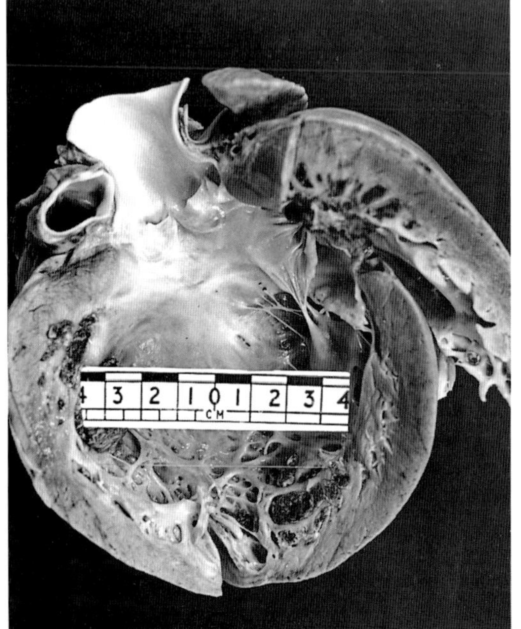

b)

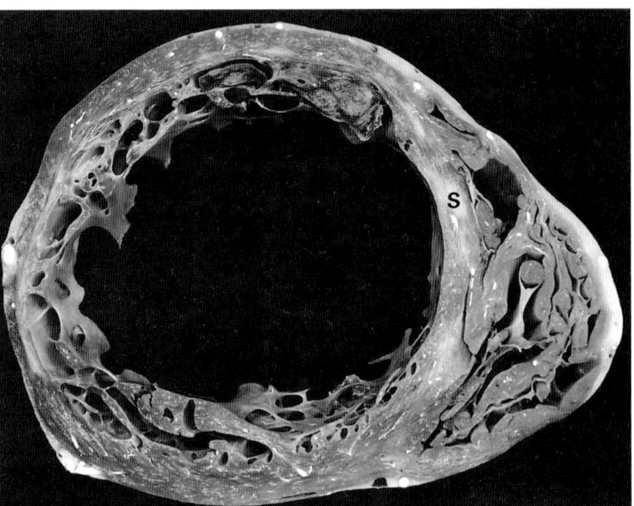

c)

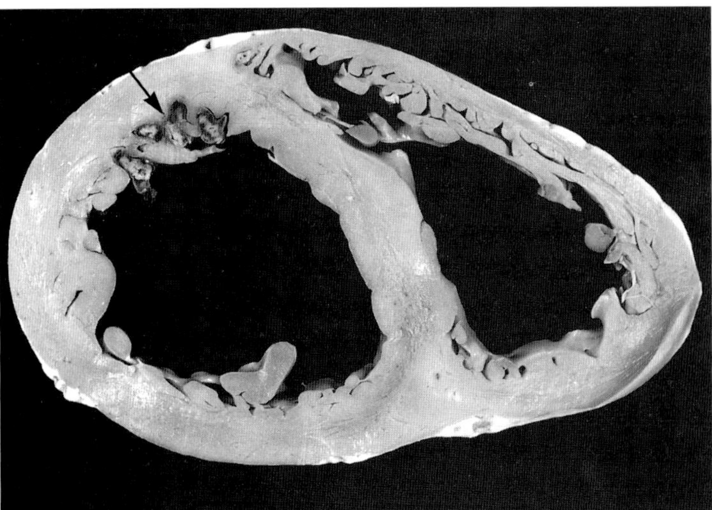

Fig. 5.28 a,b,c Dilated cardiomyopathy — macroscopic features. (**a**) Heart opened in the conventional manner to show globular shape with a dilated left ventricle containing mural thrombus. Diffuse mild endocardial thickening is also present. (**b**) Short axis transection of both ventricles. The left ventricular wall is thin with a large cavity dimension. The myocardium shows macroscopic areas of fibrosis, particularly in the septum (S) and in the lateral wall. Normal coronary arteriograms in life and at autopsy exclude ischaemic heart disease. (**c**) Short axis transection of both ventricles. The left ventricle is thin-walled with a large cavity diameter. Mural thrombus (arrow) is forming. The right ventricle is also dilated. There is no macroscopic scarring.

Table 5.3 Dilated cardiomyopathy — causes

Postviral myocarditis	
Genetic familial	– With skeletal muscle disease – Without skeletal muscle disease – Sex-linked – Mitochondrial – Metabolic defects
Toxic	– Drugs – Heavy metals – Alcohol
Peripartum	
Idiopathic	*? Familial* *? Autoimmune* *? Postviral*

terms a very diverse condition (Table 5.3) but the majority of cases fall into the idiopathic group. For this reason the idiopathic form will be taken as the standard for description. The designation of a heart as showing a dilated cardiomyopathy should be based on a concordance of several abnormal features (Table 5.4). It should not, for example, be used for hearts which to all intent and purpose are morphologically normal, but the subject died suddenly and unexpectedly of what the clinician may designate as 'acute heart failure' after an anaesthetic.

Pathological features

The overall heart weight is increased, with dilation of both ventricles. To record a heart as having a dilated cardiomyopathy with a normal total heart weight (adjusted for body size) is a negation of the terminology and should be avoided. Wall thickness is reduced in both ventricles, with obvious cavity enlargement; within either ventricle endocardial thickening in a focal or diffuse form is common. In the left ventricle diffuse endocardial thickening over the septum is often striking. The thickening is not more than 3 mm in depth and is an adaptive response by the endocardium to the abnormal volume of the ventricle. Mural thrombus formation frequently develops around the trabeculae of one or both ventricles, particularly at the apices. Atrial enlargement is almost universal, with thrombi in either appendage common. It is part of the definition of the disease that obstructive coronary lesions are absent. Many hearts with a dilated cardiomyopathy have large coronary arteries but the presence of some non-stenosing atherosclerotic plaques is inevitable in Western populations. To recognise pathologically a combination of ischaemic heart disease with a dilated cardiomyopathy would be extremely difficult if not impossible. The misleading clinical term ischaemic cardiomyopathy is used to indicate a patient who develops congestive cardiac failure without previous episodes of infarction recognised clinically, in whom there is a hypokinetic dilated left ventricle and in whom angiography or autopsy shows severe diffuse coronary stenosis. Scarring is readily recognisable macroscopically at autopsy in ischaemic cardiomyopathy. In true dilated cardiomyopathies macroscopic scarring is unusual.

Microscopic features

In dilated cardiomyopathies there is a constellation of histological abnormalities (Table 5.4) which include myocyte changes, fibrosis and interstitial inflammation (Fig. 5.29). These changes are present to differing degrees and may individually be absent. Some examples of dilated cardiomyopathy have such minimal histological changes that the diagnosis rests on knowledge of ventricular function in life.

Myocyte morphology is usually abnormal. Myocyte diameter is not increased and there is a wide scatter in size with a population of smaller fibres. This appearance is sometimes referred to as myocyte attenuation. The nuclear changes of hypertrophy are present, with a marked variation in nuclear area and DNA content. In many cases the myocytes appear abnormally vacuolated. This appearance is due to an alteration in the relative proportions of intracellular constituents with a reduction in the number of myofibrils and an

Table 5.4 Morphological features of idiopathic dilated cardiomyopathy

Macroscopic	Total heart weight ↑ LV cavity diameter ↑ LV wall thickness normal or ↓
Microscopic	Nuclear hypertrophy in myocyte Myocyte diameter normal or ↓ (attenuation) Interstitial fibrosis ↑ Myofibrillary volume ↓ Myocardial T lymphocyte density ↑ Myocardial monocyte/macrophage density ↑

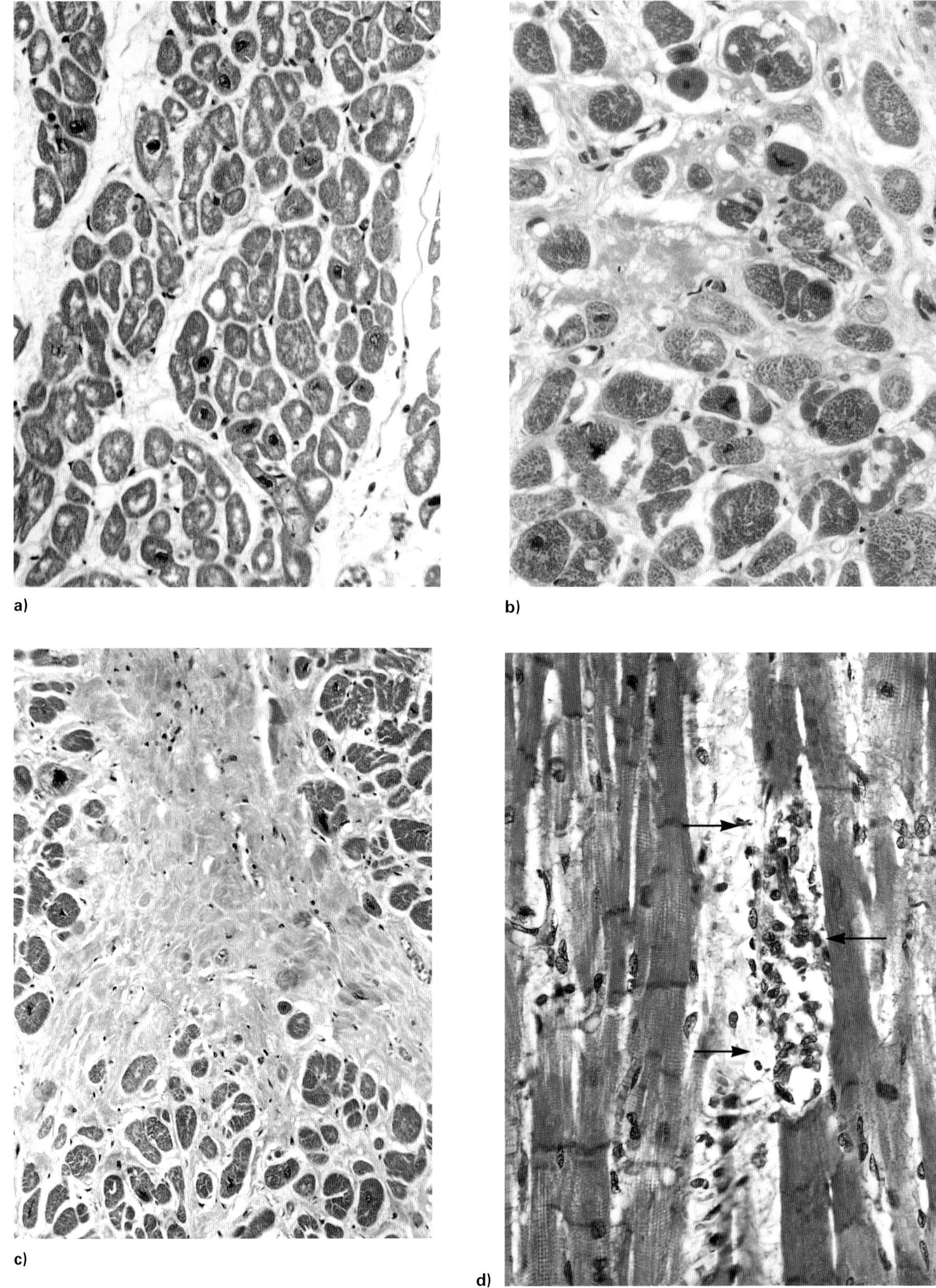
a)
b)
c)
d)

increase in the mitochondrial mass. The degree of myofibrillary loss correlates well with the decline in systolic contractile power[62] and can be used to assess prognosis in biopsy material. Formal measurement of the mean myocyte myofibrillary volume has been carried out from electronmicrographs but can be more crudely estimated by quantitative light microscopy.

The term myocytolysis is sometimes applied to this process of a reduction in myofibrillary content of the myocyte. It is a misleading term, firstly because myofibrillary reduction is a non-specific response to injury and can equally occur in chronic ischaemia, and secondly because the term is used in cardiac rejection to indicate a totally separate process of individual myocyte death.

In dilated cardiomyopathy, to a varying degree, evidence of individual myocyte death can be found. This takes the form of empty sarcolemmal sheaths containing macrophages (Fig. 52.9d) and may be recognised either in transverse or longitudinal sections of the myocytes. The process is in some ways analogous to piecemeal necrosis of hepatocytes in the liver and can be used to assess the speed of progression of the disease.

The second major microscopic feature of a dilated cardiomyopathy is an increase in myocardial fibrosis. This may take the form of a diffuse increase in interstitial fine fibrosis surrounding individual myocytes, or of coarser trabeculae of fibrous tissue. Macroscopically visible scars always require coronary disease to be rigorously excluded, and are rare. It is unknown whether the fibrosis represents the inevitable consequence of hypertrophy or reflects myocyte loss. Taken in conjunction with the histological evidence of myocyte damage and loss the latter seems likely. Overall there is no striking increase of chronic inflammatory cells in the interstitial tissues. When formally counted the number of lymphocytes and macrophages is somewhat increased in about one-third of dilated cardiomyopathies as compared with normal myocardium. In some cases of dilated cardiomyopathy focal areas of lymphocytic accumulation within the interstitial spaces occur and the term 'chronic myocarditis' is sometimes used to describe such cases. The difficult borderline between myocarditis and dilated cardiomyopathy[63,64] has been discussed earlier in this chapter but in general it is best to avoid the term chronic myocarditis unless virtually every microscopic field shows a lymphocytic infiltration.

Fig. 5.29 a,b,c,d Dilated cardiomyopathy — microscopic features. (**a**) Variation in myocyte size with myofibrillary loss producing vacuolated cells. Other abnormalities such as interstitial fibrosis are absent in this case. (**b**) Variation in myocyte size with an increase in interstitial fibrosis which was beginning to surround individual cells. (**c**) This case shows the formation of larger confluent areas of fibrous replacement of myocytes. (**d**) This case shows active loss of individual myocytes. One myocyte (arrows) has died, invoking a florid macrophage response within the sarcolemmal sheath. Adjacent myocytes appear normal.
(**a**) Haematoxylin–eosin × 42
(**b**) Haematoxylin–eosin × 65
(**c**) Haematoxylin–eosin × 42
(**d**) Haematoxylin–eosin × 165

The difficulty in the histological diagnosis of a dilated cardiomyopathy is that the relative degree of myocyte change and interstitial fibrosis differs from case to case. Ideally both should be present; in reality it may be one or the other.

Pathogenesis of idiopathic dilated cardiomyopathy

The disease is not common, but not rare. In England and Wales over the last 5 years an average of 7790 people are recorded by the Registrar General as having died of a cardiomyopathy. Most were probably the idiopathic type. The disease is almost certainly multifactorial; the current views favour direct myocyte toxicity from a number of factors such as alcohol, viral infection and altered immunity. Documented cases which develop following an episode of biopsy-proven myocarditis, although rare, do support the view that idiopathic dilated cardiomyopathy is in some way related to previous viral infection of the myocardium.

Yet another aspect of the pathogenesis of dilated cardiomyopathy is the role of autoantibodies generated against constituents of the myocyte. A familial element may be implicated in this immune response.

Finally, a significant proportion of dilated cardiomyopathies are found to be familial. When detailed echocardiographic and electrocardiographic studies are made of the families of index cases, up to 25% are found to have evidence of inherited cardiac disease. In such families many of the other members have subclinical involvement demonstrated by echocardiography.

Viral infection and idiopathic dilated cardiomyopathy

The hypothesis that persistent viral infection of myocytes can in some way lead to a dilated cardiomyopathy is entirely plausible but so far unproven.

On the positive side animal models exist, particularly in mice, in which viral infection produces an acute myocarditis with a high mortality. In survivors, however, after a long latent period cardiac failure may develop in which the heart shows all the changes associated with a dilated cardiomyopathy. This applies both to Coxsackie infection in the mouse and Papovavirus infection in the dog. In Papova infection litters may show a complete spectrum from acute myocarditis and death within days to the late onset after 2 years of cardiac failure in animals who had no apparent acute infection.

In humans who have had acute viral myocarditis, follow-up studies show that long-term ventricular dysfunction is common and that some subjects develop a dilated cardiomyopathy. In one study[64] of 20 patients with biopsy-proven myocarditis all developed subsequent fibrosis and eight (40%) had a fully expressed dilated cardiomyopathy. A follow up study of 42 patients positive for complement fixing antibodies against Coxsackie B virus during an acute attack of myocarditis showed 10 to have developed dilated cardiomyopathy by 15 years.[65] It is, however, clear that the vast majority of patients who present with dilated cardiomyopathy have no documented previous attack of acute myocarditis.

In patients with a dilated cardiomyopathy retrospective surveys have looked for serological evidence of viral infection, particularly with the Coxsackie group. Results have been mixed. This type of research is made inherently difficult by the high prevalence of neutralising antibodies against a range of enteroviruses in the population at large, making the significance of any differences very dependent on the selection of the control subjects. A recent study using specific IgM for Coxsackie virus found 33% of subjects with dilated cardiomyopathy to be positive compared with 5% of healthy unmatched control sera. This significant difference, however, vanished when comparison was made with both local community and household controls.[66] It is difficult to know what is the most applicable control group. The serological data could be interpreted as indicating that, when infection with cardioselective viruses in the household or community is high, a small proportion of those infected are at risk of developing dilated cardiomyopathy. Some studies have also looked for serological evidence of persistent virus-specific IgM in sequential blood samples from patients with dilated cardiomyopathy. Some reports indicate that persistent IgM antibodies are found in dilated cardiomyopathy; other studies report a high frequency of seroconversion in both directions with time, and long-term persistently elevated IgM antibodies as rare. It can be concluded that serological studies give some support to the role of the Coxsackie group of viruses in dilated cardiomyopathy, but are hardly conclusive.

Nucleic acid and in situ hybridisation studies have provided more direct evidence on the role of viruses in dilated cardiomyopathy. The earliest work[20] used a broad enteroviral probe in slot blotting techniques and reported up to 50% of cases of dilated cardiomyopathy to be positive. More specific and sensitive in situ hybridisation found positive myocytes containing viral RNA in up to 25% of cases of dilated cardiomyopathy.[19] Yet more specific and sensitive PCR study followed. Of five studies reported so far two found no viral RNA while three found very little difference in the incidence of positive results between cases of dilated cardiomyopathy and in controls. It is particularly relevant that viral persistence clearly does occur in hearts in which there is clinical evidence of disease. In future, distinction may have to be made between virulent and avirulent strains of cardiotropic viruses, particularly those of the Coxsackie group. It may be that whether or not the virus is virulent is what determines whether cardiac damage occurs.

Overall the view remains that viral infection plays a role in up to one-third of cases of dilated cardiomyopathy. While this may be so it remains unclear by what mechanism persistent viral infection either causes myocyte death or inhibits myocyte function. In situ studies show that the actual number of myocytes which contain viral RNA is very small considering the severe abnormality in function that is present in dilated cardiomyopathy.

Altered immunity and dilated cardiomyopathy

A significant proportion of patients with dilated cardiomyopathy develop autoantibodies to the beta-adrenergic receptor, to myosin, to a molecule (M7) and the adenine nucleotide translocator carrying ADP/ATP complexes in the mitochondria,[67] and to constituents of the intercalated disc. The problem has always been to know whether this is any way pathogenetic of the disease or merely a secondary phenomenon following myocardial damage. The frequency of autoantibodies to cardiac constituents is, however, far higher in dilated cardiomyopathy than in equivalent patients with ischaemic heart disease.[68] Along with those autoantibodies there is evidence of immune activation within the myocardium of subjects with dilated cardiomyopathies. The endothelial cells express high levels of MHC II antigens and ICAM-1 is also strongly expressed in dilated cardiomyopathies. In families with dilated cardiomyopathy, subclinical cases also show these features, suggesting that immune activation and autoantibodies may play a pathogenic role. One view is that antibodies which bind to the myocyte may gain access to the cell and reach the mitochondria or myofibrils initiating energy production or myofibrillary contraction.[69,70] During Coxsackie virus infection associated with acute myocarditis, antibodies appear that will bind both viral antigens and components of the sarcolemma of the myocyte, suggesting that antigenic mimicry is involved. Such antibodies are toxic or cytotoxic to the myocyte and may persist long after the virus has vanished from the myocardium.

Cardiotoxic causes of dilated cardiomyopathy

Alcoholic cardiomyopathy

The archetypal form of dilated cardiomyopathy due to the direct toxicity of an external agent is alcoholic cardiomyopathy. The toxicity of alcohol is probably related to its degradation to acetaldehyde. In animal models acetaldehyde derivatives cause abnormalities in calcium binding and myofibrillary ATPase as well as a decline in mitochondrial function, a decline in protein synthesis and an accumulation of lipid within the myocyte.[71]

The spectrum of morphological abnormalities of the heart is wide in alcoholism. At one extreme there is an increased risk of sudden death without obvious macroscopic abnormality of the heart in alcoholics who have fatty change in the liver. This increased risk has been observed throughout the world[72] but the mechanism is uncertain. Microscopically there may be an increase in stainable lipid within myocytes (Fig. 5.30) but no other abnormality. At the other extreme there are subjects with all the clinical and pathological features of an idiopathic dilated cardiomyopathy. There are no specific microscopic features that indicate that the aetiology is excess alcohol ingestion.[73] Myofibrillary loss with empty vacuolated myocytes is often a striking feature and one which, while not specific, should invoke the question of alcohol. Between these two extremes are hearts in which the left ventricular mass is elevated with some increase in interstitial fibrosis but without a very dilated cavity. A small subset of patients shows heavy interstitial fibrosis and some excess iron deposition in the interstitial tissues. Atrial dilatation is common and atrial arrhythmias a strong clinical feature.

Electron microscopy has reported a wide range of abnormalities including mitochondrial swelling and crystal disruption, increased membrane-bound debris and myelin figures, myofibrillary

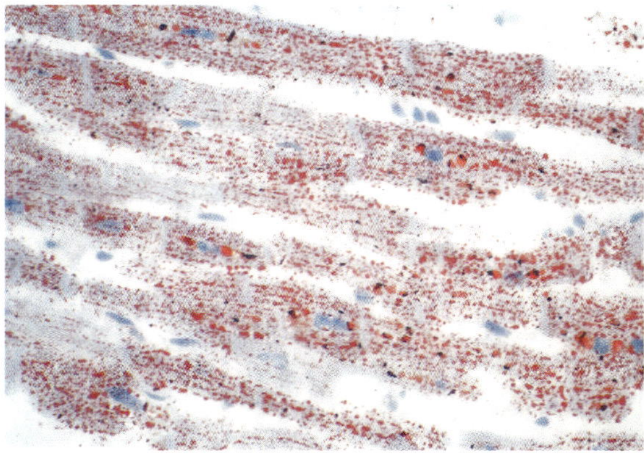

Fig. 5.30 Fat deposition within myocytes. Fine droplets of sudanophilic material are widely distributed within the myocytes. While seen in alcoholism the change like that seen in the liver is non-specific and can occur in many other conditions.

loss and lipid deposition. None are specific for alcohol induced myocyte damage.[73]

The other difficulty with the concept of alcoholic heart disease is that in the absence of specific pathological features the diagnosis depends on a clinical history of excessive alcoholic intake. The real frequency is therefore difficult to judge and claims that alcohol is the single commonest cause of a dilated cardiomyopathy[74] are hard to confirm or refute. Death certification data with regard to alcohol-related deaths are notoriously inaccurate due to the social stigma attached to the disease. It is usually stated that alcoholic cirrhosis and cardiomyopathy rarely occur together although the evidence is observational and anecdotal. There is clearly considerable variation in susceptibility of individuals to liver or cardiac involvement, which in part may depend upon genetic variations in the metabolism of alcohol. At least in the early stages of alcoholic cardiomyopathy total abstention from alcohol may lead to improvements in left ventricular function; in a small proportion of cases concomitant vitamin B deficiencies occur and left ventricular function may improve with replacement therapy.

Heavy metal toxicity

Heavy metals such as cobalt and nickel complex with the sulphotrial groups of alpha-lipoic acid and thereby interfere with oxidation of alpha-ketoglutarate in the Krebs cycle. The classic cobalt cardiomyopathy occurred as an epidemic in Quebec following the addition of trace amounts of the metal to maintain the 'head' on beer but industrial poisoning occurs sporadically. The macroscopic features are identical to any other dilated cardiomyopathy. Microscopically, myocyte changes often predominate. The myocytes appear finely vacuolated throughout, with focal areas of more pronounced myofibrillary loss resulting in almost empty cells. Fine interstitial fibrosis also develops. Thus, while it is possible to suspect a heavy-metal-induced cardiomyopathy and any case with these histological features should have a detailed industrial history taken, once again the changes are not specific.

Adriamycin cardiomyopathy

Pathogenesis

The anthracycline group of cytotoxic agents are highly effective in the treatment of a wide range of malignancies and are particularly used in children; unfortunately they are also cardiotoxic. Anthracyclines such as adriamycin and doxorubicin owe their antineoplastic activity to inhibition of nucleic acid synthesis binding to the DNA and blocking DNA and RNA polymerases. It is less clear whether this is also the mechanism of myocyte toxicity. The substances do cause a dose-dependent reduction of messenger RNA and inhibition of gene expression for both myofibrillary proteins and energy-producing enzyme systems. Anthracyclines, however, also bind to the mitochondrial membrane, inactivating the electron transport chain, and are reported to cause free radical production and lipid peroxidation within myocytes.[75]

Clinically the anthracyclines produce progressive ventricular failure associated with dilatation of the ventricles and a reduction in wall thickness comparable to any other dilated cardiomyopathy. The effect is markedly dose-related. With total doses of over 550 mg/m^2 body surface area 30% of patients will develop cardiac failure; with doses below this threshold less than 1% of patients develop cardiotoxicity. Even these lower doses, however, can be shown to reduce myocardial function without clinical symptoms. Sudden death and arrhythmias are also common in subjects without overt cardiac involvement. There is some evidence that cardiotoxicity may not be manifest for up to 10 years after treatment has stopped.

Morphological changes

Myocardial biopsies are used to monitor cardiotoxicity and are a situation where electron-microscopic examination is mandatory.[76] Light microscopic changes appear late, after cardiac damage is already established. At least three biopsies should be taken and converted in smaller fragments for fixation for electronmicroscopy. It is recommended that at least 10 electronmicroscopy blocks are cut. Two forms of ultrastructural change occur. Sarcotubular dilatation leads to finely vacuolated myocytes in which the mitochondria remain relatively normal. In the other type myofibrillary loss occurs, leaving an empty cell containing only a few oddly shaped mitochondria. The changes are regarded as of equal significance and are focal in the early stages, with normal myocytes adjacent to a very abnormal myocyte. A grading system is used on which alterations in dosage are decided.

In the later stage, years after therapy, hearts with dilated ventricles and an increase in interstitial fibrosis occur and can be difficult to distinguish from any other dilated cardiomyopathy.

Familial dilated cardiomyopathy

When large numbers of patients with idiopathic dilated cardiomyopathy are investigated, with specific search for other family members either with clinically expressed disease or with no symptoms but abnormal echocardiograms or electrocardiograms, the frequency of a familial trend is high and may reach 20%.[77] No specific morphological criteria, however, distinguish the hearts from this group when they are transplanted. The familial trend is probably due to many different genetic causes. One view is that what is inherited are particular polymorphisms of the MHC class II antigens making the individual particularly prone to generate autoimmune antibodies. Such a view sees a proportion of familial cardiomyopathies as an organ specific autoimmune disease.

In other cases the genetic trend is due to mutations in a specific gene controlling a key metabolic step or structural protein. Many of these single gene disorders involve skeletal muscle predominantly but may also involve cardiac muscle. In such cases there are always some individuals or families who reverse the process and have major cardiac and minor skeletal muscle symptoms. Yet another group of familial cardiomyopathies are due to genetic abnormalities in mitochondrial genomic material and inherited via the mother.

Cardiomyopathies associated with neuromuscular symptoms

The majority of the skeletal myopathies involve the heart to some degree and it is characteristic that conduction and rhythm abnormalities predominate over contractile abnormalities and cardiac failure. The degree of cardiac involvement is very variable; in some families the general trend is for skeletal problems to be dominant, but an occasional subject has cardiac problems alone.

Myotonic dystrophy. This autosomal dominant familial disease is characterised by muscle weakness, stiffness and atrophy combined with ocular cataracts, premature baldness, mental deficiency and cardiac conduction disturbances. It is the most common familial muscular dystrophy. In a high proportion of affected individuals (approximately 85%) the ECG is abnormal and detailed electrophysiological studies show prolonged nodal and ventricular conduction. Only about 15–20% of affected individuals, however, have cardiac symptoms including atrial fibrillation and complete heart block. Sudden death occurs and is reported to be the final event in up to 30% of individuals with myotonic dystrophy. The disorder is now known to be due to an increased number of cytosine–thymidine–guanine repeats in a protein kinase gene located on chromosome 19. The normal gene has up to 40 repeats, the mutant gene many hundreds. While in essence the abnormality is physiological and alters muscle membrane excitability, both in skeletal and cardiac muscle structural damage occurs. In skeletal muscle type II fibres atrophy and vanish; in the heart conduction fibres vanish and are replaced by fibrofatty tissue. The AV node and bundle are most severely affected but focal loss of contractile myocytes may also occur. Localised subepicardial scars may develop in the left ventricle.

Duchenne's and Becker's muscular dystrophy. Both of these familial disorders are due to abnormalities of the gene controlling synthesis of dystrophin situated on the X chromosome. An abnormal dystrophin or a total absence of dystrophin results. Dystrophin is located normally on the sarcolemma of the muscle cell and is thought to be complexed with glycoproteins and concerned with calcium ion transport. Both cardiac and skeletal muscle dystrophin are encoded by the gene and in many families the level of gene expression is similar in both tissues. Cardiac involvement clinically ultimately develops in more than 80% of cases of Duchenne's dystrophy although cardiac failure is the terminal event in only 10%.[78] While Becker's dystrophy is less severe with regard to the skeletal muscle, cardiac involvement is somewhat more common than in Duchenne's dystrophy. Cases with almost pure cardiac symptoms occur. This fact led to a search for abnormalities of the dystrophin gene among familial cardiomyopathies without any skeletal abnormality and a sex-linked purely cardiac form in which dystrophin was absent in the heart but present in skeletal muscle was found. This suggests that promoter genes exist for both tissues and absence of the cardiac promoter leads to a pure cardiomyopathy.[78]

Dystrophin is a component of the cytoskeleton of myocytes and its reduction or absence is associated with myocyte loss and fibrous replacement. This process will affect both conduction and contractile myocytes. In the left ventricle subepicardial posterobasal regional fibrosis is characteristic and is found even in asymptomatic female carriers.[79] This characteristic focal fibrosis produces a highly characteristic ECG pattern.[80]

Mitochondrial defects in cardiomyopathy

A small proportion of cases of dilated cardiomyopathy are due to defects in the mitochondrial respiratory and oxidative phosphorylation systems due to mutations of mitochondrial DNA.[81] The exact proportion of cases due to such abnormalities is not known. Such mitochondrial defects are more likely to be present in cases of dilated cardiomyopathies in which conduction defects are prominent and in those with a clear familial tendency associated with minor skeletal muscle weakness.

The mitochondrial respiratory chain system is fundamental in providing ATP for energy. The system comprises five protein complexes on the inner mitochondrial membrane. The unique mitochondrial DNA has sequences coding for 13 polypeptides making up this system. Most of the well-documented mutations of mitochondrial DNA are causes of weakness in ocular and skeletal muscle in which cardiac involvement is manifest as conduction rather than contractile abnormalities and often a relative minor part of the clinical spectrum. Attention has however now turned to the investigation of more pure dilated cardiomyopathies with both familial and sporadic occurrence and mt DNA deletions and point mutations in the respiratory chain system have been found. Among the mitochondrial mutations overall a characteristic feature is that the proportion of mutant DNA varies widely from tissue to tissue within an individual thus producing considerable phenotypic expression variability even within one family. Kearns–Sayre syndrome is characterised by progressive conduction abnormalities associated with weakness of the eye muscles developing during early life. Complete AV block by 20 years of age is common. Skeletal muscle biopsies show red ragged fibres in trichrome-stained sections but in the heart there is simple loss of conduction myocytes leaving empty spaces in nodal and atrioventricular bundle areas. The selectivity of the disease for the conduction system is probably explained by a higher proportion of mutant DNA being present rather than an inherent high energy demand by the tissue.

For the pathologist there are no morphological features of a dilated cardiomyopathy specific for mitochondrial defects. The pathology is essentially that of myocyte loss followed by fibrosis which is accentuated in the conduction tissue. In practical terms the mitochondrial DNA should be analysed in familial cases of cardiomyopathy and in those in whom a dilated cardiomyopathy appears in infancy. Mitochondrial DNA can be studied in cardiac muscle biopsies[80] to confirm the diagnosis.

Peripartum cardiomyopathy

This form of dilated cardiomyopathy is defined as the onset of left ventricular dilatation and cardiac failure which appears during the last 3 months of a pregnancy or during the first 6 months postpartum. The condition is very heterogeneous in both clinical expression and pathology.[82] On one hand the disease has been regarded as an early manifestation of a pre-existing latent cardiomyopathy, on the other as a specific disease precipitated by pregnancy which is potentially reversible. Care should be taken to use the term strictly and apply it only when there is clinical evidence of left ventricular failure. Use of the term when there is a sudden death postpartum with a morphologically normal heart leads to considerable confusion.

Functionally and morphologically the heart is indistinguishable from idiopathic dilated cardiomyopathy. The left ventricle shows combinations of hypertrophy and dilatation with or without mural thrombus. Myocyte hypertrophy and interstitial fibrosis are usually present. Several series emphasise that there is a far higher frequency of interstitial T lymphocyte infiltration than is found generally in idiopathic dilated cardiomyopathy.[83] This high frequency of 'acute myocarditis' has been thought to be the reason why at least 50% of patients recover rapidly, and immunosuppression has been recommended. Whatever the basic pathological process the pathogenesis is as controversial as that of idiopathic dilated cardiomyopathy. Viral infection, toxic or drug-induced myocardial damage, autoimmune phenomena and vitamin deficiencies have all been postulated. Series from different socio-economic groups and populations may not be comparable.

RESTRICTIVE CARDIOMYOPATHY

Restrictive patterns are the least common form of cardiomyopathy. Three distinct subgroups exist (Fig. 5.17). In one the condition is primarily an abnormality of the left ventricular myocardium and the endocardium is normal. The ventricle remains normal in size and has normal systolic function. Abnormal diastolic relaxation hinders ventricular filling, particularly late in diastole. Left atrial filling pressures rise and pulmonary hypertension with right ventricular hypertrophy develops. Another important subgroup is where the diastolic restriction is due to an endocardial abnormality such as endocardial fibroelastosis. In a final group thrombosis on the endocardium begins to obliterate the cavities of the ventricles. In this condition of endomyocardial fibrosis (EMF) subsequent organisation of the thrombus produces a thick endocardium, restricting diastolic filling.

Endomyocardial fibrosis

Sequestered within the term endomyocardial fibrosis (EMF) are two entities with similar morphological expressions but which occur in different geographic areas. In the tropical areas of Africa, South America and India there is a disease characterised by marked endocardial fibrosis often extending into the myocardium. In non-tropical areas there is a disease with an acute phase of endocardial thrombosis associated with systemic eosinophilia followed by a healed or latent phase of dense endocardial fibrosis. There can be no argument that the final stages of the two diseases look identical. What is hotly debated is whether the two diseases are really one seen at different stages or totally separate in pathogenesis. At any particular point in time over the last 30 years either the unitarian or the dual view has been in the ascendant.

Tropical endomyocardial fibrosis

The typical macroscopic feature of the disease is extreme endocardial fibrosis forming a dense

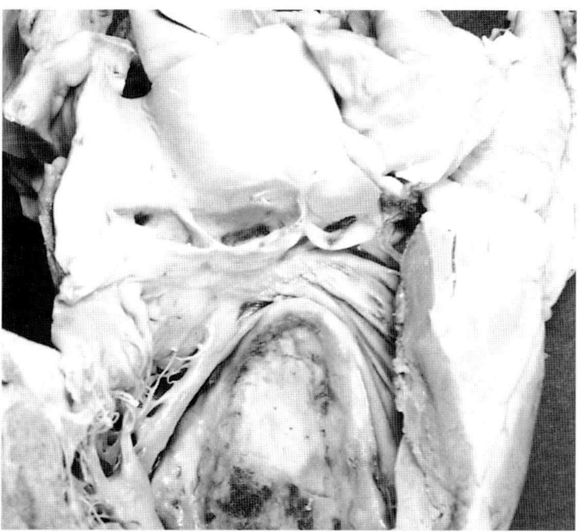

Fig. 5.31 Tropical endomyocardial fibrosis. The apical portion of the ventricle is obliterated by a layer of dense hyaline fibrous tissue which extends up onto the septum.

white layer effacing the trabecular pattern of the interior of the ventricle (Fig. 5.31). Endocardial fibrosis may be focal or diffuse and involve either or both ventricles. When it is focal the inflow portions of the ventricles are usually involved and fibrosis surrounds and incorporates the papillary muscles and reduces the cavity size. Apical obliteration of the ventricular cavity is common. The histological appearances[84] are of a layer of dense collagen with hyaline change and calcification; separating this from the underlying myocardium is a layer of more loosely arranged vascular connective tissue. Lymphocytic infiltration is common and fibrosis extends down into the underlying myocardium. Striking by their absence in descriptions of the pathology of tropical EMF are eosinophils and surface thrombus on the endocardium. This is true even of biopsies taken apparently early in the disease. Any relation between tropical endomyocardial fibrosis and eosinophilia is hotly denied by some authorities.[85]

Pathogenesis of tropical endomyocardial fibrosis. The disease has a striking geographic restriction to within a 12° latitude band on either side of the equator in the continents of Africa, India and America. The subject has been recently reviewed in an international symposium[86] and one theory is that the disease is a late result of circulating hypereosinophilia related to previous parasitic infections. Alternatively it may be an enhanced immunological response to streptococci and thus analogous in some ways to chronic rheumatic disease, or a late immune response with cardiac autoantibodies to malaria, or to nutritional deficiencies, or finally due to high concentrations or deficiencies of some trace elements in tropical soil.

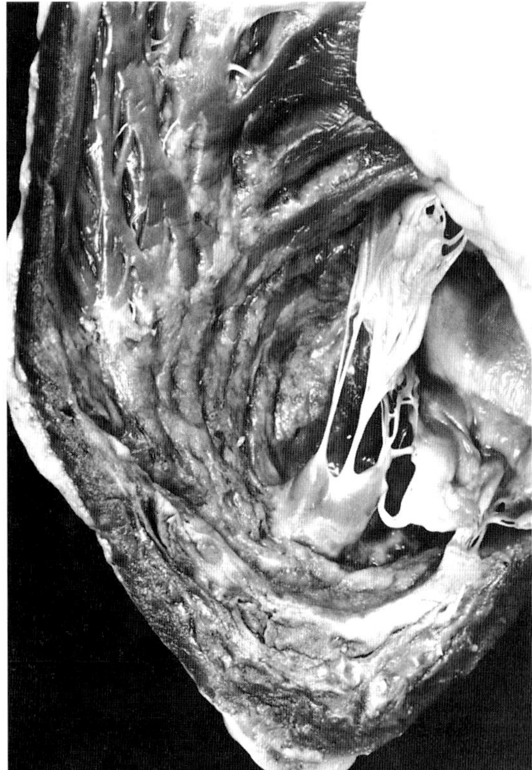

Fig. 5.32 Eosinophilia related endocardial thrombosis — early stage. The endocardium over the apex and around the inflow tract of the right ventricle is covered by a shaggy coat of thrombus. Fibrous white endocardial thickening has not yet developed. Circulating eosinophilia with lung shadowing was present.

Temperate zone endomyocardial fibrosis

There are many morphological similarities of temperate zone endomyocardial fibrosis with the

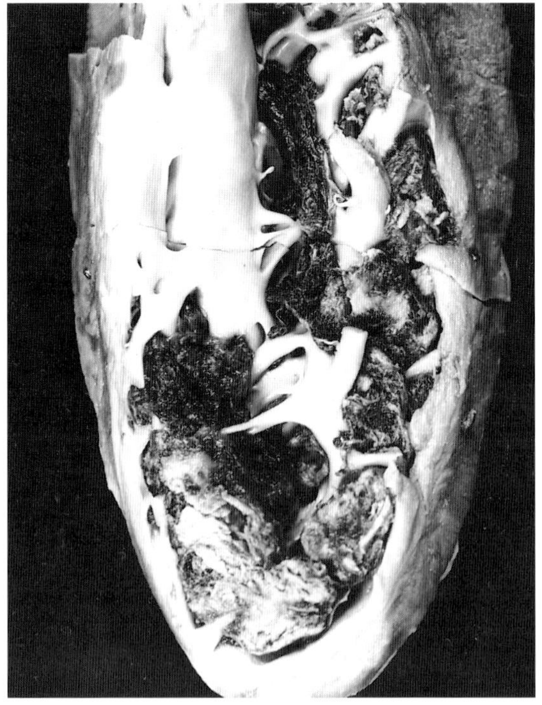

Fig. 5.33 Eosinophilia related EMF — late stage. There is dense white endocardial thickening surrounding a papillary muscle. More recent thrombus formation has also occurred. Long-standing hypereosinophilia with ulcerative colitis.

tropical form; however, the main distinguishing feature is that it is far more common outside the tropics to see an acute thrombotic phase. Thrombus forms over the endocardium as a flat, rather shaggy coat (Fig. 5.32). Later, dense white endocardial thickening occurs (Fig. 5.33). The distribution is reminiscent of the endocardial abnormality in the tropical form in that one or other or both ventricles are involved, with a predilection for the inflow tracts and apical regions. Thrombosis surrounds the papillary muscles and effaces trabeculae. The histological appearance shows clearly defined stratification with superficial thrombus beneath which there is organisation and vascular connective tissue beneath which is more dense fibrous tissue (Fig. 5.34). Cases which present in the acute phase have intense eosinophilic infiltration of the thrombus and underlying myocardium. Inflammation often extends into the underlying myocardium and this type of case is often known as Löffler's eosinophilic endomyocarditis. Many cases, however, when seen at autopsy or in surgical specimens, are in a less acute phase and eosinophils are scanty or absent. The ultimate burnt out phase of the disease leaves the endocardium converted into a fibrous sheet up to a centimetre thick.

Cases may present clinically in the acute phase, when a circulating eosinophilia is still present, with embolic phenomena and thrombus demonstrated on echocardiography. Cases also present later after the eosinophilia has long vanished with restrictive ventricular function and mitral or tricuspid regurgitation due to fibrosis around the chordae and papillary muscles. Surgical decortication of the fibrous sheet and valve replacement is often carried out with a relatively high frequency of postoperative A-V conduction disturbances. In such chronic cases the previous occurrence of eosinophilia can often only be surmised from the clinical history of previous diseases.

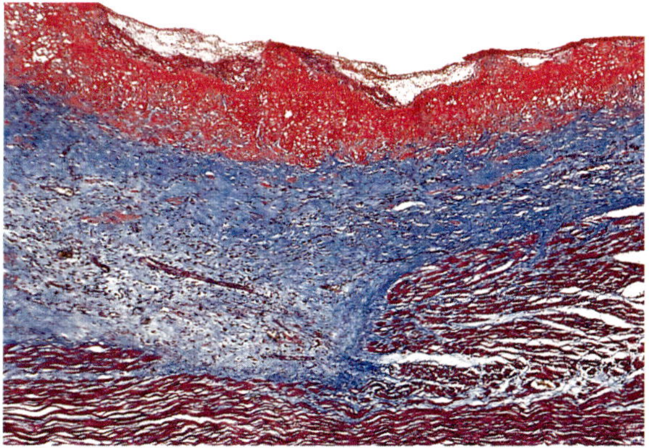

Fig. 5.34 Eosinophilia related EMF — histology. There is very distinct stratification of the endocardial thickening with a layer of fibrous tissue adjacent to the endocardium (blue) covered by a layer of recent thrombus (red). Picro–Mallory trichrome stain × 54

Pathogenesis of temperate zone EMF. The disease is now clearly recognised as being due to endomyocardial damage mediated by circulating activated eosinophils. While many cases do have a local tissue eosinophilia the disease can also be caused by a high proportion of the circulating eosinophils being activated without an increase in total numbers. Every disease causing eosinophilia has the potential to induce EMF and reported cases include hypereosinophilia associated with T cell proliferations, chronic parasitic infection, Löffler's pneumonitis, eosinophilic leukaemias, Behçet's disease and ulcerative colitis. Endocardial damage is mediated by the local and systemic release of eosinophilic granule basic proteins which are cytotoxic to a wide range of cells.[87] The toxicity is not necessarily dependent on eosinophils being present at the site of injury. In temperate zones the whole spectrum of the disease from acute endocardial thrombosis to end-stage endocardial fibrosis is now known as eosinophil-related endomyocardial disease.

Endocardial fibroelastosis (EFE)

This condition is heterogeneous and probably the end stage of a number of insults to the endocardium. In descriptive terms the endocardium is white and opaque and histologically shows parallel arrays of new elastic laminae (Figs 5.35–5.39). Endocardial fibroelastosis is most commonly seen in two circumstances. In the first it is part of other congenital abnormalities including congenital aortic valve stenosis, congenital mitral valve stenosis, and hypoplastic and anomalous coronary arteries. The left ventricle may be small and hypo-

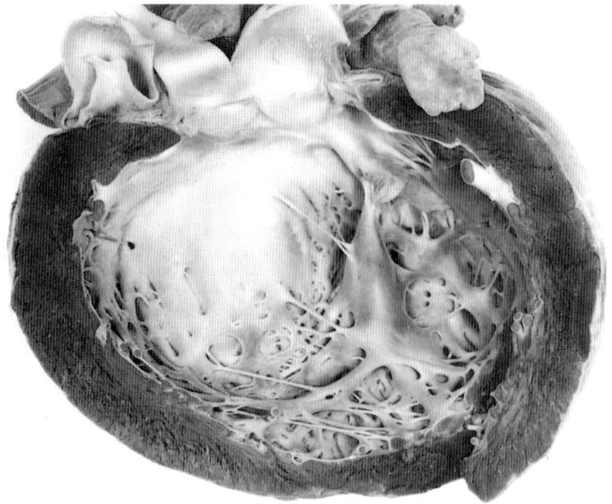

Fig. 5.35 Endocardial fibroelastosis. The left ventricle is dilated and globular with even white endocardial thickening. Macroscopically there is no evidence of myocardial scarring.

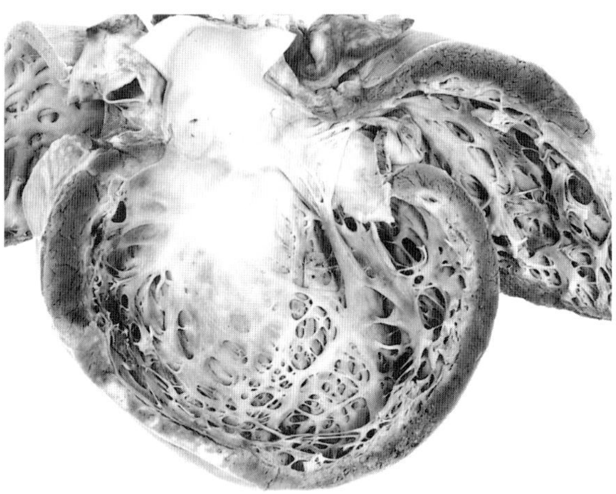

Fig. 5.36 Endocardial fibroelastosis. The left ventricle is globular with endocardial white thickening. The underlying myocardium shows widespread fibrosis.

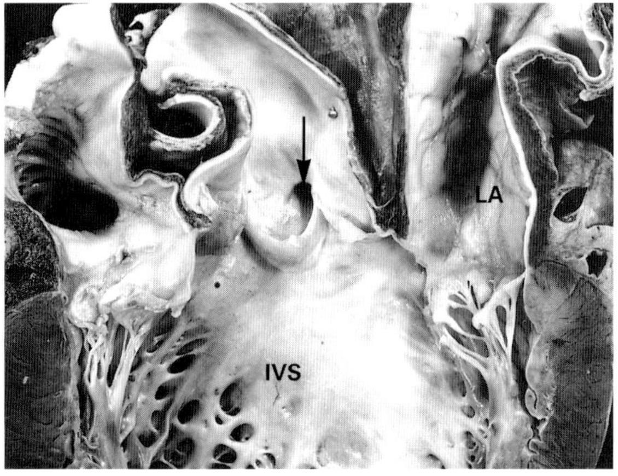

Fig. 5.37 Endocardial fibroelastosis. The dilated left ventricle shows white endocardial thickening over the interventricular septum (IVS); the endocardial thickening is also pronounced in the left atrium (LA). One coronary orifice is present (arrow). The right coronary artery opened from the pulmonary trunk.

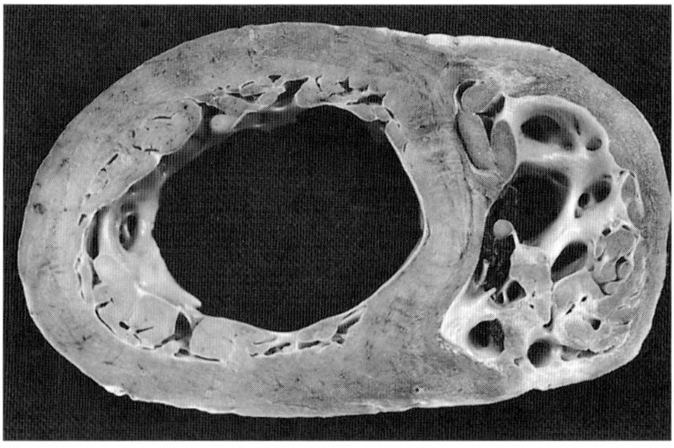

Fig. 5.38 Childhood cardiomyopathy with fibroelastosis. A familial cardiomyopathy, probably mitochondrial, based on pattern of inheritance. Death at 2 years. The left ventricle is dilated with some endocardial thickening. The right ventricle is hypertrophied also with marked endocardial thickening.

plastic or large and dilated. In severe congenital abnormalities the endocardial thickening may play a role in preventing return to normal after correction. The second circumstance is endocardial fibroelastosis in association with chronic dysfunction or damage to the left ventricular muscle by diseases in early childhood. What is produced in children is a dilated-type cardiomyopathy on which endocardial restriction is superimposed. Functionally a combination of dilated and restrictive physiology is produced. Sudden death is a feature of the condition even in young subjects with reasonable exercise capacity. Some semantic difficulties are created. Some authorities would classify cases such as those in Figures 5.35 and 5.36 as infantile or juvenile dilated cardiomyopathy, arguing that the endocardial response is simply secondary. Others would label in particular Figure 5.35 as primary dilated endocardial fibroelastosis. It is questionable whether fibroelastosis is anything more than a response to a heterogeneous group of con-

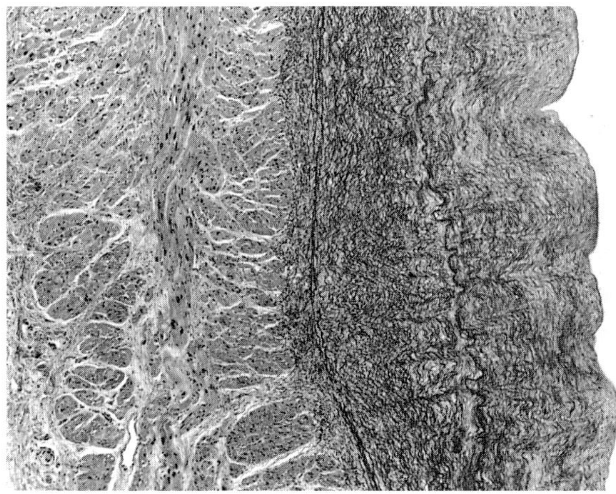

Fig. 5.39 Endocardial fibroelastosis. The endocardium of the left atrium is thickened at least ten times normal and contains numerous parallel elastic laminae
EVG × 10

ditions which damage the myocardium in early life.

Myocardial restrictive cardiomyopathy

Where the endocardium and pericardium are normal and restriction in diastole is present the abnormality lies within the myocardium itself (Fig. 5.40). In common with the other pathophysiological forms of cardiomyopathy several disease processes can produce an identical restrictive physiology. Series of cases with the diagnosis based on biopsy or transplant specimens show the commonest form to be amyloid deposition.[88] Another form has diffuse perimyocyte interstitial fibrosis while often having a morphologically normal myocardium. Individual case reports suggest that restriction can develop in haemochromatosis, sarcoidosis, myocarditis and in a familial form in which the myocytes have an abnormal arrangement. The macroscopic features of a restrictive cardiomyopathy are a small left ventricle with a normal endocardium without mural thrombus (Fig. 5.40). In amyloid the ventricle may or may not be enlarged. Left atrial pressures are high to compensate for impaired filling and the atrial wall becomes very thick. Severe right ventricular hypertrophy develops in long standing cases.

Amyloid heart disease

Amyloid fibrils of all known derivations can be deposited in the myocardium but there is a wide variation in the morphological and clinical expressions.[89]

Ventricular involvement with the production of

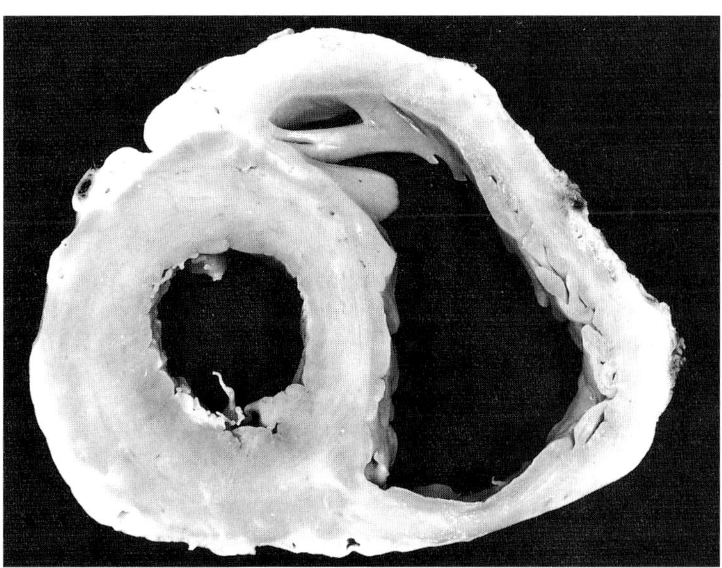

Fig. 5.40 Restrictive cardiomyopathy due to amyloid. The left ventricular shape is normal. The right ventricle is both dilated and thick walled. Total heart size was not increased when transplantation was performed for severe restriction.

a restrictive cardiomyopathy is seen in immunoglobulin-type primary amyloidosis (amyloid AL), where the derivation is immunoglobulin light chain, in chronic generalised infection (secondary amyloid), where the derivation is a fragment of the acute phase serum amyloid A (amyloid AA), and in genetic familial forms in which variants of the prealbumin transthyretin protein which normally binds thyroxin are deposited (amyloid AF). Familial forms often have concomitant involvement of peripheral nerves. All of these forms produce identical ventricular lesions. The size of the left ventricle is very variable.[90] It may remain small (Fig. 5.40) or be very considerably increased in mass. In the latter case the ventricular wall is thick and involvement is often asymmetric with the septum being disproportionally thick. Clinical misdiagnosis of hypertrophic cardiomyopathy is common on echocardiography (Fig. 5.41). The cut surface of the myocardium is at autopsy smooth and featureless in contrast to the whorled, fibrous appearance of hypertrophic cardiomyopathy. Histologically the characteristic lesion is amyloid material forming a lattice in the interstices of which some myocytes survive (Fig. 5.42). Myocyte loss occurs with the tissue condensing to produce focal aggregates of amyloid material which can invoke a giant cell reaction. Involvement of the walls of small intramyocardial vessels may or may not be prominent.[91] Electronmicroscopy (Fig. 5.43) shows that the early lesions consist of even deposition of fibrillary protein on the sarcolemma of myocytes splinting the cell externally. Concomitant atrial involvement is usual. The sinus node is often heavily involved and atrial arrhythmias are a prominent clinical feature of cardiac amyloid.

Over the age of 70 amyloid deposits in the heart become increasingly common and are often coincidental findings.[91] Two forms of such 'senile' cardiac amyloid exist. In one, isolated deposits of amyloid are confined to the atria (amyloid IAA). Deposits can be seen as small translucent nodules on the endocardium (Fig. 5.44) by the naked eye in formalin-fixed hearts and histologically both intramyocardial and intraendocardial foci can be found. The number of these foci is very variable. Most hearts from subjects over 70 will contain at least one deposit if the search is assiduous.[92]

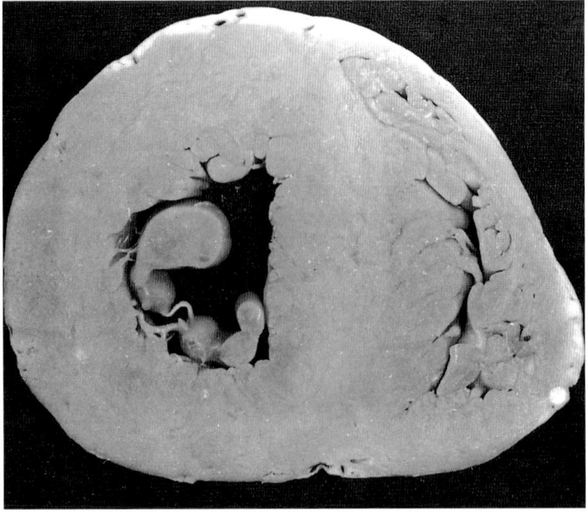

Fig. 5.41 Restrictive cardiomyopathy due to amyloid. The total heart size at transplantation was very large (810 g). The left ventricle was thick walled with marked septal asymmetric hypertrophy leading to an erroneous initial echo diagnosis initially of HCM.

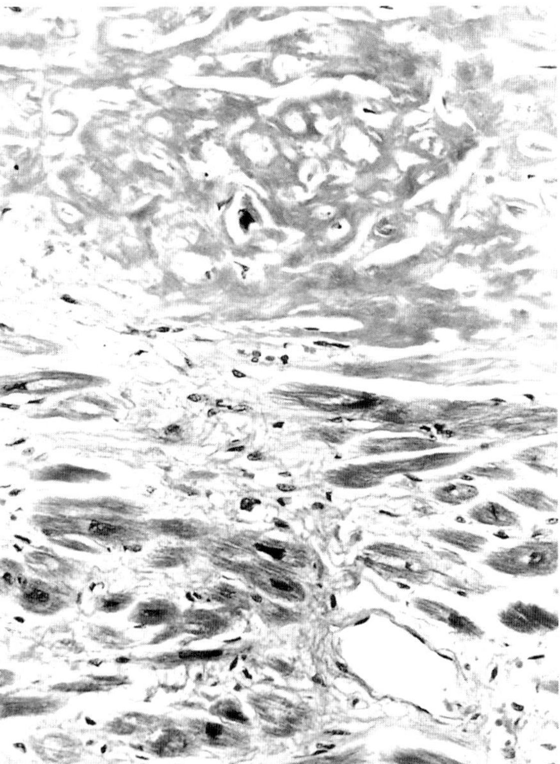

Fig. 5.42 Amyloid deposition in the myocardium. Amyloid is deposited around each myocyte, producing a honeycomb-like appearance. Myocytes initially are present in each cell but many vanish, leaving empty spaces. Ultimately the tissue collapses, leaving a nodule of amyloid material. Haematoxylin–eosin × 105

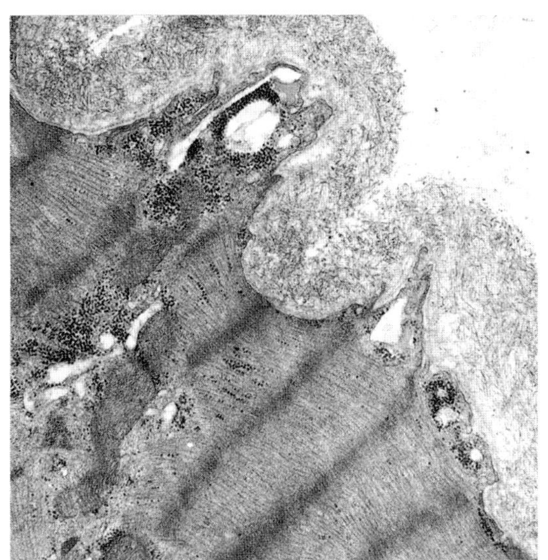

Fig. 5.43 Amyloid deposition in the myocardium. Amyloid is initially deposited as a layer of fibrillary material applied to the outside of each myocyte.
Haematoxylin–eosin × 10 400

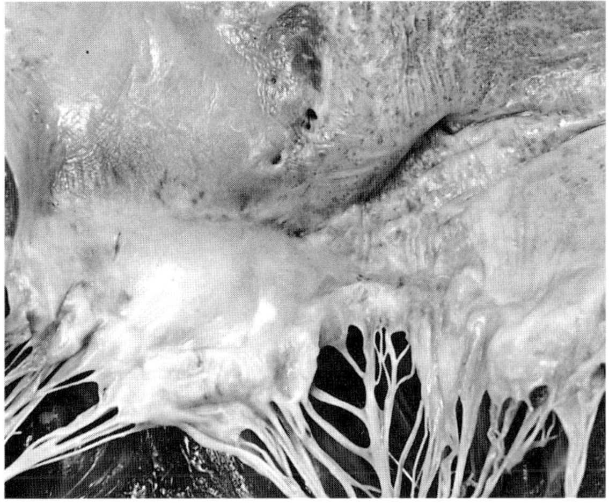

Fig. 5.44 Amyloid deposition in atria and valve. Nodules can be seen beneath the endocardium of the left atrium. These spread down on to the mitral valve.

The variation in the reported frequency of senile isolated cardiac amyloid reflects different degrees of obsession in the search. The origin of isolated atrial amyloid is thought to be atrial natriuretic factor produced by atrial myocytes.

Another form of senile cardiac amyloid (amyloid SCA) has a very similar distribution of deposits in the atria to amyloid IAA but also has foci in the ventricular muscle. This form is thought to be one form of transthyretin protein of which more than 30 variants are known.[89]

The clinical significance of both forms of senile cardiac amyloid is often difficult to establish. Neither form produces classic restriction and they are usually regarded as an incidental autopsy finding. Study of elderly subjects, however, shows that deposition of amyloid is associated with an increased frequency of atrial arrhythmias and cardiac failure. Such clinical manifestations are probably multifactorial in old people but it is difficult to escape the view that atrial amyloid deposition contributes to some extent.

Other forms of restrictive cardiomyopathy — biopsy interpretation

Cardiac biopsy is used as the means of elucidating the cause of restriction and confirming or refuting the presence of amyloid. In biopsies, due to the focal nature of amyloid deposition, considerable care has to be taken in interpretation and false negatives occur. Personal experience suggests that examining a Congo red stain in a 10–15 μm thick section under polarised light is as sensitive as any other light microscopy technique. When a 'honeycomb' of amyloid is seen in which myocytes are incorporated the diagnosis is clear. Electronmicroscopy is however the most sensitive method for minimal deposits and should be routinely carried out in restrictive cardiomyopathy. In about a quarter of cases of restrictive cardiomyopathy due to amyloid deposition the amount of collagen exceeds that of the actual amyloid. In such cases vascular deposition or electronmicroscopy confirmation of fibrillary material applied closely and evenly to myocytes is a valuable confirmation that amyloid is the initiating factor in restriction.

Most series record that amyloid deposition causes 40–60% of pure restrictive cardiomyopathy. The remainder make up a rather heterogeneous group. In one form there is intense and even perimyocyte fibrosis in the inner third of the left ventricular myocardium. The 'honeycomb' appearance seen in amyloid is reproduced by pure connective tissue. The origin of this form of fibrosis is unknown. In another form, although the left ventricular mass is normal, the individual myocytes show hypertrophy with some disarray.

Some of these cases are familial and possibly are the extreme end of the spectrum of hypertrophic cardiomyopathy. Finally, there are cases in which the left ventricle is histologically normal even though function is abnormal.

ARRHYTHMOGENIC CARDIOMYOPATHIES

A small subgroup of cardiomyopathies present with arrhythmias alone and contractile function is preserved. The best defined is right ventricular dysplasia. In its fully expressed form the disease is readily recognised at autopsy. The right ventricle is dilated and thin-walled (Figs 5.17, 5.45, 5.46). Segments of the right ventricle show replacement of the ventricular wall by fibrous and adipose tissue. In most cases transmural loss of myocytes is present in at least some segments with the site of predilection being the anterior wall of the right ventricular outflow tract. Fibrosis appears to surround and isolate individual myocytes (Fig. 5.47) and a chronic inflammatory cell/lymphocytic infiltrate is present in most cases. Some endocardial focal thickening may occur but mural thrombus is absent and the pericardium is normal. The disease predominantly affects the right ventricle but some fibrosis in the subendocardial and subepicardial left ventricle is present in many cases.

The disease has come to prominence because of sudden death on exercise in apparently fit individuals and its familial nature.[93] Cardiac failure is very rare. Study of several generations in families in which there have been sudden deaths from fully expressed cases show that subclinical involvement with minor conduction abnormalities, ventricular arrhythmias particularly arising in the right ventricular outflow and echocardiographic contraction abnormalities in the right ventricle are common. Progression occurs over many years although sudden death is a complication at all ages. Deaths which occur suddenly in such subclinical cases, unless the family history is known, may be misdiagnosed at autopsy. Histological sections of at least three segments of the right ventricular myocardium, including the right ventricular outflow, must be examined in any apparently unexplained sudden death. Care must be

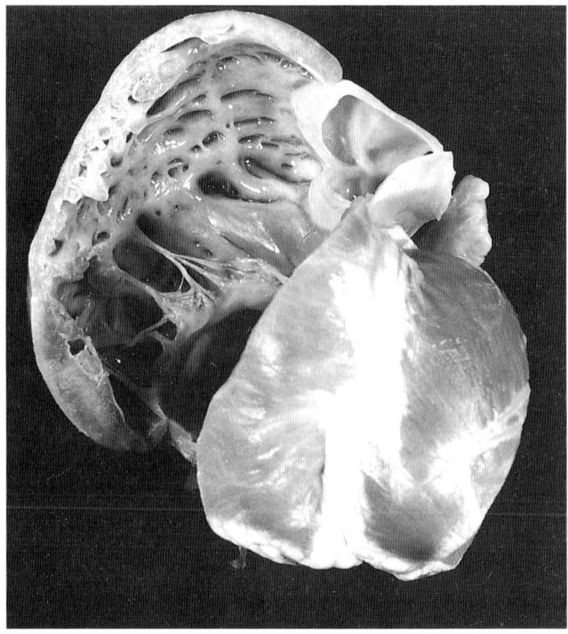

Fig. 5.45 Right ventricular dysplasia. The right ventricle is hugely dilated with marked thinning with fibrosis and fat at one point.

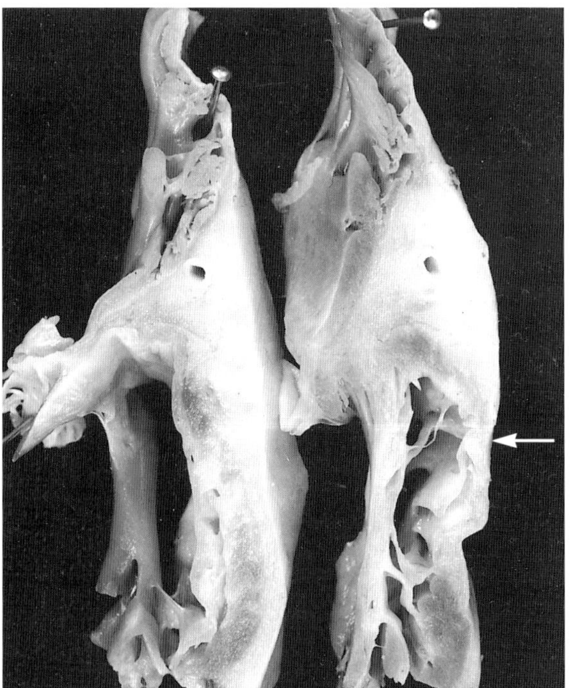

Fig. 5.46 Right ventricular dysplasia. Two segments of the right ventricle show marked adipose tissue infiltration associated with wall thinning (arrow). Sudden death at 35 with a history of syncope but good exercise tolerance.

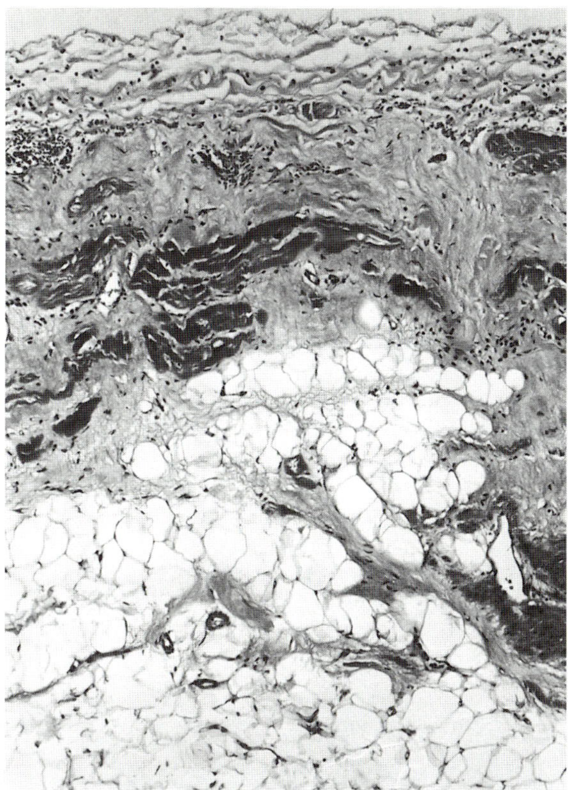

Fig. 5.47 Right ventricular dysplasia — histology. The right ventricular wall shows fibrous replacement of muscle associated with adipose infiltration. It is the fibrous replacement of muscle that is the important diagnostic feature. Fatty infiltration alone is a very common and unimportant phenomenon which is age-related, particularly in women.

taken not to overinterpret adipose tissue infiltration between the myocytes, which is a normal age-related change, particularly in women. In right ventricular dysplasia there is transmural replacement of myocardial tissue with fat and fibrous tissue.

The pathogenesis of the disease is unknown. On one hand the inflammatory cell infiltrate has been interpreted as a major factor causing progression of myocyte loss and a link has been made to the autoimmune-mediated left ventricular damage seen in the most usual form of dilated cardiomyopathy which involves the left ventricle. On the other hand others have regarded the disease as a partial failure of right ventricular development — the fully developed form of which is Uhl's disease — in which from birth there is a total absence of right ventricular myocardial tissue.[94]

MYOCARDIAL STORAGE DISORDERS

Deposition of a wide range of substances in the myocardium, either due to exogenous intake or endogenous overproduction of a particular product, leads to diseases which can produce cardiomyopathies of the dilated, restrictive or hypertrophic form.

IRON STORAGE DISEASE

In haemochromatosis the myocardium is simply the recipient of an excess of iron and the pathology is produced by the genetic form, with a defect in intestinal transferrin receptor, or by multiple transfusions for chronic anaemias due to haemolysis. Iron is deposited in both the atria and ventricles, producing a clinical picture of a dilated or a restrictive cardiomyopathy. Atrial arrhythmias are common as in atrioventricular block due to deposition of iron in the AV node.

The heart is macroscopically mahogany brown in colour with a dilated left ventricle, often containing mural thrombus. Histologically (Fig. 5.48), iron is present both within myocytes, particularly in the perinuclear zone, and in macrophages in the interstitial spaces.[95,96] Free

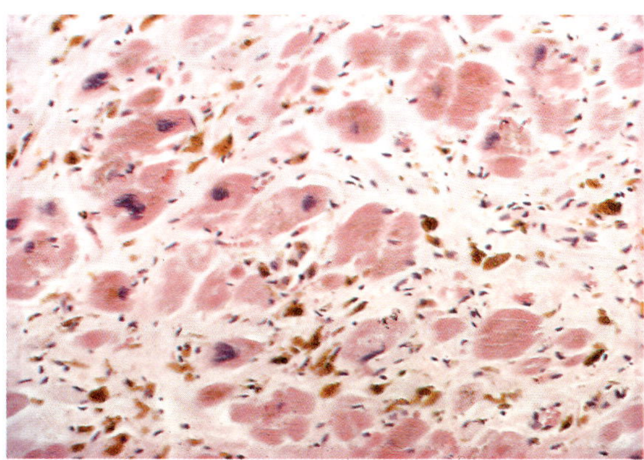

Fig. 5.48 Haemochromatosis. Iron pigment is present within myocytes and within macrophages in the interstitial tissues. There is heavy interstitial fibrosis. Haematoxylin–eosin × 345

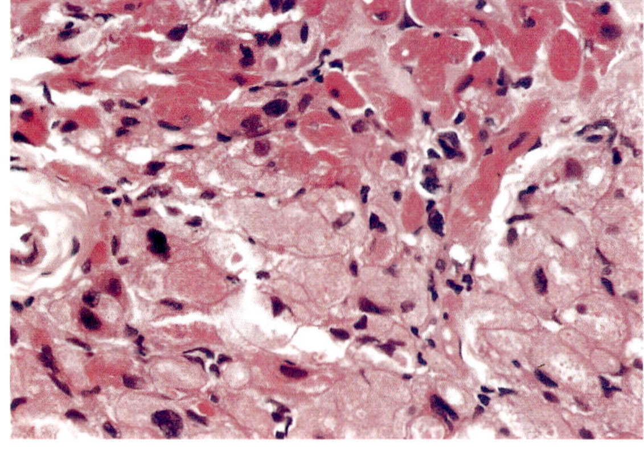

a)

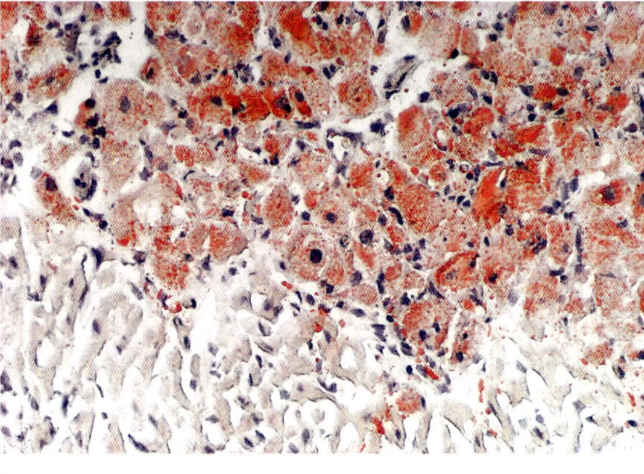

b)

iron deposits are also present in the interstitial tissues, which show a very considerable increase in diffuse interstitial fibrosis. The sequence of progress is probably that the death of myocytes releases iron into the interstitial tissues, followed by fibrosis.

HYPEROXALURIA

In primary oxalosis and in secondary oxalosis due to renal failure, calcium oxalate crystals may be widely distributed in many tissues including the myocardium.[97] Both conduction abnormalities and cardiac failure may develop, usually in conjunction with atrophy and neuropathy. Calcium oxalate crystals can be easily identified as light brown, strongly birefringent, hedgehog-shaped bodies in routine haematoxylin–eosin-stained sections. Considerable inflammatory response is initiated, often with giant cells, and myocardial

Fig. 5.49 a,b Histiocytoid cardiomyopathy. (**a**) Clusters of myocytes in focal areas have a vacuolated clear cytoplasma. Adjacent myocytes are normal. (**b**) The abnormal myocytes contain fine droplets of sudanophilic material.
(**a**) Haematoxylin–eosin × 215
(**b**) Sudan × 215

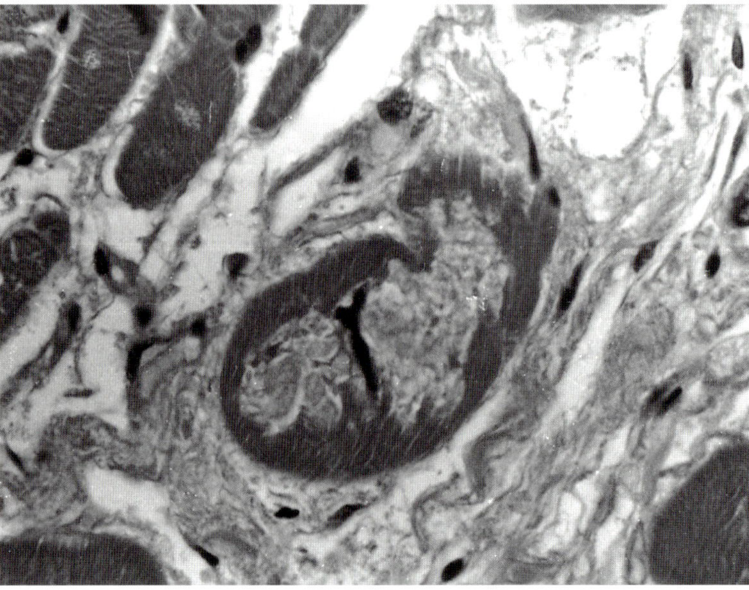

Fig. 5.50 Mucoid change in myocytes. A myocyte contains abundant blue mucoid material.

fibrosis occurs. AV block is due to nodal and His bundle destruction.

HISTIOCYTOID CARDIOMYOPATHY

In infants a rare entity may cause sudden death. Macroscopically there are yellow nodules up to 4 mm across particularly beneath the endocardium. Histologically (Fig. 5.49) the nodules consist of myocytes distended by fine vacuoles which are both PAS- and Sudan-positive. The entity is variously regarded as a storage disease in which the abnormal metabolite is not known or as a histiocytosis.[98]

MUCOID DEGENERATION

With increasing age and particularly in subjects over 70 occasional myocytes show accumulation of a mucinous material within the cell (Fig. 5.50). The material, which is PAS-positive, fills the cell, displacing the myofibrils. The number of such cells is higher in subjects with diabetes and myxoedema but is by no means specific for these conditions. The change is not known to have any functional correlate and even in hearts showing the change extensively the number of myocytes involved is only a tiny proportion of those in the myocardium.

REFERENCES

1. Vliegen H, van der Laarse A, Cornelisse C, Eulderink F. Myocardial changes in pressure overload-induced left ventricular hypertrophy. A study on tissue composition, polyploidization and multinucleation. Eur Heart J 1991; 12: 488–494.
2. Olivetti G, Melissan M, Balbi T, Quaini F, Sonnenblick EH, Anversa P. Myocyte nuclear and possible cellular hyperplasia contribute to ventricular remodelling in the hypertrophic senescent heart in humans. J Am Coll Cardiol 1994; 24: 140–149.
3. Shozawa T, Kawamura K, Okada E, Sageshima M, Masuda H. Development of binucleated myocytes in normal and hypertrophied human hearts. Am J Cardiovasc Pathol 1990; 3: 27–36.
4. Mann J, Jennison S, Moss E, Davies M. Assessment of rejection in orthotopic human heart transplantation using proliferating cell nuclear antigen (PCNA) as an index of cell proliferation. J Path 1992; 167: 385–391.
5. Saito Y, Nakao K, Arai H, Nishimura K, Okumura K, Obata K. Augmented expression of atrial natriuretic polypeptide gene in ventricle of human failing heart. J Clin Invest 1989; 83: 298–305.
6. Roberts R. Molecular biology of the cardiovascular system. In: Roberts R, ed. Molecular biology series. Hamden, CT: Blackwell, 1992: 1–14.
7. Komuro I, Kaida T, Shibazaki Y, et al. Stretching cardiac myocytes stimulates protooncogene expression. J Biol Chem 1990; 265: 3595–3598.
8. Huysman J, Vliegen H, VanderLaarse A, Eulderink F. Changes in non-myocyte tissue composition associated with pressure overload of hypertrophic human hearts. Pathol Res Pract 1989; 184: 577–581.
9. Weber K, Brilla C. Pathological hypertrophy and cardiac interstitium — fibrosis and renin–angiotensin–aldosterone system. Circulation 1991; 83: 1849–1865.
10. Gerdes A, Kellerman S, Moore J et al. Structural remodelling of cardiac myocytes in patients with ischemic cardiomyopathy. Circulation 1992; 86: 426–430.
11. Anversa P, Olivetti G, Capasso JM. Cellular basis of ventricular remodeling after myocardial infarction. Am J Cardiol 1991; 68: 7D–16D.
12. Zimmer G, Zimmermann R, Hess O et al. Decreased concentration of myofibrils and myofiber hypertrophy are structural determinants of impaired left ventricular function in patients with chronic heart diseases: a multiple logistic regression analysis. J Am Coll Cardiol 1992; 20: 1135–1142.
13. Schlant R, Sonnenblick E. Pathophysiology of heart failure. In: Schlant R, Alexander R, ed. The heart, arteries and veins, 8th ed. New York: McGraw-Hill, 1994: 557–572.
14. O'Connell J, Renlund D. Myocarditis and specific myocardial diseases. In: Schlant R, Alexander R, ed. The heart, arteries and veins, 8th ed. New York: McGraw-Hill, 1994: 1591–1608.
15. Aretz H. Myocarditis: the Dallas criteria. Hum Pathol 1987; 18: 619–624.
16. Woodruff J. Viral myocarditis – a review. Am J Pathol 1980; 101: 425–479.
17. Grist N, Reid D. Epidemiology of viral infections of the heart. In: Banatvala J, ed. Viral infections of the heart. London: Edward Arnold, 1992: 23–31.
18. Huber S. Animal models: immunological aspects. In: Banatvala J, ed. Viral infections of the heart. London: Edward Arnold, 1993: 82–103.
19. Kandolf R, Ameis D, Kirschner P, Canu A, Hofschneider P. In situ detection of enteroviral genomes in myocardial cells by nucleic acid hybridization: an approach to the diagnosis of viral heart disease. Proc Natl Acad Sci USA 1987; 84: 6272–6276.
20. Archard L, Bowies N, Cunningham L et al. Molecular probe for detection of persisting enterovirus infection of human heart and their prognostic value. Eur Heart J 1991; 12: 56–59.
21. Tracy S, Wiegand V, McManus B et al. Molecular approaches to enteroviral diagnosis in idiopathic cardiomyopathy and myocarditis. J Am Coll Cardiol 1990; 15: 1688–1694.
22. Neu N, Rose N, Beisel K, Herskowitz A, Gurri-Glass G, Craig S. Cardiac myosin induces myocarditis in genetically predisposed mice. J Immunol 1987; 139: 3630–3636.
23. Gonwa T, Capehart J, Pilcher J, Alivizatos P.

Cytomegalovirus myocarditis as a cause of cardiac dysfunction in a heart transplant recipient. Transplantation 1989; 47: 197–199.
24. Van der Linde MR, de Koning J, Hoogkamp-Korstanje JAA et al. Range of atrioventricular conduction disturbances in Lyme borreliosis: a report of four cases and review of other published reports. Br Heart J 1990; 63: 162–168.
25. Higuchi M, De Morais C, Narreto A, Lopes E, Stolf N, Bellotti G. The role of active myocarditis in the development of heart failure in chronic Chagas' disease. A study based on endomyocardial biopsies. Clin Cardiol 1987; 10: 665–670.
26. Koberle F. Chagas' disease and Chagas' syndrome: the pathology of the trypanosomiasis. Adv Parasit 1968; 6: 63–116.
27. Luft B, Billingham M, Remington J. Endomyocardial biopsy in the diagnosis of toxoplasmic myocarditis. Transplant Proc 1986; 18: 1871–1873.
28. Billingham M. Pharmacotoxic myocardial disease: an endomyocardial study. In: Sekiguchi M, Olsen E, Goodwin J, ed. Myocarditis and related disorders. Heidelberg: Springer-Verlag, 1985: 282.
29. Buja L, Ferrans W, Roberts W. Drug-induced cardiomyopathies. Adv Cardiol 1974; 13: 330–348.
30. Fenoglio J, Ursell P, Kellog C, Drusin F, Weiss M. Diagnosis and classification of myocarditis by endomyocardial biopsy. N Engl J Med 1983; 308: 12–18.
31. Shammas R, Movahed A. Sarcoidosis of the heart. Clin Cardiol 1993; 16: 462–472.
32. Valantine H, McKenna W, Nihoyannopoulos P et al. Sarcoidosis: a pattern of clinical and morphological presentation. Br Heart J 1987; 57: 256–263.
33. Silverman K, Hutchins G, Bulkley B. Cardiac sarcoid: a clinicopathological study of 84 unselected patients with systemic sarcoidosis. Circulation 1978; 58: 1204–1211.
34. Roberts W, McAllister H, Ferrans V. Sarcoidosis of the heart – a clinicopathological review of 35 necropsy patients and review of 78 previously described cases. Am J Med 1977; 63: 86–108.
35. Shiff A, Blatt C, Colp C. Recurrent pericardial effusion secondary to sarcoidosis of the pericardium: a biopsy proved case. N Engl J Med 1969; 28: 141–143.
36. Garrett J, O'Neill H, Blake S. Constrictive pericarditis associated with sarcoidosis. Am Heart J 1984; 107: 393–394.
37. Fleming H, Bailey S. Sarcoidosis of the heart. J R Coll Physicians 1981; 15: 245–253.
38. Ratner S, Fenoglio JJ, Ursell P. Utility of endomyocardial biopsy in the diagnosis of cardiac sarcoidosis. Chest 1986; 90: 528–533.
39. Davies M, Pomerance A, Teare R. Idiopathic giant cell myocarditis — a distinctive clinico-pathologic entity. Br Heart J 1975; 37: 192–195.
40. Theaker J, Gatter K, Evans D, McGee J. Giant cell myocarditis: evidence for the macrophage origin of the giant cells. J Clin Pathol 1985; 38: 160–164.
41. Burke J, Medline N, Katz A. Giant cell myocarditis and myositis associated with thymoma and myasthenia gravis. Arch Pathol 1969; 88: 359–366.
42. Kodama M, Matsumoto Y, Fujiwara M et al. Characteristics of giant cells and factors related to the formation of giant cells in myocarditis. Circ Res 1991; 69: 1042–1050.
43. Gries W. Giant cell myocarditis: first report of recurrence in the transplanted heart. J Heart Lung Transplantation 1992; 11: 370–374.
44. World Health Organization. Report of the WHO/ISFC task force on the definition and classification of cardiomyopathies. Br Heart J 1980; 44: 672–673.
45. Keren A, Popp R. Assignment of patients into the classification of cardiomyopathies. Circulation 1992; 86: 1622–1633.
46. Teare D. Asymmetrical hypertrophy of the heart in young patients. Br Heart J 1958; 20: 1–8.
47. Solomon S, Wolff S, Watkins H et al. Left ventricular hypertrophy and morphology in familial hypertrophic cardiomyopathy associated with mutations of the beta-myosin heavy chain gene. J Am Coll Cardiol 1993; 22: 498–505.
48. Chikamori T, Doi Y, Yonezawa Y, Dickie S, Ozawa T, McKenna W. Comparison of clinical features in patients >60 years of age to those <40 years of age with hypertrophic cardiomyopathy. Am J Cardiol 1990; 66: 875–877.
49. Hecht G, Klues H, Roberts W, Maron B. Coexistence of sudden cardiac death and end-stage heart failure in familial hypertrophic cardiomyopathy. J Am Coll Cardiol 1993; 22: 489–497.
50. Spirito P, Maron B. Patterns of systolic anterior motion of the mitral valve in hypertrophic cardiomyopathy: assessment by two-dimensional echocardiography. Am J Cardiol 1984; 54: 1039–1046.
51. Webb J, Sasson Z, Rakowski H, Lui P, Wigle E. Apical hypertrophic cardiomyopathy: clinical follow-up and diagnostic correlates. J Am Coll Cardiol 1990; 15: 83–90.
52. Davies M. The current status of myocardial disarray in hypertrophic cardiomyopathy. Br Heart J 1984; 51: 361–363.
53. Becker A, Caruso G. Myocardial disarray. A critical review. Br Heart J 1982; 47: 527–538.
54. Maron B, Anan T, Roberts W. Quantitative analysis of the distribution of cardiac muscle cell disorganisation in the left ventricular wall of patients with hypertrophic cardiomyopathy. Circulation 1981; 63: 882–894.
55. Tanaka M, Fujiwara H, Onodera T et al. Quantitative analysis of narrowings of intramyocardial small arteries in normal hearts, hypertensive hearts and hearts with hypertrophic cardiomyopathy. Circulation 1987; 75: 1130–1139.
56. Maron B, Spirito P, Wesley Y, Arce J. Development and progression of left ventricular hypertrophy in children with hypertrophic cardiomyopathy. N Engl J Med 1986; 315: 610–614.
57. McKenna W, Stewart J, Niyannopoulos P, McGinty F, Davies M. Hypertrophic cardiomyopathy without hypertrophy: two families with myocardial disarray in the absence of increased myocardial mass. Br Heart J 1990; 63: 287–290.
58. Harding A, Langton A. The heart disease of Friedreich's ataxia: a clinical and electrocardiographic study of 115 patients with an analysis of serial electrocardiographic changes in 30 cases. Q J Med 1983; 52: 489–502.
59. Bordiuk J, Legato M, Lovelace R, Blumenthal S. Pompe's disease: electromyographic, electron

microscopic, and cardiovascular aspects. Arch Neurol 1970; 23: 113–119.
60. Goldman M, Cantor R, Schwartz M, Baker M, Desnick R. Echocardiographic abnormalities and disease severity in Fabry's disease. J Am Coll Cardiol 1986; 7: 1157–1161.
61. Broadbent J, Edwards W, Gordon H, Hartzler G, Krawisz J. Fabry cardiomyopathy in the female confirmed by endomyocardial biopsy. Mayo Clin Proc 1981; 56: 623–628.
62. Figulla H, Rahlf G, Nieger M, Luig H, Kreuzer H. Spontaneous hemodynamic improvement or stabilization and associated biopsy findings in patients with congestive cardiomyopathy. Circulation 1985; 71: 1095–1104.
63. Deck W, Palacios I, Fallon J et al. Active myocarditis in the spectrum of acute dilated cardiomyopathies. N Engl J Med 1985; 342: 885–897.
64. Tazelaar H, Billingham M. Myocardial lymphocytes (fact, fancy or myocarditis?). Am J Cardiovasc Pathol 1986; 1: 47–50.
65. Levi G, Scalvini S, Voeterrani M, Marangoni S, Arosio G, Quadri A. Coxsackie virus disease: 15 years later. Eur Heart J 1988; 12: 1303–1307.
66. Keeling PJ, Tracey S. The link between enterovirus and DCM, serological molecular. Br Heart J 1994; 72(Supp): 25–29.
67. Schultheiss H-P. Disturbance of the myocardial energy metabolism in dilated cardiomyopathy due to autoimmunological mechanisms. Circulation 1993; 87: IV43–IV48.
68. Latif N, Baker C, Dunn M, Rose M, Brady B, Yacoub M. Frequency and specificity of antiheart antibodies in patients with dilated cardiomyopathy detected using SDS-PAGE and Western blotting. J Am Coll Cardiol 1993; 22: 1378–1384.
69. Schulze K, Becker B, Schultheiss H-P. Antibodies to the ADP/ATP carrier — an autoantigen in myocarditis and dilated cardiomyopathy — penetrate into myocardial cells and disturb energy metabolism in vivo. Circ Res 1989; 64: 179–192.
70. Maisch B, Bauer E, Cirsi M, Kochsiek K. Cytolytic cross-reactive antibodies directed against the cardiac membrane and viral proteins in coxsackievirus B3 and B4 myocarditis. Characterization and pathogenetic relevance. Circulation 1993; 87: IV49–IV65.
71. Preedy V, Atkinson L, Richardson P, Peters T. Mechanisms of ethanol-induced cardiac damage. Br Heart J 1993; 69: 197–200.
72. Thomas A, Knapman P, Krikler D, Davies M. A community study of the causes of 'natural' sudden death. BMJ 1988; 297: 1453–1455.
73. Olsen E. The pathology of cardiomyopathy: a critical analysis. Am Heart J 1979; 98: 385–392.
74. Regan T. Alcohol and nutritional disease. In: Schlant R, Alexander R, ed. The heart, arteries and veins, 8th ed. New York: McGraw–Hill, 1994: 1943–1948.
75. Rhoden W, Hasleton P, Brooks N. Anthracyclines and the heart. Br Heart J 1993; 70: 499–502.
76. Billingham. M, Bristow M. Evaluation of anthracycline cardiotoxicity: predictive ability and functional correlation of endomyocardial biopsy. Cancer Treat Symp 1984; 3: 71–76.
77. Michels W, Mills P, Miller F, Tajik A, Chu J, Driscoll D. The frequency of familial dilated cardiomyopathy in a series of patients with idiopathic dilated cardiomyopathy. N Engl J Med 1992; 326: 77–82.
78. Muntoni F, Cau M, Ganau A et al. Brief report: deletion of the dystrophin muscle-promoter region associated with X-linked dilated cardiomyopathy. N Engl J Med 1993; 329: 921–925.
79. Sanyal S, Johnson W. Cardiac conduction abnormalities in children with Duchenne's progressive muscular dystrophy – electrocardiographic features and morphologic correlates. Circulation 1982; 66: 853–863.
80. Perloff J, Roberts W, Deleon A, O'Doherty D. The distinctive electrocardiogram of Duchenne's progressive muscular dystrophy. Am J Med 1967; 42: 179–188.
81. Remes A, Hassinen I, Majamaa K, Peuhkurinen K. Mitochondrial DNA deletion diagnosed by analysis of an endomyocardial biopsy specimen from a patient with Kearns–Sayre syndrome and complete heart block. Br Heart J 1992; 68: 408–411.
82. O'Connell J, Costanzo-Nordin M, Subramanian R et al. Peripartum cardiomyopathy: clinical, hemodynamic, histologic and prognostic characteristics. J Am Coll Cardiol 1986; 8: 52–56.
83. Midei M, DeMent S, Feldman A, Hutchins G, Baughman K. Peripartum myocarditis and cardiomyopathy. Circulation 1990; 81: 922–928.
84. Kartha C, Gupta N. Pathological spectrum and possible pathogenesis of endomyocardial fibrosis. In: Valiathan M, Somers K, Chandrasekharan Kartha C, ed. Endomyocardial fibrosis. Delhi: Oxford University Press, 1993: 125–140.
85. Shaper A. The aetiology of endomyocardial fibrosis. In: Valiathan M, Somers K, Chandrasekharan Kartha C, ed. Endomyocardial fibrosis. Delhi: Oxford University Press, 1993: 121–124.
86. Valiathan M, Somers K, Chandrasekharan Kartha C, ed. Endomyocardial fibrosis. Delhi: Oxford University Press, 1993: 1–302.
87. Sasano HRV. Eosinophilic products lead to myocardial damage. Hum Pathol 1989; 20: 850–857.
88. Katritsis D, Wilmshurst P, Wendon J, Davies M, Webb-Peploe M. Primary restrictive cardiomyopathy: clinical and pathologic characteristics. J Am Coll Cardiol 1991; 18: 1230–1235.
89. Hesse A, Altland K, Linke RP et al. Cardiac amyloidosis: a review and report of a new transthyretin (prealbumin) variant. Br Heart J 1993; 70: 111–115.
90. Roberts W, Waller B. Cardiac amyloidosis causing cardiac dysfunction: analysis of 54 necropsy patients. Am J Cardiol 1983; 52: 137–146.
91. Steiner I. The prevalence of isolated atrial amyloid. J Pathol 1987; 153: 395–398.
92. Cornwell G, Murdoch W, Kyle R, Westermark P, Pitkanen P. Frequency and distribution of senile cardiovascular amyloid. Am J Med 1983; 75: 618–623.
93. Thiene G, Nava A, Corrado D, Rossi L, Pennelli N. Right ventricular cardiomyopathy and sudden death in young people. N Engl J Med 1988; 318: 129–133.
94. Gerlis LM, Schnidt-Ott SC, Ho SY, Anderson RH. Dysplastic conditions of the right ventricular myocardium: Uhl's anomaly v. arrhythmogenic right ventricular dysplasia. Br Heart J 1993; 69: 142–150.
95. Olson L, Edwards W, Holmes D, Miller F, Nordstrom L,

Baldus W. Endomyocardial biopsy in hemochromatosis: clinicopathologic correlates in six cases. J Am Coll Cardiol 1989; 13: 116–120.
96. Barosi G, Arbustini E, Gavazzi A, Grasso M, Pucci A. Myocardial iron grading by endomyocardial biopsy. A clinicopathologic study on iron overloaded patients. Eur J Haematol 1989; 42: 383–388.
97. Coltart DJ, Hudson REB. Primary oxalosis of the heart: a cause of heart block. Br Heart J 1971; 33: 315–319.
98. Saffitz J, Ferrans V, Rodriguez E, Lewis F, Roberts W. Histiocytoid cardiomyopathy: a cause of sudden death in apparently healthy infants. Am J Cardiol 1983; 52: 215–216.

6

The pathology of the cardiac valves

INTRODUCTION

The structure and function of the aortic and pulmonary valves are essentially identical, as are those of the mitral and tricuspid valves. In the aortic and pulmonary valves competence depends on the semilunar shape of the cusps themselves. In addition, part of the ventricular faces of the cusps abut, thus preventing prolapse of the cusps when the aortic and pulmonary pressures are higher than those in the ventricular cavity. In the mitral and tricuspid valves prolapse of the cusps into the atria is prevented by the chordae attached to the cusp. The chordae and papillary muscles control the correct apposition of the cusps as the ventricles change in shape.

When examining the cardiac valves at autopsy it is best not to cut the valve ring because once this is done any real appreciation of valve function, whether this be stenosis or regurgitation, is lost.

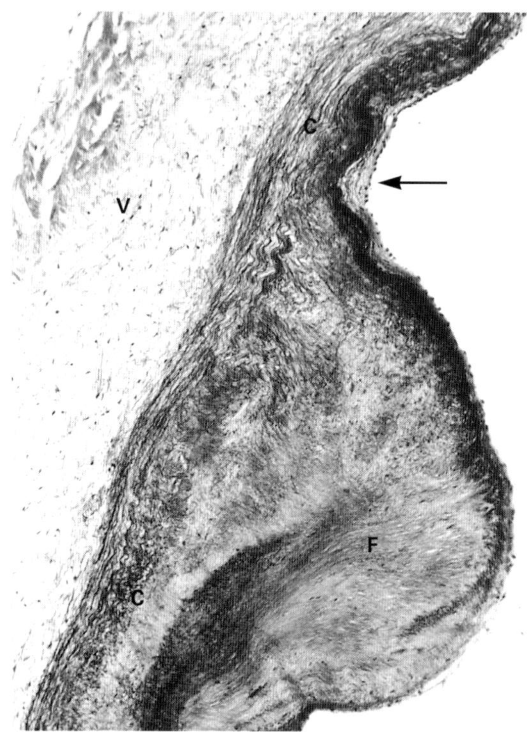

Fig. 6.1 Normal aortic valve. There is a dense core of collagen in the cusp (C) with a well-formed, more superficial layer of connective tissue on the ventricular face (V). On the aortic face there is only a thin layer of connective tissue covered by endothelium (arrow). A dense nodule of fibrosis (F) marks the apposition point of the cusp with its neighbours. EVG × 16

TISSUE RESPONSES IN VALVE CUSPS

The basic structure of valve cusps, whether atrio-ventricular or semilunar (Figs 6.1, 6.2), is a core of dense collagen (valve fibrosa) continuous with the valve ring and covered on both aspects by a layer of loosely arranged collagen rich in glycosaminoglycans (valve spongiosa). Each aspect of the cusp is covered by endothelium. Normal valve cusps are avascular but there is considerable turnover of the connective tissue within the cusps and they cannot be considered as inert structures. The range of tissue responses that can occur in a predominantly collagenous tissue is however limited.

The tissue processes within valve cusps can be categorised as mechanically induced, inflammatory or degenerative in nature.

Mechanically induced changes

The connective tissue of the spongiosa proliferates following mechanical trauma to produce a more dense collagenous layer. Whether this direct response is due directly to mechanical forces acting on fibroblasts in the valve spongiosa or to endothelial denudation and platelet adhesion re-

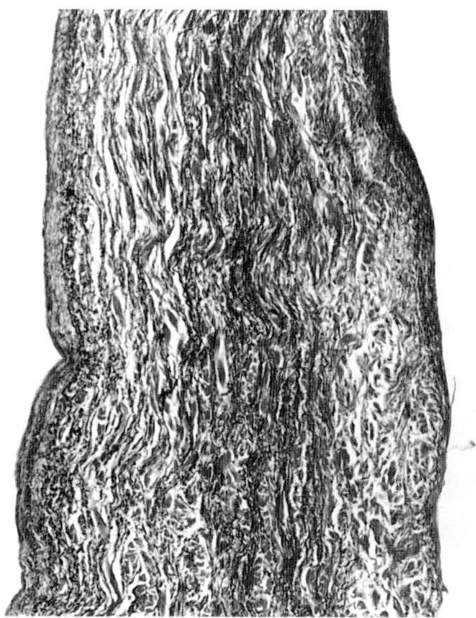

Fig. 6.2 Normal mitral valve. In the body of the anterior cusp there is a trilaminar appearance with a central dense collagenous layer and on either side more loosely organised connective tissue.
EVG × 16

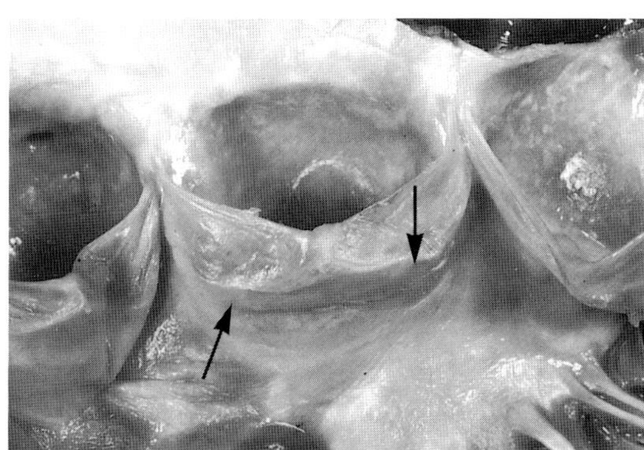

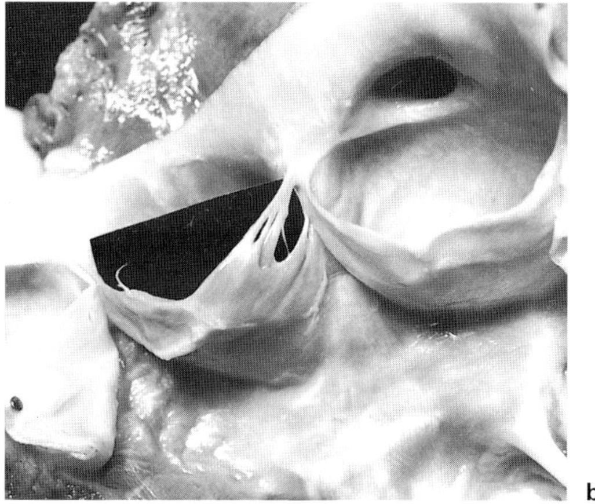

Fig. 6.3 a,b Aortic valve — age-related mechanical change. (**a**) Viewed en face the valve has a central nodule from which two ridges (arrows) pass laterally. These ridges mark the apposition line of the cusps and are due to mechanical trauma over the years. (**b**) This valve has fenestrations at the lateral margins of the cusps but these defects are above the closure line and cannot cause regurgitation.

leasing growth factors is not clear. These mechanical impact lesions are a tissue response common both to valve cusps and the endocardium. Mechanical trauma produces accentuation with increasing age of the closure lines on the cusps (Fig. 6.3), regurgitant jet or impact lesions (Fig. 6.4) on the endocardium. Within this secondary fibrous endocardial thickening fine elastic laminae may develop. The characteristic of all these mechanical injuries to cusps and endocardium is that the fibrous thickening is superficial and superimposed on the underlying structure of the valve.

Fig. 6.4 Jet and friction lesions on endocardium. The anterior cusp of the mitral valve shows very thickened yet long and tortuous chordae. The basic lesion was a floppy mitral valve in which excessive movement of the cusp led to chordae constantly hitting each other. In the atrium there is a jet lesion (arrows), indicating where a mitral regurgitant jet hit the left atrial endocardium.

Inflammatory changes

Inflammatory changes are associated with vascu-

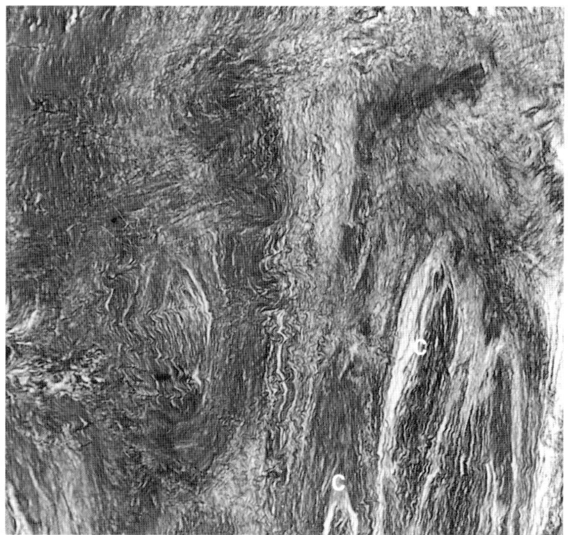

Fig. 6.5 Postinflammatory (rheumatic) valve disease. The trilaminar architecture of the mitral cusp is totally obliterated by fibrosis; chordae (C) are incorporated into the fibrosis. EVG × 16

larisation of the cusps from the base. Associated with the ingrowth of new vessels chronic inflammatory cells appear and there is enhanced fibrous proliferation within all layers of the cusp which finally obliterates its laminar architecture (Fig. 6.5). The surface area of the cusp is usually reduced but the cusp becomes thicker. Inflammatory valve disease (valvulitis) is due either to immune mediated damage, examples being rheumatic heart disease and ankylosing spondylitis, or direct infection with microorganisms. The latter condition, infective endocarditis, is considered in Chapter 7.

Degenerative changes

The degenerative changes which occur in valves are either calcification within the fibrous tissue of the cusp and valve rings or replacement of the fibrous core of the cusp by more loosely arranged collagen with myxomatous areas rich in glycosaminoglycans (mucoid degeneration).

Myxomatous or myxoid degeneration occurs particularly in the mitral valve (floppy valve) and is associated with a reduction in the tensile strength of cusps and chordae leading to their expansion (Figs 6.4, 6.6) with an increase in both cusp area and length. Such enlarged cusps contrast strikingly with the retracted and shrunken cusps of rheumatic disease. The archetypal form of myxoid change occurs in Marfan's disease, due to abnormalities of the fibrillin molecule and thus the binding of collagen fibres in the cusp.

Calcification may either be age-related, occurring in otherwise morphologically normal valves, or affect valves in which there is pre-existing disease such as postinflammatory chronic valvulitis. The calcification develops within dense collagen (Fig. 6.7), particularly when this is under mechanical stress. The deposition of calcium is in some way related to the exposure of calcium binding sites on the collagen. Cellular mechanisms (Chapter 2) may also be involved. When the calcium/phosphate levels in the blood are altered,

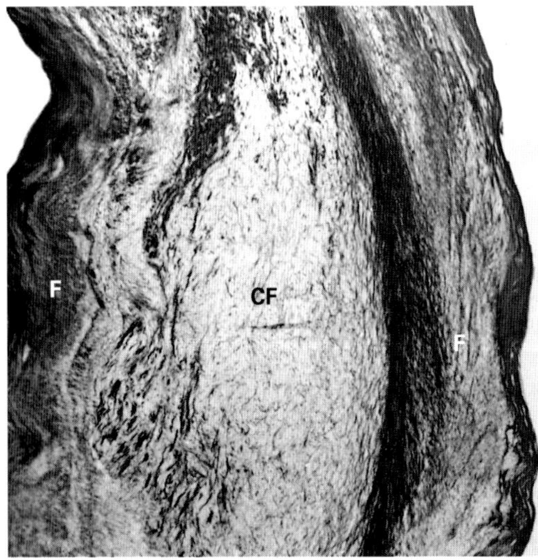

Fig. 6.6 Myxoid change in mitral valve. The trilaminar architecture of the cusp is retained but overall cusp thickness is increased. The collagen of the central fibrosa (CF) is irregularly arranged with many clear areas containing connective tissue mucin. Both the atrial and ventricular faces of the cusp show secondary fibrosis (F).
EVG × 16

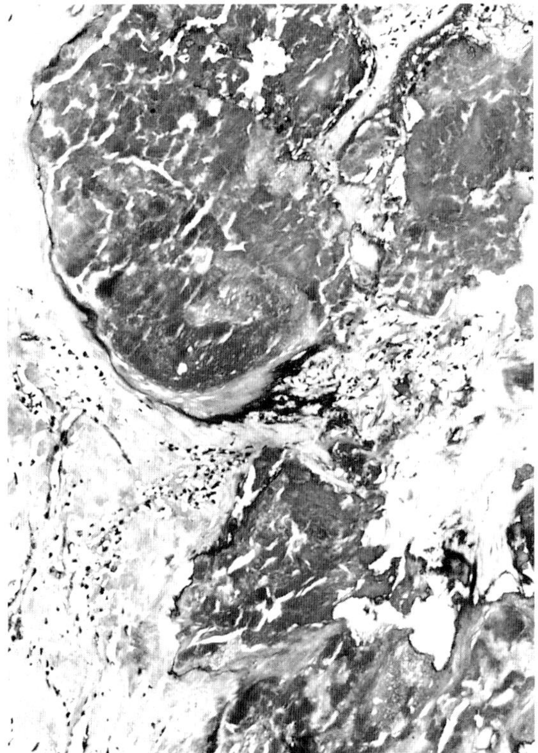

Fig. 6.7 Calcification in valve cusps. Calcification develops as nodular masses. These masses often have brightly eosinophilic crumbly centres while at the periphery the tissue outline is retained and basophilic due to calcium deposition. Some chronic inflammatory cells are almost ubiquitous whatever the basic underlying valve abnormality. Foreign body giant cells may also occur.
Haematoxylin–eosin × 45

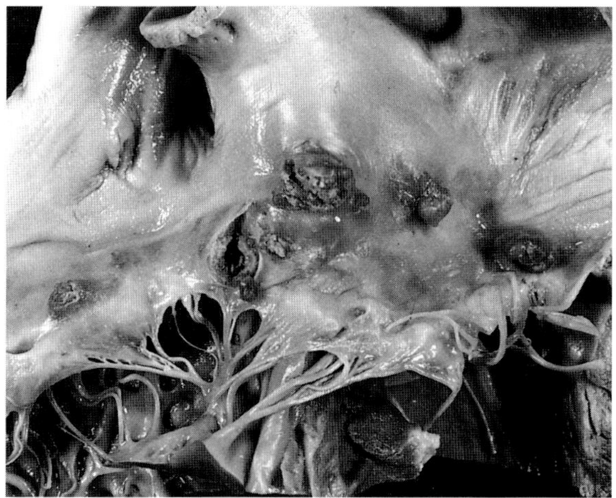

Fig. 6.8 Mitral calcification in chronic renal failure. Along the bases of the cusps of the mitral valve nodular masses of calcification project through the overlying endocardium.

as in, for instance, chronic renal failure, valve calcification may be greatly enhanced (Fig. 6.8) although the pattern of calcification is identical to that seen in pure age-related change.[1]

RHEUMATIC VALVE DISEASE

Rheumatic valve disease affects all four valves in various combinations and will be considered as a process before describing the functional abnormalities which cause stenosis or regurgitation in individual valves.

Chronic rheumatic valve disease occurs long after an attack of acute valvulitis due to acute rheumatic fever. Chronic rheumatic valve disease is thus a long-term sequela of immune-mediated cusp injury. In the chronic stage three processes, cusp fibrosis, cusp calcification and commissural fusion act together to give any combination of stenosis and regurgitation in the aortic, mitral and tricuspid valves.

ACUTE RHEUMATIC FEVER

In acute rheumatic fever a group A streptococcal pharyngitis is followed after a latent period of 2–4 weeks by a febrile illness associated with skin rashes, flitting transient arthritis, a pancarditis and on occasion chorea. The term pancarditis means that all three layers of the heart, pericardium, myocardium and endocardium, are involved. The pericarditis is the most obvious clinically, with effusions and a pericardial friction rub being commonly heard. Pericarditis is usually transitory and does not lead to long-term sequelae. The myocarditis is clinically important in that it is responsible for ventricular dilatation, heart failure and the acute mortality of acute rheumatic fever. In the acute phase valvulitis is the least of the problems. Valve regurgitation during the acute attack is due to the ventricular dilatation consequent on myocarditis rather than to the cusp lesions themselves.

Acute rheumatic fever is predominantly a disease of childhood but repeated attacks continuing into adolescence are common. A first attack of rheumatic fever in adults should be regarded as a clinical diagnosis needing stringent review.

PATHOLOGY OF ACUTE RHEUMATIC FEVER

The disease has declined dramatically in the Western world. This decline has, however, to be viewed both against the remaining high frequency in Third World countries with warm climates, such as Egypt and the sub-continent of India, and a minor resurgence in developed countries.[2] Fatal cases allow the full expression of the pancarditis to be observed. The pericarditis is acute and fibrinous with no specific histological features. The myocarditis, in contrast, has very specific histological features. The myocarditis is characterised by the appearance of small giant cell granulomata, the Aschoff bodies, in the connective tissue of the myocardium (Fig. 6.9). In the acute phase each Aschoff body has a small central focus of collagen which appears hyper-eosinophilic and 'smudgy'. Around this central focus are gathered epithelioid-like and spindle-shaped cells. The former are almost certainly macrophage-derived. Various names have been given to these cells, including Anitschow cells for those with a central bar of chromatin within the nucleus and Aschoff giant cells for small multinucleated cells.

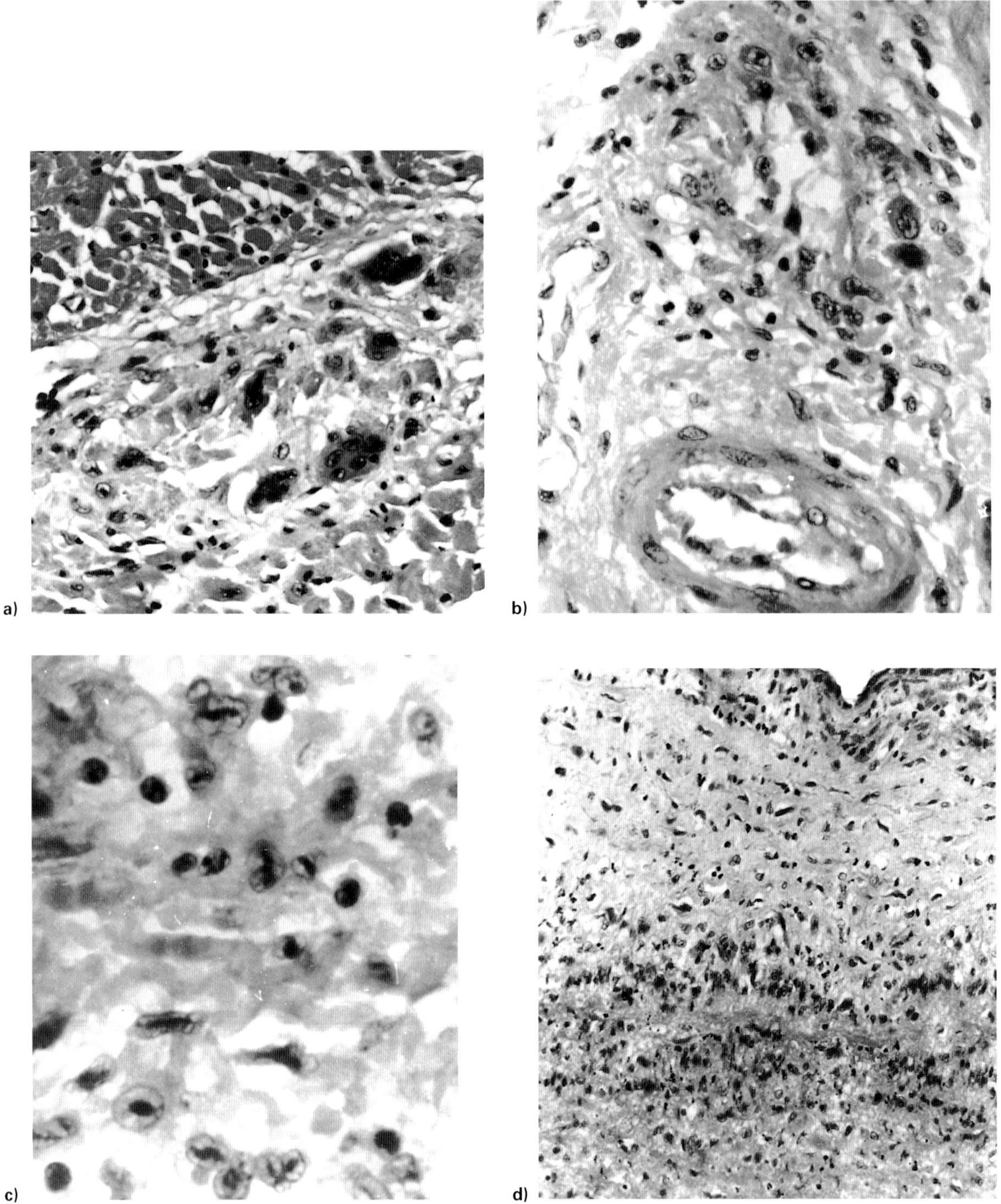

Fig. 6.9 a,b,c,d Aschoff bodies. (**a**) An oval Aschoff body is situated in the interstitial tissue of the myocardium. It has a central focus of altered collagen surrounded by Aschoff giant cells. (**b**) A perivascular Aschoff body in which giant cells are less prominent than in (**a**). The small artery shows endothelial swelling. (**c**) A loosely formed Aschoff body in which the predominant cell type is the Anitschow cell, with an open vesicular nucleus with a central bar of chromatin. (**d**) A linear subendocardial Aschoff body with a palisade of cells around altered collagen. This type may be mistaken for a rheumatoid nodule. (**a**) Haematoxylin–eosin × 105 (**b**) Haematoxylin–eosin × 165 (**c**) Haematoxylin–eosin × 260 (**d**) Haematoxylin–eosin × 160

Anitschow cells in isolation have no specificity for acute rheumatic fever. They are a variety of mesenchymal cell readily induced in the connective tissue of the heart in young individuals by a wide range of insults. While originally regarded as being myogenic and derived in some way from smooth muscle cells or even myocytes, immunohistochemical studies suggest a mesenchymal fibroblastic cell origin.

Aschoff bodies are in general small, being at the most 0.5 mm in diameter and visible only microscopically. They must not be confused with much larger rheumatic nodules that develop in the skin in acute rheumatic fever or the rheumatoid nodule of rheumatoid arthritis, both of which can be visible macroscopically. Aschoff bodies occur in the connective tissue of the heart, which often appears somewhat oedematous and has a diffuse infiltrate of mononuclear inflammatory cells. In the subendocardial connective tissue Aschoff bodies also abound and in the left atrium there may be a continuous layer to form a giant single Aschoff body some centimetres in length but only a fraction of a millimetre in width.

The myocarditis is the most sinister of the acute components of the pancarditis. The ventricles in some cases become dilated, leading to functional mitral regurgitation; congestive cardiac failure, arrhythmias and atrioventricular heart block may develop. While Aschoff bodies are often widespread the degree of myocardial dysfunction is often out of all proportion to the histological changes, particularly given that myocyte necrosis is not present.

Specific criteria exist for the definitive diagnosis of acute rheumatic fever[3] in which there must be evidence of prior streptococcal infection with one major and two minor or two major criteria present (Table 6.1). These criteria, modified by the AHA from those of Duckett & Jones in 1944, define a standard for comparative epidemiological studies of the disease. Those who wish to make the diagnosis of a first attack of rheumatic fever in adults should adhere to these standards.

Following the subsidence of the acute phase of rheumatic fever Aschoff bodies enter a healing phase in which fibrosis replaces the cellular element. This process is, however, very prolonged. Recognisable Aschoff bodies may persist for up to 20 years after the original acute attack. Thus the finding of Aschoff bodies in the left atrial appendage in a subject undergoing mitral valve surgery many years after an attack of acute rheumatic fever, does not suggest that there is current active disease but merely confirms that the subject has had acute rheumatic fever in the past. In subjects who survive the acute phase of rheumatic fever long-term myocardial damage is not a recognised clinical problem.

Table 6.1 Criteria for the clinical diagnosis of acute rheumatic fever

Major criteria	Carditis
	Polyarthritis (particularly if flitting — joint to joint)
	Chorea
	Erythema marginatum
	Subcutaneous nodules
Minor criteria	Fever
	Acute phase proteins raised
	ESR raised
	Rising ASO

In the acute phase of rheumatic fever the valvulitis is the least striking aspect pathologically, albeit the most important for ultimately causing chronic rheumatic valve disease. The cusps, particularly those of the mitral valve, appear slightly swollen and along the apposition lines small, flat, brown, translucent vegetations form. These vegetations are small and sessile, measuring less than 2 mm in thickness, and do not lead to systemic emboli. Histologically the valve appears slightly oedematous, with a scattering of chronic inflammatory cells. The vegetations are predominantly composed of platelets. Beneath the vegetations fibroblastic proliferation is present in the valve tissue. While in general Aschoff bodies do not occur within the cups there are well-characterised cases in which Aschoff bodies have occurred.

PATHOGENESIS OF ACUTE RHEUMATIC FEVER

The link between rheumatic fever and group A streptococcal infection 2–4 weeks previously is very clear from the epidemiology of the disease. The decline of the disease in the Western world over the last 40 years, to a point at which most medical students will not see a case, has brought research into the disease to a virtual standstill.

Rheumatic fever is, however, still rampant in the underdeveloped world.

The declining interest in the disease means that the exact mechanisms by which a pancarditis is caused remain unclear.

At its simplest level the disease is immune in nature. There is clear evidence that streptococcal antigens invoke a wide range of circulating antibodies. Some of these antibodies are an exaggerated response to streptococcal antigens, an example being the antistreptolysin O (ASO) titre. Most of the antibodies, however, have no direct pathogenetic function. A minority of the antibodies induced do cross-react with cardiac and other connective tissues.[4] The rather simplistic view therefore emerged that rheumatic fever was due to fortuitous sharing of an antigen by the streptococcus and cardiac tissue, and that antibodies caused the tissue damage. The name molecular or antigenic mimicry highlights this view.[5] Many of the cardiac autoantibodies generated in acute rheumatic fever, however, for example those against myosin, also occur in many other cardiac conditions and may be simply a response to myocardial damage. Whether such antibodies perpetuate damage or inhibit function is discussed in Chapter 5. The hypothesis does however indicate that the immune mechanism is not mediated by circulating antigen/antibody complexes comparable to the mechanism which produces poststreptococcal glomerulonephritis or polyarteritis nodosa.

This simple humoral antibody view of the immune basis of acute rheumatic carditis is not entirely in accord with some of the facts. The Aschoff body has histological features that suggest cell-based immune damage. The centres of the Aschoff bodies do not contain bound immunoglobulins and the cells are of macrophage derivation. The level of circulating antibodies does not correlate well with the clinical severity of the disease although it is true that in subjects with rheumatic fever the ASO titres are often higher than in subjects with an identical streptococcal pharyngitis but without rheumatic fever. The rather unsatisfactory state at the moment is that cell-based immunity probably plays a major role and that a gene related to the antigens of the HLA types confers susceptibility to acute rheumatic fever. Research is hindered by the lack of an animal model which exactly mimics the disease; inoculation of streptococcal antigens with Freund's adjuvant in rodents will produce a myocarditis but Aschoff bodies are lacking.

CHRONIC RHEUMATIC VALVE DISEASE

The importance of acute rheumatic fever is that chronic valve lesions may develop after a latent period of up to 30 years. In rheumatic-fever-related disease there are therefore two latent periods. The first is short, between the streptococcal pharyngitis and the acute systemic manifestations. Reports vary widely as to the exact proportion of cases of group A streptococcal pharyngitis with joint and skin manifestations who develop an acute pancarditis, but it is no more than 5%. The second, longer, latent period is between the resolution of the acute phase of the valvulitis and the clinical detection of chronic valve lesions.

The pathological hallmarks of chronic rheumatic valve disease (Figs 6.10, 6.11) are commissural fusion, cusp fibrosis with retraction (i.e. reduction in cusp area) and calcification. Combinations of these three processes in the aortic, mitral and tricuspid valves will produce all permutations of stenosis and/or regurgitation in these valves. It is characteristic of chronic rheumatic valve disease that more than one valve is involved, with mixed functional abnormalities. It is rare for any other pathological process to achieve this mixed haemodynamic picture.

Histologically the salient feature of chronic rheumatic valve disease is dense fibrosis which obliterates valve architecture with loss of the distinction between the fibrosa and spongiosa. Another feature, particularly in the mitral valve, is vascularisation of the cusps from their bases. Along with this vascularisation, focal collections of lymphocytes are common. Over the cusp surface, particularly at points of cusp apposition, small sessile microscopic thrombi are common. These must not be taken to indicate residual rheumatic activity; they merely indicate trauma due to abnormal valve function and are found in all disrupted valves, whatever the cause.

Not all subjects who develop acute rheumatic

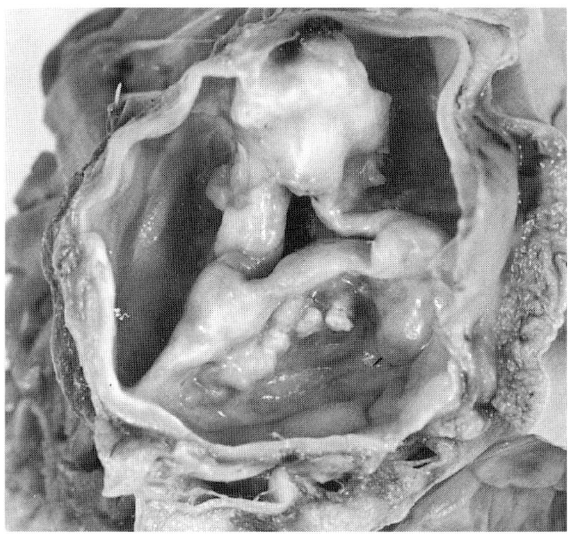

Fig. 6.10 Aortic valve stenosis — chronic rheumatic disease. Viewed from the aortic aspect there is fusion of all three commissures associated with heavy dystrophic calcification. The valve aperture is central and triangular in shape.

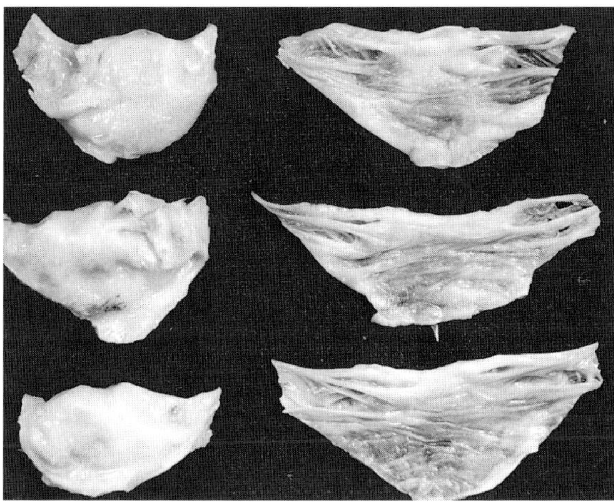

Fig. 6.11 Aortic valve regurgitation — chronic rheumatic disease. The cusps excised at valve replacement for pure rheumatic aortic regurgitation are shown alongside normal cusps. The rheumatic disease produces thick fibrotic cusps which are reduced in area as compared with normal.

carditis in childhood ultimately develop chronic valve lesions. The proportion of those who do not may be as high as 90%. It is an unresolved question what processes take place during the second long latent period. On the one hand there is a hypothesis that during this latent period repeated subclinical attacks of further rheumatic carditis are occurring. Evidence for this view is based on the episodic increases in antibodies to streptococcal antigens found in asymptomatic subjects who have had a previous attack of rheumatic fever. Further evidence comes from the fact that recurrent episodes of clinically expressed rheumatic fever dramatically increase the subsequent risk of chronic valve disease and reduce the latent period. In geographic areas where acute rheumatic fever is still endemic and severe this mechanism almost certainly operates. In adolescents in such populations mitral stenosis may occur within a year or two of the acute attack.

In geographic areas in which the acute disease is less rampant the latent periods are much longer. It is possible that here secondary mechanisms entirely unrelated to the rheumatic process are operating. Once collagen synthesis is enhanced in a mechanically damaged valve it appears to continue. Once a large amount of collagen is laid down, in time, calcification will develop.

The diagnosis of chronic rheumatic disease in its late stage is dependent entirely on the presence of combinations of commissural fusion and cusp fibrosis. The subject ideally will give a history of rheumatic fever in childhood. In geographic areas where acute rheumatic fever has declined a high proportion of subjects found to have valve lesions which fit the pathological features of chronic rheumatic disease have no clinical history of acute rheumatic fever. These cases can either be regarded as being due to prior forgotten or subclinical acute rheumatic fever, or categorised simply as post inflammatory in nature, implying that there may be other causes of an acute valvulitis that can lead to an identical end-stage valve. The most frequently postulated cause is a viral valvulitis, but proof of this view is lacking.

STRUCTURE, FUNCTION AND PATHOLOGY OF INDIVIDUAL VALVES

AORTIC VALVE

NORMAL STRUCTURE AND FUNCTION

The concept that there is a ring or annulus to which the cusps are attached is often applied to

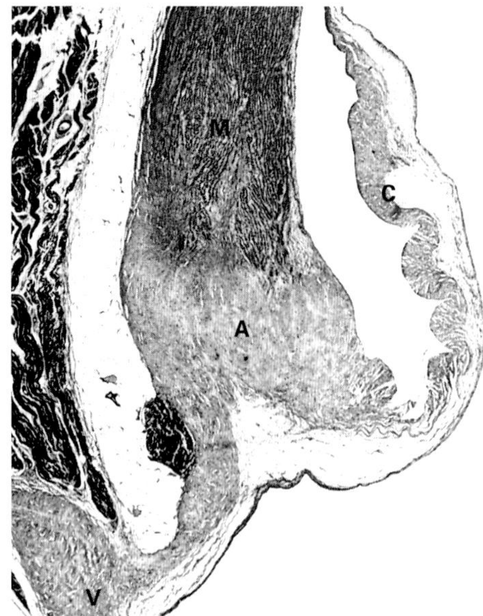

Fig. 6.12 Normal aortic root and valve. The aortic media (M) interdigitates with the fibrous tissue of the aortic valve sleeve (A). This collagenous structure is continuous with the collagenous core of the valve cusp (C). The aortic valve is attached to the fibrous skeleton of the heart and the mitral valve (V).
Trichrome × 6

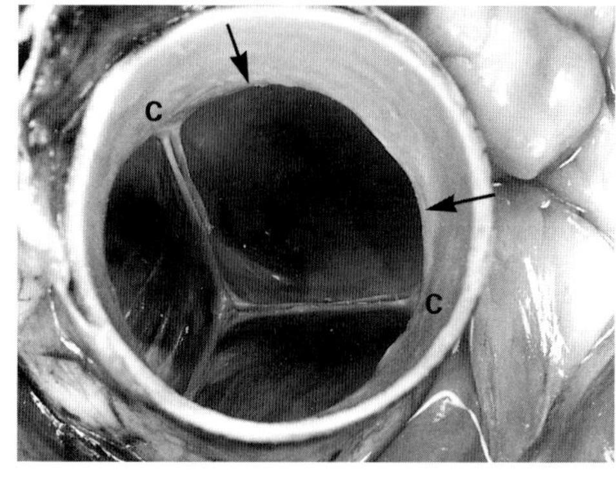

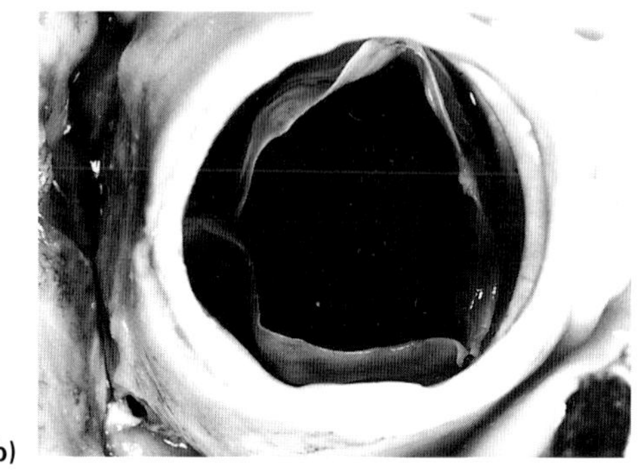

Fig. 6.13 a,b Normal aortic valve. (**a**) The valve is viewed from above in its closed position. The three cusps are approximately equal in size and juxtapose on their ventricular faces. The junction between the aortic valve tube and the aorta is marked by a ridge (arrows) on which the commissures (C) lie. In a normal competent valve the cusps close the whole orifice of the valve. (**b**) In the fully open position normal cusps fold back into their respective sinuses.

valves. In the aortic valve this view is an oversimplification. The aortic valve cusps are contained within a short fibrous tube (Fig. 6.12) which has three points at its upper margin forming a coronet. The cusps meet at the commissures, which are attached to the points of the coronet. Behind each cusp the tube forms the wall of the sinus of Valsalva. The tube is some 1–1.5 cm long and its upper border interdigitates with the media of the aortic root (Fig. 6.12). Its lower border is fused to the base of the mitral valve and the muscular interventricular septum. An increase in the diameter of the upper border of the sleeve is of considerable functional importance because it decreases the degree of cusp abutment; thus mutual cusp support in the closed position is reduced, leading potentially to regurgitation. The boundary between the aorta and the aortic sleeve is marked by a distinct ridge at the level of the commissures (supra-aortic ridge) (Figs 6.13, 6.14). The diameter of the lower border of the sleeve is not important in functional terms but does determine the ring size of any prosthetic valve that has to be surgically inserted.

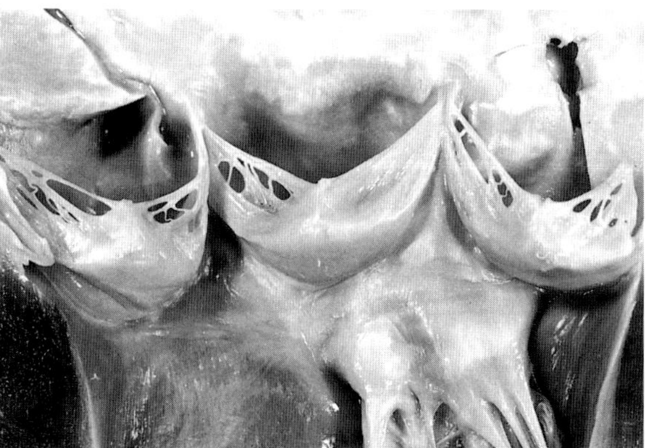

Fig. 6.14 Normal aortic valve. The valve has been opened to show the ventricular faces of the cusps. Each cusp has a central nodule from which ridges pass laterally. These are the apposition lines of the cusp. Above these lines the cusp may be extensively fenestrated without functional abnormality.

When viewed from the aorta in the closed position the cusps are seen to abut over a large proportion of their ventricular faces (Fig. 6.13); this mutual support is vital in maintaining competence. The combined surface area of the cusps exceeds that of the aortic root itself by some 40%. When the ventricular faces of the aortic cusps are inspected each is seen to have a nodule at the centre point of the free edge (noduli Arantii). From this nodule a ridge extends laterally in each direction. This ridge marks the apposition line of the cusps. Above this ridge the cusp tissue separates sinus from sinus, not sinus from ventricle, in the closed position. There are often fenestrations in this lunular area (Fig. 6.14) and they must not be mistaken for clinically significant perforations through the cusp body. Perforations through the cusp body are always pathological, and lead to regurgitation. The fibrous tissue of the lunular area of the cusps has a role in supporting the main body of the cusp in the closed position.

In normal aortic valves the cusps are freely mobile and fold back into the sinus during each ventricular ejection.

MECHANICAL AND AGE-RELATED AORTIC VALVE CHANGES

With increasing age the central nodule and the apposition lines of the cusps become accentuated as a result of proliferation of fibrous tissue on the ventricular aspect of the cusp. This is a response to constant mechanical impact over years. Constant mechanical flexion of the connective tissue in the cusp fibrosa also leads to calcification. This calcification (Fig. 6.15) occurs in a C-shaped band at the point of maximal cusp flexion. Together these age/mechanically-related changes produce what is known as aortic valve sclerosis in older subjects. The changes are responsible for the mid-systolic ejection murmur so common in older people, reflecting the slight rigidity of the cusps, which fail to fold back completely into the sinuses of Valsalva. Minor degrees of calcification do not produce a significant pressure gradient in life across the outflow tract of the left ventricle but more severe degrees are an important cause of stenosis in patients over 65 years of age.

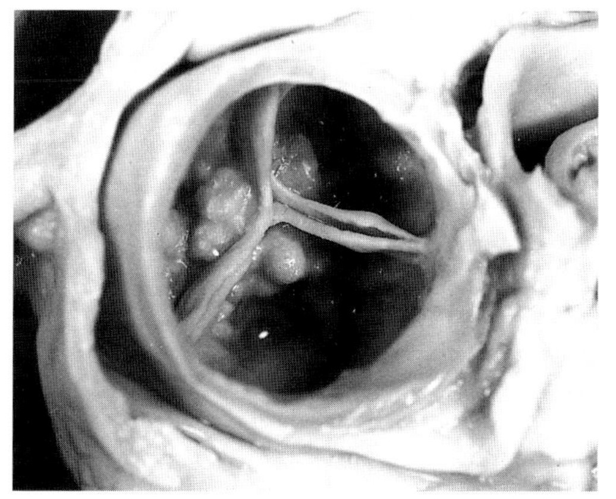

Fig. 6.15 Age-related aortic valve calcification. Viewed from the aorta the valve is tricuspid without commissural fusion. Each cusp has nodules of calcium projecting into the sinus.

VARIATION IN AORTIC VALVE STRUCTURE

The ideal normal aortic valve has three cusps of equal size; the closure lines are symmetric and each cusp abuts to the same degree. In reality many tricuspid aortic valves show some inequality in cusp size and in consequence the closure lines are not symmetrical.[6] Modern methods of detecting aortic regurgitation in life using Doppler ultrasound confirm that in the normal population trivial degrees of aortic regurgitation are not uncommon and are probably due to these minor variations in aortic cusp morphology.

A significant proportion of normal subjects have a minor congenital abnormality in that there are two (Figs 6.16, 6.17) rather than three aortic cusps. The frequency reported is around 1–2% of the general population. There is a considerable morphological spectrum within bicuspid aortic valves.[7] At one extreme the two cusps are equal in size and each appears to have a normal cusp shape. At the other extreme one cusp is much larger than the other and has a deeply indented free edge forming a bilobed cusp. This notch is often associated with a ridge running across the aortic aspect of the cusp to the sinus. Such ridges, or raphes, are thought to represent a rudimentary malformed commissure. Occasional bicuspid

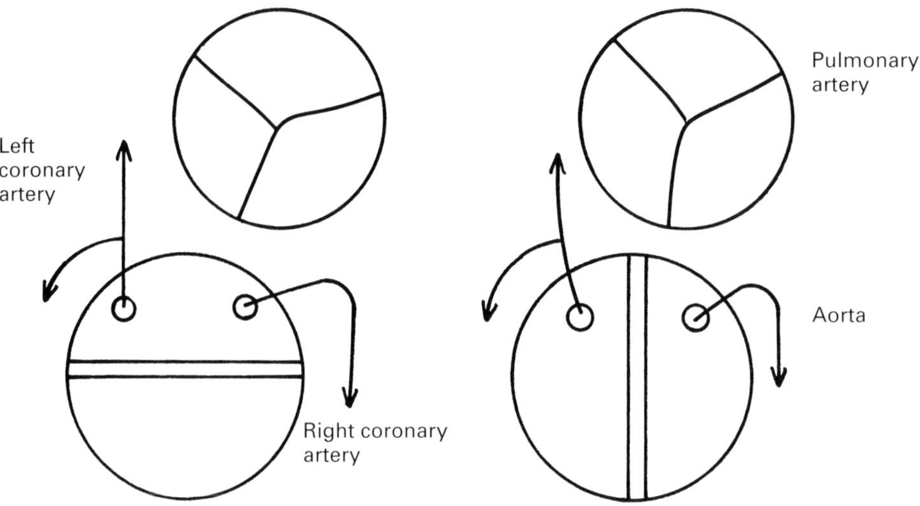

Fig. 6.16 Variants of bicuspid aortic valves. The two variants of coronary artery anatomy in relation to the cusps are shown. The relative proportion of each type is very variable in different reported series.

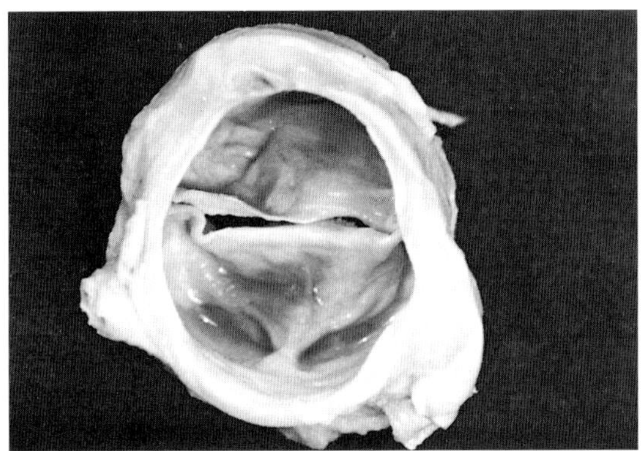

Fig. 6.17 Bicuspid aortic valve. This bicuspid valve has not undergone calcification, has two cusps of approximately equal size and has a small raphe. It was an incidental finding at autopsy.

valves have a discrete fibrous chord running from the indented free edge to the aortic wall; such chords support the cusp in the closed position. Bicuspid valves are strongly associated with aortic coarctation, being found in between 40% and 50% of cases.[8] The coronary arteries may both arise from an anterior sinus or from a right and left sinus. There is work suggesting that valves which are genuinely genetic have two interleaflet triangles. In adults it is more common to find three interleaflet triangles with bicuspid valves, suggesting that in utero either the right and left coronary cusps fused or the right or left fused with the non-coronary cusp after the formation of the commissures. They are in fact abnormalities acquired in utero.[9]

Quadricuspid aortic valves are rare (< 1/1000) but subject to the same variation in cusp structure as bicuspid valves.[10] As far back as Leonardo da Vinci the efficiency of the aortic valve with regard to bicuspid, tricuspid and quadricuspid designs has been considered. The tricuspid design is the most efficient functionally. Subjects with bicuspid and quadricuspid valves, therefore, although having no functional abnormality at birth, are at an increased risk of developing further abnormal valve function in later life.

AORTIC VALVE STENOSIS

When examining a heart with aortic stenosis at autopsy the valve should be kept intact and should be viewed from above. The valve can be dissected out from the heart intact and retained if need be. In such specimens the degree of obstruction can be assessed and the cause of the stenosis can be ascertained by noting the number of cusps, their shape, the shape of the residual opening and the presence of calcification (Fig. 6.18).

The commonest cause of isolated aortic stenosis

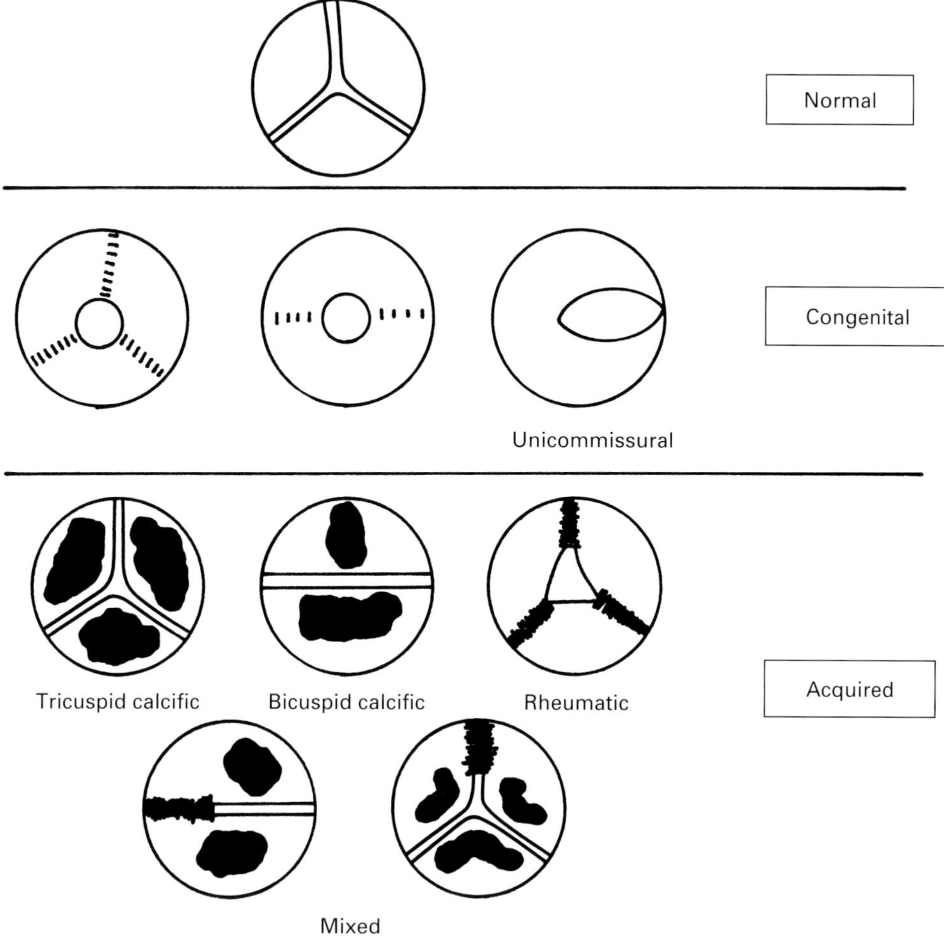

Fig. 6.18 Different types of aortic valve stenosis

in adults is calcification of a bicuspid valve.[11,12] This applies in all geographic populations irrespective of the frequency of acute rheumatic fever because rheumatic disease more usually causes mixed rather than isolated valve lesions. Calcification develops in the cusps by around the age of 30 and as it progresses leads to increasing cusp rigidity, with stenosis developing at any age from 35 to over 80. The majority of cases become symptomatic in the age range 45–60. The best terminology for the condition is calcific bicuspid aortic stenosis.

Even when calcification is advanced in bicuspid valves it is usually possible to see that the valve opening is essentially transverse. Fusion of the two commissures does not occur with pure bicuspid calcific aortic stenosis. The calcification develops as linear deposits and nodules within the valve fibrosa and tends to protrude out into the sinus. Ulceration and thrombosis on the aortic surface of the nodules is common. Bicuspid valves which have a well defined raphe in the larger cusp tend to calcify early and a bar of calcification in the raphe holds the cusp out into the outflow tract, causing obstruction (Fig. 6.19). In the advanced stages both cusps may become totally calcified and replaced by nodules of calcium (Figs 6.20, 6.21). The degree of left ven-

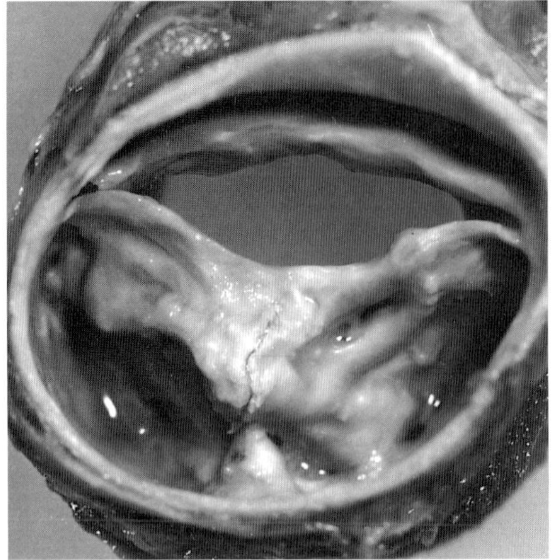

Fig. 6.19 Bicuspid calcific aortic valve stenosis. There is heavy calcification in the raphe of one cusp. This cusp is held across the outflow while the other cusp remains mobile. The valve opening is transverse and oval in shape.

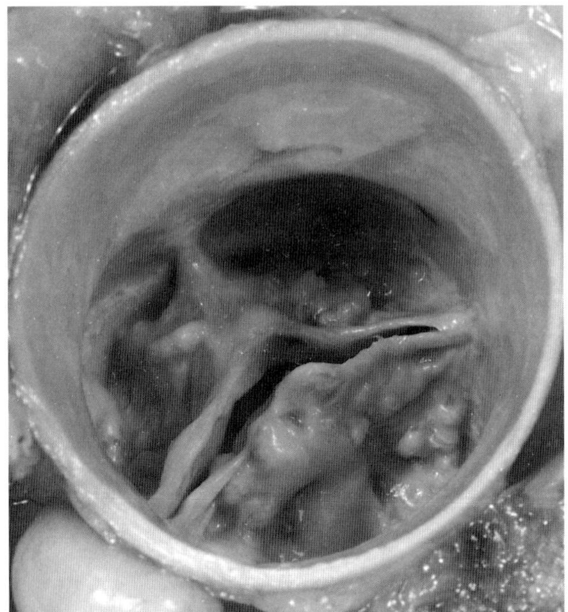

Fig. 6.20 Bicuspid calcific aortic valve stenosis. There is heavy calcification in both cusps, with the opening being a transverse slit.

tricular outflow obstruction in bicuspid valves relates directly to the amount of calcification.

The calcification is of the dystrophic type and the valve cusps are usually not vascularised. With

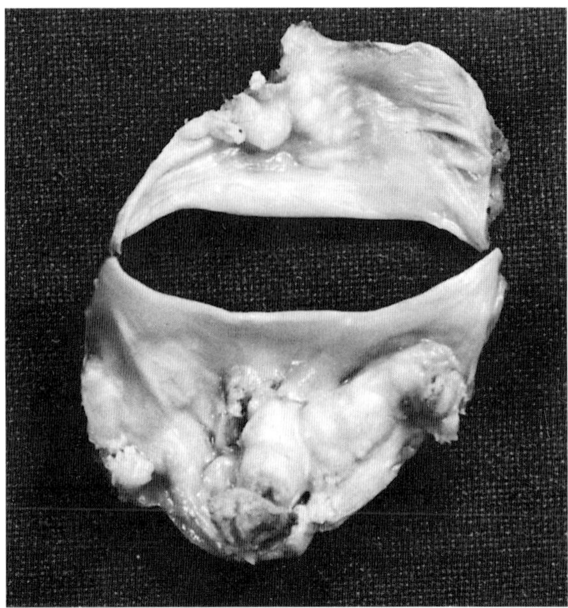

Fig. 6.21 Bicuspid calcific aortic valve stenosis — surgical specimen. In such surgical excisions the cusps can often be aligned in the position they occupied in life to illustrate the transverse opening. Both cusps are calcified. There is no fusion of the commissures.

advanced calcification some chronic inflammatory cells may be found, however, and the centre of the nodules often undergoes eosinophilic degeneration and cavitation. Some vascularisation from the base may occur in such valves, as may a giant cell response to the calcium.

Rheumatic aortic valve stenosis is characterised by symmetric fusion of all three commissures, producing a central triangular valve orifice (Fig. 6.22). While stenosis may be the dominant functional abnormality, rheumatic aortic valves often have a degree of concomitant regurgitation. Cusp calcification may be superimposed on the underlying rheumatic process. As an isolated entity rheumatic aortic valve disease is rare, mitral disease usually being present also.

The third cause of isolated aortic valve stenosis is cusp calcification developing in a tricuspid aortic valve (Fig. 6.23). With age many aortic valve cusps undergo sclerosis; in the extreme expression of this process sufficient calcium accumulates to cause cusp rigidity and stenosis. The condition is often called 'senile' tricuspid calcific aortic valve stenosis, highlighting the fact that symptoms are rare before 75 years of age. In

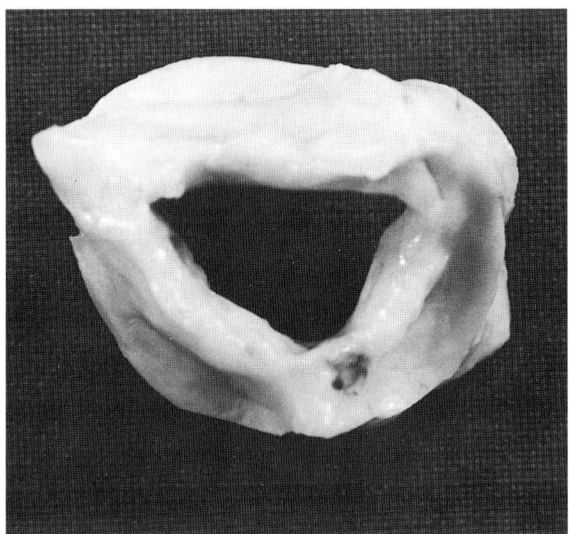

Fig. 6.22 Rheumatic aortic stenosis – surgical excision. There are three valve cusps, all reduced in area and fused at the commissures to produce a triangular orifice.

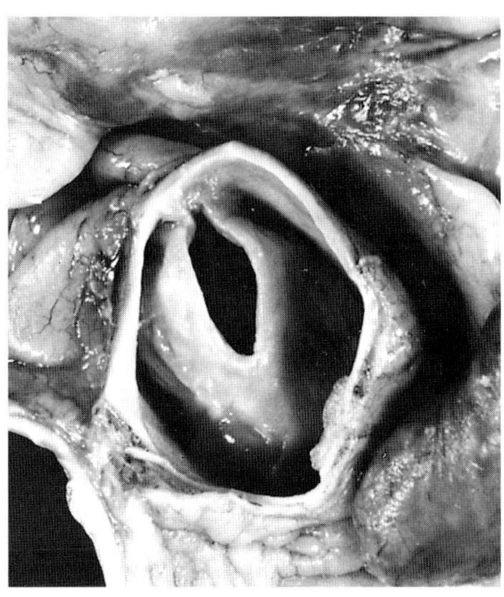

Fig. 6.24 Uncommissural congenital aortic valve stenosis. Viewed from the aortic aspect the orifice is eccentric and tear-drop in shape, taking origin from the only commissure present.

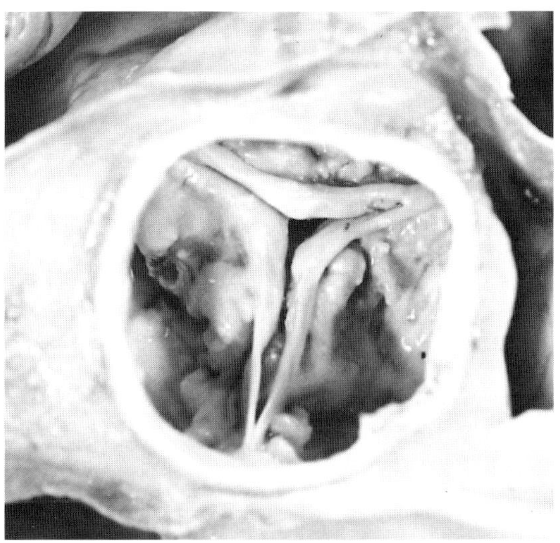

Fig. 6.23 Tricuspid calcific aortic valve stenosis. All three cusps contain nodules of calcium. There is no commissural fusion.

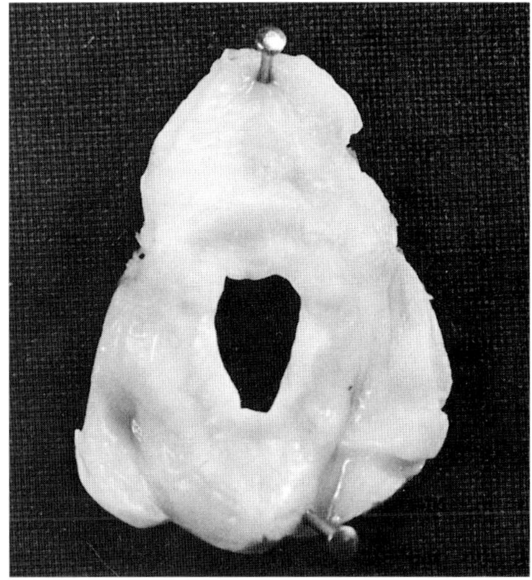

Fig. 6.25 Congenital aortic valve stenosis. The valve viewed from above is a fibrous diaphragm with a central aperture. There is a hint of commissural formation in the presence of ridges but no clear separation into cusps exists.

reality the age distribution curves of bicuspid and tricuspid aortic valve stenosis overlap in the age range 60–80 and the descriptive names of the valve morphology are best. The age-related calcification in tricuspid aortic valves is more symmetric and regular than that which occurs in bicuspid valves. The calcification develops as C-shaped masses along the line of maximum cusp flexion. In common with bicuspid aortic valves the calcium bulges out from the aortic face of the valve into the sinus, and ulceration with overlying thrombus formation may occur.

All three conditions described so far cause isolated aortic stenosis in adult life and are acquired, although the calcification in the bicuspid valve is based on a congenital anomaly which initially causes no symptoms.

The term congenital aortic valve stenosis is applied when left ventricular outflow obstruction is present at or shortly after birth. A range of malformed valves are responsible in which commissural and cusp formation is defective. In so-called unicommissural valves (Fig. 6.24) there is a fibrous diaphragm with an eccentric elliptical orifice.[13] Other valves have a transverse orifice or are a diaphragm with a central hole (Fig. 6.25). In aortic valve dysplasia the cusps are represented by nodular masses of proliferating fibroblasts without any attempt to form normal cusp structure. Many of these conditions cause severe obstruction early in life or in utero and are associated with other cardiac abnormalities such as left ventricular hypoplasia and endocardial fibroelastosis. Unicommissural valves in particular are, however, sometimes encountered in young adults with isolated aortic stenosis.

The majority of aortic valves with stenosis can be fitted into the categories described. A small proportion fall into a 'mixed' category.[14] In one form there is fusion of one commissure in what appears to have been originally a tricuspid valve (Fig. 6.26). There may be association with calcification in one or more cusps. The pathogenesis of such valve lesions is uncertain. Commissural fusion is the hallmark of inflammatory disease and if there is associated mitral disease the aortic valve can be confidently ascribed to a previous valvulitis, most probably rheumatic in origin. Many valves of this type, however, occur in isolation. They have been described as pseudobicuspid aortic valve stenosis. As this name implies, the asymmetric commissural fusion leaves a valve that behaves as if it were bicuspid in the context of developing calcification. In practise the distinction between a true congenital bicuspid valve with a deep cleft in the free edge and the acquired bicuspid valve is far from easy. In the former the commissure failed to divide or become fused in utero, in the latter the commissure became fused in adult life. A useful guide is whether both cusp edges can be traced up to the commissure. If they can, the lesion is acquired. Some of these valves would, however, be classified differently by equally experienced pathologists.

A second form of mixed stenosis is bicuspid valves in which there is additional commissural fusion (Fig. 6.27). These can be associated with mitral disease but even when they are not the assumption is made that they represent previous rheumatic disease.[15]

Demographics of isolated aortic valve stenosis

In 465 valves removed surgically at St Georges Hospital over a ten year period 63.7% were bicuspid, 26.9% tricuspid and 5.3% rheumatic. The male/female ratio for bicuspid valves was 1.9 for tricuspid valves 0.8. The mean age for bicuspid valves was 64.9 (31–93) for tricuspid

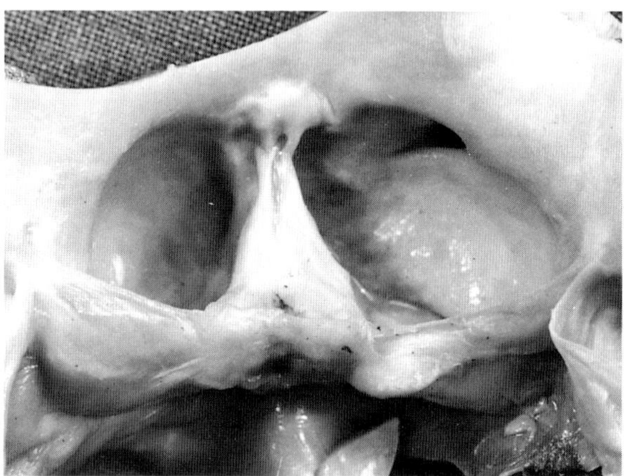

Fig. 6.26 Mixed aortic valve stenosis. One commissure only shows fusion and the edge of each cusp can be traced up to the aortic wall, suggesting this was acquired in adult life.

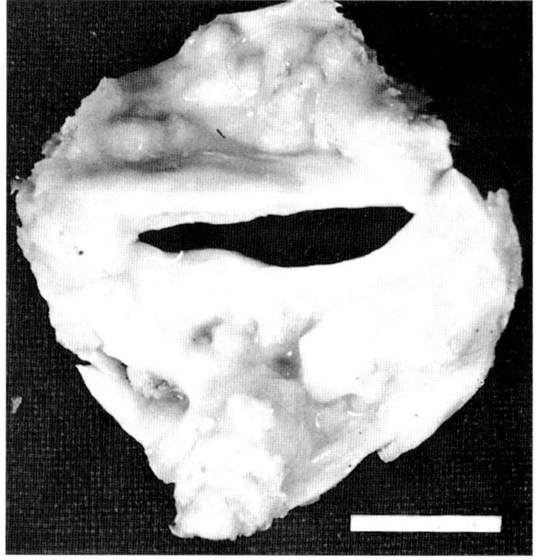

Fig. 6.27 Mixed aortic valve stenosis. The valve is bicuspid but there is fusion of both commissures.

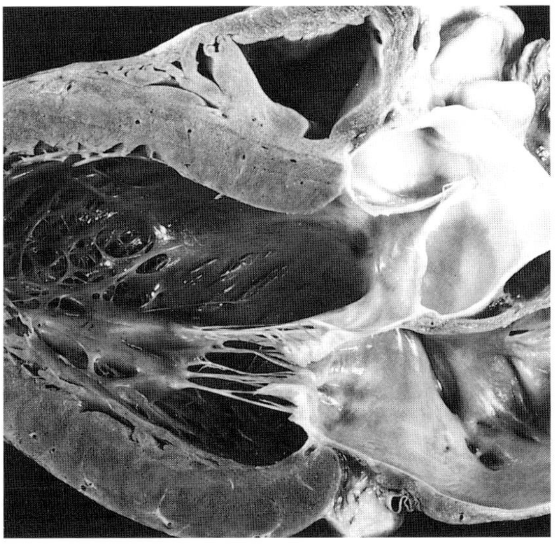

a)

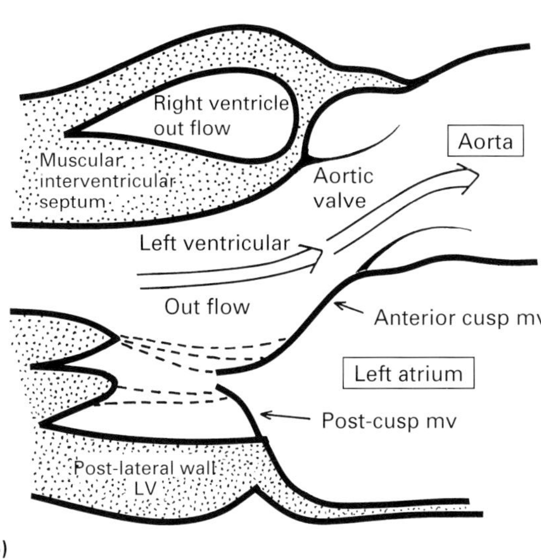

b)

Fig. 6.28 a,b The normal left ventricular outflow. It has three components. Below the valve the outflow tract is bordered by the anterior cusp of the mitral valve and by the muscular interventricular septum. The sinus and valve cusps are the middle component, while above the valve there is the aorta itself.

valves 73.4 (55–95) emphasising the overlapping age range reported previously (ref 11). Coronary artery grafts were needed twice as frequently (22.3% v 44.8%) in tricuspid valves. The frequency of concomittant atherosclerosis in the coronary arteries and the presence of macrophages producing osteopontin in cusp tissue suggests hyperlipidaemia may enhance cusp calcification. Hypercalcaemia is known to produce tricuspid aortic stenosis in chronic renal failure. Enhanced calcium mobilisation due to osteoporosis has been postulated to cause the female propensity to tricuspid calcific stenosis in the absence of high serum calcium levels.

Supra- and subaortic stenosis

The anatomy of the left ventricular outflow tract is best appreciated in long axis sections (Fig. 6.28). It can be seen that there is a subvalve component bound by the anterior cusp of the mitral valve and the muscular interventricular septum, a valve component at the level of the cusps and a supravalve component comprising the root of the aorta. Obstruction can occur at any of the three levels (Fig. 6.29) and has an identical effect on left ventricular function. Valvar stenosis is by far the most common. The other two, while not strictly valvar, are considered here because of their functional comparability with valvar stenosis.

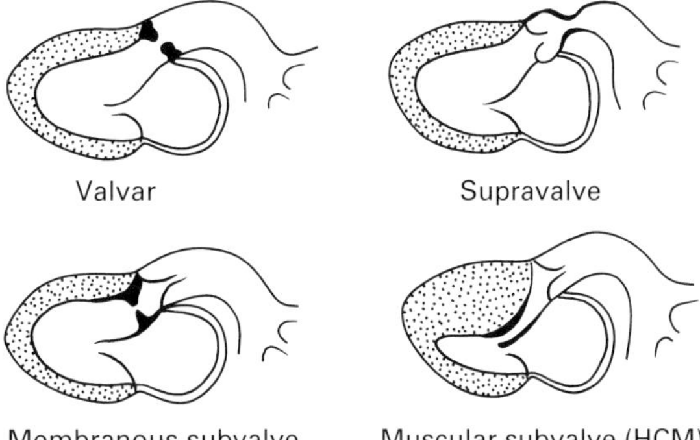

Fig. 6.29 Diagram of sites of LV outflow obstruction

Subaortic stenosis

One form of subaortic stenosis is caused by a congenital discrete fibrous membrane, another by excess myocardial muscle in the upper ventricular septum. There is, however, a spectrum between these two conditions and the matter is further complicated by the development of subaortic endocardial lesions in hypertrophic cardiomyopathy (Chapter 5).

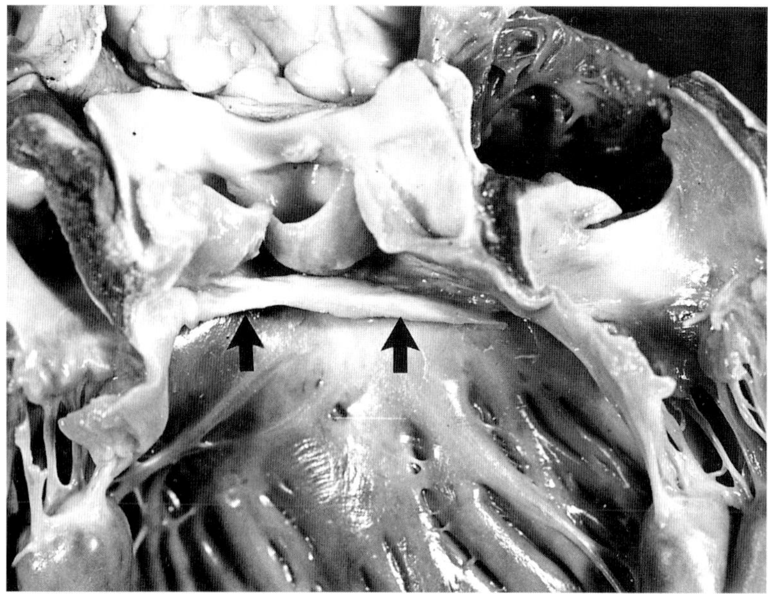

Fig. 6.30 Membranous subaortic stenosis. A fibrous shelf passes from the base of the mitral valve across the interventricular septum below the aortic valve (arrows).

Discrete membranous sub-aortic stenosis. This condition is more common in males and forms about 10% of congenital aortic stenosis, i.e. obstruction present at birth. A white fibrous membrane a few millimetres thick runs from the anterior cusp of the mitral valve on to the interventricular septum just below its membranous portion (Fig. 6.30). The membrane may be crescentic in shape or form a collar around the whole outflow tract, being a diaphragm with a central hole. Material from these membranes is usually seen by pathologists after surgical excision. The membrane consists of fibrous tissue with collagen, elastin and smooth muscle cells but is usually avascular. It appears to be formed within the endocardium rather than just being superimposed on normal underlying endocardium. Membranous subaortic lesions are usually excised in early life. Examples of the crescentic form not causing significant obstruction are occasionally found coincidentally at autopsy.

Muscular subaortic stenosis. There is a major difficulty both clinically and pathologically in distinguishing between muscle hypertrophy in the upper septum with some superimposed endocardial thickening occurring as a congenital defect and hypertrophic cardiomyopathy. Both cause the upper septum to bulge out into the outflow tract below the valve. In general, hypertrophic cardiomyopathy does not present until adolescence (Chapter 5) and muscular subaortic stenosis in infants is probably a developmental abnormality

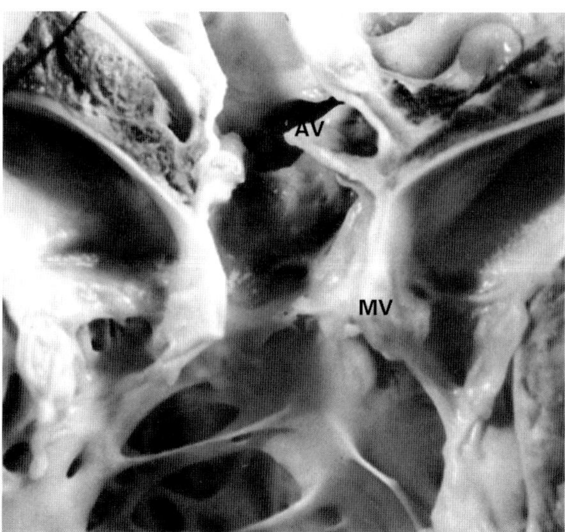

Fig. 6.31 Tunnel subaortic stenosis. Beneath the aortic valve (AV) there is a narrow tunnel formed in part by muscle bundles and in part by fibrous tissue which distorts and incorporates the anterior cusp of the mitral valve (MV).

analogous to the condition found more commonly in the right ventricular infundibulum. The muscle bulge may be quite discrete or form a long tunnel beneath the valve. Macroscopically, muscle bundles and an increase in fibrosis with endocardial thickening form a tunnel beneath the aortic valve (Fig. 6.31). The histological picture mimics true hypertrophic cardiomyopathy in that fibrosis and hypertrophic cardiac muscle are mixed in a disorganised way. It may be impossible to separate the two conditions in material reamed out from the outflow to surgically relieve obstruction. The clinical history, the age of the subject and gene analysis are better ways of making the distinction.

Supra-aortic stenosis

This condition is inherited as an autosomal dominant condition, although sporadic cases due either to new mutations or to very variable degrees of phenotypic expression in the family are common. The aortic lesion may be a discrete waist in the whole aortic wall just above the supra-aortic ridge (Fig. 6.32), a simple fibrous diaphragm on the intima or a long tubular section of hypoplasia. In the last instance there may be discontinuous segments of similar hypoplasia in other parts of the aorta or pulmonary arteries. Proximal to the obstruction the aorta dilates, accentuating an hourglass appearance. The coronary arteries also dilate and become tortuous. Abnormal flow across the aortic valve and turbulence in the sinuses of Valsalva often lead to sclerosis of the valve cusps, sometimes adding a component of valve obstruction.

It is often difficult clinically both to gauge the exact degree of obstruction and if it is haemodynamically significant to decide what to do surgically. Very discrete lesions can be excised but the commonest hourglass type is just above the valve and may necessitate replacement of the whole aortic root with reimplantation of the coronary arteries into a graft. Surgical replacement is made even more difficult by the fact that the aortic wall disease is seldom confined to the apparent area of stenosis. Even in cases without apparent valve obstruction sudden death is a risk in both adolescents and adults. The striking histological feature in the aortic wall is extreme disorganisation of the normal regular arrangement (Fig. 6.33) of the elastic lamina and layers of smooth muscle cells in the media. This higgledy-piggledy arrangement may be confined to short segments or involve virtually the whole aorta. A proportion of cases of supra-aortic stenosis are associated with characteristic facies, minor mental retardation and hypercalcaemia (Williams's syndrome). Such patients often have

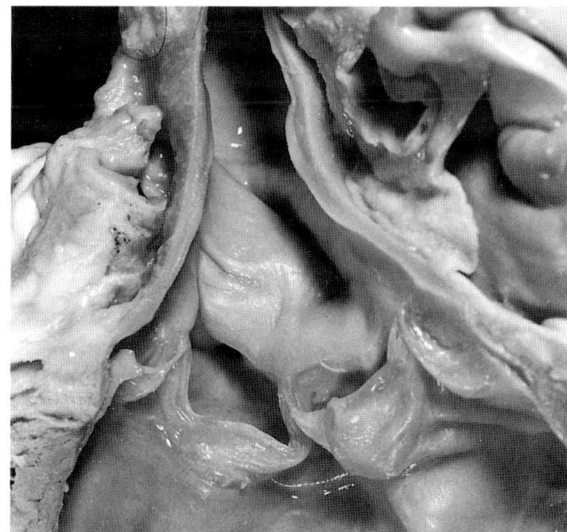

Fig. 6.32 Supra-aortic stenosis. There is a constriction of the aorta with a thick wall immediately above the valve.

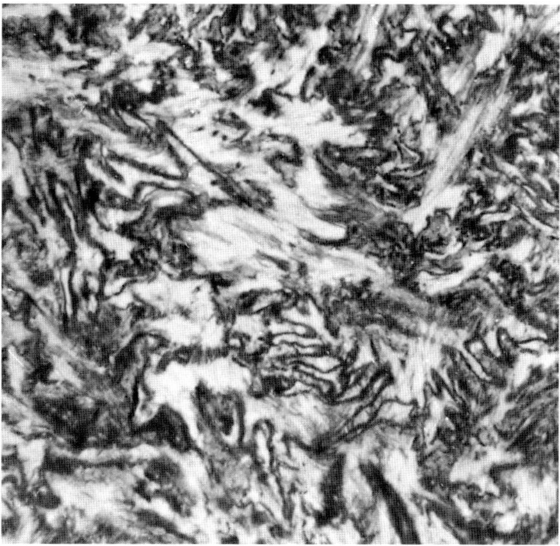

Fig. 6.33 Aortic media in supra-aortic stenosis. The medial elastic tissue, instead of being in parallel arrays, is disorganised and arranged in a criss-cross manner. EVG × 165

more widespread arterial disease, whereas non-familial isolated supra-aortic stenosis is more restricted to the ascending aorta. No linkage or genetic data exist on the families with fully expressed Williams's disease but linkage to a site near the elastin gene on chromosome 7[16] has been found in families with aortic lesions as the sole manifestation.

Angiodysplasia in aortic valve stenosis

Recurrent gastrointestinal bleeding is a feature of a small minority of patients with aortic valve stenosis. The cause appears to be small arterio-venous malformations in the mucosa, particularly of the stomach. The exact relation of these gastric mucosal lesions to aortic stenosis is unknown but valve replacement alleviates the bleeding.[17] The lack of any mechanistic explanation for the association has led to doubts over its existence[18] and a suggestion that the vascular lesions are an age-related phenomenon and that, this being so, it is fortuitously associated with aortic valve sclerosis.

The coronary arteries in aortic valve stenosis

In bicuspid aortic valves the coronary arteries more frequently show a left dominant pattern and the orifices may be higher in the aorta.[19] In common with other conditions causing left ventricular hypertrophy in aortic valve stenosis the lumen of the major epicardial arteries is increased[20] when compared to normal hearts. There are anecdotal suggestions that aortic valve stenosis protects the coronary arteries from atheroma. Clinical experience, however, suggests that patients with bicuspid aortic stenosis may have coronary stenosis. Insertion of coronary bypass grafts at the time of aortic valve surgery is needed in up to 25% of cases. In tricuspid aortic stenosis it is twice as high.

AORTIC VALVE REGURGITATION

Competence in the aortic valve depends on a very critical relation between the total area of the cusps and that of the aortic root. It also depends on the structural integrity of the cusps and their being firmly supported at the commissures. Competence can be demonstrable only if the valve is kept intact and even then is not easy. Perfusion fixation at systemic pressures within the aorta sufficient to close the valve gives the ideal perception of the presence and cause of regurgitation but requires special apparatus and is time-consuming.

With increasing age the ascending aorta dilates and with this the diameter of the upper border of the aortic valve sleeve (supra-aortic ridge) also increases. Potentially this disturbs the critical relation between cusp and root area but remodelling of the cusps occurs and total aortic

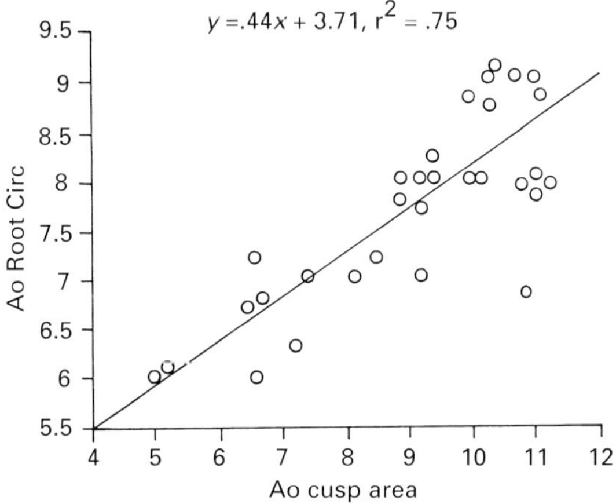

Fig. 6.34 Relation of cusp area and root circumference in normal aortic valves.

Table 6.2 Causes of pure aortic regurgitation

Cusp disease	
Cusp contraction (rheumatic)	
Cusp perforation (infective endocarditis)	
Cusp tears (trauma)	
Bicuspid valve	
Myxoid change in cusp	
Rheumatoid nodules in cusp	
Aortic root disease	
Aortitis	Syphilis HLA-B27-related disease Giant cell aortitis Rheumatoid
Non-inflammatory (ectasia aortic root)	Marfan's syndrome Other genetic defects in connective tissue synthesis Idiopathic Bicuspid valve
Loss of cusp support (aortic intimal tear)	Marfan's syndrome Dissection Trauma

cusp area increases (Fig. 6.34). There will, however, be a point at which the aortic root area increases either rapidly or to a degree for which cusp remodelling cannot compensate. The degree to which the cusps abut on their ventricular faces is reduced. Ultimately one cusp slips under the edge of the others in diastole, and regurgitation occurs. The pathological processes potentially causing aortic regurgitation are shown in Table 6.2.

Individual causes of aortic regurgitation — cusp abnormalities

Rheumatic disease

The simplest cause of aortic regurgitation is rheumatic disease. In its pure form there is no commissural fusion and therefore no stenosis. Each cusp is reduced in area and thickened; in extreme cases the cusps are represented by fibrous ridges. Such small immobile cusps cannot close and cover even an aortic root of normal dimensions (Fig. 6.11).

Rheumatoid disease occasionally involves the aortic valve, producing dense fibrous thickening of one or more cusps.[21] Histological examination shows the typical palisaded granulomas. The valve lesions are often misdiagnosed as rheumatic until histology is performed.

Bacterial endocarditis

Another very simple cause of pure regurgitation, occurring in both bicuspid and tricuspid aortic valves, is perforation through the body of a cusp following bacterial endocarditis (Fig. 6.35). Such perforations allow direct communication between the aortic root and left ventricular cavity. In the

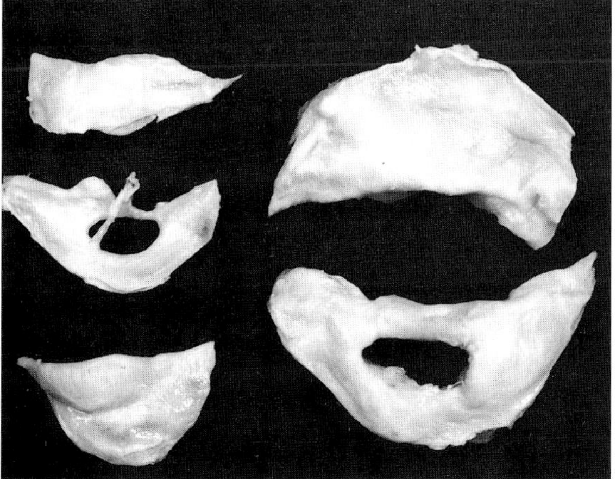

Fig. 6.35 Aortic regurgitation — post bacterial endocarditis. In each case, one with a bicuspid the other with a tricuspid valve, there are defects with smooth edges through the centre of a cusp.

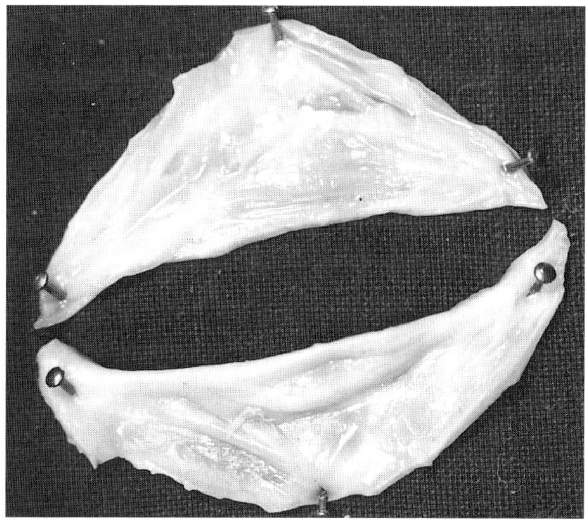

Fig. 6.36 Aortic regurgitation due to a bicuspid aortic valve. One cusp is larger than the other but neither has a raphe or notch in the free edge. The edge of the more elongated cusp has a linear thickening as a consequence of regurgitant flow. No calcification or commissural fusion is present.

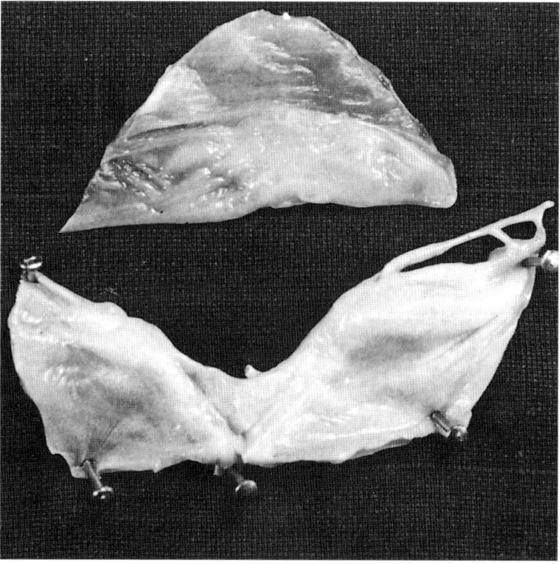

Fig. 6.37 Aortic regurgitation due to a bicuspid aortic valve. There are two cusps. The larger has a deep notch in its free edge. This valve represents the extreme end of the range of bicuspid valves. The notch represents the site of abortive commissure formation.

acute phase the hole is surrounded by vegetations; less commonly destruction of the free edge of the cusp has occurred. In the healing phase considerable fibrosis and thickening of the cusps occur as vegetations are organised leaving a hole with clean-cut, smooth edges. Fibrotic changes further diminish cusp mobility and normal apposition.

Bicuspid aortic valves

The predominant risk for an individual with a bicuspid aortic valve is that of developing isolated aortic stenosis or bacterial endocarditis. A minority of subjects, however, develop pure aortic regurgitation.[22–24] The risk is greatest in those valves in which there is considerable inequality in cusp size and those in which there is a cleft in the free edge of the larger cusp (Figs 6.36, 6.37). Such cusps seem inherently unable to support each other adequately in the closed position, allowing the free edge of one to slip under the other. In a small minority of bicuspid valves the free edge of the large cusp depends for its support on a fibrous chord joined to the aorta. Spontaneous rupture of this chord may precipitate sudden regurgitation (Fig. 6.38).

A further factor enhancing the risk of aortic regurgitation is an association of enlargement of the root of the aorta with bicuspid aortic valves. Any such dilatation will further jeopardise the inherent need of the two cusps to abut and support each other. The association of aortic root dilatation with bicuspid valves is thought to be a coexisting primary defect in the aortic media. Dilatation precedes the development of regurgitation rather than being secondary to it. Supporting evidence for this comes from the increased risk of aortic dissection in subjects with bicuspid aortic valves.[25]

Myxoid change in aortic valve cusps

Some surgical series of cases of aortic regurgitation record a significant number of cases

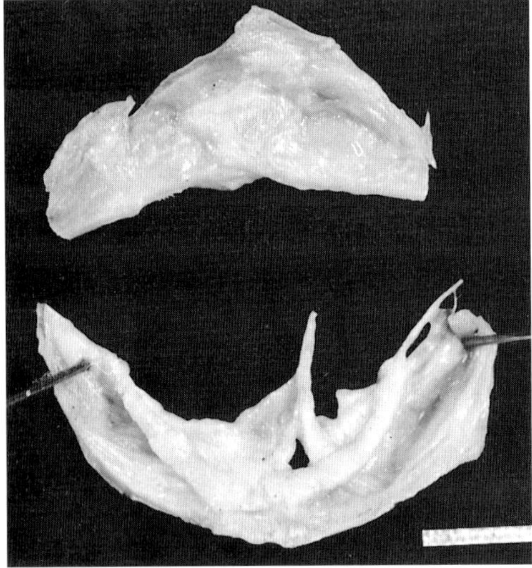

Fig. 6.38 Aortic regurgitation due to a bicuspid aortic valve. The free edge of the larger cusp was supported by a fibrous chord attached to the aorta. This broke, leading to sudden aortic regurgitation and emergency surgery.

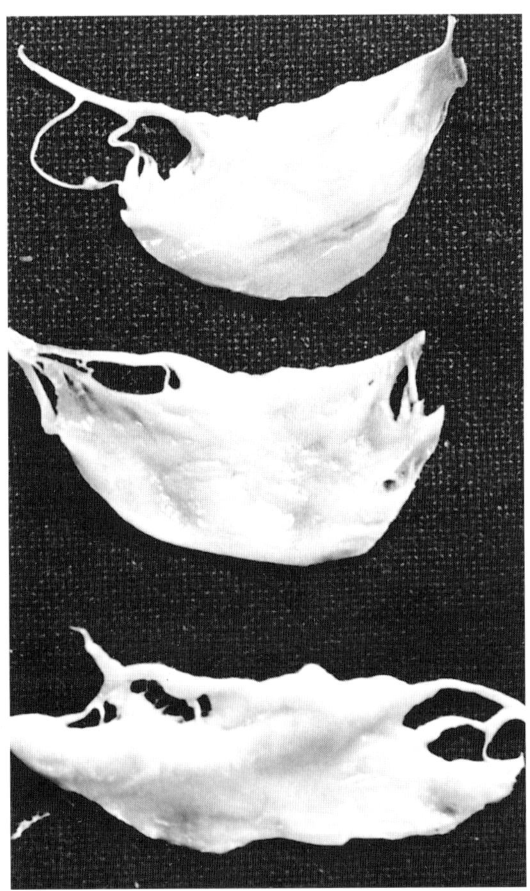

Fig. 6.39 Myxoid aortic cusps and aortic regurgitation. There are three cusps; all are thickened but felt soft to the touch. The lunular area of the cusp is expanded and stretched, producing chord-like structures. The aortic root was normal in size. Reproduced from Pathology of Cardiac Valves (1980) with permission of M. J. Davies and publishers Butterworth–Heinemann Ltd.

as being due to myxomatous degeneration with destruction of the valve fibrosa leading to cusp expansion. The process is regarded as being an analogue to the floppy mitral valve. Using the criteria of more than 50% of the valve showing excess acid mucopolysaccharide deposition, 12 of 37 (33%)[26] and 13 of 55 (24%)[27] of cases of surgical replacement of the valve for pure aortic regurgitation were ascribed to myxomatous valves. Our own experience suggests the condition to be much rarer. The differences in frequency are probably artificial rather than real. It is our belief that the cause of aortic regurgitation can be only ascertained by knowledge of the full constellation of the cusp morphology, echo-measured aortic root diameter at the level of the commissures, and an aortic wall biopsy. When all this data is available the great majority of cases of aortic regurgitation with somewhat stretched cusps have significant root dilatation. Nevertheless an occasional case of expanded myxoid aortic cusps with a normal root does occur (Fig. 6.39).

Individual causes of aortic regurgitation — aortic root abnormalities

Both dilatation and distortion of the aortic root, acting together or separately, will cause regurgitation. The basic cause may be either degenerative non-inflammatory disease or an inflammatory aortitis.

Aortitis

In both syphilis and HLA-B27-related disease there is a florid inflammatory process in the media of the root of the aorta. Both look similar histologically, with a marked adventitial accumulation of lymphocytes and plasma cells; inflammation extends into the media along vasa vasorum which show marked endothelial proliferation and lumen obliteration. Medial elastic and muscle destruction occurs initially within focal areas related to the vasa vasorum but later becomes a uniform destruction of much of the media (Chapter 4).

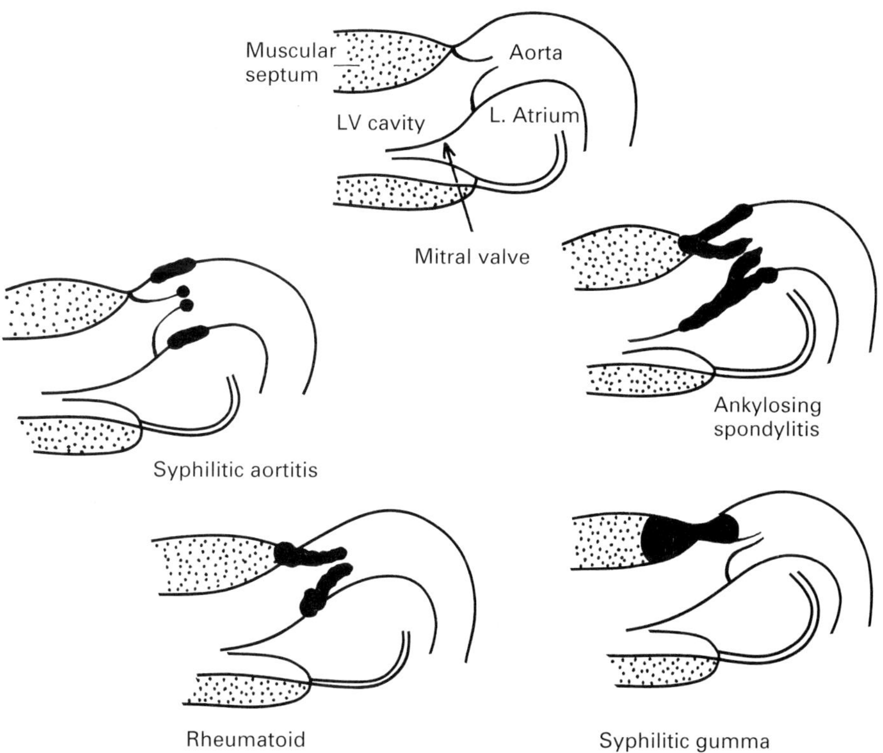

Fig. 6.40 Aortic root involvement in aortitis. The pattern of involvement is shown for syphilis, ankylosing spondylitis and rheumatoid.

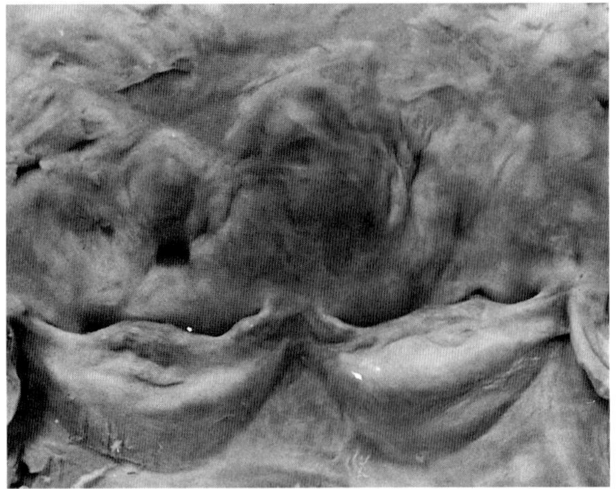

Fig. 6.41 Syphilitic aortic regurgitation. The hallmark of syphilis is separation of the commissures at their insertion into the aortic wall.

Despite the microscopic appearances of luetic and HLA-B27-related aortic disease being so similar the diseases can readily be distinguished by their macroscopic features (Fig. 6.40).

In syphilis the aortic root is moderately dilated, with separation of the commissures. Syphilitic aortitis often occurs in a well-demarcated band confined to the first 4–6 cm of the ascending aorta (Fig. 6.41). In this band the intimal surface, viewed en face, is wrinkled and puckered (tree bark scarring). This appearance has no specificity for any particular form of inflammatory aortitis or indeed for inflammation. An identical appearance is seen following non-inflammatory medial destruction but in this case is more widespread. Syphilis does not involve the aortic valve cusps themselves. The free edges of the cusps may have a linear thickening but this is the ubiquitous response to regurgitant flow rather than having any direct link with syphilis. Syphilis does not involve the base of the anterior cusp of the mitral valve, extend into the upper interventricular septum or involve the atrial septum. The only exception to this rule is if there is gumma formation in the upper interventricular septum (Chapter 4). Syphilitic aortitis may also involve the coronary ostia, leading to their reduction to pinpoint openings.

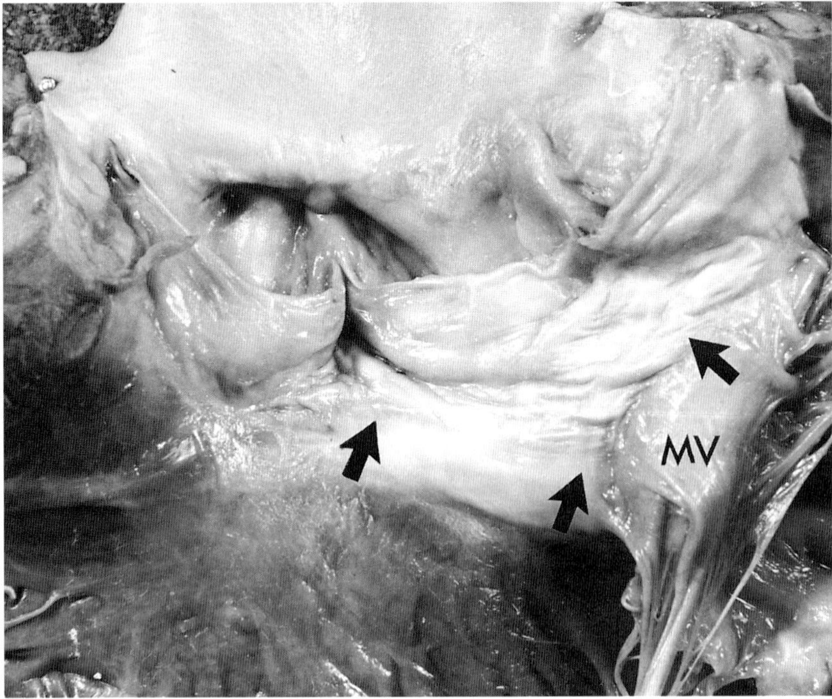

Fig. 6.42 Aortic regurgitation due to ankylosing spondylitis. The whole aortic root, including the sinuses, the base of the mitral valve (MV) and the membranous septum, is thickened and white (arrows). The commissures are stretched and distorted but not separated. Reproduced from Pathology of Cardiac Valves (1980) with permission of M. J. Davies and publishers Butterworth–Heinemann Ltd.

In contrast, in HLA-B27-related aortitis[28,29] the aortic root is less dilated and the commissures are not separated. The aortic root is thickened, with white fibrous tissue extending into the sinuses and on to the bases of the aortic valve cusps (Fig. 6.42). Fibrous thickening extends downward on to the base of the anterior cusp of the mitral valve. Fibrosis and intense chronic inflammation with endarteritis obliterans of small arteries also extend into the atrial septum to involve the atrioventricular node. Heart block with aortic regurgitation is therefore strongly suggestive of HLA-B27-related cardiac disease[29] but does occur with syphilitic gummas, which have a predilection for the upper interventricular septum.

HLA-B27-related cardiac disease may develop in subjects with clinically expressed joint disease of the ankylosing spondylitis type, or precede the appearance of joint disease. Less commonly the cardiac disease occurs in isolation in individuals who are HLA-B27-positive. There is also an association with Reiter's syndrome and psoriasis.[30]

Another form of aortitis, giant cell aortitis (Chapter 4), also causes regurgitation. The aortic root is dilated, with the wall thinned rather than thickened. There is no commissural fusion, cusp involvement or mitral involvement. The characteristic histology is in the media of the ascending aorta. Within the media are flat plates of necrotic smooth muscle and fragmented elastic tissue; at the margins giant cells are applied to the broken elastic tissue. The degree of inflammation in the adventitia is less than that found in the other inflammatory conditions causing regurgitation.

Characteristically, patients with giant cell aortitis are more likely to be female, are elderly and have an increased risk of aortic rupture, either immediately after surgical replacement of the valve or after a long period. These patients can usually be identified by the association of a raised ESR, the characteristic age and gender, the presence of aortic regurgitation and the absence of serological evidence of syphilis or HLA B27 group prior to valve replacement or autopsy.

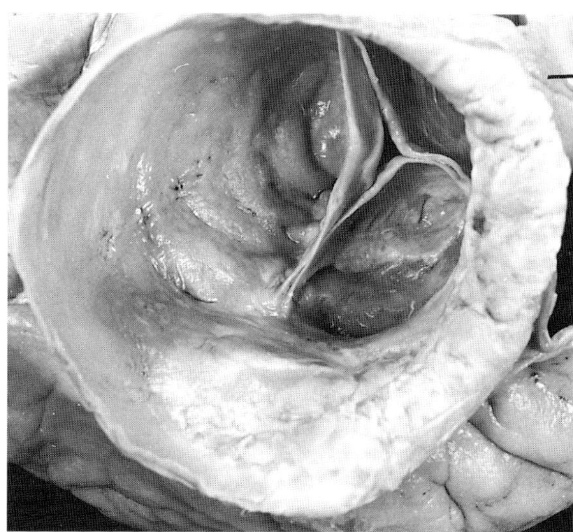

Fig. 6.43 Non-inflammatory aortic root dilatation — aortic regurgitation. The root of the aorta is widened with effacement of the supra-aortic ridge. There is widespread wrinkling and folding of the intima but histology showed no evidence of inflammation. Two cusps have prolapsed beneath the third, leaving a small central defect in the closed valve leading to mild aortic regurgitation.

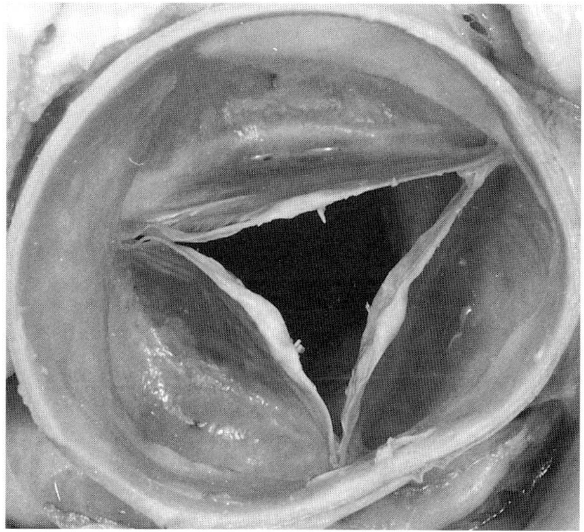

Fig. 6.44 Non-inflammatory aortic root dilatation — severe regurgitation. The aortic root is widened and the supra-aortic ridge is lost. The cusps do not meet in the closed position, leaving a large central aperture. All three cusps have nodular thickening along their free edges as a consequence of regurgitation.

Non-inflammatory aortic root dilatation

The characteristic macroscopic findings are a dilated aortic root and a dilated, thin-walled ascending aorta. Intimal wrinkling may be pronounced or absent. The usual supra-aortic ridge at the level of the commissures is effaced and the whole root is opened out, making it very easy to see the cusps from above (Figs 6.43, 6.44).

When the disease is symmetrical, the cusps fail to meet, leaving a central defect in the closed position. The root involvement, however, is often not symmetrical and the supra-aortic ridge may be lost to a greater degree in one sinus. In such cases the associated cusp may slip beneath its fellow cusps in the closed position, leading to regurgitation. Cusps which prolapse and have regurgitant flow over their edge develop a linear thickening confined to the edge, the cusp body being normal (Fig. 6.45). Histological sections in the long axis of the cusp (Fig. 6.46) show a typical tadpole shape. Non-inflammatory root dilatation is associated with a range of histological abnormalities in the media of the ascending aorta. It seems that the diameter of the upper border of the aortic sleeve is dependent on the media of the root of the aorta being normal rather than on the tissue of the aortic valve itself.

An additional mechanism producing aortic regurgitation in association with root dilatation is elongation of the commissural attachments themselves (Fig. 6.47). The histological changes are very variable and do not have to be very striking. For example, in hypertension there is clinical

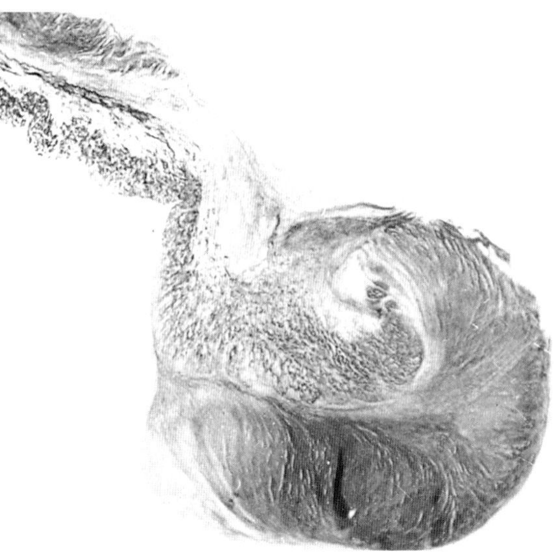

Fig. 6.46 Non-inflammatory aortic regurgitation — cusp morphology. In histological sections taken in the vertical axis the cusp body can be seen to be normal while at the free edge there is a nodule of dense fibrosis superimposed on the underlying valve. There is no vascularisation. This nodular thickening is the result of mechanical injury due to regurgitant flow. Reproduced from Pathology of Cardiac Valves (1980) with permission of M. J. Davies and publishers Butterworth–Heinemann Ltd.

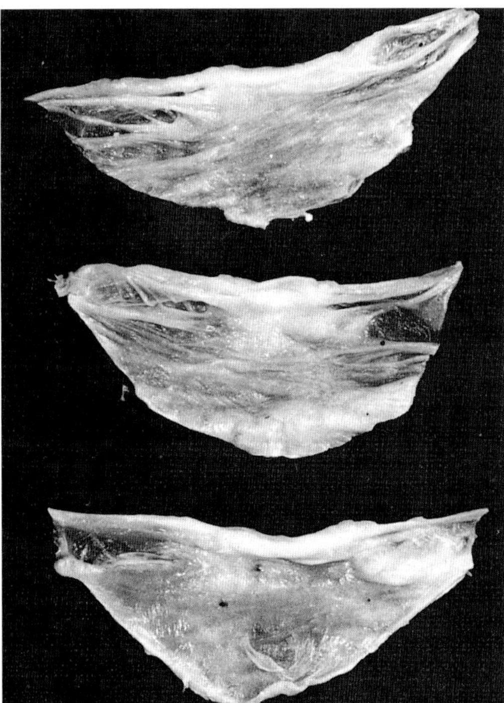

Fig. 6.45 Non-inflammatory aortic root dilatation — surgical replacement for regurgitation. In surgically excised valve cusps it is possible to recognise root dilatation by the normality of the cusps in term of size and by the rolled free edge, indicating regurgitant flow.

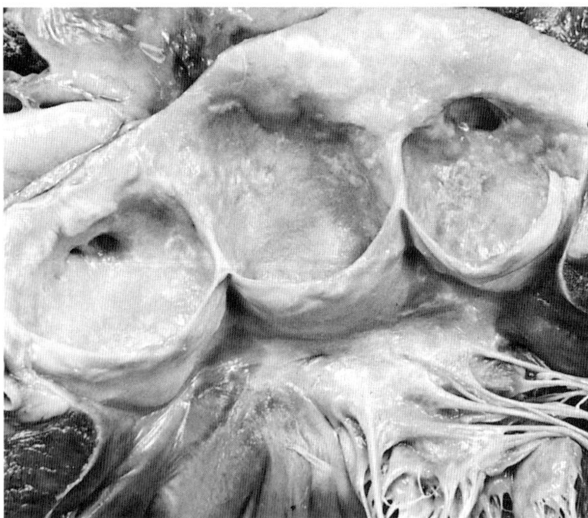

Fig. 6.47 Non-inflammatory aortic regurgitation. The aortic root is increased in size but the commissural attachments are stretched, allowing cusp prolapse. Stretching of the commissural attachments is present in variable degrees in aortic root dilatation and also occurs in old age.

evidence that minor degrees of aortic regurgitation are common. The diameter of the aortic root at the supra-aortic ridge is increased to a modest extent and the media shows some loss of smooth muscle, the elastic laminae becoming straighter and closer together than usual. At the other extreme there is advanced fragmentation and loss of the elastic laminae, with cystic medial change. The medial thickness is drastically reduced.

The terminology of non-inflammatory aortic root dilation is confusing and several names are used. Aortic root dilation is a feature of Marfan's syndrome. Cases of idiopathic root dilatation without any other stigmata of Marfan's have been regarded as a *forme fruste*, i.e. partial phenotypic expression of that disease. There is no genetic study as yet which confirms abnormalities of the fibrillin in the aortic wall. Others use the terms annulo-aortic ectasia,[31] idiopathic medial aortopathy or idiopathic aortic root dilatation.[32] Part of the terminological problem arises from the fact that age-related changes in the aortic media are common and lead to root dilatation.[33] Genetic defects in connective tissue synthesis in the media also lead to root dilatation.

Supra-aortic intimal tears

In dissection of the ascending aorta when the intimal tear is transverse, localised and just above the supra-aortic ridge, prolapse of a portion of aortic wall with an attached commissure leads to aortic incompetence. If the patient survives the cusp may be attached at a lower level permanently, leading to chronic regurgitation. Tears in the ascending aorta that are more superficial and do not cause dissection lead to the cusp becoming permanently attached at a lower level than the other cusps and chronic regurgitation develops (Fig. 6.48). Such partial aortic wall tears can occur in hypertension, in Marfan's disease, in any aortic medial degeneration and after closed chest trauma.[34]

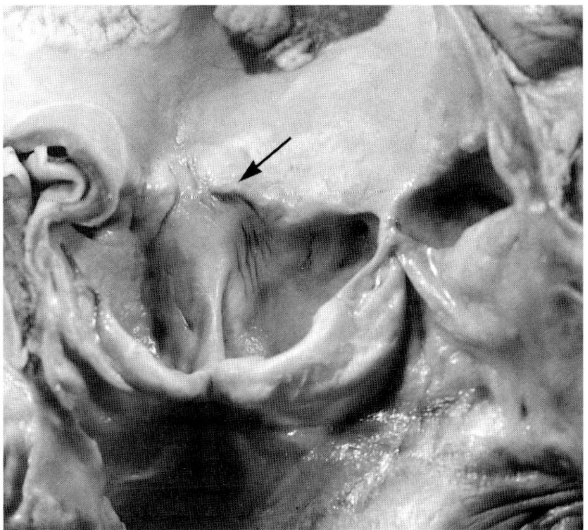

Fig. 6.48 Aortic regurgitation due to old aortic dissection. There is a healed tear (arrow) just above one commissure which has led to downward displacement of the whole commissure and two cusps.

Quantification of cusps and aortic root in regurgitation

In a number of studies the cusp area has been measured and plotted against the area of the aortic root at the level of the commissures (Fig. 6.34). In this way the exact relation of the two parameters can be seen and compared to normal valves. For routine use this method is too tedious. All that can be done is to inspect the valve from above and make a judgement as to whether the cusps will oppose. The presence of nodular thickening on the free edge of one or more cusps is valuable confirmation that regurgitation occurred in life. In a similar manner the presence of a jet lesion, i.e. a patch of localised thickening where regurgitant flow hits the endocardium, on the upper interventricular septum or the ventricular face of the anterior cusp of the mitral valve is confirmation of the presence of regurgitation in life. If the valve ring is opened the only measurement worth making is the circumference of the aortic root at the commissural level. Values of over 11 cm and under 13 cm may be associated with regurgitation; with values above 13 cm regurgitation is almost certain. The most effective way of convincingly demonstrating regurgitation remains to fix the valve shut by perfusion of the ascending aorta with formalin.

MITRAL VALVE

STRUCTURE AND FUNCTION

In their fully open position both mitral and

tricuspid valves have large orifices. The normal open mitral valve has an orifice measuring between 4 and 6 cm^2. When ventricular pressure rises the cusps are lifted to meet and close these orifices (Figs 6.1–6.8). Competence is aided by a reduction in the size of the valve orifices in ventricular systole. The cusps are prevented from being forced into the atria by chordae attached to their free edges. In turn the chordae insert into the papillary muscles, which control both the tension and the position of the cusps as the ventricle changes shape in systole. It is therefore clear that mitral competence is a complex mechanism depending more on active muscle contraction than does the function of the aortic valve. It is accordingly not easy to judge minor degrees of incompetence of the mitral valve at autopsy.

Viewed from above the closed mitral valve forms a flat floor to the left atrium (Fig. 6.49). The majority of this floor is made up of the anterior cusp while the smaller crescentic shaped posterior cusp is often divided into three scallops — lateral, central and medial. In the normal valve the cusps form a flat surface without any bulge into the atria. The cusps abut over their atrial surfaces by up to 0.5 cm in their short axis. The cusps meet at lateral and medial commissures which do not show any fusion.

The anterior cusp of the mitral valve is strikingly larger and thicker than the posterior cusp and hangs into the left ventricle, dividing it into an inflow and outflow portion (Fig. 6.50). The base of the anterior cusp is attached to the aortic valve and the membranous interventricular septum. The shape of the anterior cusp is roughly semicircular while the posterior cusp, if excised, is roughly rectangular in shape.

The chordae are inserted into the ventricular surfaces (rough zones) of both cusps, or on to the free edge. Chordal anatomy is highly variable and very complex classifications into order of importance exist. It is simplest to bear in mind that chordae vary widely in the amount of cusp tissue they support. In the anterior cusp the chordae insert mainly into the margins of the cusp, leaving a central free area. A very common variant, however, is to have an extra flap of central cusp tissue into which fine chordae are inserted. Special fan chordae mark each commissure. Some chordae are muscularised, containing a core of myocardial muscle tissue.

The papillary muscles are divided into an anterolateral and a posteromedial group, each with a variable number of subheads. Each papillary

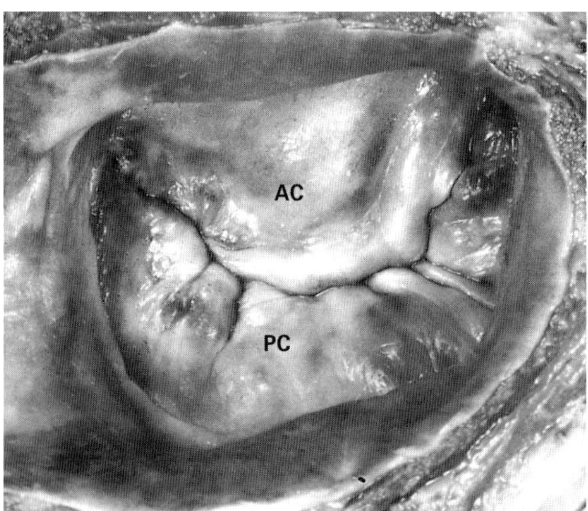

Fig. 6.49 Normal closed mitral valve. The closed mitral is viewed from the left atrium. The anterior cusp (AC) is D shaped while the posterior cusp (PC) is crescentic and subdivided. Both cusps appose and neither has prolapsed into the atrium. The slight degree of ballooning of the anterior cusp is normal with increasing age.

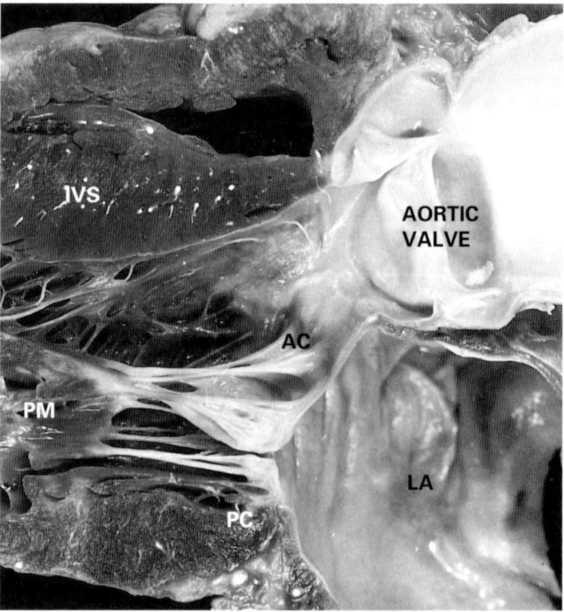

Fig. 6.50 Normal mitral valve — long axis view. The anterior cusp (AC) and posterior cusp (PC) meet and are held at the same level by the chordae and papillary muscles (PM). Neither cusp prolapses into the atrium (LA).

muscle group gives chordae to both cusps. Each muscle head has a central artery running in its long axis. These arteries are the terminal portions of straight, relatively unbranched, penetrating vessels derived from the left circumflex artery (anterolateral group) or right coronary artery (posteromedial group).

The mitral valve cusps have a core of densely arranged collagen (valve fibrosa) which is continuous with the connective tissue core of the chordae and is attached to the atrioventricular ring. The fibrosa is covered on each aspect by a layer of more loosely arranged connective tissue rich in acid mucopolysaccharides (valve spongiosa). This spongiosa layer is accentuated around the chordal insertions. The atrioventricular rings are often regarded as dense collagenous structures. In fact, particularly on the lateral aspects of the atrioventricular rings, there is merely an accentuation of the collagen at the cusp base, which is loosely attached to the atrial and ventricular endocardium. Normal muscle contraction in the adjacent ventricular myocardium rather than dense collagen seems to be the major factor in retaining normal atrioventricular ring size.

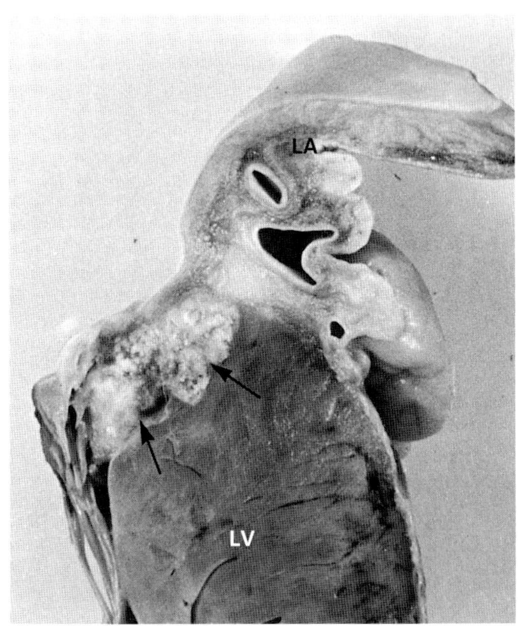

Fig. 6.51 Mitral valve ring calcification due to age. In so-called mitral ring calcification the process (arrows) develops on the endocardium just beneath the posterior cusp and protrudes upwards, lifting the base of the cusp. LA = left atrium, LV = left ventricle.

AGE-RELATED CHANGES IN THE MITRAL VALVE

With increasing age minor degrees of bulging into the atria by either one scallop of the posterior cusp or multiple small, dome-shaped protrusions along the free edge between chordal insertions ('hooding') become increasingly common. It is often difficult to determine at exactly what point such upward protrusions should be designated mitral valve prolapse. In practical terms, unless the free edge of a portion of cusp is exposed in the closed position regurgitation would not be present.

The valve cusps also thicken with age, associated with a loss of the translucency of the posterior cusp that is seen in young hearts. Nodular thickening develops along the apposition lines of both cusps and some thickening of isolated chordae often occurs. Lipid deposition occurs on the ventricular surface of the mitral valve but does not have any pathological sequelae. Calcification in the valve ring (Fig. 6.51) becomes increasingly common with age. Depending on how assiduously calcification is looked for the frequency is very variably reported but a figure of 10% of individuals over 50 years of age is likely to be reasonably accurate.[35] Calcification visible by the naked eye is rare before the age of 70 unless there are reasons for enhanced connective tissue calcification.[1] Although the process is traditionally called ring calcification it actually begins in the angle between the ventricular endocardium and the cusp, i.e. it is subvalvar. The calcium forms as aggregates which ultimately coalesce to form a bar 2–5 cm long beneath the posterior cusp. The posterior cusp is lifted into the atria but is otherwise normal. In a few cases the centre of the calcific mass breaks down and becomes pultaceous (Fig. 6.52). Such lesions must not be mistaken for syphilis or tuberculosis. Inflammatory infiltrates and foreign-body giant cells occur around such breaking-down ring calcification, compounding the chance of misinterpretation. Symptoms from mitral ring calcification are rare and it is usually a coincidental autopsy finding.[36] Cases in which the calcification completely surrounds the valve orifice may develop minor degrees of stenosis and

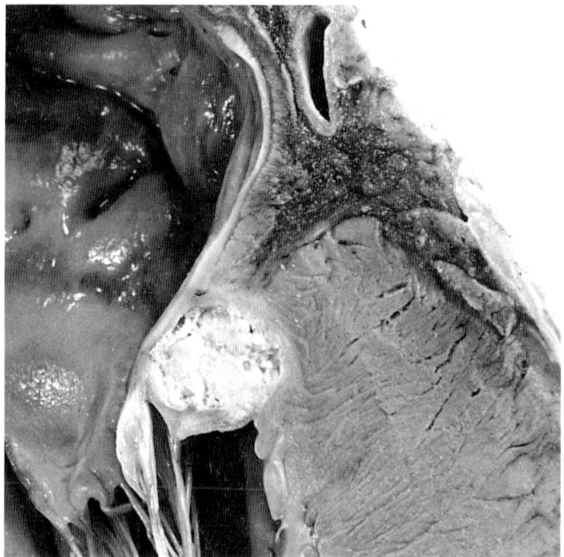

Fig. 6.52 Mitral valve ring calcification due to age. In this case the ring calcification has degenerated into a nodule of white, caseous-like material.

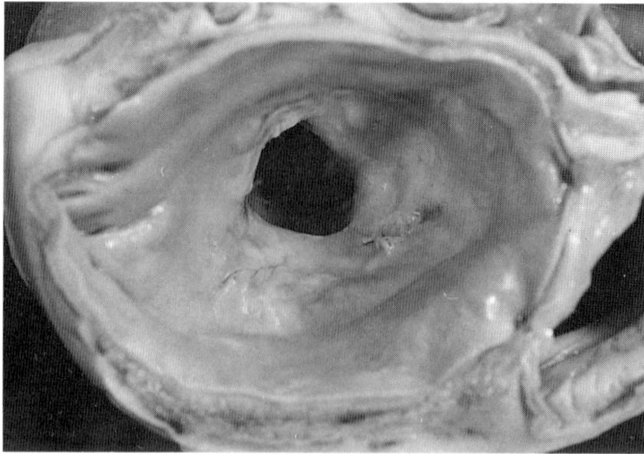

Fig. 6.53 Rheumatic mitral stenosis. Viewed from above the valve aperture is reduced in size due to fusion of both commissures but calcification is not present.

regurgitation. Calcium may also extend on to the interventricular septum, transecting the atrioventricular bundle and causing complete heart block. This association is known as Rytand's syndrome.

MITRAL STENOSIS

For all practical purposes the sole cause of mitral stenosis in adults is chronic rheumatic valve disease. Mitral stenosis is more common in women, reported ratios ranging from 1.5–4 in excess of males. In the simplest and most common form of mitral stenosis in younger individuals, commissural fusion is the dominant mechanism (Figs 6.53, 6.54).

Cusp thickening may be minimal and the valve becomes a mobile diaphragm with a small central, oval, 'fish mouth' opening. Clinical signs of severe obstruction occur at valve orifice areas of less than 1.5 cm^2. This form of stenosis is very amenable to closed valvotomy in which, via the left atrium, the commissures are split by the finger, a dilator or a knife. Such operations do not allow direct visual examination of the valve but can be performed without cardiac bypass, thus being quick, cheap and low-risk. In older subjects cusp fibrosis and calcification play a more major part in obstruction (Fig. 6.55) and

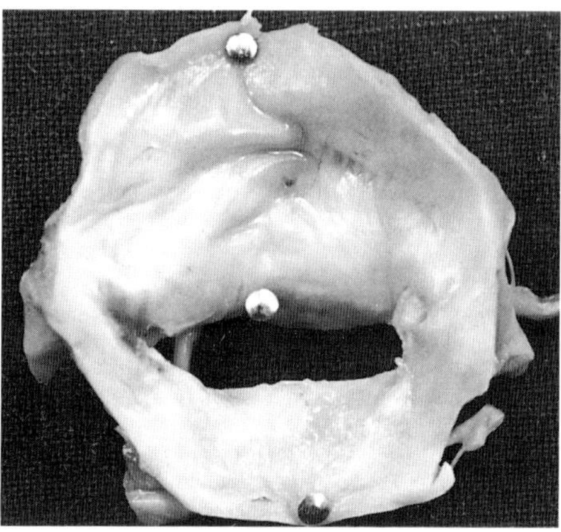

Fig. 6.54 Rheumatic mitral stenosis — surgical excision. The valve orifice is small and oval in shape due to commissural fusion. No calcification is present.

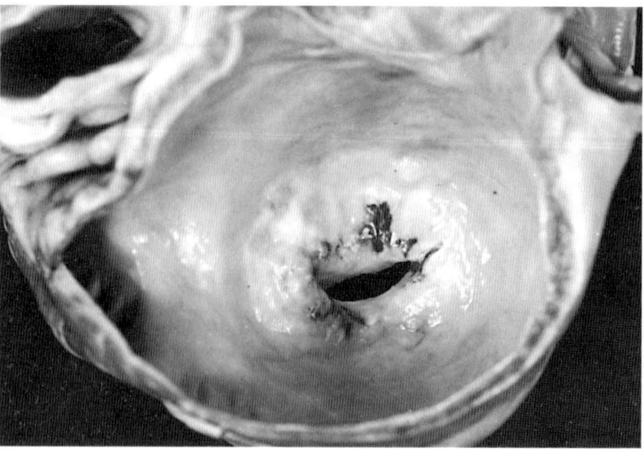

Fig. 6.55 Rheumatic mitral stenosis. Viewed from the left atrium the orifice of the valve is oval due to commissural fusion associated with nodular calcification.

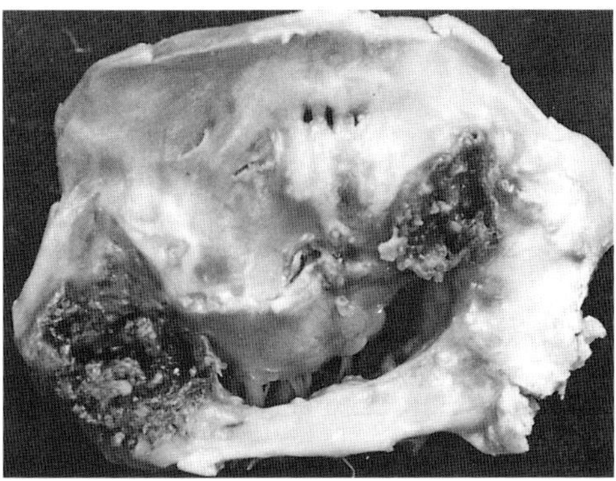

Fig. 6.56 Rheumatic mitral stenosis — surgical excision. Both commissures are fused and contain ulcerated nodules of calcium. The aperture is crescentic in shape.

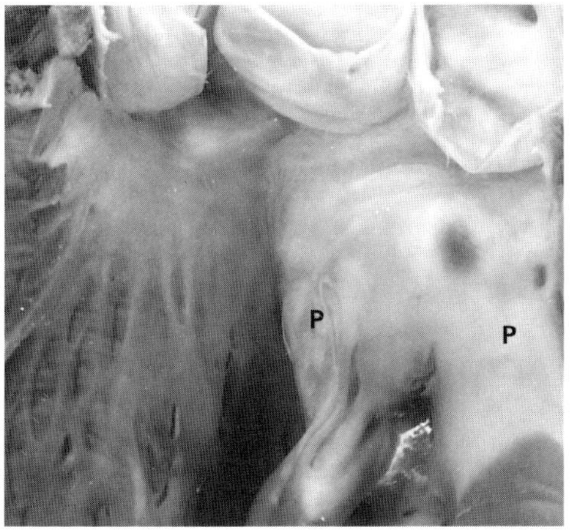

Fig. 6.57 Mitral stenosis – subvalve obstruction. The fusion of the chordae and papillary muscles in fibrous pillars (P) narrows the orifice (arrow) of the mitral valve below cusp level.

commissural fusion may even be absent.[37,38] Calcification develops as linear or nodular masses either within the cusp or at the commissures. Ulceration and thrombosis over these nodules occurs (Fig. 6.56). A further element to mitral stenosis occurs below the valve, when chordae fuse to form a fixed fibrous tunnel obstructing flow from the inflow into the outflow portions of the left ventricle (Fig. 6.57). All these more complex forms of mitral stenosis require valve replacement for alleviation.

Left atrial size in mitral stenosis is very variable. No cavity enlargement may be present with a thick, hypertrophied atrial wall; at the other extreme massive dilation may occur with a very thin wall from which atrial muscle has vanished. Factors determining atrial size include concomitant regurgitation, atrial fibrillation and increasing age, all of which are associated with large atria. Very large left atria may displace the left main bronchus and compress the recurrent laryngeal nerve causing laryngeal paralysis. Compression of the oesophagus also occurs and has been associated with stricture formation caused by impediment of the passage of potassium tablets. The presence (Fig. 6.58) or absence of thrombus in the atria is also unpredictable but is associated with atrial fibrillation and larger atria. Thrombus most commonly protrudes from the atrial appendage but may also extend as a sheet over the posterior wall and roof of the atria. The deepest layers of such diffuse thrombi often calcify. Systemic emboli are common in mitral stenosis, occurring in up to 30% of cases and being strongly linked to episodic atrial fibrillation.

Bacterial endocarditis is a rare complication of pure mitral stenosis and when it occurs indicates some degree of co-existing regurgitation (Chapter 7).

The clinical picture of pure mitral stenosis is dominated by pulmonary hypertension as a consequence of high pulmonary venous pressure. Right ventricular hypertrophy is pronounced

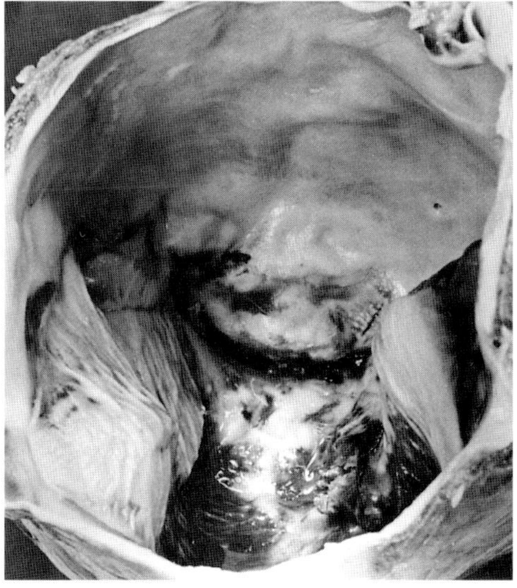

Fig. 6.58 Rheumatic mitral stenosis. In contrast to Figures 6.48 and 6.50, where the atrium was small, here the atrium is enlarged and contains a large amount of mural thrombus. The valve aperture is a crescent-shaped slit.

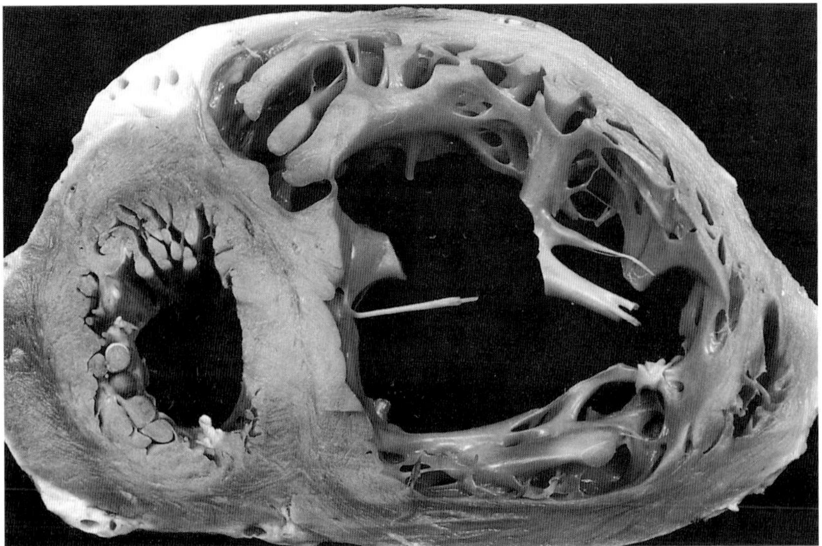

Fig. 6.59 Right ventricular hypertrophy in mitral stenosis. In a cross-section of both ventricles the left is seen to be normal while the right ventricle is dilated and very thick-walled. The right ventricular morphology shows the effect of severe pulmonary hypertension and concomitant tricuspid regurgitation.

while the left ventricle is small (Fig. 6.59). A brown, solid lung with very large numbers of alveolar macrophages containing iron and deposits of haemosiderin in the interstitial tissues is the striking feature of long-standing mitral stenosis. This degree of haemosiderosis reflects the elevation of pulmonary venous pressure over long periods. In mitral stenosis survival for years is possible, reflecting the fact that the left ventricle is protected.

Supravalve mitral stenosis

Stenosis due to a fibrous diaphragm crossing the atrium just above the mitral valve itself (Fig. 6.60) is a congenital anomaly unrelated to rheumatic disease. Most cases are diagnosed in childhood but occasionally are not discovered until adult life.

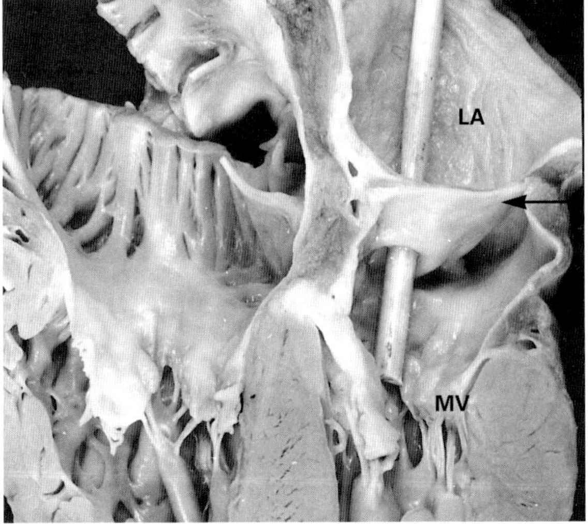

Fig. 6.60 Mitral stenosis — supravalve level. There is a fibrous diaphragm with a central hole just above the mitral valve (MV) itself. LA = left atrium. The valve is normal.

MITRAL REGURGITATION

It is very difficult to assess regurgitation of the mitral valve at autopsy with any degree of certainty. This reflects that normal valve function has many components, some of which depend on muscle contraction and are impossible to simulate in the dead heart.[38] Nevertheless, pressure volume loads placed on the left ventricle by perfusion across the aorta will passively close the valve and allow gross disruption to be identified. The valve should always be inspected first from the left atrium with the valve ring intact. Squeezing the left ventricle or filling the ventricle with water and then squeezing will show cusp prolapse, chordal rupture and papillary muscle rupture in a manner impossible to reproduce once the ring is opened. Malfunction of many different components of the valve can cause regurgitation (Table 6.3; Fig. 6.61).

Ring abnormalities

As discussed previously, the mitral valve ring is not a rigid structure and the size of the atrioventricular orifice is dependent on the normality of the ventricular myocardium. The size of the mitral orifice is markedly reduced in systole. Any cause of left ventricular dilation can cause mitral regurgitation. In part this is due to dilation of the mitral valve orifice, which can be assessed by measuring the circumference of the mitral orifice

Table 6.3 Causes of pure mitral regurgitation

Cusp abnormality	
Cusp expanded	Floppy mitral valve, Marfan's syndrome
Cusp perforated	Infective endocarditis
Cusp retracted	Rheumatic disease, systemic lupus
Chordal abnormality	
Chordae long	Floppy mitral valve, Marfan's syndrome
Chordae ruptured	Floppy mitral valve, infective endocarditis
Chordae short	Rheumatic disease
Ring abnormality	
Dilated	Marfan's syndrome, floppy mitral valve
Calcified	Age-related
Ventricular abnormality	
Dilated left ventricle	'Functional', Marfan's syndrome
Papillary muscle abnormality	
Ruptured	Ischaemic disease
Fibrotic	Ischaemic disease

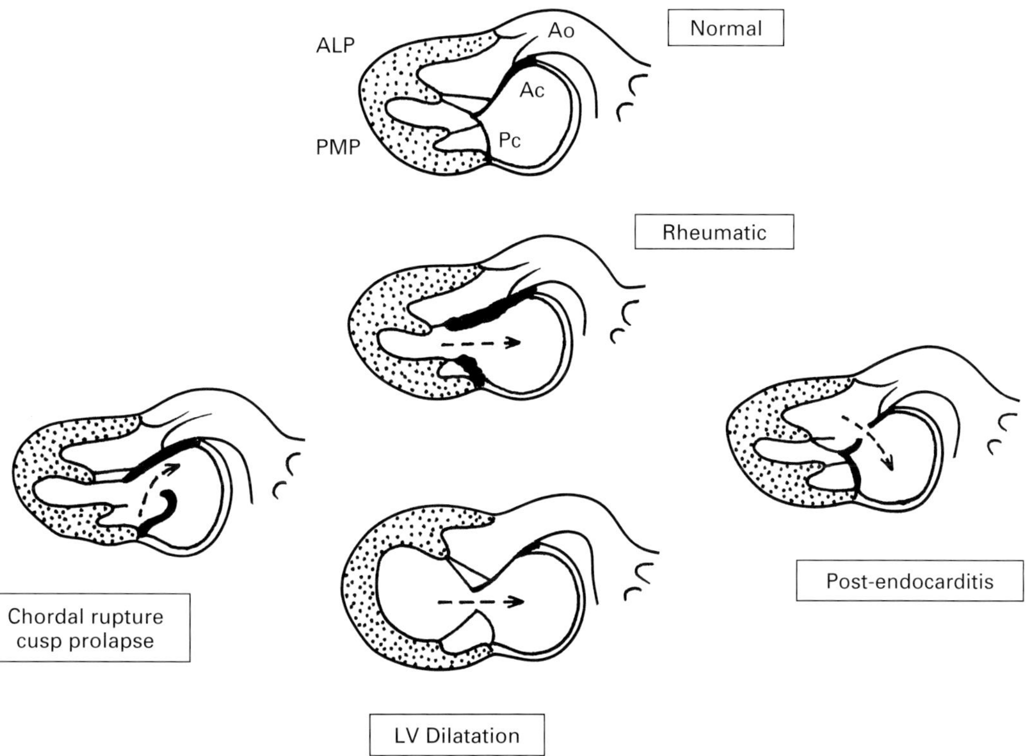

Fig. 6.61 Mechanisms of mitral regurgitation. In the normal valve the bases of the anterolateral (ALP) and posteromedial (PMP) papillary muscles subtend a narrow angle. The anterior (AC) and posterior cusps (PC) meet and neither moves up into the atria when closed. In rheumatic disease the cusps do not meet. In a dilated ventricle the angle subtended by the papillary muscles increases and the cusps do not meet. In the floppy valve cusp prolapses. In bacterial endocarditis there is a cusp defect. The direction of the regurgitant jet (→) varies with aetiology.

at autopsy. In part, however, it is due to alteration in the axis of the papillary muscle, and thus chordal tension on the cusps, as the bases of the papillary muscles move apart. Ring size may not necessarily be increased.[39] Mitral regurgitation that waxes and wanes as left ventricular shape alters with treatment is known as functional mitral regurgitation. Fixed dilation of the left ventricle will lead to chronic mitral regurgitation. In patients with any of the genetic defects of connective tissue synthesis, including Ehlers–Danlos and Marfan's syndrome, such fixed dilation may occur. A vicious cycle is probably initiated in which weakness of the mitral ring and myocardial collagen allows dilation to develop which progresses as mitral regurgitation progresses.

Mitral regurgitation due to cusp and chordal abnormalities

Rheumatic mitral regurgitation

Regurgitation in chronic rheumatic disease is associated with cusp retraction and reduction in area leading to a reduction in cusp mobility due to chordal fusion and shortening (Figs 6.62–6.64). The most frequent pattern is for the posterior cusp to be reduced in area and tethered to the posterior wall of the left ventricle by shortened thick chordae (Fig. 6.65).[40]

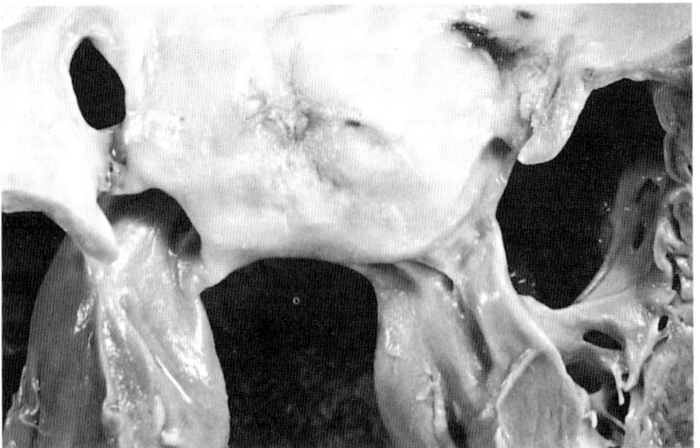

Fig. 6.63 Rheumatic mitral regurgitation. The chordae to the cusp are fused into fibrous pillars and are drastically shortened, tethering the cusp to the apex of the papillary muscle, preventing any cusp movement and causing severe regurgitation.

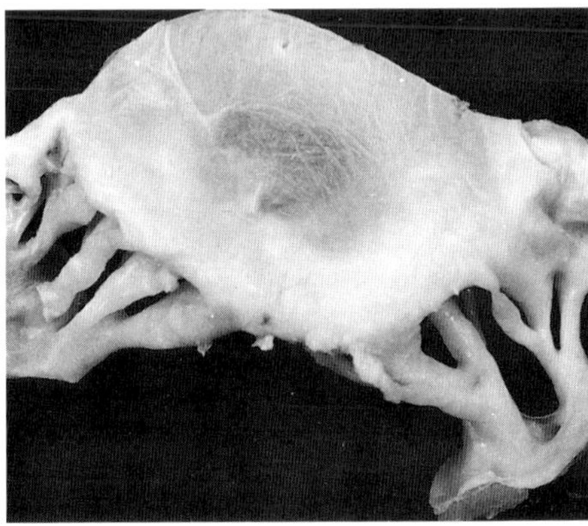

Fig. 6.64 Rheumatic mitral regurgitation. In this surgically excised valve the chordae are short and thick. Their number appears reduced because each represents several chordae fused together.

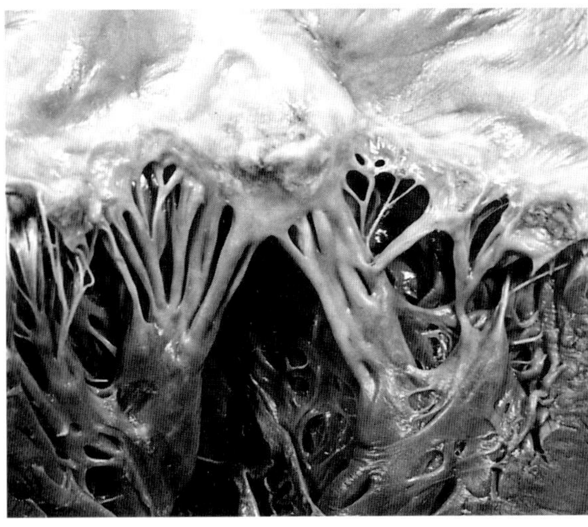

Fig. 6.62 Rheumatic mitral regurgitation. The chordae of both the anterior and posterior cusp are thickened and fused together although their length is not reduced. Such thickening reduces cusp mobility and causes moderate regurgitation.

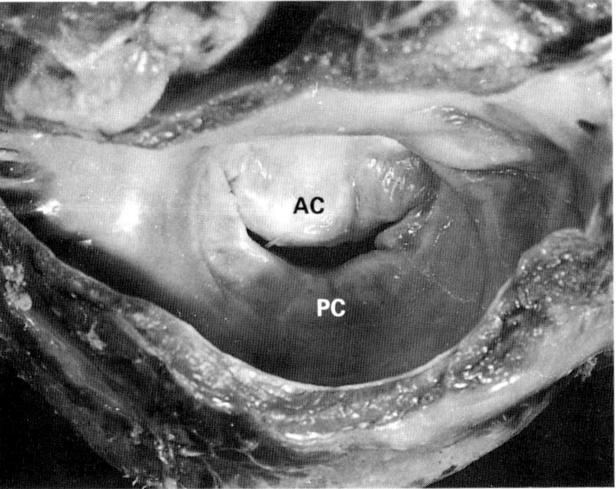

Fig. 6.65 Rheumatic mitral regurgitation. The valve has been fixed in the closed position and is viewed from the atrium. Although the anterior cusp (AC) is thick it was mobile. No clinical evidence of stenosis. The valve does not close because of retraction and tethering of the posterior cusp (PC).

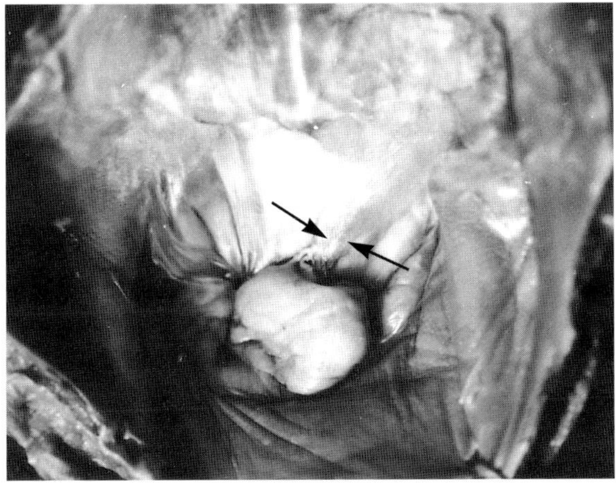

Fig. 6.66 Mitral regurgitation due to floppy mitral valve. The mitral valve is viewed from the left atrium with the ventricle perfused through the aorta at 100 mmHg with formalin. A dome-shaped portion of the cusp has prolapsed into the atria and fluid is jetting (arrows) from beneath this portion of the cusp.

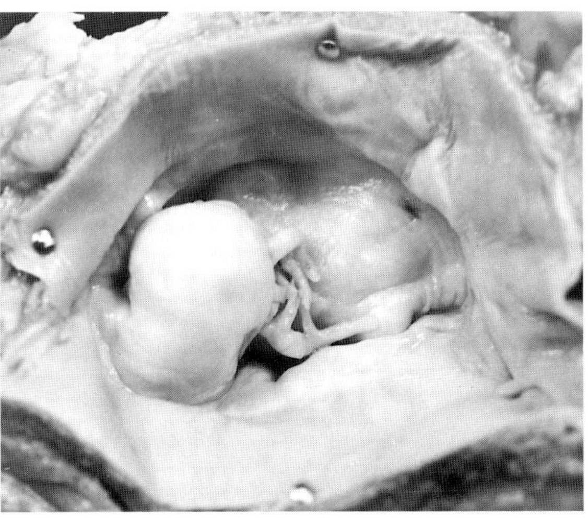

Fig. 6.67 Floppy mitral valve. Viewed from the left atrium the greater part of both cusps bulges upward in the closed position. The stumps of ruptured chordae project into the atrium. The absence of any papillary muscle excludes the possibility of this rupture being due to ischaemic disease.

a)

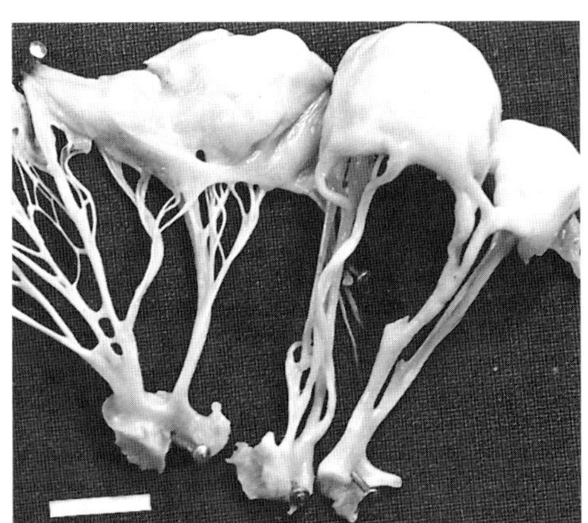

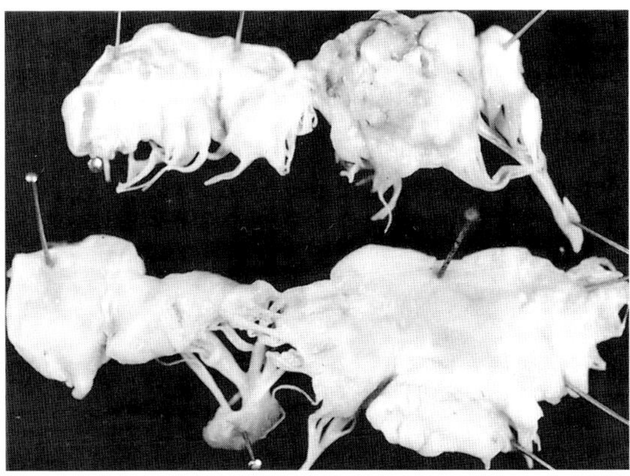

b)

c)

Fig. 6.68 a,b,c Mitral regurgitation due to floppy valve — surgical specimens. (**a**) There is a dome-shaped, white, opaque segment in the posterior cusp and the chordae are long. While the appearances are unlike rheumatic disease it is the soft feel of the valve that is most striking and contrasts with the hard fibrous rheumatic valve. (**b**) In this valve both the anterior and posterior cusps are folded and convoluted rather than dome-shaped. Again the soft feel of the valve cusps is a useful diagnostic point. (**c**) In this patient with Marfan's syndrome the anterior cusp (AC) of the mitral valve is expanded and convoluted with chordal rupture (arrow). The aortic root was also dilated leading to aortic regurgitation. The free edges of the aortic cusps have nodular thickening.

The floppy mitral valve

In this condition the valve cusps increase in area and the chordae elongate and may rupture. This allows prolapse of a portion of a cusp into the atria in systole and regurgitation occurs. The cusps develop a very characteristic dome shape at autopsy (Figs 6.66, 6.67) which can also be recognised in valves excised surgically (Fig. 6.68).

The entity has many names. The expanded, dome-shaped cusps when felt at surgery are soft and hypermobile, leading to the term floppy valve. Pathologists have used the names myxomatous, mucinous, hooded or ballooned mitral valve. Clinicians have used the term redundant or prolapsing mitral valve. The clinical recognition of prolapse of the mitral valve into the atria has been made very easy by echocardiography. Even so, the ease by which such prolapse can be recognised creates its own difficulties. There is no exact definition of normality. Under certain conditions a significant proportion of normal young individuals show minor cusp prolapse. It is very far from sure whether this is a physiological variant or a modification in function due to structural and pathological alterations in the cusp. Cusp prolapse can occur in association with ischaemic damage to the papillary muscles. It is certain therefore that cusp prolapse in life with an isolated late systolic click is not necessarily an indication of the presence of a floppy valve, i.e. a pathological change in the cusp itself (Table 6.4).

Table 6.4 Mitral valve prolapse — causes

Physiological	
Structural	
Chordae long	Floppy valve, Marfan's syndrome
Cusp expanded	Floppy valve, Marfan's syndrome
Chordae ruptured	Floppy valve, postendocarditis, Marfan's syndrome
Papillary muscle fibrosis	Ischaemic heart disease Dilated cardiomyopathy

The essential lesion of the floppy valve is disintegration of the valve fibrosa (Figs 6.6, 6.69). Collagen bundles appear to be fragmented and cystic spaces, which contain acid mucopolysaccharides, appear. The posterior cusp appears to be particularly prone to this change. Similar changes are also seen in the chordae. The resultant weakness of the cusp and chordae, coupled with the haemodynamic stress, leads to elongation and stretching of the valve. On histological examination, minor degrees of the change are almost universal and normality merges into abnormality. The changes also show a marked

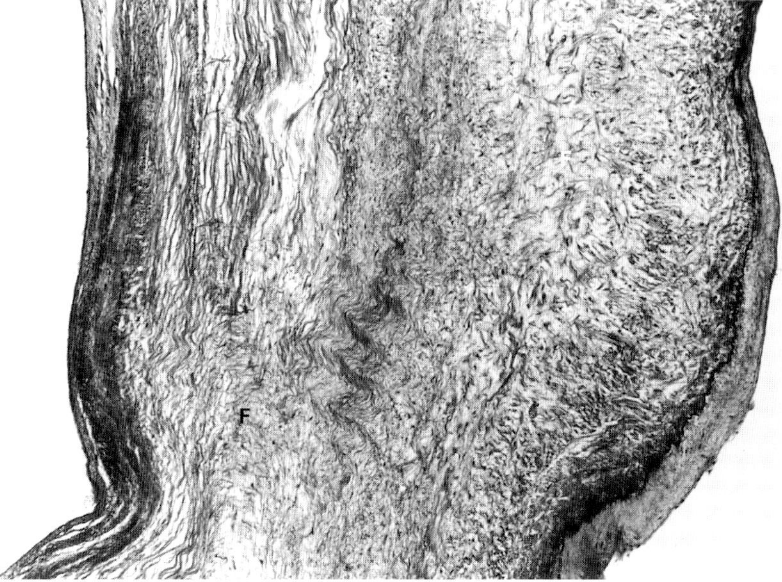

Fig. 6.69 Floppy valve — histology. The fibrosa (F) is widened but instead of dense collagen is formed of irregular arranged loose connective tissue.
EVG × 160

increased frequency with age.[41] The valve is not vascularised and inflammatory cells are absent, although the presence of mast cells is not unusual. Calcification is not present unless age-related ring calcification is present incidentally.

Minor degrees of myxoid change are associated with some hooding of the posterior cusp between chordal insertions. More extensive change allows the posterior cusp to expand in area and the chordae to elongate; the medial, lateral or middle scallop of the valve, or any combination, may be involved. The first clinical indication of this process is a systolic click which later becomes associated with a late systolic murmur. Angiocardiography and echocardiography show the click to be associated with a tensing of chordae as the expanded cusp is suddenly halted; regurgitation produces a murmur in late systole. As the cusp prolapse worsens, the murmur becomes pansystolic, indicating more significant mitral regurgitation throughout systole.

Late systolic murmurs thought to indicate minor cusp prolapse were found in 74 of 1169 healthy young females, giving an incidence of 6.3%.[42] An autopsy study of 1984 hospital patients showed that the overall incidence of finding at least part of the mitral valve prolapsing due to a floppy valve was 5%, with an increase in old age.[41]

In the majority of these patients the floppy valve is only an auscultatory phenomenon and, at worst, minor mitral regurgitation occurs late in systole. The prognosis of minor degrees of cusp prolapse due to floppy valves is good and little different from subjects without a valve abnormality. Nevertheless, in a small proportion of patients the regurgitation increases in severity, but how commonly such a progression occurs remains uncertain. Certainly the floppy valve has become a major cause of valve surgery for isolated mitral regurgitation.[40] On the other hand, in an autopsy study of 91 floppy valves only 14 directly caused death and an additional 36 may have contributed to death.[41]

Symptomatic disease is associated with a number of complications superimposed on the floppy valve (Fig. 6.70). Chordal rupture results from the expanded cusp exerting increased stress on the chordae and from actual dissolution of collagen in the chordae. It is the single most common complication producing clinically important regurgitation. Chordal rupture is seen most frequently in the posterior cusp; it allows a far greater cusp prolapse and an increase in mitral regurgitation. Sequential rupture of minor chordae over months leads to gradual increase of clinical disability, while a major chordal rupture leads to sudden, even catastrophic, regurgitation. Anterior

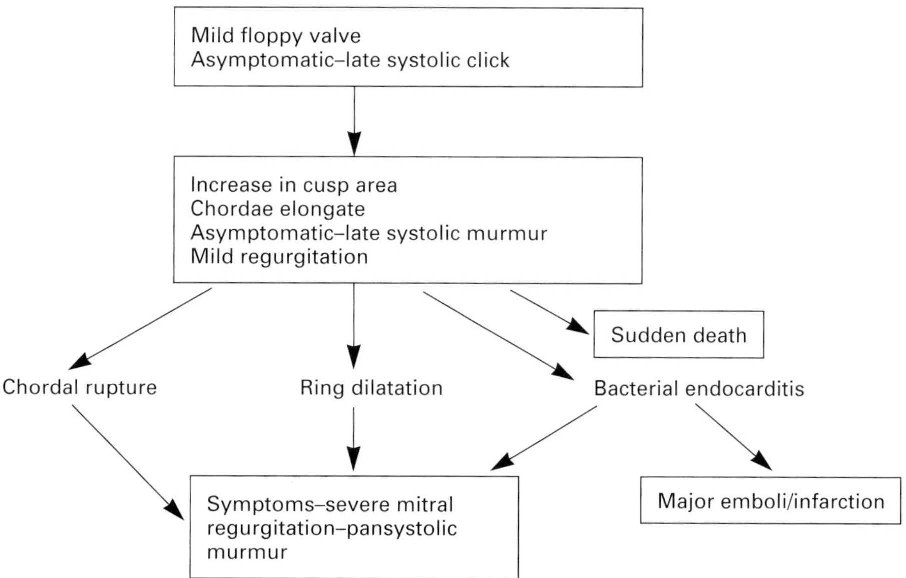

Fig. 6.70 Progression in floppy mitral valve

chordal rupture also has more serious consequences. A study of 44 surgically excised valves showed posterior chordal rupture in 24, anterior rupture in 10 and rupture of anterior as well as posterior chordae in two.[41] Significant mitral regurgitation when cusp involvement is advanced in both cusps or the mitral annulus is dilated may occasionally occur without chordal rupture.

In the floppy valve, the cusp and chordae are excessively mobile and hit both adjacent chordae and the endocardium of the posterior wall of the left ventricle. This commonly leads to thickening of the cusp and chordae and to linear endocardial thickening (friction lesions) under the posterior cusp (Fig. 6.71). Very occasionally this results in a fibrous mass encasing the chordae (Fig. 6.72), as first noted by Salazar & Edwards.[43] The anterior cusp may also just reach the interventricular septum, producing a more diffuse patch of endocardial fibrosis. Thickening and fusion of adjacent chordae following this mechanical trauma are not uncommon in association with the floppy valve and must not be mistaken for rheumatic disease (Fig. 6.4).

Histological examination of floppy valves shows, as a constant feature, an increase of surface fibrosis over the atrial aspect of the cusps, where contact and friction occur. This fibrosis is associated macroscopically with a rather crumpled, apparently thickened valve, which has often been mistaken for an indication of rheumatic disease. The cusps, however, feel soft, unlike the leathery consistency of rheumatic valves. More important is the frequent finding of small, predominantly platelet thrombi at the sites of cusp contact. Occasionally, papillary Lambl's excrescences develop. Thrombus incorporation also occurs in the friction

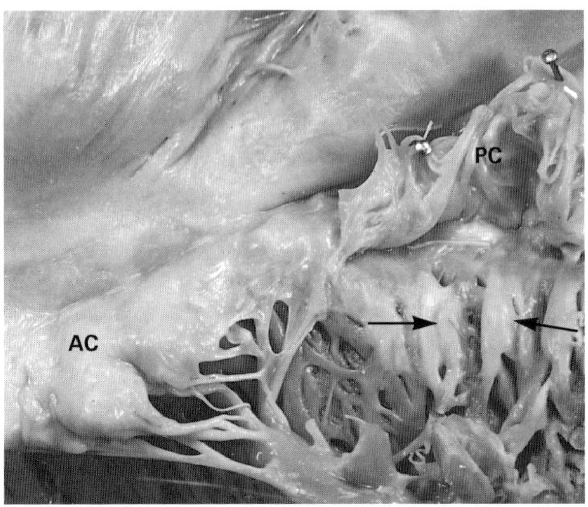

Fig. 6.71 Floppy mitral valve. The anterior cusp (AC) shows the typical expanded and folded appearance of a floppy valve. The posterior cusp (PC) has been turned up to show vertical linear endocardial thickening on the posterior wall of the ventricle (arrows).

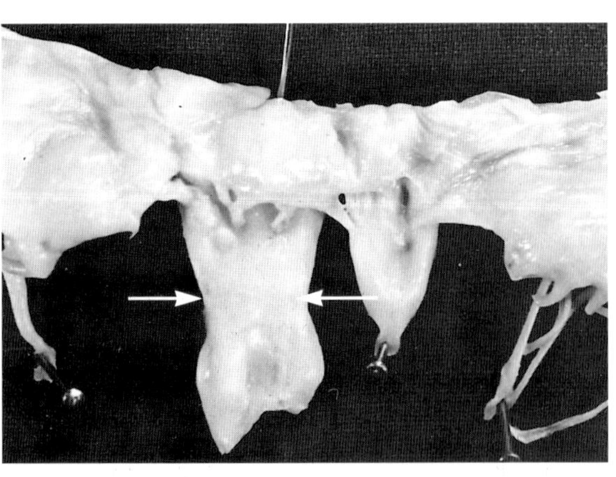

a)

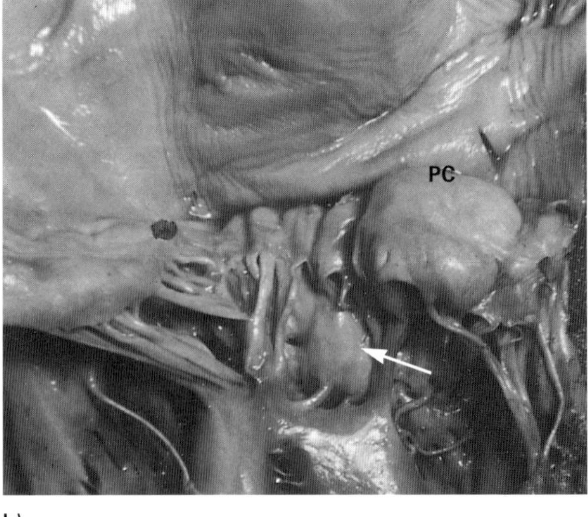

b)

Fig. 6.72 a,b Floppy mitral valve — chordal fusion. (**a**) The posterior cusp chordae are fused together in a plate of fibrous tissue (arrows) which had to be dissected away from the wall of the ventricle during valve replacement. (**b**) In this post-mortem specimen there is a typical dome-shaped segment of the posterior cusp (PC). In another segment of the posterior cusp chordae are fused onto the ventricular wall (arrow).

lesions behind the posterior cusp. On both of these areas of thrombus deposition, bacterial endocarditis may develop. It usually occurs on the atrial surface of the cusps[36] but also more rarely on the posterior ventricular wall. The precise risk of any individual with a floppy valve developing endocarditis is uncertain, but it is low. An autopsy study of 91 cases showed bacterial endocarditis in only five, and clinical accounts of the late systolic murmur syndrome all stress an excellent prognosis. Despite this, in patients with bacterial endocarditis in the developed world a floppy mitral valve is the commonest predisposing abnormality. The risk of bacterial endocarditis becomes greater when some mitral regurgitation is present. It is debatable whether patients with a late systolic click due to a floppy valve should be given prophylactic antibiotic therapy, but clear that those with a late systolic murmur due to regurgitation should.

An association between transient loss of vision due to small peripheral retinal emboli and the floppy valve exists.[44] Small platelet emboli are probably knocked from the contact surfaces of the valve. Large thrombi capable of causing major embolic strokes occur only with bacterial endocarditis on floppy valves.

A small proportion of patients with floppy valves have an unexplained tendency to ventricular premature contractions.[45] In rare cases, sudden death is seen without another apparent cause than a floppy valve. In a long-term follow-up of 23 patients with mild mitral prolapse six died suddenly.[46] Evidence is emerging that patients with floppy valves who run this risk of death have an abnormal electrocardiogram characterised by inverted T waves in the posterolateral leads. This electrocardiographic abnormality may be familial. Numerous explanations have been put forward for the phenomenon, including abnormal pull on the papillary muscles, mechanical interference with the left circumflex coronary artery, mechanical stimulation of the myocardium from chordal impact and an associated myocardial interstitial fibrosis.

Mitral valve prolapse may be familial and may or may not be associated with minor skeletal abnormalities, including joint hypermobility and thoracic skeletal abnormalities such as pectus excavatum. A number of other familial conditions are associated with the floppy valve. In Marfan's syndrome there is cusp involvement identical to that in the floppy valve, but with superimposed ring dilatation. Similar valve appearances are seen in osteogenesis imperfecta and pseudoxanthoma elasticum. In approximately one-third of patients with floppy mitral valves, the tricuspid valve is similarly involved, although this is only very rarely clinically significant because of the lower pressures in the right side of the heart.[47]

The exact pathogenesis of the floppy valve remains uncertain. The very strong association with known genetic disturbances of collagen and elastin synthesis such as Marfan's, Ehlers–Danlos and osteogenesis imperfecta clearly shows that malformed or poorly adherent connective tissue fibrillary proteins do cause floppy valves. It is far less clear what the pathogenesis is in subjects with purely valve abnormalities. The genetic status of familial floppy valves without skeletal abnormalities is not known. It is not impossible for gene expression to vary from tissue to tissue and there may still be abnormalities of the fibrillin gene. Age and mechanical stress clearly play a role in leading to the expression of the disease and could be operating against the genetic background of minor defects in connective tissue synthesis. Inflammatory destruction does not appear to be a factor but among other putative mechanisms are exposure to a toxic agent in pregnancy, operating on the 35th to 42nd day of fetal life when valves and vertebrae are forming, and a purely mechanical breakdown of collagen due to excess stresses imposed by abnormal and decreased chordal support to the cusp.[48]

Other causes of chordal rupture

In our experience, the vast majority of ruptured chordae are in association with the abnormally expanded cusps of the floppy valve.

On rare occasions, spontaneous chordal rupture occurs where the cusp is otherwise normal. Such cases are usually encountered in relatively young individuals and come to surgery. The phenomenon is particularly prone to occur in pregnancy. Occasionally, the condition follows closed chest trauma.

In rheumatic disease, rupture of the anterior cusp chordae may occur in young subjects with active valvulitis. Chordal rupture is not a feature of chronic rheumatic disease in the UK.

Bacterial endocarditis in the acute phase leads to considerable necrosis of collagen; chordal rupture and cusp perforation are natural sequelae.

Direct mechanical trauma may lead to chordal rupture. It occurs in two rare situations: repeated prolapse of an atrial myxoma through the orifice leads to a 'ball-wrecking' action on the valve; in hypertrophic obstructive cardiomyopathy there is repeated impact of the anterior cusp on the thickened septum. It must be stressed that the chordae are avascular and are not subject to ischaemia and rupture in coronary heart disease.

Mitral regurgitation from papillary muscle abnormalities

Ischaemic papillary muscle damage is now probably the single most frequent overall cause of mitral regurgitation, although it is often not clinically severe and infrequently leads to surgical intervention.

Every grade of severity of regurgitation is seen.

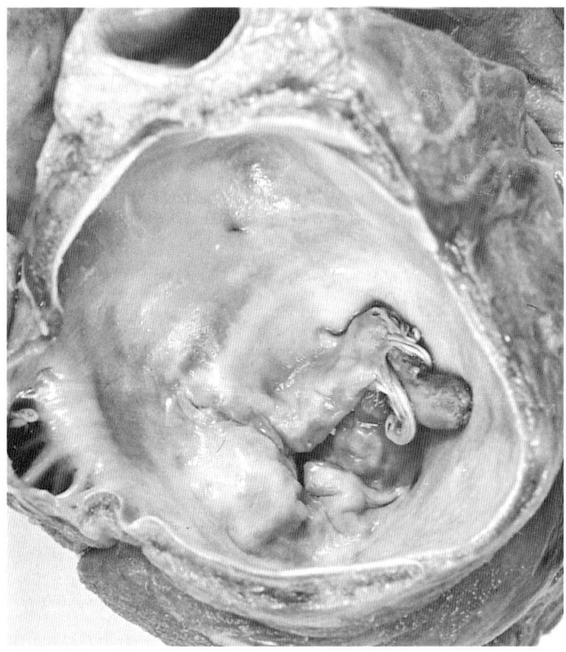

Fig. 6.73 Papillary muscle rupture — ischaemic heart disease. Viewed from the left atrium there is a stump of a papillary muscle attached to chordae which has prolapsed. In life this stump crosses and recrosses the mitral valve, leading to severe regurgitation.

The papillary muscles show necrosis in 20–50% of patients with acute regional myocardial infarcts at autopsy. Mitral regurgitation occurs in the acute phase in about 15% of anterior infarcts and in up to 40% of posterior infarcts, presumably because of loss of contractile papillary function. Most cases resolve within a short period.[49] Sudden catastrophic regurgitation occurs following papillary muscle rupture (Fig. 6.73). The clinical picture is dramatic, with a suddenly acquired pansystolic murmur and rapid deterioration in the patient's clinical state. Clinical differentiation from an acquired ventricular septum defect is often difficult. At autopsy, the papillary muscle stump is found in the left atrium but during life echocardiography shows it to be continually crossing the orifice as the cusp flails. Rupture may be of the whole muscle or may affect only one head. In the latter instance the patient may survive for some days and a complex knot of chordae tangled round the papillary muscle may be found in the atrium.

Regurgitation may also persist after acute infarction or develop slowly in the next few months following an acute episode of infarction. All grades of severity of mitral regurgitation are seen. In these cases, replacement of necrotic

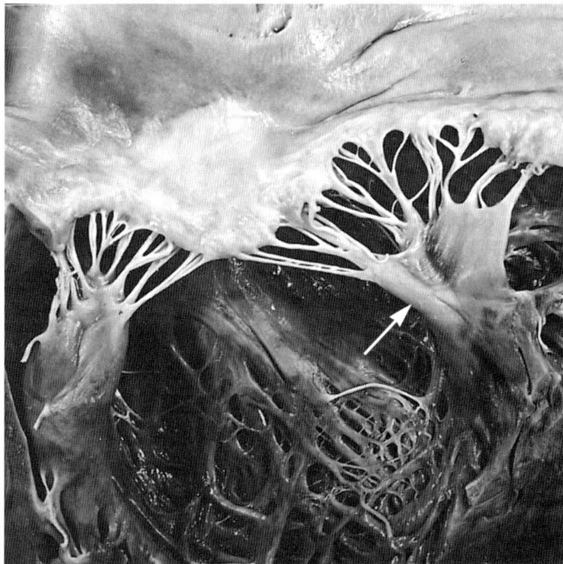

Fig. 6.74 Ischaemic mitral regurgitation. The papillary muscle has an apical segment which is thinned and elongated (arrow) following the fibrous replacement of an area of acute infarction.

muscle by fibrous tissue leads to thinned papillary muscles. The apex of the papillary muscle may become a thin, calcified bar (Fig. 6.74). In most instances the apex of the papillary muscle elongates, allowing prolapse of part of a cusp upward.[50]

Mitral regurgitation due to bacterial endocarditis

Bacterial endocarditis can involve the posterior cusp of mitral valve predominantly and lead to destruction of cusp tissue and chordal rupture. In untreated cases, vegetations extend on to the posterior wall of the atrium following the line of the regurgitant jet. A wide range of conditions predispose to bacterial endocarditis on the posterior cusp, among the most frequent being floppy valves and rheumatic mitral regurgitation. Infection of mitral ring calcification is rare, but can lead to an abscess burrowing into the posterior aspect of the valve ring. Anterior cusp bacterial endocarditis may occur in both floppy and rheumatic valves, but also on the regurgitant jet lesion of aortic incompetence and by direct spread from the aortic valve. In the anterior cusp, aneurysm formation and central perforation are as common as chordal rupture. Infection high on the ventricular aspect of the anterior cusp may lead to an aneurysm burrowing beneath the aortic valve cusps.

TRICUSPID VALVE

TRICUSPID VALVE PATHOLOGY

The anatomy of the tricuspid valve is very variable. It is conventionally described as having three cusps, anterior, posterolateral and septal. The septal cusp is small, often rudimentary and can even be absent without apparent clinical consequences. The septal cusp is, however, a useful landmark because its base is inserted diagonally across the membranous interventricular septum. The anterior cusp is large and is suspended across the right ventricular cavity in a manner analogous to the anterior cusp of the mitral valve in the left ventricle. The posterior cusp is inserted along the posterior and lateral portions of the ring, meeting the septal and anterior cusps respectively. The commissures are marked by fan chordae. The chordal and papillary muscle patterns are highly variable but this variation is of no clinical consequence. Only the conal papillary muscle complex on the septum is relatively constant, although small.

With increasing age, expansion and doming of the tricuspid valve cusps are not infrequent (Fig. 6.75). The lesion is exactly analogous to the floppy mitral valve but is even more common. 30% of patients with floppy mitral valves have equivalent tricuspid valve lesions. In the tricuspid valve, significant degrees of the change are more frequent in chronic bronchitis, suggesting that increased right ventricular pressure exacerbates the doming, but it is also strikingly age-related. Little, if any, significant tricuspid regurgitation arises from pure cusp abnormality. Chordal rupture does not occur. Friction lesions occur on the septum in relation to chordae but again are of no functional consequence.

Ulceration of the inflow surface of the anterior cusp is relatively common (Fig. 6.76). The lesions range in appearance from shallow erosions to deep punched ulcers with raised margins. The ulcer base is yellowish. The lesion occurred in 6% of 2647 autopsy hearts studied by Pomerance;[51] in 97% of the 156 cases pulmonary pathology was present. The lesion is a good indicator of

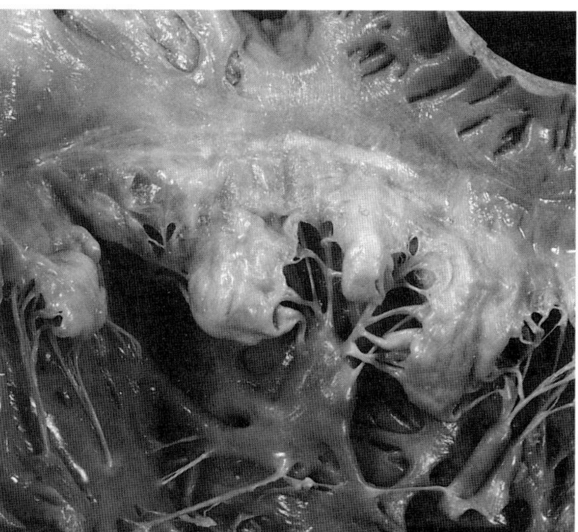

Fig. 6.75 Tricuspid valve in old age. All of the cusps of the valve are expanded and domed. This change, while associated with floppy mitral valves, is also a common isolated finding in old hearts.

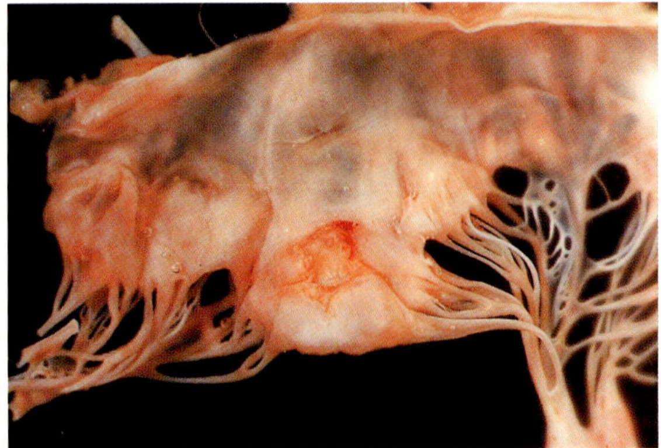

Fig. 6.76 Tricuspid valve ulceration. Isolated ulcers occur as yellow, sharply demarcated pits on the anterior cusp.

acute or chronic pulmonary hypertension and is almost certainly mechanical in origin.

In infants, small pinpoint-sized cysts containing blood are common on the atrial surface of the tricuspid valve cusps. Begg[52] found that 56% of infant and fetal hearts showed such cysts, particularly in association with hypoxia before death. Sectioning shows that the cysts are lined with endothelium and are in communication with the ventricular cavity. Occasionally, one becomes large enough to obstruct flow.[53] Similar cysts on the tricuspid or mitral valves of adults are occasionally reported.[54] A network of white strands joining the region of the foramen ovale in the atrium to the coronary sinus and inferior cava just above the tricuspid valve is often found in normal hearts. These so-called Chiari nets are remnants of the sinus venosus valve.

In Ebstein's anomaly of the tricuspid valve, its insertion on the septum and posterior wall is shifted downwards towards the ventricle (Fig. 6.77). A portion of the ventricular muscle is therefore 'atrialised'. All degrees of abnormality exist,[55] from simple downward shift by 1 cm of relatively normal cusps to a sheet of tissue without obvious commissures, low in the ventricle. In these cases where the valve cusps do not separate and remain as a diaphragm with small peripheral apertures, stenosis results. While most cases are diagnosed in infancy a few remain undetected until adult life. Right bundle branch block is a constant feature, while pre-excitation, due to downward shift of the normal tricuspid ring allowing abnormal atrial-ventricular continuity, is common.

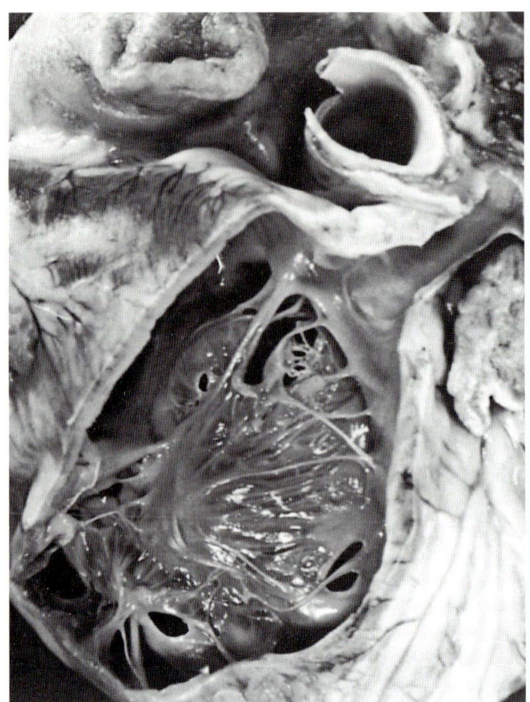

Fig. 6.77 Ebstein's anomaly — tricuspid valve. Viewed from the outflow tract of the right ventricle the tricuspid valve is a fibrous diaphragm with peripheral fenestrations inserted at a level well below the atrioventricular junction.

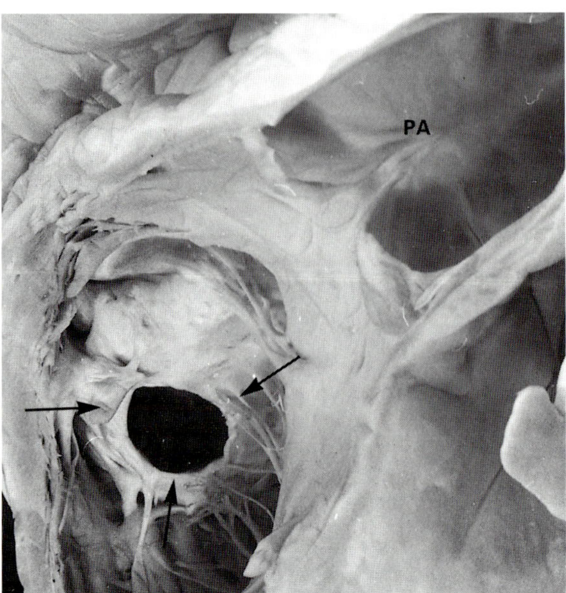

Fig. 6.78 Tricuspid valve stenosis — rheumatic disease. There is commissural fusion producing a fibrous diaphragm (arrows) with a central aperture. PA = pulmonary artery.

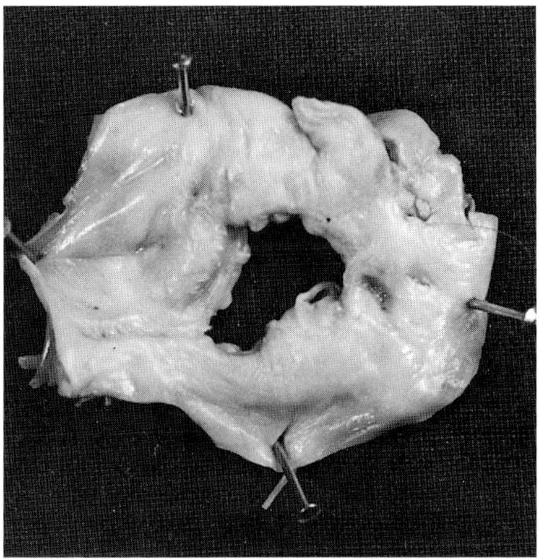

Fig. 6.79 Tricuspid valve stenosis. The valve excised surgically is a fibrous diaphragm with a central hole due to fusion of all three commissures. There is concomitant aortic and mitral disease.

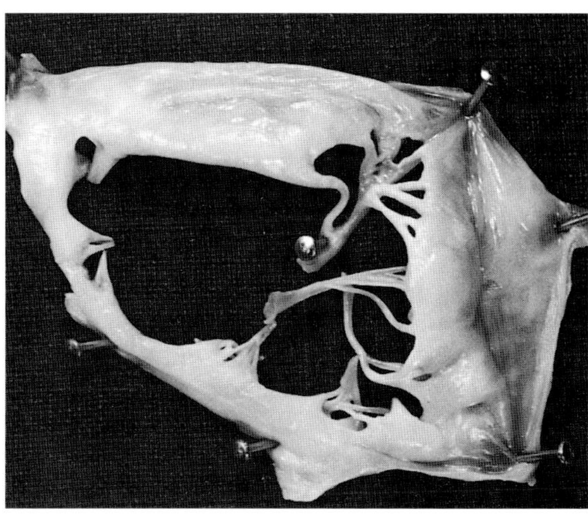

Fig. 6.80 Rheumatic tricuspid regurgitation. In this surgical specimen the cusps, particularly the anterior, are slightly thick; the dominant cause of regurgitation was ring dilatation.

TRICUSPID VALVE STENOSIS

Fusion of the three commissures in rheumatic disease produces a diaphragm with a fixed central aperture (Figs 6.78, 6.79). The valve remains mobile and significant degrees of cusp fibrosis or calcification are very rare. Tricuspid rheumatic disease, for all practical purposes, does not occur without co-existent aortic or mitral disease.

TRICUSPID REGURGITATION

Although rheumatic disease does cause some cusp fibrosis in the tricuspid valve, the predominant cause of regurgitation is ring dilatation. It seems that, even with gross cusp destruction, unless the valve ring dilates no really significant haemodynamic result occurs. For these reasons perhaps the single most useful quantitative observation on valve dimensions to make at autopsy is the tricuspid ring circumference. Values over 13 cm are abnormal.

The commonest cause of tricuspid regurgitation is ring dilatation secondary to right ventricular failure. This may be reversible if ventricular performance can be improved; the term 'functional' is used to indicate that the condition is analogous to the mitral regurgitation occurring in left ventricular failure.

Ring dilatation due to basic connective tissue weakness occurs in Marfan's syndrome. In rheumatic disease, the tricuspid valve cusps may become thickened and retracted but significant regurgitation occurs only if the ventricle dilates (Fig. 6.80).

PULMONARY VALVE

The structure and function of the pulmonary valve are similar to those of the aortic valve, with an identical physiology but a little less robust morphology.

The cusps are named in relation to the aortic cusps — right, left and anterior.

In pulmonary hypertension the valve cusps become somewhat more opaque and thickened by a surface layer of fibrosis. This does not appear to be of any clinical consequence. With age, fenestrations of the cusp lunulae appear but, as in the aortic valve, have no functional effect.

Bicuspid and quadricuspid pulmonary valves are far rarer than in the aortic valve and abnormalities at the two sites are not linked.

PULMONARY VALVE STENOSIS

At valve level, the most frequent cause of stenosis is a congenital defect. Isolated pulmonary stenosis is found in 1.5–6.5/10 000 live births, forming 2–13% of all congenital heart lesions.[56] The valve is usually a diaphragm with a central aperture which is highly variable in size from case to case. Ridges often mark the commissural sites. The lesion is very easily correctable, simply by splitting the diaphragm, and this should be done at an early age. If encountered at autopsy in adult life the late results of pulmonary valve dilatation or commissurotomy are strands or chords of fibrous tissue but no recognisable cusp. Untreated or unrecognised cases of congenital pulmonary stenosis may survive to adult life, developing increasing right ventricular hypertrophy. Pulmonary valve stenosis may or may not be accompanied by fibromuscular stenosis of the infundibular outflow portion of the right ventricle. Infundibular stenosis may also develop, purely as a secondary phenomenon, in extreme hypertrophy due to stenosis at valve level. In Fallot's tetralogy (pulmonary stenosis, overriding aorta and ventricular septal defect with right ventricular hypertrophy) a combination of valvar and infundibular stenosis is usual.

PULMONARY INCOMPETENCE

Dilatation of the main pulmonary artery may occur in high-flow pulmonary hypertension such as is associated with atrial septal defects. It may lead to ring dilatation and murmurs indicating pulmonary incompetence. Some secondary, flow-related cusp fibrosis may develop. Isolated cusp abnormalities producing significant regurgitation are rare. In patients with cusps virtually destroyed following relief of congenital stenosis, the murmur of regurgitation is present but haemodynamic consequences are unusual. Treated bacterial endocarditis leaves clean-cut cusp perforations but again the haemodynamic consequences are slight. For all practical purposes rheumatic pulmonary disease does not exist except as a very minor component of disease of all four valves. There is a hint in the literature that in countries where rheumatic disease is very common congenital heart disease with high flow and pressure in the pulmonary artery accentuates the pulmonary lesions of chronic rheumatic valve disease.

CARCINOID VALVE DISEASE

Up to 50% of patients with widespread deposits of a functional carcinoid tumour develop various combinations of pulmonary incompetence and stenosis, and of tricuspid regurgitation.

The lesions are very characteristic.[57,58] The pulmonary valve cusps become shrunken, white and thick (Fig. 6.81). An indrawing of the valve at the commissural level leads to a degree of stenosis. The tricuspid valve leaflets become white, opaque and reduced in area. Patches of white endocardial thickening also occur in the right atrium and ventricle.

On histological examination the lesion is seen to be a proliferation of young fibrous tissue on both surfaces of the cusps. There is no destruction of the underlying cusp fibrosa.

The lesion is thought to reflect a direct effect on the endocardium of vasoactive amines, including serotonin, produced by the tumour. Because the lung deactivates these products, the left-sided valves are spared.

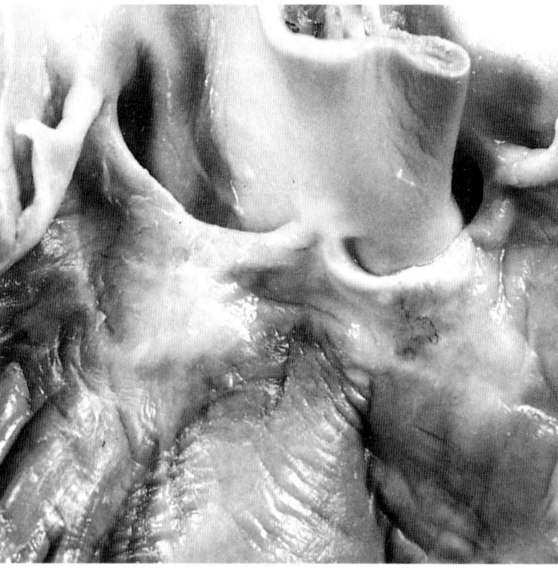

Fig. 6.81 Pulmonary valve in carcinoid disease. The valve cusps are white, fibrotic and reduced in area with an indrawing of the valve to narrow the orifice.

In patients with hepatic secondaries from ileal, gastric, pancreatic and ovarian carcinoid tumours, 49 of 79 cases collected by Grahame-Smith[58] had valve lesions.

Left-sided valve lesions are very rare but are described in a few cases with a shunt bypassing the lungs, or with tumours in the lung.[58] The precise pathogenesis of the endocardial fibrosis is not clear. Direct damage by serotonin, followed by insudation of fibrinogen and proliferation of young fibroblasts, is thought to be the most likely mechanism.

MISCELLANEOUS VALVE CONDITIONS

VALVE DISEASE IN SYSTEMIC LUPUS ERYTHEMATOSUS

The original accounts of the pathology of systemic lupus by Libmann[59] stressed that over 50% of acute fatal cases had a distinctive form of endocarditis on the mitral valve. Flat vegetations covered both cusp surfaces, extended on to atrial and ventricular endocardium and were found in the angles between cusp and ventricular endocardium. Occasional cases with large vegetations simulating infective endocarditis were described. Fibrinoid necrosis is present throughout the valve, with an inflammatory infiltrate and haematoxyphil bodies. Longer survival of patients treated for systemic lupus has led to the recognition that a valve morphologically indistinguishable from chronic rheumatic mitral stenosis or incompetence and aortic incompetence can occur. The only unique feature about such valves is continuing fibrinoid necrosis and an inflammatory infiltrate heavier than that usually seen in chronic rheumatic disease.

VALVE LESIONS IN RHEUMATOID ARTHRITIS

Rheumatoid granulomata may occur in the ring and cusps of the aortic and mitral valves. The commonest manifestation is aortic regurgitation due to valve cusp distortion, but very occasionally the distortion is sufficient to produce stenosis. About 5% of patients with severe rheumatoid arthritis are reported as having cardiac granulomata but of these very few have valve malfunction.[60]

In up to 66% of rheumatoid patients without clinical heart disease, the aortic and mitral valves show a variable degree of non-specific thickening and scarring, very closely resembling rheumatic disease but without commissural fusion or calcification. This high incidence suggests that these minor changes are a true rheumatoid manifestation rather than co-existent mild chronic rheumatic disease.[60]

ATRIAL SEPTAL DEFECT

With atrial septal defects of secundum type, three different abnormalities of the mitral valve are described. In the first place, floppy mitral valves seem to be unduly associated with the septal defect. Secondly, co-existent rheumatic mitral stenosis and atrial septal defect are the basis of so-called Lutembacher's syndrome. In fact, both conditions are frequently diagnosed in error when the third, most common, abnormality is present.[61] In this unnamed but commonest of these conditions, the portions of both cusps related to the medial commissure and directly underneath the atrial defect show surface thick-

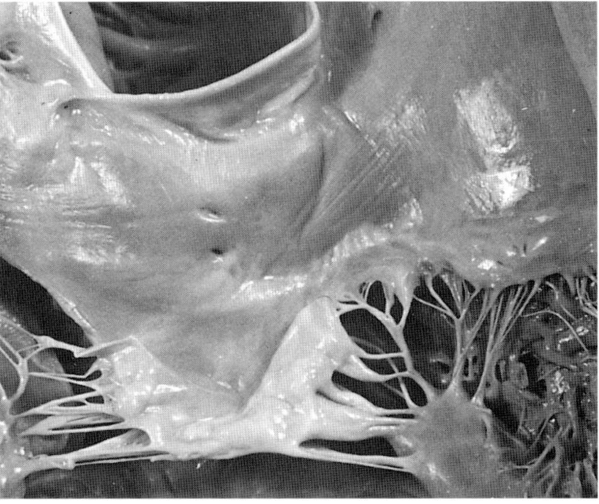

Fig. 6.82 Mitral valve in secundum atrial septal defect. The medial half of the anterior cusp and its attached chordae show fibrous thickening. Some chordae are fused. The changes are confined to the portions of the valve that lie directly underneath the septal defect.

ening but no contraction (Fig. 6.82). The cusp may appear somewhat domed upward. Thickening often involves the medial fan chordae. Histological examination shows surface fibrosis but no vascularisation, scarring or destruction of the valve fibrosa. The lesion is not seen in early life but is an almost constant feature in patients with unclosed secundum atrial defects who survive into later life. The lesion represents a haemodynamic effect, possibly an upward movement, resulting from a Venturi effect caused by blood flow across the defect. The effect of atrioventricular septal defects of the primum type on the mitral valve is described in Volume 10.

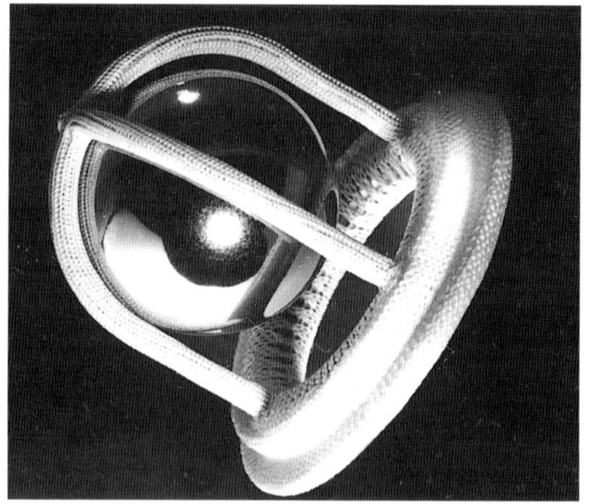

Fig. 6.83 Cage and ball Starr-type prosthetic valve. The valve function depends on the free movement of the ball within the cage and on it being able to fit exactly into the ring in the closed position. The ball shown here is steel — some models have propylene balls. The ring is covered by Teflon and this is sown into the original valve orifice. The struts of the cage here are covered in Teflon — some models have bare metal struts.

PROSTHETIC HEART VALVES

The first replacement of a human heart valve with a mechanical prosthesis was performed in 1952; the subsequent improvements in the quality of the prosthetic material as well as in the processing of human and animal tissues have been enormous. All these improvements have led to a significant decrease in morbidity and mortality rates related to prosthetic valve complications. Even pathologists who do not work in specialised centres will encounter prosthetic valves which have been in situ for some years, and knowledge of the type of valves inserted and the potential complications is necessary for an audit of long-term results of valve replacement.

Valve prostheses can be divided into two main types (Table 6.5). Mechanical prostheses can be divided into cage and ball prostheses, of which the prototype is the Starr–Edwards (Fig. 6.83), and low-profile prostheses (caged disk, bileaflet and hinged), which include the St Jude, Medtronic–Hall and Bjork–Shiley (Fig. 6.84). The second type are bioprostheses made of biological material such as fascia lata, dura mater, bovine or porcine pericardium, porcine aortic valve (Fig. 6.85) or human aortic valve (homograft) (Fig. 6.86).

Table 6.5 Prosthetic valves

Mechanical
Ball and cage
Tilting disc
Disc and cage
Hinged bileaflet
Tissue
Natural
Human aortic homograft
Porcine aortic valve
Constructed
Pericardial valve
Fascia lata valve

MECHANICAL PROSTHESES

Numerous mechanical prostheses exist.[62] The Starr–Edwards valve is the prototype of the caged ball mechanical prosthesis and has been in use since 1960. It consists of a metal frame and a silicone ball (poppet), with a Teflon sewing ring. The prosthesis designed to be in the aortic position has three struts, whereas the one going into the mitral position has four struts. The Smeloff–Cutter is the other type of caged ball prosthesis currently available.

Among the low-profile (i.e. not protruding into the ventricular cavity) prostheses, most belong to the tilting disk group. This includes the Bjork–Shiley model, which has two different types of occluder: a spherical disk or a convexo-concave disk. The spherical disk is made of

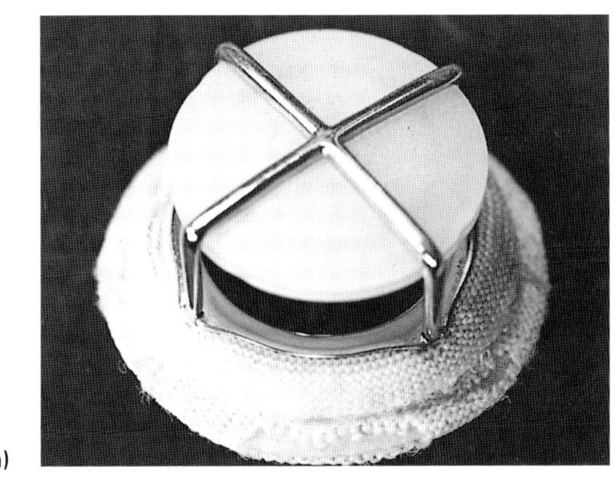

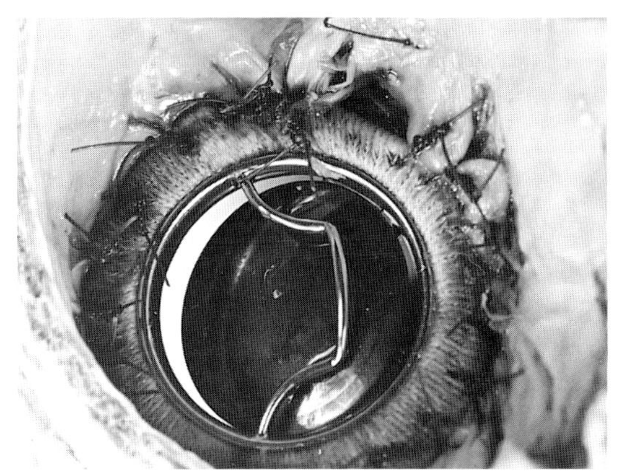

Fig. 6.84 a,b Low-profile disc and hinged prosthetic valves. In (**a**) the valve has a flat disc moving inside a cage and in (**b**) there is a tilting disc controlled by a spring. Both valve prostheses project into the LV cavity far less than cage and ball valves.

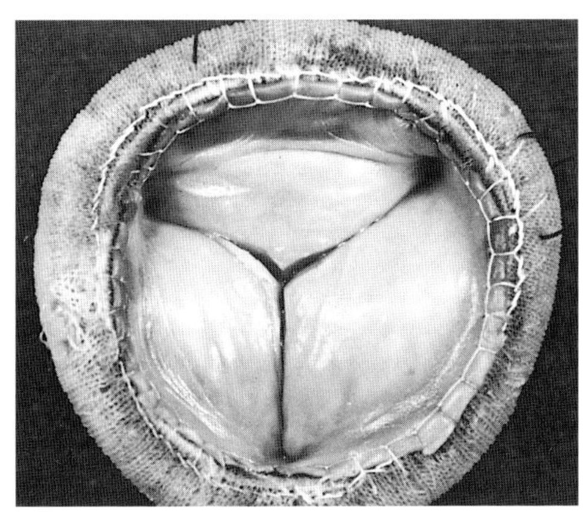

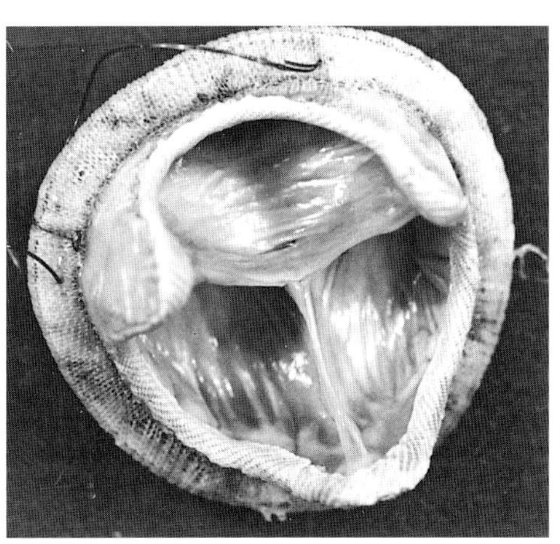

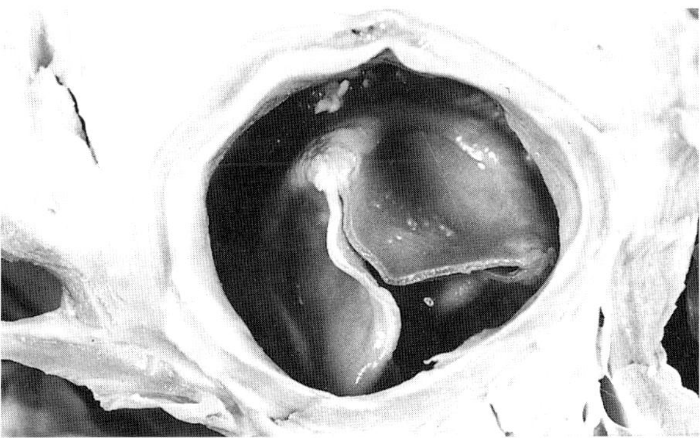

Fig. 6.85 a,b,c Tissue prosthetic valve. (**a,b**) The valve has a three-pronged stent and a frame within which is attached a gluteraldehyde fixed pig aortic valve.
(**c**) Valves constructed out of pericardium or fascia lata can be recognised by the absence of the normal anatomical landmarks seen in cusps.

pyrolytic carbon and is suspended in a metal cage with two struts. The convexo-concave model has a single strut which is part of the metal cage; this design modification results in a 40% increase in blood flow through the prosthesis. Other tilting disk prostheses include the Lillehei–Kaster, the Omniscience and the Medtronic–Hall types. The other group of low-profile prostheses includes hinged bileaflet prostheses, of which the St Jude is the prototype. The frame of the prosthesis is

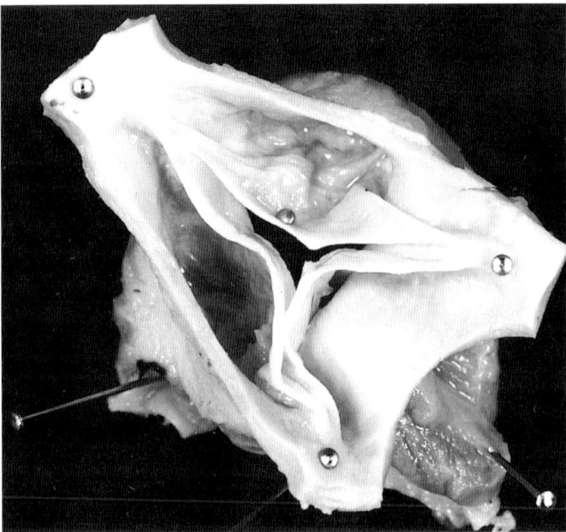

Fig. 6.86 Human aortic homograft prepared for use. This tissue valve is prepared by dissecting out a cadaver aortic valve. It can be used after fixation in gluteraldehyde or fresh after sterilisation with a disinfectant.

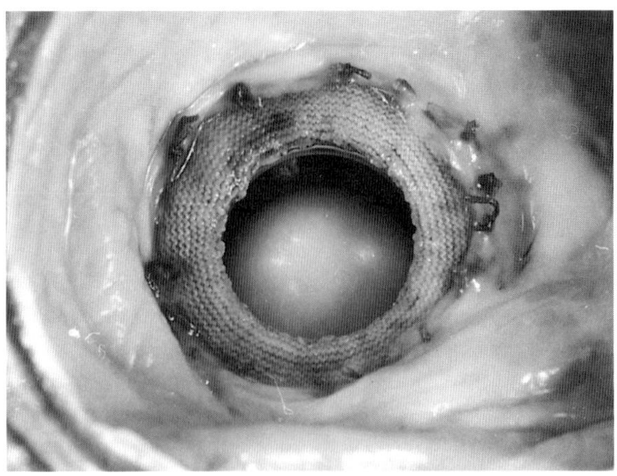

Fig. 6.87 Starr-type prosthetic valve — normal function. Viewed from the left atrium this valve, which had been in situ for 2 years, showed none of the sutures impinging on the orifice. The sutures are partially covered by white fibrous tissue but much of the valve sewing ring is uncovered. No paraprosthetic leak is present. No thrombus is present.

made of pyrolytic carbon-coated graphite and the leaflets of pyrolytic carbon and tungsten. The St Jude prosthesis is the one with the lowest haemodynamic profile.

Data from the Valve Registry Office at the Royal Postgraduate Medical School in London for the year 1990 show that the most commonly used mechanical prostheses in the United Kingdom are the Bjork–Shiley (20.39%) and the St Jude Medical (17.64%) models.

The morphological and radiological appearances of all the prosthetic heart valves commercially available have been reviewed.[62] They have been classified according to the presence or absence of a radio-opaque ring, the level of the projections of the ring itself and other features such as the height of the stents. Considering that the name of the prosthetic device changes from one country to the other, this is an excellent review which includes nearly all, if not all, the models available.

The examination of a valve prosthesis starts with the examination of the heart itself. The size of the cardiac chambers, the presence or absence of left ventricular hypertrophy, left ventricular scarring, thrombi and morphological appearances of the remaining native valves and the great vessels should all be assessed.

At autopsy, once post-mortem clot has been removed, it is possible to check prosthetic function by manually opening and closing the valve. The attachment of the ring of the prosthesis into the valve orifice should be checked for the integrity of the sutures. The ring of the valve usually becomes covered by layers of white fibrous tissue (Figs 6.87, 6.88) but this may not be complete even after some years. This tissue should not extend across the orifice itself. Gentle washing is usually effective in removing post-mortem clot, allowing the presence of ante-mortem thrombus to be identified.

When the original valve lesion was regurgitation, the ventricular cavity, the mitral annulus and/or the aortic root will be dilated. The dilatation of the valvular orifice allows the insertion of a relatively big prosthesis. If there is discordance between the size of the prosthesis and the size of the valvular orifice or the cardiac chamber this may lead to problems such as entrapment of a portion of the struts into the myocardium and subsequent overgrowth of fibrous tissue, or bending of the struts resulting in turbulent flow. In more severe cases, obstruction to the left ventricular outflow tract by a caged ball prosthesis has been described, especially in patients with hypertrophic cardiomyopathy or any other entity resulting in a thickened ventricular septum. Bioprostheses in the aortic position can obstruct a coronary ostium if one of the stents struts is over an ostium.[63]

The sutures attaching the prosthesis to the myocardium or the aortic wall should also be assessed. Trapping of untrimmed long sutures into a tilting disc prosthesis has been described. In some cases, where sutures have cut through the tissue, it is possible to pass a probe between the ring of the valve and the wall of the cavity to demonstrate a perivalvular leak (Fig. 6.88). Perivalvular leaks have also been reported in patients with connective tissue diseases such as Marfan's syndrome, in whom the annuli appear to be weaker than in the normal population.

Once the integrity of the prosthetic ring has been assessed, the amount of local fibrous tissue can be evaluated. Some authors call this overgrowth of fibrous tissue on to the prosthetic orifice pannus formation (Fig. 6.89). Others call it 'neointimal proliferation' or 'fibrous sheath'. This overgrowth of fibrous tissue appears to be time-related and is only an indication that the valve has been implanted for some time. In some cases, however, this benign tissue growth can invade the prosthetic structure and impede the movement of the ball or disc or cause stenosis.

Anticoagulation and the risk of haemolysis have always been closely related. The first models of mechanical prostheses were associated with considerable mechanical damage to the red blood cells and resulted in haemolysis, leading to a second valve replacement. Today the frequency of haemolysis as a complication is quite low in big surgical series, but it still can be seen (Fig.

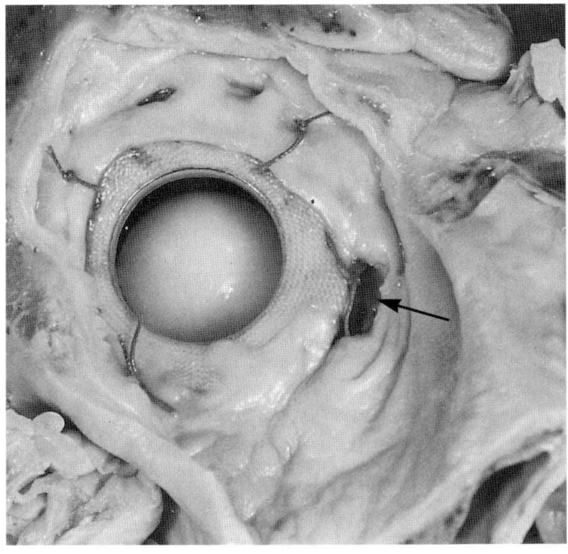

a)

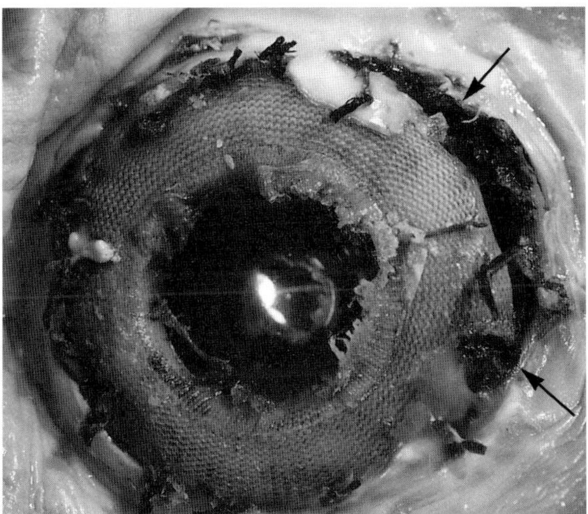

b)

Fig. 6.88 a,b Starr-type prosthetic valve — paraprosthetic leaks. (**a**) Viewed from the left atrium this valve, which had been in situ for some years, shows considerable covering of the sewing ring but fibrous tissue does not encroach on the orifice. A small paraprosthetic leak (arrow) is present, due to one of the ring sutures cutting out or breaking. (**b**) This valve has dehisced from the atrioventricular tissue over a large segment of the ring (arrows). Severe regurgitation occurred.

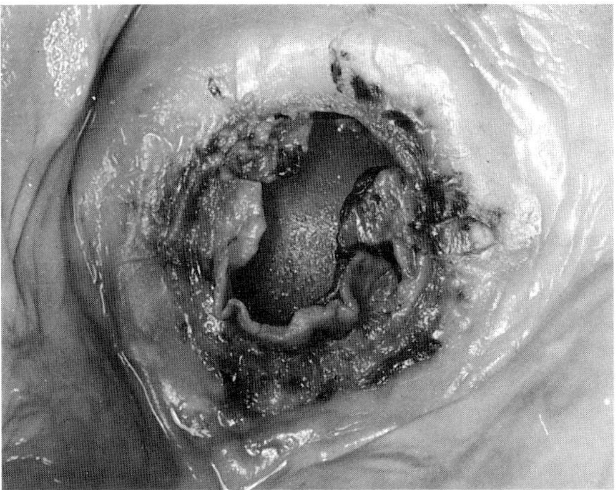

Fig. 6.89 Starr-type prosthesis — pannus formation. Viewed from the left atrium the valve ring is covered by white fibrous tissue. This tissue is however beginning to extend across the valve orifice as a 'pannus'. With such extension thrombus formation is often present.

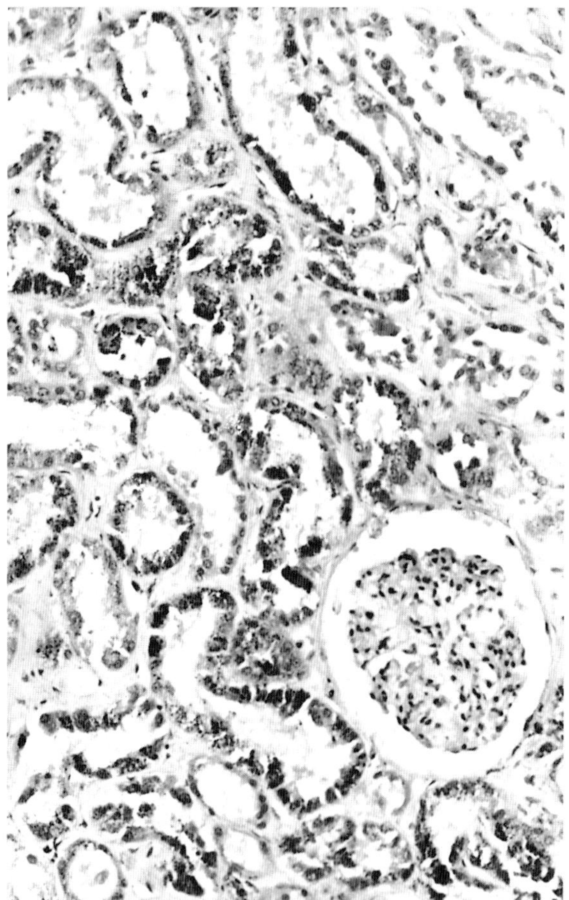

Fig. 6.90 Renal tubular haemosiderosis with a mechanical valve. The patient had a severe persistent haemolytic anaemia associated with a paraprosthetic leak of a Starr valve in the mitral position. The renal tubules are loaded with iron pigment.

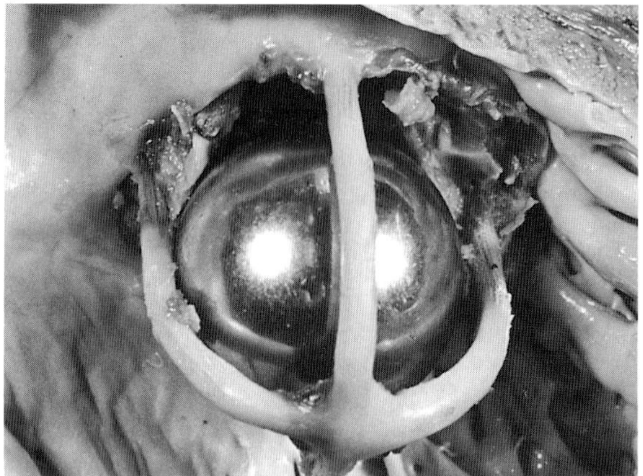

Fig. 6.91 Bacterial endocarditis on a Starr prosthesis. Vegetations cover a shallow cavity which is developing adjacent to the ring. The cage was Teflon covered and this has allowed white fibrous tissue to cover in the struts. Metal struts often remain bare.

6.90), especially with tilting disc prostheses and whenever a paraprosthetic leak appears.[64] Up to 15% of patients with a prosthesis have been shown to have iron-deficiency anaemia.[65]

Infective endocarditis on valve prostheses has traditionally been divided into early — up to 60 days after the operation — and late. Although the prognosis is poor in both cases, early prosthetic endocarditis on a mechanical valve has the highest mortality rate. The infective process generally results in variable degrees of periprosthetic regurgitation, since it tends to break sutures loose and thus render the prosthetic ring unstable. Occasional instances of prosthetic stenosis due to a vegetation have been reported. In the case of a mechanical prosthesis, the sutures tend to disappear progressively as a result of the infection and the prosthesis may end up 'hanging on one suture'. Since synthetic materials do not favour bacterial growth, the microorganisms tend to stay at the prosthesis–myocardium interface, resulting in a ring abscess (Fig. 6.91). Atrioventricular conduction disturbances are not uncommon at this stage. The vegetations may grow and lead to the progressive occlusion of the disc or result in sudden impedance to its movement and sudden death. The complications of prosthetic endocarditis are similar to those observed in native valve endocarditis, with cerebral emboli being the most serious. Overall rates for prosthetic valve endocarditis are around 1–6%, but the mortality rate reaches 50% or even more.[63]

Treatment for prosthetic endocarditis may include urgent prosthetic valve re-replacement. Culture of part of the cloth-covered ring or of the bioprosthetic cusps may yield evidence of a microorganism. However, since many cases will have received antibiotic treatment, the results are not always reliable.

The resistance to flow caused by the ball or the disc has always been difficult to determine. Most manufacturers will test the prostheses in vitro under variable haemodynamic conditions, such as different heart rates and different blood pressure values. The overall performance of the prostheses will be assessed in vitro by measuring the pressure drop or gradient, the effective orifice area, the regurgitant fraction and the turbulence. These tests have shown that the St Jude Medical prosthesis has the best haemodynamic profile, with the largest orifice area, and that the Bjork–Shiley monostrut model has the lowest regurgitant fraction, whereas the Starr–Edwards prosthesis is the most stenotic one because of the central location of the poppet. In most cases, these tests are satisfactory, but in some specific models of mechanical prostheses they have not been helpful to detect complications at a frequency higher than expected: in patients with a Starr–Edwards prosthesis and cloth-covered cage stents the cloth tends to wear out and the naked metal results in a higher number of thrombotic complications than other Starr–Edwards models. Another well-recognised complication is the fracture of the poppet, which has been mostly seen with the Starr-Edwards model 6120. The Silastic ball becomes yellow, probably as a result of lipid infiltration, and breaks. This can lead to the poppet getting stuck in one of the stents or coming out of the cage into the circulatory system, either intact or in embolising small fragments. In some rare instances, it has been the site of thrombosis. This complication of the Silastic poppet has been called 'ball variance'. Fracture of the strut in the Bjork–Shiley convex–concave 60° and 70° prostheses has become another well-recognised complication, seen only with these models of Bjork–Shiley prosthesis and requiring emergency surgery. The mortality rate for emergency valve replacement due to strut fracture was reported as being as high as 84% in a multicentre study. Metal wear occurring in the Lillehei–Kaster has also been seen occasionally. The pyrolytic carbon leaflet of the St Jude prosthesis has been reported to fracture and cause embolism.

TISSUE PROSTHESES

Bioprostheses, being made of biological material, present with different complications. The materials used are bovine pericardium (Ionescu–Shiley bioprosthesis) or porcine aortic valve (Hancock or Carpentier–Edwards bioprosthesis). Bioprostheses made of fascia lata and of dura mater are no longer available because of their high failure rate.

The animal tissue used to construct valves is treated with glutaraldehyde and thus there is no question of viability or indeed of an immune response to the prosthesis. These forms of bioprosthesis therefore depend on the long-term mechanical properties of fixed, dead collagenous

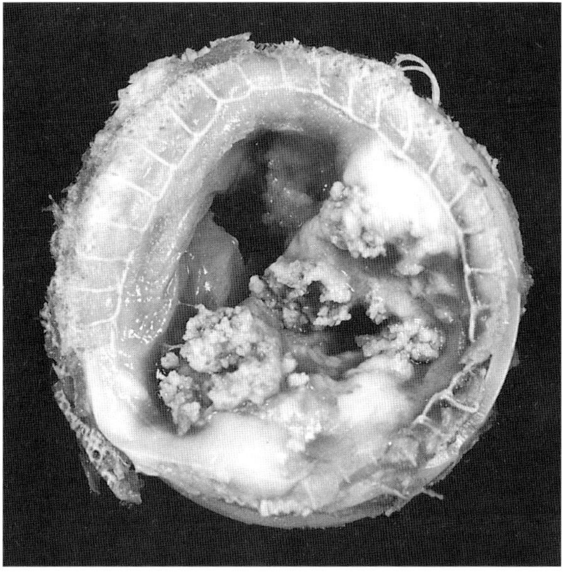

a)

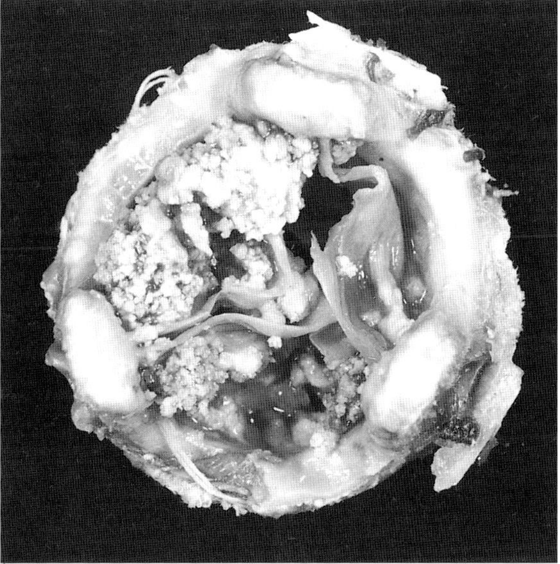

b)

Fig. 6.92 Tissue valve failure — cusp tear and calcification. In this Carpentier–Edwards-type pig valve both calcification and cusp tearing led to a combination of stenosis and regurgitation, requiring a second valve replacement.

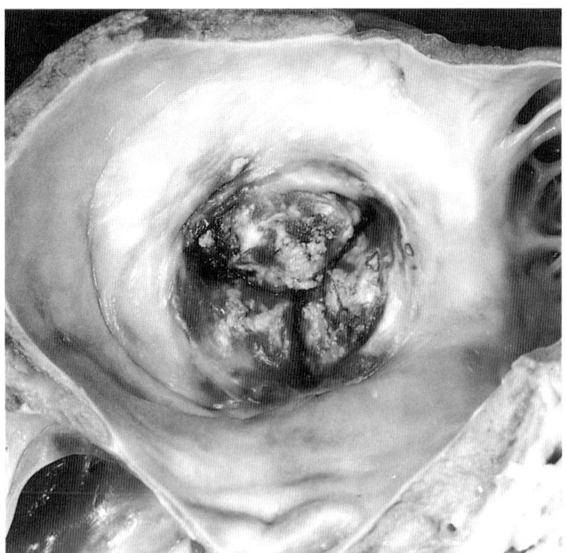

Fig. 6.93 Tissue valve failure — cusp calcification. In this tissue valve viewed from the left atrium all three cusps are heavily calcified. The valve, inserted into a girl aged 13, produced fatal severe mitral obstruction 3 years later.

tissue. Such tissue has two inherent problems: firstly it will ultimately tear (Fig. 6.92) and secondly it will calcify (Fig. 6.93).

These difficulties led to the use of human homograft aortic valves. Valves are harvested from autopsies and the fresh aortic valve and a cuff of aortic root used as a bioprosthesis without use of glutaraldehyde. Thus the collagen has not been subject to fixation. It has always been a debated matter whether viable fibroblasts in the donor valve survive and replicate the collagen. It seems likely they do not when derived from autopsies. Aortic valves obtained for use as homograft from living donors undergoing transplantation and pulmonary valves switched into the aortic position in the same individual do contain viable fibroblasts and synthesise collagen.

The rationale of the switch procedure is that a viable valve is placed in the aorta, whereas the tissue prosthesis inserted into the pulmonary position is likely to last longer in the low-pressure system.

The Hancock bioprosthesis was the first commercially available bioprosthesis, in the early 1970s. It consists of a porcine aortic valve mounted on a stent, with a sewing ring covered in cloth. Both the stents and the cloth are covered in knitted polyester. The valves were originally fixed in formalin, but glutaraldehyde, which results in a more stable cross-linking of collagen and improves the flexibility and the duration of the cuspal tissue, has been used since 1973. All porcine aortic valves have a septal shelf, which is part of the myocardium of the ventricular septum, in their right coronary cusp, which makes it slightly larger than the other two cusps. This shelf can result in decreased blood flow and a gradient through the bioprosthesis if it is big enough to protrude into the valve orifice. It also is one of the most frequent sites for calcification. The newest Hancock model (Hancock II) has resolved the problem of the septal shelf by re-implanting three porcine aortic cusps instead of using an intact porcine aortic valve; the manufacturers have also replaced the polypropylene frame with an acetal resin frame that is much more resistant to wear.

The Carpentier–Edwards bioprosthesis has been available since 1976. Porcine aortic valves are also used in its manufacture but it has a distinctive wire stent, made of cobalt and nickel, which is flexible. The stents are asymmetrical, like the cusps of a normal porcine aortic valve.

The Ionescu–Shiley bioprosthesis is made out of bovine pericardium. It was developed by Dr M. Ionescu in 1971 and has been commercially available since 1976. The pericardium is fixed in glutaraldehyde and the bioprosthetic cusps are cut and mounted on a titanium stent, thus eliminating the problem of the septal shelf resulting in decreased blood flow through the bioprosthesis.

All bioprostheses other than the homograft have a cloth-covered ring, which will be covered by fibrous tissue to different degrees, depending on the length of time the bioprosthesis has been implanted. This fibrous tissue growth can involve the stents of the bioprosthesis and even invade it and involve the commissures of the bioprosthetic cusps, but only rarely will this fibrous tissue result in significant haemodynamic changes.

Reviews regarding the long-term performance of porcine bioprostheses[66] have shown that primary tissue failure (tearing) has been the major indication for re-operation, mostly after a symptom-free interval of approximately 8 years. Infective endocarditis was seen at a rate of 0.5%

per patient-year, but the mortality rate related to it was extremely high, up to 67% in some series.[67] The frequency of primary tissue failure correlates with the age of the patient, bearing a direct relationship with low age and an inverse relationship with old age (over 70 years). Freedom from primary tissue failure has been reported as 27% at 10 years for patients under 30 years, increasing to 83% for patients above 60 years of age.

Although primary tissue failure is the main cause of failure of bioprostheses, especially in children, there are a few reports of cuspal retraction without stenosis,[68] in which the bioprosthetic cusps have been incorporated into the valve ring because of fibrous tissue overgrowth. Histological examination of these cusps showed extensive deposits of amorphous material with cholesterol clefts and neovessels in the fibrous tissue, together with a mild inflammatory reaction.

Mismatches between the size of the bioprosthesis and the size of the valvular orifice will result in the stents of the bioprosthesis bending inwards. Although this does not generally result in any haemodynamic alteration, the odd case with a severe mismatch can result in turbulent flow and an increased risk of thrombosis. Obstruction of the left ventricular outflow tract has also been reported in cases of bioprosthetic replacement in the mitral position in patients with a small left ventricular cavity. This stent deformity has been called 'stent creep' and has been occasionally associated with prosthetic malfunction. Although the mechanism behind the stent creep deformity is not known, some authors believe[69] that it is related to the size of the prosthesis and not to the type of bioprosthesis. Stent creep has been seen with increasing frequency in bioprosthesis with a flexible polypropylene stent. It has been shown that the stent creep tends to be more significant with time and in hearts with smaller left ventricular end-systolic volumes, which would support the theory that relates it to secondary compression caused by size mismatch between the prosthesis and the orifice or the cavity in which it has been placed.

Primary tissue failure, wear-and-tear or structural valve deterioration/degeneration is the name given by both cardiovascular pathologists and surgeons to the presence of calcium deposits on the bioprosthetic cusps resulting in dysfunction of the bioprosthesis and requiring a second valve replacement. In general, the wear and tear effect is haemodynamically noticeable and requiring replacement around 8–10 years after operation. Around 20–30% of bioprostheses fail at 10 years and more than 25% fail at 15 years. In some cases, however, this calcification process seems to be accelerated. Children have a very high calcium turnover and thus bioprostheses are not used in this age group. Diabetes mellitus, pregnancy and renal disease are all relative contraindications to the use of bioprostheses, since all of them increase the frequency of the wear and tear phenomenon. An occasional young adult will require a second valve replacement only a few years — even months — after operation and some postmenopausal women who are taking calcium supplements will also calcify their bioprostheses much faster than usual. The structural dysfunction rates are similar for the aortic valve homograft.

Porcine aortic bioprostheses consist histologically of three layers: a ventricularis, composed of collagen fibrils; a spongiosa or middle layer, consisting of proteoglycan and loose collagen; and a fibrosa which is only collagen. The predominant types of collagen are types I and II, with a ratio of 2.3:1. The pericardial bioprostheses, on the other hand, consist of a homogeneous surface of collagen which is nearly all type I. Thus normal structures show changes after implantation, as early as a few days postoperatively. The changes start with fibrin and platelet deposition on the bioprosthetic cusps and may evolve into a full-blown picture of mild chronic inflammation with lymphocytic infiltrates, giant cells and areas with focal disruption of the collagen fibrils. Neutrophils are never present except in the case of infective endocarditis. The lack of endothelium allows the insudation of plasma proteins and favours the presence of platelet aggregates.

Amongst the plasma proteins that infiltrate the bioprosthetic tissue is osteocalcin, which contains gamma-carboxyglutamic acid; this acid has been frequently found in calcified bioprostheses. The role of osteocalcin in primary tissue failure is still unclear; it has been shown that the administration of vitamin K antagonists decreases the level of gamma-carboxyglutamic acid in the tissues, but does not decrease calcification.[70]

The mode of failure differs between the porcine and the pericardial bioprostheses, probably because of their different design and manufacturing processes. The porcine bioprosthesis will have calcific nodules at the commissures whereas the pericardial bioprosthesis tends to have tears associated with the commissural sutures or 'alignment stitches' used to hold the cusp close to the stent. Morphological studies have shown[71–73] that the tears tend to start at the commissure and extend towards the base of the cusp, resulting in prolapse of the torn cusp and valvular regurgitation. Histological examination of the explanted bioprosthesis has shown disorganisation of the collagen bundles, together with lipid and protein infiltration. The Dacron ring was never endothelialised. Whenever there is fibrous tissue growth on to the area of contact between the cusp and the stent the frequency of tissue failure decreases. However, instances of functional impairment due to this fibrous tissue overgrowth have also been reported. No significant differences have been found in the failure rates of the Ionescu–Shiley pericardial valve compared to the Hancock pericardial valve.

The lack of endothelial covering seems to be a constant finding in different series of explanted pericardial bioprostheses,[74] together with exposure of the components of the pericardial cusps in the abraded areas. The presence of calcific deposits leading to cuspal tears varies between the series; it has been reported to be slightly more frequent with bioprostheses in the aortic than in the mitral position. It has been suggested that the differences between the Ionescu–Shiley model and the Hancock one may be due to the different concentration of glutaraldehyde used for fixation of the valve (0.2% versus 0.5% respectively). Most of the tears were close to the stent and could be classified as belonging to the Ishihara I group. Histological examination of these pericardial bioprostheses showed a significant decrease in the birefringent properties of collagen, together with loss of its usual spatial pattern, and the presence of calcific deposits. Scanning electron microscopy studies have confirmed the absence of endothelial cells covering the pericardial cusps. Others have shown that there is also thickening of the explanted pericardial cusps, probably due to infiltration by plasma proteins and lipids; this would lead to a decrease in elasticity, altering the local balance of stress forces and resulting in long-term disruption of the collagen fibres, since the thickened cusps do not bear stresses as well as the non-infiltrated cusps. This accumulation of lipids and plasma proteins has also been considered to be partially responsible for the different response of the pericardial bioprostheses to anti-mineralisation treatments when compared to porcine bioprostheses.[73]

Aortic valve homografts

Aortic valve homografts were in use as early as 1962 but their use was discontinued in the mid-1970s because of a very high incidence of cusp tears. This was probably a result of the preservation technique available at that time, which was either chemical sterilisation or valve irradiation. Today most homografts are removed with a sterile technique, kept in an antibiotic solution and frozen for storage. The results are often excellent (Fig. 6.94).

Early failure of an aortic valve homograft is generally due to aortic dilatation or to technical problems such as malposition of the valve itself.

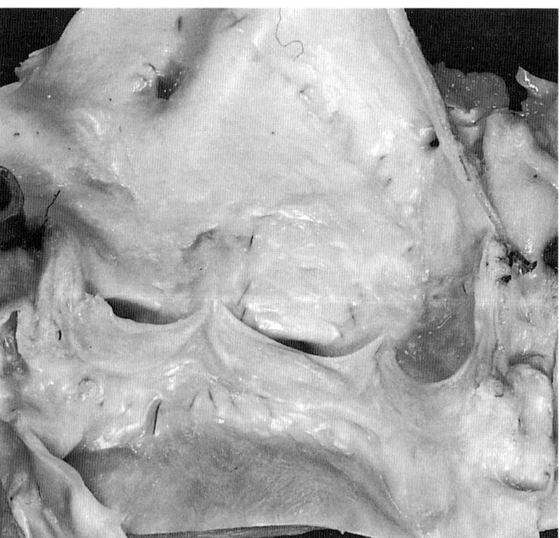

Fig. 6.94 Aortic homograft — normal function. This homograft had been inserted 8 years before death from non-cardiac cause. The cusps are intact, thin and mobile without calcification. Both the upper and lower suture lines are barely visible, having been covered by fibrous tissue.

Insertion of the soft homograft valve is inherently a more difficult procedure than sewing in a prosthetic valve with a rigid stent. The major cause for late valve failure is cusp rupture resulting in progressive aortic regurgitation or, less frequently, infective endocarditis.

The use of antibiotics for sterilisation has resulted in significant improvements in the duration of use of the homograft. The aortic valve cusps are infiltrated by fibrous tissue from the host, resulting in an increased support for the cusps. This had not been observed in chemically treated valves. Histological studies have shown loss of the endothelium on the donor cusps and this fact has been considered to be responsible for the tissue failure as well as for the increased frequency of thrombi and the decrease in fibroblast function.

Several factors have been implicated in the appearance of aortic regurgitation in homografts: the length of implantation is important, since follow-up studies have shown an increased incidence of aortic regurgitation with time. Systemic hypertension can increase the frequency of cuspal rupture, and aortic root dilatation will result in a higher frequency of aortic regurgitation. In general the frequency of infective endocarditis is low with aortic valve homografts, and thromboembolic complications are rare. A recent review of 555 aortic homografts[75] showed that primary tissue failure was the most common complication, with an incidence of around 5% per patient-year at 20 years. The rate of thromboembolic events was extremely low (0.034% per patient-year) and the incidence of infective endocarditis was also very low, at 1.1% per patient-year.

Stent-mounted allografts have been used for mitral valve replacement.[76] Both marginal and central ruptures have been observed, in approximately 50% of the allografts. Histological examination showed lack of endothelialisation, together with a thin layer of fibrin overlying the cusps. The host's fibrous tissue was shown to be present in all allografts. This fibrous tissue layer consisted of fibroblasts and collagen fibrils, with no blood vessels, and was covered by endothelium. The areas covered by this fibrous tissue did not show cuspal detachment.

OTHER SURGICAL PROCEDURES IN VALVE DISEASE

When mitral stenosis is due to dominant commissural fusion without calcification the valve orifice can be mechanically enlarged from the left atrium with a finger or dilator. The aim is to split the valve cusps along the line of the original commissure. Refusion of the commissures may occur leading to reoccurrence of stenosis (Fig. 6.87). Splits that enter the body of the cusp may produce significant regurgitation. The surgical approach to mitral regurgitation due to floppy mitral valve has become more conservative over the last 5 years. It is now common to excise the prolapsed segments of cusp and suture the remaining cusp tissue together. The sutures become buried in the valve and are difficult to see after some years. In severe mitral or tricuspid regurgitation due to dilatation of the valve ring, annuloplasty may be carried out. A purse-string suture is passed round the orifice, drawn tight and tied over a wedge of Teflon (Fig. 6.95).

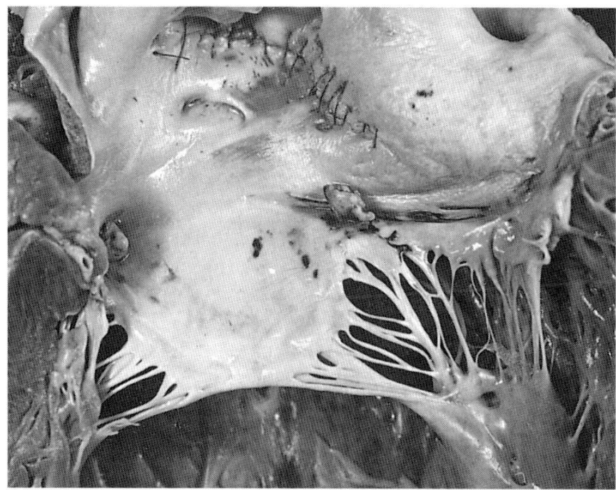

Fig. 6.95 Mitral annuloplasty. A suture has been placed around the annulus and tied over a wedge of Teflon in the atrium. The ring size has been reduced, thus diminishing the degree of regurgitation.

REFERENCES

1. Nestico P, DePace N, Kotler M, Rose L, Brezin J, Swartz C. Calcium phosphorus metabolism in dialysis patients with and without mitral annular calcium. Analysis of 30 patients. Am J Cardiol 1983; 51: 497–500.
2. Kavey R, Kaplan E. Resurgence of rheumatic fever. Pediatrics 1989; 84: 585–586.
3. American Heart Association Group of the Committee on Rheumatic Fever, Endocarditis and Kawasaki Disease. Guidelines for the diagnosis of rheumatic fever. Jones Criteria 1992 Update. JAMA 1992; 268: 2069–2073.
4. Cunningham M, McCormack J, Fenderson P. Human and murine antibodies cross-reactive with streptococcal M protein and myosin recognise the sequence GLN-LYS-SER-LYS-GLN I in M protein. J Immunol 1989; 143: 2677–2683.
5. William R. Molecular mimicry and rheumatic fever. Clin Rheum Dis 1985; 11: 573–591.
6. Vollebergh F, Becker A. Minor congenital variations of cusp size in aortic valves. Possible link with isolated aortic stenosis. Br Heart J 1977; 39: 1006–1010.
7. Edwards J. The congenital bicuspid aortic valve. Circulation 1961; 23: 485–488.
8. Becker A, Becker M, Edwards J. Anomalies associated with coarctation of the aorta: particular reference to infancy. Circulation 1970; 41: 1067–1976.
9. Angelini A, Ho S, Anderson R et al. The morphology of the normal aortic valve as compared with the aortic valve having two leaflets. J Thorac Cardiovasc Surg 1989; 89: 363–367.
10. Hurwitz L, Roberts W. Quadricuspid semilunar valve. Am J Cardiol 1973; 31: 623–626.
11. Passik C, Ackermann D, Pluth J, Edwards W. Temporal changes in the causes of aortic stenosis: a surgical pathological study of 646 cases. Mayo Clin Proc 1987; 62: 119–123.
12. Peterson M, Roach R, Edwards J. Types of aortic stenosis in surgically removed valves. Arch Pathol Lab Med 1985; 109: 829–832.
13. Falcone M, Roberts W, Morrow A, Perloff J. Congenital aortic stenosis resulting from an uncommissural valve. Clinical and anatomic features in 21 adult patients. Circulation 1971; 44: 272–280.
14. Waller B, Carter J, Williams HJ, Wang K, Je E. Clinicopathologic correlations. Bicuspid aortic valve, comparison of congenital and acquired types. Circulation 1973; 48: 1140–1150.
15. Sadee AS, Becker AE, Verheul JA. The congenital bicuspid aortic valve with post-inflammatory disease — a neglected pathological diagnosis of clinical relevance. Eur Heart J 1994; 15: 503–506.
16. Ewart A, Morris C, Ensing G et al. A human vascular disorder, supravalvular aortic stenosis, maps to chromosome 7. Proc Natl Acad Sci USA 1993; 90: 3226–3230.
17. Scheffer S, Leatherman L. Resolution of Heyde's syndrome of aortic stenosis and gastrointestinal bleeding after aortic valve replacement. Ann Thorac Surg 1986; 42: 477–480.
18. Mehta P, Heinsimer J, Bryg R. Reassessment of the association between gastrointestinal arteriovenous malformation and aortic stenosis. Am J Med 1989; 86: 275–277.
19. Lerer P, Edwards W. Coronary arterial anatomy in bicuspid aortic valve. Necropsy study of 100 hearts. Br Heart J 1981; 45: 142–147.
20. Abdalali S, Baliga G, Clayden A, Smith D. Coronary artery luminal diameter in aortic stenosis. Am J Cardiol 1985; 55: 450–453.
21. Roberts W, Kehoe J, Carpenter D. Cardiac valvular lesions in rheumatoid arthritis. Arch Intern Med 1968; 122: 144–156.
22. Sadee A, Becker A, Verheul H, Bouma B, Hoedemaker G. Aortic valve regurgitation and the congenitally bicuspid aortic valve: a clinico-pathological correlation. Br Heart J 1992; 67: 439–442.
23. Olsen L, Subramanian R, Edwards W. Surgical pathology of pure aortic insufficiency — a study of 225 cases. Mayo Clin Proc 1984; 59: 835–841.
24. Roberts W, Morrow A, McIntosh C. Congenitally bicuspid aortic valve causing pure aortic regurgitation without superimposed infective endocarditis: analysis of 13 patients requiring aortic valve replacement. Am J Cardiol 1981; 47: 206–209.
25. Larson E, Edwards W. Risk factors for aortic dissection: necropsy study of 161 cases. Am J Cardiol 1984; 53: 849–855.
26. Tonnemacher D, Reid C, Kawanishi D. Frequency of myxomatous degeneration of the aortic valve as a cause of isolated aortic regurgitation severe enough to warrant aortic valve replacement. Am J Cardiol 1987; 60: 1194–1196.
27. Allen W, Matloff J, Fishbein M. Myxoid degeneration of the aortic valve and isolated severe aortic regurgitation. Am J Cardiol 1985; 55: 439–444.
28. Bulkley B, Roberts W. Ankylosing spondylitis and aortic regurgitation – description of the characteristic cardiovascular lesion from study of eight necropsy patients. Circulation 1973; 68: 1914–1927.
29. Liu S, Alexander C. Complete heart block and aortic insufficiency in rheumatoid spondylitis. Am J Cardiol 1969; 23: 888–892.
30. Paulus H, Pearson C, Pitts W. Aortic insufficiency in 5 patients with Reiter's syndrome: a detailed clinical and pathological study. Am J Med 1972; 53: 464–472.
31. Lemon D, White C. Annulaortic ectasia: angiographic, haemodynamic and clinical comparison with aortic valve insufficiency. Am J Cardiol 1978; 41: 482–486.
32. Marquis Y, Richardson J, Ritchie A, Wigle E. Idiopathic medial aortopathy and arteriopathy. Am J Med 1968; 4: 939–954.
33. Schlatmann T, Becker A. Pathogenesis of dissecting aneurysms of aorta. Comparative histopathologic study of significance of medial changes. Am J Cardiol 1977; 39: 21–26.
34. Murray C, Edwards J. Spontaneous laceration of ascending aorta. Circulation 1973; 47: 848–858.
35. Pomerance A. Pathological and clinical study of calcification of the mitral valve ring. J Clin Pathol 1970; 23: 354–361.
36. Lachman A, Roberts W. Calcific deposits in stenotic mitral valves – extent and relation to age, sex, degree of stenosis in a study of 164 operatively excised valves. Circulation 1978; 57: 808–815.
37. Hanson T, Edwards B, Edwards J. Pathology of surgically excised mitral valves. One hundred consecutive cases. Arch Pathol Lab Med 1985; 109: 823–828.
38. Roberts W, Perloff J. Mitral valvular disease. A clinicopathological survey of the conditions causing the mitral valve to function abnormally. Ann Intern Med 1972; 77: 939–975.

39. Burch G, Giles T. Angle of traction of the papillary muscles in normal and dilated hearts. A theoretical analysis of its importance in mitral valve dynamics. Am Heart J 1972; 84: 141–144.
40. Waller B, Morrow A, Maron B. Etiology of clinically isolated severe, chronic, pure mitral regurgitation: analysis of 97 patients over 30 years of age having mitral valve replacement. Am Heart J 1982; 104: 276–288.
41. Davies M, Moore B, Braimbridge M. The floppy mitral valve: study of incidence, pathology and complications in surgical, necropsy and forensic material. Br Heart J 1978; 40: 468–481.
42. Iskandrian A, Kotler M, Kimbiris D, et al. Prolapse of the mitral valve: clinical, hemodynamic, angiographic and electrocardiographic correlations. Cardiology 1978; 63: 321–326.
43. Salazar A, Edwards J. Friction lesions of ventricular endocardium: relation to tendineae of mitral valve. Arch Pathol 1970; 90: 364–376.
44. Wilson L, Keeling P, Malcolm A, Russell R, Webb-Peploe M. Visual complications of mitral leaflet prolapse. Br Med J 1977; 2: 86–88.
45. Winkle R, Lopes M, Fitzgerald J, Goodman D, Schroeder J, Harrison D. Arrhythmias in patients with mitral valve prolapse. Circulation 1975; 52: 73–81.
46 Nishimura R, McGood M, Shub C, Miller FJ, Ilstrup D, Tajik A. Echocardiographically documented mitral-valve prolapse: long-term follow-up of 237 patients. N Engl J Med 1985; 313: 1305–1309.
47. Lucas RJ, Edwards J. The floppy mitral valve. Curr Probl Cardiol 1982; 7: 1–48.
48. Gaasch W, O'Rourke R, Cohn L, Rackley C. Mitral valve disease. In: Schlant R, Alexander R, ed. The heart, arteries and veins, 8th ed. New York: McGraw-Hill, 1994: 1483–1518.
49. Perloff J, Roberts W. The mitral apparatus. Functional anatomy of mitral regurgitation. Circulation 1972; 46: 227–239.
50. Raizada V, Benchimol A, Desser K, Reich F, Sheasby C, Graves C. Mitral valve prolapse in patients with coronary artery disease. Echocardiographic–angiographic correlation. Br Heart J 1977; 39: 53–60.
51. Pomerance A. Pathological and clinical study of calcification of the mitral valve ring. J Clin Pathol 1970; 23: 354–361.
52. Begg J. Blood-filled cysts in the cardiac valve cusps in foetal life and infancy. J Path Bact 1964; 87: 177–178.
53. Gallucci V, Stritoni P, Fasoli G, Thiene G. Case Reports. Giant blood cyst of tricuspid valve. Successful excision in an infant. Br Heart J 1976; 38: 990–992.
54. Liese G, Brainard S, Goto U. Giant blood cyst of the pulmonary valve. Report of a case. N Engl J Med 1963; 269: 465–467.
55. Anderson K, Lie J. Ebstein's anomaly of the heart revisited. Am J Cardiol 1978; 41: 739–745.
56. Hoffman J, Christianson R. Congenital heart disease in a cohort of 19 502 births with long-term follow-up. Am J Cardiol 1978; 42: 641–647.
57. Roberts W, Sjoerdsma A. The cardiac disease associated with the carcinoid syndrome (carcinoid heart disease). Am J Med 1964; 36: 5–34.
58. Grahame-Smith DG. The carcinoid syndrome. Am J Cardiol 1968; 21: 376–387.
59. Libman E, Sacks B. A hitherto undescribed form of valvular and mural endocarditis. Arch Intern Med 1924; 33: 701–738.
60. Sokoloff I. Cardiac involvement in rheumatoid arthritis and allied disorders: current concepts. Mod Concepts Cardiovasc Dis 1964; 33: 847–850.
61. Davies MJ. Mitral valve in secundum atrial septal defects. Br Heart J 1981; 46: 126–128.
62. Mehlem DJ. A pictorial and radiographic guide for identification of prosthetic heart valve devices. Prog Cardiovasc Dis 1988; 30: 441–464.
63. Schoen FJ. The first step to understanding valve failure: an overview of the pathology. Eur J Cardiothorac Surg 1992; 6: S50–S53.
64. Schoen FJ. Cardiac valve prostheses: pathological and bioengineering considerations. J Card Surg 1987; 2: 65–108.
65. Silver MD, Butany J. Mechanical heart valves – methods of examination, complications and modes of failure. Hum Path 1987; 18: 577–585.
66. Valente M, Minarini M, Thiene G, Bortolotti U, Milano A, Talenti E, Gallucci V. The pathology of Hancock Standard porcine valve prosthesis: a 20 year span of experience. J Card Surg 1990; 5: 328–335.
67. Milano AD, Bortolotti U, Mazzucco A, Guerra F, Stellin G, Talenti E, Thiene G, Gallucci V. Performance of the Hancock porcine bioprosthesis following aortic valve replacement: Considerations based on a 15-year experience. Ann Thorac Surg 1988; 46: 216–222.
68. Murphy SK, Roger WC, Fleming WH, McManus BM. Retraction of bioprosthetic heart valve cusps. Hum Pathol 1988; 19: 140–147.
69. Akiyama K, Sawatani O, Imamura E, Endo M, Hashimoto A, Koyanagi H. Stent creep of porcine bioprosthesis in the mitral position. Ann Thorac Surg 1988; 46: 73–78.
70. Levy RJ, Schoen FJ, Clarke Anderson H, Harasaki H, Koch TH, Brown W, Lian JB, Cumming R, Gavin JB. Cardiovascular implant calcification: a survey and update. Biomater 1991; 12: 707–714.
71. Thiene G, Bortolotti V, Valente M, Milano A, Calabrese F, Talenti E, Mazzucco A, Gallucci V. Mode of failure of the Hancock pericardial valve xenograft. Am J Cardiol 1989; 63: 129–133.
72. Walley VM, Rubens FD, Campagna M, Pipe AL, Keon WJ. Patterns of failure in Hancock pericardial bioprostheses. J Thorac Cardiovasc Surg 1991: 102: 187–194.
73. Hilbert SL, Ferrans VJ, McAllister HA, Cooley DA. Ionescu–Shiley bovine pericardial bioprostheses — histological and ultrastructural studies. Am J Pathol 1992; 140: 1195–1204.
74. Nistal F, Garcia-Martinez V, Fernandez D, Artinano E, Mazorra F, Gallo I. Degenerative pathologic findings after long-term implantation of bovine pericardial bioprosthetic heart valves. J Thorac Cardiovasc Surg 1988; 96: 642–651.
75. Matsuki O, Robles A, Gibbs S, Bodnar E, Ross DN. Long-term performance of 555 aortic homografts in the aortic position. Ann Thorac Surg 1988; 46: 187–191.
76. Maxwell L, Gavin JB, Barrat-Boyes BG. Uneven host tissue ongrowth and tissue detachment in stent mounted heart valve allografts and xenografts. Cardiovasc Res 1989; 23: 709–714.

7

Infective endocarditis

INTRODUCTION

Infective endocarditis is the growth of micro-organisms, usually bacteria, on the endocardium, or on a valve, within the heart. The organism can be recovered by culture from masses of thrombus, known as vegetations, on the valve (Fig. 7.1). Infective endocarditis contrasts with the endocarditis of acute rheumatic fever where neither bacteria nor their antigens are present in the valve. Recognition that rickettsiae and fungi can also grow on endocardial surfaces has led to the term bacterial endocarditis being superseded by the term infective endocarditis.

Previously, emphasis was placed on the contrast between the clinical and pathological features of acute bacterial endocarditis and those of subacute or chronic endocarditis. The former, typically caused by *Staphylococcus aureus*, developed in patients without previous known valve disease, progressed rapidly and septic emboli led to pyaemic abscesses. The latter, classically caused by *Streptococcus viridans*, was slower in onset and was usually associated with pre-existing valve disease; cardiac murmurs changed slowly over a period of weeks and emboli led to bland infarction. Before the advent of antibiotics both diseases inevitably led to death, either within a week in the acute form or within 1–2 months in the subacute form. A small minority of patients lived for longer periods but Horder in 1909 recorded a 100% mortality of proven cases of bacterial endocarditis within 18 months of diagnosis.

It is now recognised that a wide range of microorganisms can cause infective endocarditis

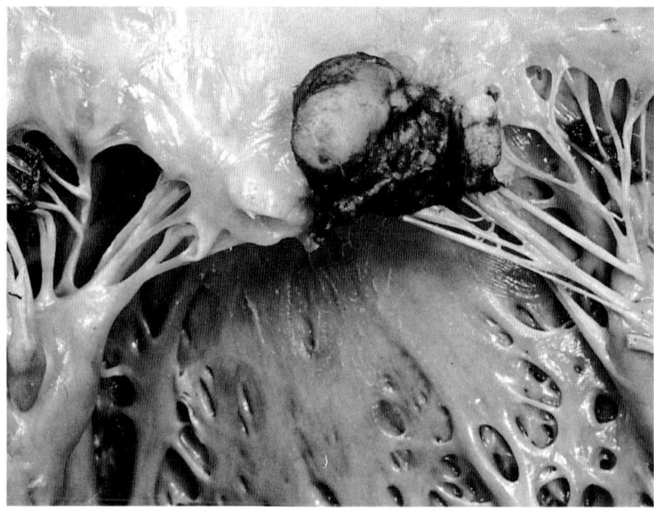

Fig. 7.1 Bacterial endocarditis — vegetations. The anterior cusp of the mitral valve has a large vegetation attached to its atrial aspect. The large size of the vegetation and its lack of relation to the cusp apposition line mark it as an example of infective endocarditis — in this case *Staphylococcus aureus*. The underlying valve was not abnormal prior to infection. Reproduced from Pathology of Cardiac Valves (1980) with permission of M. J. Davies and publishers Butterworth–Heinemann Ltd.

and there is a broad clinical spectrum between the two original extremes; it is largely the characteristics of the infecting organism that determine the clinical features. It is therefore now more usual to qualify the term infective endocarditis by the name of the organism and to gauge the resultant clinical picture accordingly rather than to apply the terms acute, subacute or chronic.

PATHOGENESIS OF BACTERIAL ENDOCARDITIS

Experimental models

Two factors, small thrombi on an endocardial surface and a concurrent episode of bacteraemia, are prerequisites of bacterial endocarditis. In the most frequently used animal models[1] an intravenous catheter is passed into the right atrium of a rabbit to induce endothelial damage on the leaflets of the tricuspid valve with the consequent formation of small platelet thrombi. Organisms are subsequently injected intravenously and the frequency with which bacterial endocarditis results is assessed. Both processes, valve damage and bacteraemia, prove to be essential; neither alone will lead to bacterial endocarditis (Fig. 7.2). If the intra-atrial catheter is removed the frequency with which bacterial endocarditis can be induced falls with time, and once the platelet thrombi are covered by endothelium infection does not supervene. The rate of occurrence of bacterial endocarditis is directly related to the numbers and the virulence of the organism which is injected.

Highly virulent organisms such as *Staphylococcus aureus* can establish infection on the tricuspid valve at lower dosages than the much less virulent *Streptococcus viridans*. In the context of causing bacterial endocarditis virulence depends in part on the ability of the organism to bind to substances or components that are not normally present on undamaged endocardium or valves. Organisms, such as *Staphylococcus aureus*, streptococci of groups A, C and G and *Candida albicans*, having the ability to bind to fibronectin by specific receptors will readily cause endocarditis. Variants of these organisms which have lost the ability to bind to fibronectin will not.[2] The ability to bind to platelets and glycoproteins is an important determinant of virulence in streptococci of the viridans group.[3] A further factor in virulence is the ability of the organism, once incorporated

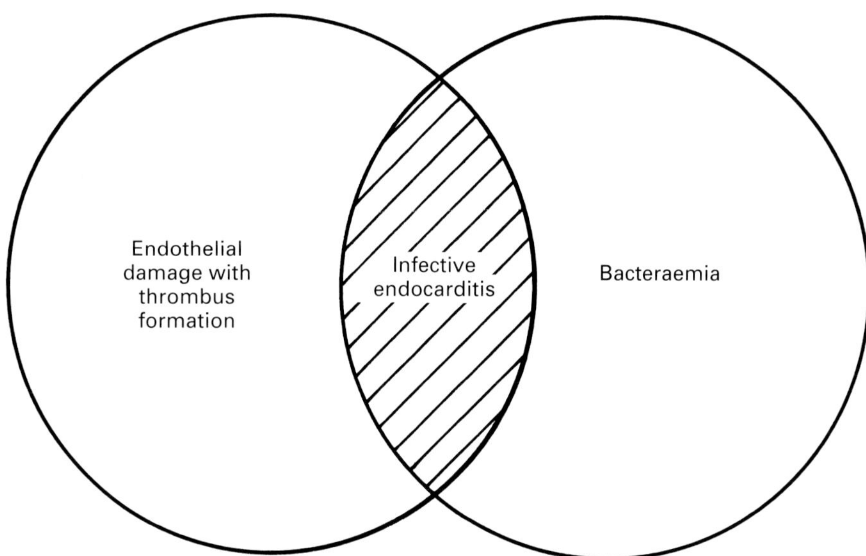

Fig. 7.2 Pathogenesis of bacterial endocarditis. A Venn diagram illustrating that a concordance of bacteraemia and endocardial damage is needed to produce bacterial endocarditis.

into a small thrombus, to produce glycosides and proteases allowing breakdown of plasma components to sustain bacterial growth; possession of such enzyme systems may explain the high frequency of certain viridans streptococci (*Streptococcus oralis* and *sanguis*) in bacterial endocarditis.[4] There is experimental evidence that the presence of agglutinating antibodies enhances the ability of an organism to cause endocarditis.[5]

Studies of the progression of infection[6] show that initially organisms are deposited on the surface of the thrombus in numbers identical to those sequestered by the spleen. There is then a lag phase of some 24 hours before rapid bacterial replication occurs within the thrombus. The lag phase has been attributed to the incorporation of the organism into a surface layer of fibrin, thus providing a protected site, free from phagocytic neutrophils, to which the term localised agranulocytosis has been applied.

Predisposing factors in human bacterial endocarditis

Many aspects of bacterial endocarditis in man suggest that these experimental models accurately reflect the natural disease. Some organisms, for example *Streptococcus viridans*, virtually only become established on a previously damaged cardiac valve. The valve lesions at particular risk of infection all involve high pressure jets and turbulent flow likely to lead to endocardial damage and therefore the formation of small platelet thrombi. Regurgitant valves constitute a far higher risk than those with pure stenosis; high pressure shunts, such as occur with ventricular septal defects, are commonly at risk; low pressure shunts, such as in secundum atrial septal defects, are virtually never associated with infective endocarditis.

The full list of potential predisposing lesions in the heart is large. Previously valves damaged by chronic rheumatic disease were responsible for the bulk of endocarditis due to streptococci of the *viridans* type.

In aortic regurgitation the first site of infection is often the ventricular aspect of the anterior cusp of the mitral valve, or the septum where the regurgitant jet flowing back across the aortic valve hits the endocardium. Bicuspid aortic valves are subject to infection due to their frequent association with mild aortic regurgitation. Mitral valve prolapse in the 'floppy valve' syndrome is a predisposing cause but because it is present in up to 5% of the normal population, the risk to any individual must be very small and probably is confined to those who have mitral regurgitation.[7]

Once again, as with aortic regurgitation, the primary site may be the consequent jet lesion on the left atrial wall rather than on the valve itself. Infection which begins on a jet lesion, rather than the valve or shunt site itself, is sometimes known as mural bacterial endocarditis.

Among the various forms of congenital heart disease patent ductus arteriosus (strictly infectious endaortitis) and ventricular septal defects predispose to infection at the site of the shunt. Small defects with high pressure jets insufficient to be haemodynamically significant carry an equal or higher risk than larger defects. In coarctation of the aorta infection develops on the aortic wall just distal to the obstruction where a high pressure jet leads to endothelial damage. Primum atrial septal defects also constitute a risk due to the associated cleft mitral valve and mitral regurgitation.

Other organisms, such as *Staphylococcus aureus*, can infect apparently normal valves. In this context it is pertinent to remember that even apparently normal valves undergo age-related thickening along the cusp apposition lines and histological examination may reveal an occasional small deposit of platelets. Thus even valves which are normal in the clinical sense may be at risk.

In man a potential cause for bacteraemia preceding the development of bacterial endocarditis may be found. Many years ago it was realised that streptococcal endocarditis on valves previously damaged by rheumatic fever was often preceded by dental work that had induced bacteraemia. Despite this knowledge and the knowledge that prophylactic antibiotics are needed to cover dental work in patients with cardiac lesions, 86 of 262 (32%) cases of endocarditis due to *Streptococcus viridans* either had had dental work within the previous 3 months or had dental sepsis.[8] There has been little change in practice, and dental treatment within the previous 3 months is still the most common source of infection.[9]

Apart from prior dental work approximately 40% of patients with bacterial endocarditis will have an obvious portal of entry for the organism into the blood stream. The origins of infection include skin lesions, wounds and lung infections preceding staphylococcal endocarditis, urogenital instrumentation, prostatectomy and intestinal surgery preceding enterococcal endocarditis and pneumonia or meningitis preceding pneumococcal endocarditis.

Any form of intravenous investigation such as cardiac catheterisation carries a risk of invoking endocarditis and this risk is very high in drug addicts who practise intravenous self-administration. Such infections are frequently contaminated by particulate material which may damage endothelial surfaces, as well as microorganisms introduced from the skin or from contaminated syringes and needles. Addicts usually develop tricuspid or pulmonary valve endocarditis, with *S. aureus* being the most commonly found microorganism, but in subjects with predisposing mitral or aortic valve lesions, left-sided endocarditis also is very common.[10] Comparison of HIV-positive and HIV-negative drug abusers with infective endocarditis yielded no differences concerning type of microorganism, embolic events and morbidity, although the HIV-positive patients had a slightly higher mortality rate.[11]

Although 60% of patients who develop bacterial endocarditis have no obvious portal of entry it is considered that previous bacteraemia must have occurred but went unrecognised or was transient. This view depends heavily on the animal work referred to above.

INCIDENCE AND PROGNOSIS OF BACTERIAL ENDOCARDITIS

In recent reviews of bacterial endocarditis considerable emphasis has been placed on comparison of the disease encountered 40 years ago with the situation today. There have been changes: the mortality has decreased from 100% to between 10% and 30%, the mean age of the patients has risen and the relative proportion of cases involving the mitral valve as compared to the aortic valve has fallen. It seems, however, that the overall number of cases has not altered appreciably.[9] Before 1918, on average, there were 573 deaths per year from infective endocarditis in England and Wales. Between 1968 and 1978, on average, there were 252 deaths annually but in a larger population; after allowing for a much reduced mortality the actual numbers of cases had probably not fallen significantly. It seems likely that the decline in numbers of patients at risk because of chronic rheumatic disease has been matched by the increasing number of patients at risk from a variety of factors relating to modern life and medical practice. It is estimated that in the USA two cases of infective endocarditis per 1000 drug addicts will occur every year.[12] All types of prosthetic cardiac valves in current use pose an increased risk for the patients,[13] as do all forms of indwelling foreign material, including pacing catheters and shunts used in renal dialysis. Any investigation involving intravascular procedures such as cardiac catheterisation may also be followed by infective endocarditis. Alcoholics, diabetics and immunosuppressed patients are particularly predisposed and the combination of this with other risk factors, such as a prosthetic valve, is more than simply additive. Not only is the risk of infection increased in such patients — for example, it is estimated that between 2% and 6% of patients on chronic renal dialysis will ultimately develop infective endocarditis — but the causative organisms are often unusual and the cases include a high proportion with fungal infection.

Table 7.1 Microorganisms isolated in infective endocarditis (approximate proportions in eight series)

Microorganism	%	
Streptococcus viridans		
S. sanguis I & II	0–25	40–50
S. mitis	0–10	
S. milleri / *S. mutans* / *S. salivarius*	0–15	
Streptococcus nutritional variant	<5	
S. haemolytica (unspecified)	10–35	
Group D streptococci		
Enterococci (unspecified)	0–15	10–20
S. bovis	1–5	
S. faecalis	5–10	
S. faecium	<1	
Staphylococcus aureus	10–15	15–25
S. epidermidis	5–10	
Gram-negative bacilli		6–8
Other		2–5
Coxiella		<1
Fungi		1–5
Negative blood cultures		8–12

CAUSATIVE ORGANISMS OF INFECTIVE ENDOCARDITIS

Bacterial infection

Many series report the relative incidence of the different organisms known to cause infective endocarditis.[5,9,13–15] The selection processes for inclusion of cases in the different series mean inevitably that one series is rarely directly comparable with another. Some consistent points, however, emerge about native valve infection (Table 7.1). The proportion of cases due to streptococci has declined over the last three decades but still accounts for between 30% and 60% of cases. The range of types of beta-haemolytic streptococcus that occur as agents is, however, far wider then previously. The incidence of staphylococcal endocarditis has increased but is still responsible for only 10–25% of cases overall. There is now a vast range of less common organisms known to cause infective endocarditis, the reports varying from single cases of rare infective agents to those more consistently noting unusual organisms to represent 1–5% of large series of cases. Among the latter group of organisms are enterococci, coagulase-negative staphylococci, Gram-negative bacilli, *Haemophilus* species and corynebacteria.

A full list of every organism now recorded to have caused infective endocarditis is virtually a catalogue of every known human pathogen as well as a considerable number of organisms found usually in veterinary practice. Patients with prosthetic cardiac valves and drug addicts both introduce a bias into any general list of causative organisms. In cases involving prosthetic valves, infection is divided into that occurring early (within 2 months) after insertion and late. The early cases are predominantly due to staphylococci but over half of these are coagulase-negative types (*S. albus*). In late onset cases just over 40% are due to streptococci of various types but there is an almost equal number of staphylococci, with coagulase-negative types predominating. Endocarditis due to Gram-negative bacteria is also far more common on prosthetic valves. The predominant microorganisms found in drug addicts are coagulase-positive staphylococci. There is a high incidence of infective endocarditis in drug addicts, 59% being caused by *Pseudomonas aeruginosa* or *Pseudomonas cepacia*, the latter organism being almost unique to endocarditis in addicts.[15] Fungi account for 5–10% of infections in drug addicts.

Bacteraemia is well known to follow cystoscopy or catheterisation of an infected bladder[16] and it is therefore not surprising that bacterial endocarditis specifically due to enterococci (*Streptococcus faecalis*) and the coliform species *Proteus* and *Pseudomonas* may result.

Pneumococcal endocarditis makes up 1–4% of all large general series and is usually consequent upon pneumonia, otitis media or meningitis. One third of cases are associated with alcoholism, which may be responsible for an apparent rising incidence of pneumococcal endocarditis.[17]

Gonococcal endocarditis, formerly responsible for up to 10% of all cases of infective endocarditis, is now rare but is still reported.[18]

Fungal endocarditis

Increasing numbers of cases of fungal endocarditis are being recorded, the approximate order of frequency of causative organism being *Candida*, *Aspergillus*, *Cryptococcus neoformans* and *Histoplasma capsulatum*, the last only being reported from geographical areas where the organism is endemic. Endocardial candidiasis occurs particularly in drug addicts, in association with long-term intravenous catheterisation, with prosthetic valves and in immunosuppressed patients.[19]

Q fever endocarditis

This form of infective endocarditis, caused by the Rickettsia-like organism *Coxiella burnetii*, is probably transmitted to man by sheep and cattle. Initially an influenza-like illness results, followed by infective endocarditis after a latent period which may be as long as 5 years.[20] A predisposing valve abnormality or a prosthetic valve is almost always present. Of 839 cases of confirmed Q fever in England and Wales between 1975 and 1981, 11% ultimately developed endocarditis.[21]

BLOOD CULTURES IN DIAGNOSIS OF INFECTIVE ENDOCARDITIS

The foundation of a firm clinical diagnosis of infective endocarditis remains the positive blood culture and actual isolation of the organism. Specific bactericidal antibiotic therapy can then be instituted. Virtually all series record, however, an appreciable number, 10%, of cases where the blood culture is sterile but in which the clinical diagnosis of infective endocarditis is strongly suspected and acted upon.[22] It is mandatory, at this point in clinical management, to consider whether the organism has fastidious growth requirements which are not being met. Some of the bacteria which cause endocarditis require specialised cultural techniques for their demonstration. The major advance has been in the isolation of streptococci of the *mutans* and nutritionally variant groups, which require the enrichment of conventional media with L-cysteine, pyridoxal or a peptide growth factor. Slow growing Gram-negative bacilli may require up to 3 weeks for isolation and include what has become known as the HACEK group (*Haemophilus* spp., *Actinobacillus* spp., *Cardiobacterium hominis*, *Eikenella corrodens* and *Kingella kingii*) to those working in this field.[14]

Some organisms, for example *Staphylococcus albus*, may be regarded in the laboratory as mere contaminants of the blood culture bottle but if consistently grown must be regarded as causative. *Coxiella* and fungal endocarditis also must be considered when routine culture yields negative or debatable results. Isolation of fungi is greatly accelerated by lysing the red cells of the blood sample and culturing the spun-down deposit. *Coxiella* infection is diagnosed by detection of serum antibodies against two polysaccharide antigens, phase I and II, present on the organism. Antibody titres of over 1/200 to phase I antigen are found in cases of *Coxiella* endocarditis. After excluding these possibilities the clinician is faced with either treating the patients empirically for bacterial endocarditis or regarding the clinical diagnosis as wrong. Surveys suggest that the vast majority of culture-negative bacterial endocarditis is, in reality, due to earlier treatment with inadequate doses of antibiotics. In patients who come to autopsy, or surgery, the organism can be grown from the valve tissue or be seen to be present in the tissues by electron microscopy even if not grown.[14] A single dose of penicillin will render the blood culture sterile for up to 2 weeks in cases due to a sensitive organism, but is totally ineffective as a cure.

THE CARDIAC LESIONS IN INFECTIVE ENDOCARDITIS

Gross appearances

The pathognomonic lesion of infective endocarditis is the vegetation, a large crumbling mass of thrombus adherent to the endocardial surface of a valve cusp or the mural endocardium. The vegetation may be either a single mass (Fig. 7.1) or multiple polypoidal masses (Fig. 7.3). Vegetations may be flatter and more sessile (Fig. 7.4). The distribution of vegetations on the cusps is neither symmetrical nor confined to the cusp apposition lines. The vegetations vary widely in size; those on the tricuspid valve, whatever the infecting organism, are often attached to the anterior cusp, are very large and swing as a pedunculated mass projecting into the right ventricular outflow tract (Fig. 7.5). Tricuspid vegetations may be yellow or white in colour (Fig. 7.6) rather than red, irrespective of whether the organism is a bacterium or a fungus.

Vegetations on the aortic valve are usually smaller. This variation in size is to some extent mediated by the different haemodynamic pressures and cavity sizes between the right and left sides of the heart rather than by the characteristics of the organism. Microorganisms of slower growth do, however, produce smaller, flatter vegetations and those of *Coxiella* (Q fever) endocarditis are in

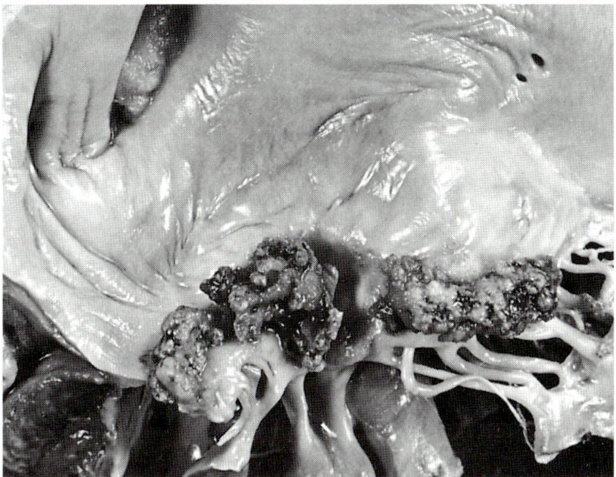

Fig. 7.3 Bacterial endocarditis — vegetations. Multiple polypoidal vegetations on the anterior and posterior cusp of the mitral valve.

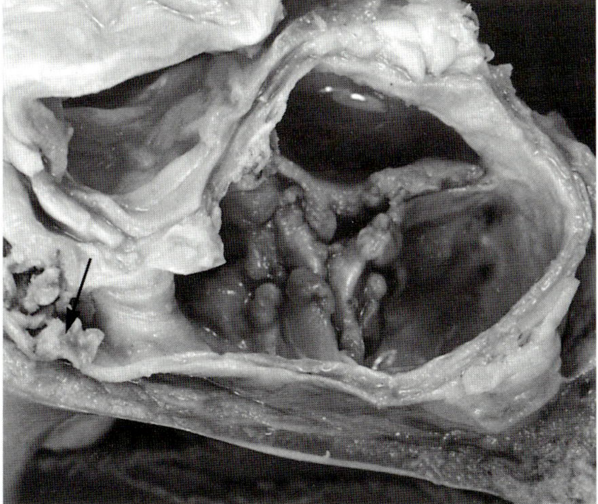

Fig. 7.4 Bacterial endocarditis vegetations — aortic valve. The aortic surface of the valve cusps, particularly the left coronary cusp, is covered by sessile vegetations. The main left coronary artery (arrow) is occluded by embolic thrombus. Reproduced from Pathology of Cardiac Valves (1980) with permission of M. J. Davies and publishers Butterworth–Heinemann Ltd.

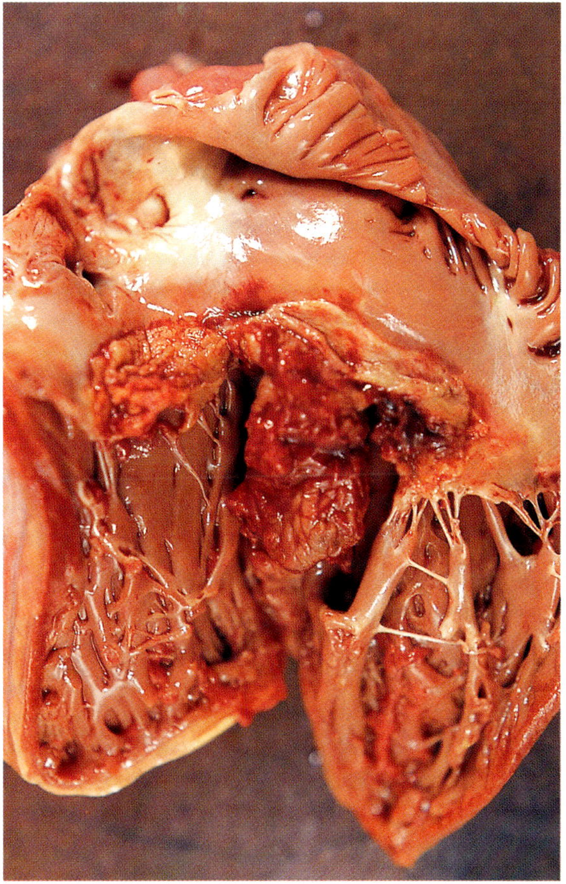

Fig. 7.5 Bacterial endocarditis vegetations — tricuspid valve. A large red pedunculated thrombus is attached to the anterior cusp of the valve.

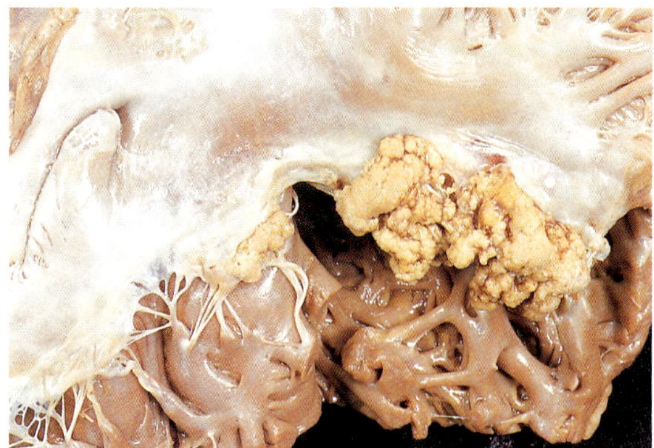

Fig. 7.6 Bacterial endocarditis vegetations — tricuspid valve. Polypoidal yellow vegetations are attached to the anterior cusp of the valve.

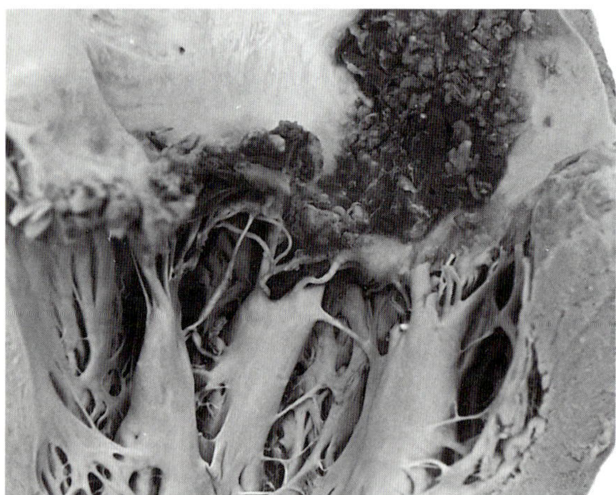

Fig. 7.7 Bacterial endocarditis — mitral valve. Vegetations have spread up on to the posterior wall of the left atrium.

particular very flat, small and somewhat unimpressive as seen by the naked eye. In advanced cases of bacterial endocarditis the vegetations may extend from the mitral valve upwards to cover the posterior wall of the left atrium. Vegetations also spread from the anterior cusp of the mitral valve up on to the aortic valve or, in the reverse situation, from aortic to mitral valve. This expansion of vegetations usually follows the line of a regurgitant jet along the endocardial surface (Fig. 7.7). Infection may also spread inward from the valve ring into adjacent myocardium.[23] This process particularly occurs in infections of the aortic valve which have extended into one of the sinuses of Valsalva. From each sinus there are natural tissue planes along which either a solid mass of thrombus burrows or a pus-filled cavity forms. Depending on which aortic sinus is involved and due to their anatomical relations, atrioventricular block or shunts between the aortic root and both atria or ventricles may develop. In mitral valve infection abscesses form around the valve ring while intramyocardial thrombotic masses are usually confined to cases of prosthetic valve infection where a potential space exists behind the sewing ring of the valve, that is the ring used by the surgeon to anchor the prosthesis to cardiac tissue. The exception is bacterial endocarditis involving mitral ring calcification where the infection spreads into the bar of calcification behind the base of the posterior cusp and thence out into the myocardium (Fig. 7.8).

The colour of the vegetations is very variable (Figs 7.5, 7.6); some are dark red, others a paler red, yellow or in some cases with a greenish tinge. Fungal endocarditis tends to produce vegetations that are paler than those of bacterial endocarditis.

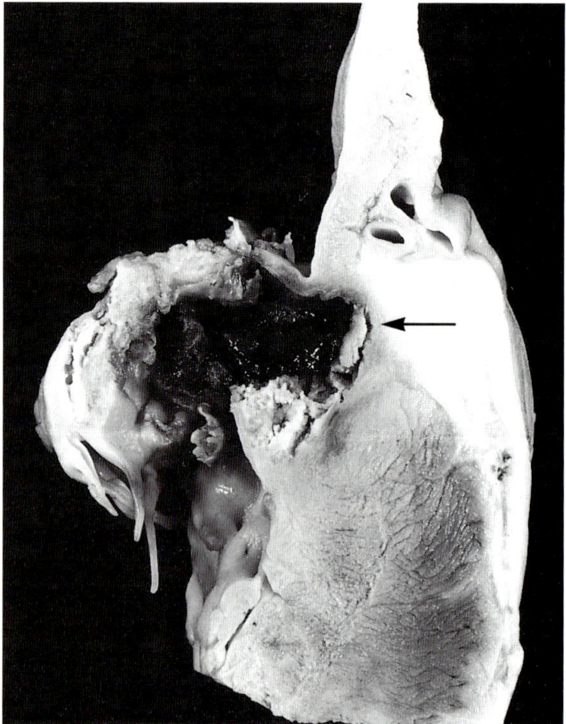

Fig. 7.8 Bacterial endocarditis — mitral valve infection developed on mitral ring calcification and burrowed into ventricular muscle (arrow) just below the insertion of the cusp.

There should be no difficulty distinguishing the vegetations of infective endocarditis from the far smaller, sessile and predominantly platelet thrombi occurring along the cusp apposition lines that are so typical of acute rheumatic endocarditis. The distinction from non-bacterial thrombotic endocarditis (NBTE) is discussed later.

Organisms toward the more virulent end of the spectrum may destroy the cusp structure. Perforations develop through the body of the cusp itself; in the acute phase these holes are ragged and surrounded by vegetations (Figs 7.9, 7.10). Large aneurysmal sacs may occur in either the aortic or mitral valve prior to cusp perforation. The opening of such an aneurysmal sac faces the aorta in the aortic valve and the left ventricular outflow in the case of the anterior cusp of the mitral valve (Figs 7.10, 7.11). Destruction and erosion of the cusp edges may lead to tears, with flailing of a whole portion of cusp; in the mitral valve, chordae may rupture (Fig. 7.12). Infections with less virulent organisms, even before treatment with antibiotics, may provoke considerable reparative fibrosis in the cusp beneath the vegetations. Both cusp and chordae may thus thicken and shorten even during the acute phase. *Coxiella* endocarditis also induces cusp fibrosis and, in the aortic valve,

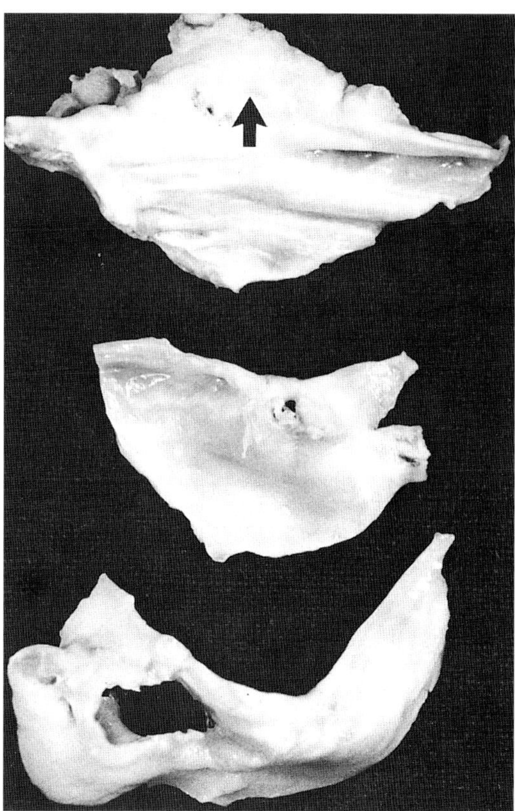

Fig. 7.10 Bacterial endocarditis — aortic valve. In this surgically excised tricuspid aortic valve one cusp has residual vegetations (arrow). Another has a perforation and an aneurysmal segment ('wind-sock').

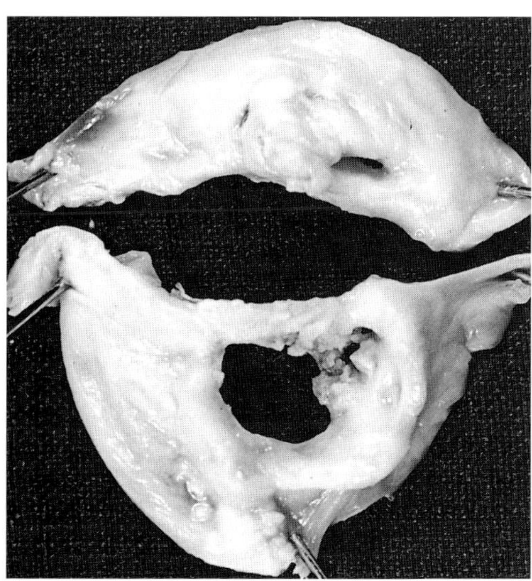

Fig. 7.9 Bacterial endocarditis — aortic valve. In this surgically excised bicuspid valve there is a large central perforation in one cusp with some residual vegetations on its rim. The other cusp is thickened with a small perforation.

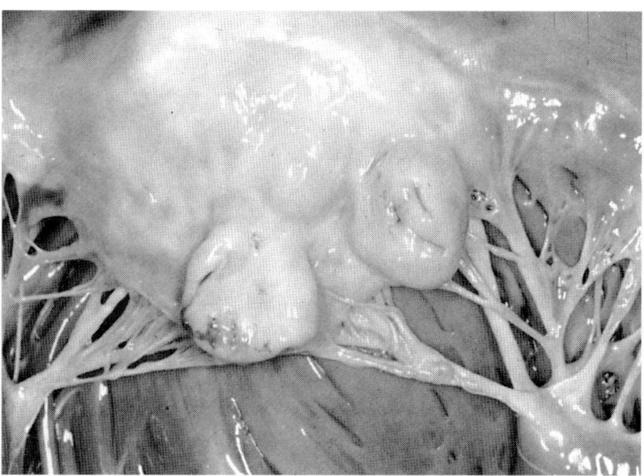

Fig. 7.11 Bacterial endocarditis — late sequela, mitral valve. The anterior cusp of the mitral valve shows two aneurysmal sacs without perforation. The opening of the sacs faces the LV outflow.

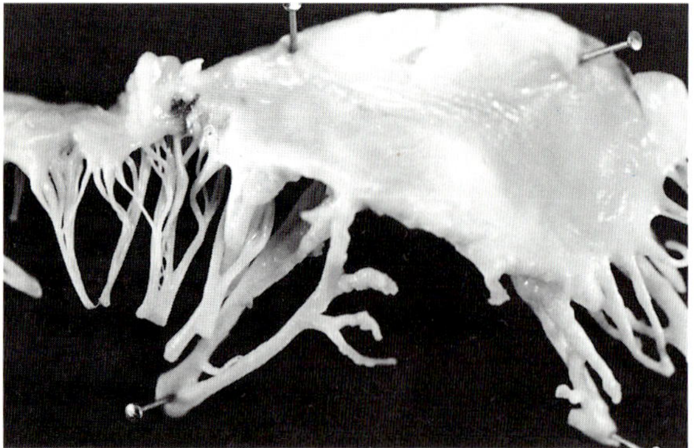

Fig. 7.12 Bacterial endocarditis — mitral valve. In this surgically excised mitral valve removed some weeks after antibiotic therapy there is erosion of the free edge of the anterior cusp of the mitral valve with several ruptured chordae covered with small calcified nodules representing previous vegetations.

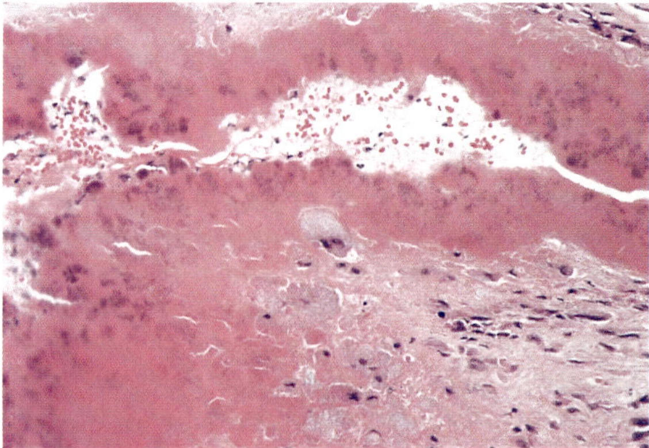

Fig. 7.13 Bacterial endocarditis — histology of vegetation. A band of amorphous bright pink fibrin and platelets is the most striking feature. On one side this contains multiple colonies of small basophilic bacteria. On the other side there is a fibroblastic and inflammatory response in the underlying valve.
Haematoxylin–eosin × 64

small aneurysmal bulges in the cusp and base of the sinus.

Following treatment with antibiotics further reparative changes take place and the vegetations diminish in size or vanish but a degree of valve disorganisation is inevitable. The vegetations may undergo almost complete lysis, leaving the underlying cusp thickened by fibrosis. Vegetations may also organise and, particularly when present between the chordae and in the angle between the posterior cusp and left ventricular wall, the resulting mass of fibrous tissue seriously restricts cusp movement. More rarely, vegetations remain as calcified nodules adherent to the cusp or chordae. In patients who survive cusp perforation the defects become smooth-edged holes through the body of the cusp.

It may or may not be possible to recognise that a valve with bacterial endocarditis has previously been abnormal. It is usually possible to recognise bicuspid aortic valves and floppy mitral valves by their characteristic dome shape in portions of cusp tissue uninvolved in the acute process. Major difficulties arise over the identification of chronic rheumatic disease. The cusp fibrosis, commissural and chordal fusion resulting from organisation of vegetations in infective endocarditis can very closely mimic the end stage of chronic rheumatic disease. In fatal cases of active bacterial endocarditis commissural fusion found at autopsy is more likely to indicate previous rheumatic disease but with valves excised surgically some months after treatment there are no criteria by which the pathologist can give a dogmatic opinion as to whether or not the valve was normal before the infective episode.

Microscopic changes in infected cusp tissue

The vegetations in bacterial endocarditis are composed of several structurally distinct zones (Fig. 7.13). The most superficial outer layer consists of finely granular eosinophilic material made up predominantly of agglutinated platelets with a few strands of fibrin. This layer is a major source of the small platelet emboli that arise in bacterial endocarditis. Immediately beneath this outer layer is a zone of densely packed fibrin containing colonies of the causative organism recognised in the case of bacteria by their punctate basophilic staining in routine haematoxylin-stained histological sections. There is experimental evidence[24] that the most superficial microorganisms are those actively dividing while the deeper colonies are metabolically inert but still viable and more resistant to antibiotics. Amid the fibrin are a few polymorphonuclear leucocytes but the striking feature is the paucity of these cells and it is clear that the bacteria are in a privileged site relatively protected from any effective cellular response. Beneath the vegetation is the cusp tissue itself which does become intensely inflamed. In the cusp vascularisation becomes a prominent feature and there is an intense fibroblastic proliferation along the base of the vegetation. The nuclei of these fibroblasts become very pleomorphic and may develop a chromatin pattern identical to the Anitschkow myocyte. The cellular exudate at the base of the vegetation contains a wide range of cells. In staphylococcal infections the number of polymorphs is high and there is considerable fibrinoid necrosis of the cusp connective tissue. This may, in part, be caused by proteases derived from the organisms but since the destruction is some distance from the vegetation itself it is more likely to be mediated by proteases released from monocytes and polymorphs. With less virulent organisms, such as *Streptococcus viridans*, the underlying cusp shows an intense fibroblastic response but no necrosis and with fewer inflammatory cells than in virulent infections. This inflammatory infiltrate is very pleomorphic and multinucleated histiocytic cells are common, particularly after treatment has been instituted. Such cells must neither be mistaken for Aschoff bodies nor taken to indicate *Coxiella* infection.

The dynamic state seems to be that proliferation of the organism occurs in the superficial layer of the vegetation; in the middle portion the organism persists for some time but is inert; while in the deepest layer, devoid of organisms, organisation develops. The reparative process, however, merely pushes the infected part of the vegetation outward into the blood flow and, in the absence of bactericidal therapy, can never effect a cure.

In fungal endocarditis the appearances are very similar to those of bacterial infections but with hyphae and/or spores easily identifiable within the centre of the vegetations. Hyphae may also extend more deeply into the underlying cusp tissue, often without a marked inflammatory response.

In *Coxiella* endocarditis the inflammatory cell infiltration is pleomorphic but with relatively small numbers of polymorphs and focal collections of large macrophages, some multinucleated, within whose cytoplasm the organism can be identified.

COMPLICATIONS AND COURSE OF THE DISEASE

Three distinct processes are collectively responsible for the clinical signs, symptoms, complications and mortality in infective endocarditis. These are first the disturbance of valve function, second embolic phenomena resulting from the friability of the vegetations, and third the consequences of the formation of circulating antigen/antibody complexes (Table 7.2).

Table 7.2 Complications of infective endocarditis

Clinical complication	Mechanism
Cardiac failure	Sudden volume overload due to regurgitation Immune-mediated intramyocardial vasculitis
Renal failure	Immune-mediated glomerulonephritis
Skin manifestations	Immune vasculitis — minor embolic component
Stroke	'Mycotic' aneurysm bleed Embolic infarcts
Gut infarction	Embolic
Splenic infarction	Embolic
Myocardial infarction	Embolic
Renal infarction	Embolic

Cardiac failure

A major contribution toward the mortality in both treated and untreated cases comes from cardiac failure. In the acute phase of bacterial endocarditis large vegetations may obstruct the valve orifice but this is only common in prosthetic valves. In native valves the destructive nature of bacterial endocarditis predominates to produce cusp fibrosis, perforation, tearing or rupture, all of which induce regurgitation whose speed of progression relates to the virulence of the organism. With prosthetic valves the Silastic and metal discs or balls and the glutaraldehyde-fixed cusps of tissue valves are not as susceptible to destruction. Vegetations form on the prosthetic valve ring and extend out across the valve orifice, obstructing flow. Some regurgitation may result from vegetations hindering movement of the disc or ball of prosthetic valves.

In bacterial endocarditis not only may there be progressive valve regurgitation but myocardial function and structure become abnormal. Small emboli in the myocardium, consisting predominantly of platelets derived from the surface of the vegetations, are particularly found in aortic valve infections. Impaction of such microemboli leads to multiple small areas of myocardial necrosis. Emboli that contain pyogenic organisms form small intramyocardial microabscesses. Even when there are no recognisable small emboli there is a generalised increase in neutrophils, eosinophils and histiocytes within the interstitial tissues of the myocardium and often tiny foci of necrosis involving two or three muscle cells. Such foci surrounded by inflammatory cells are what were described as Bracht–Wächter bodies in the older literature. Small vessels within the interstitial tissue often show a vasculitis, in that the media and perivascular tissue are infiltrated by chronic inflammatory cells; frank fibrinoid vascular necrosis is less common. The myocardial lesions are regarded as a combination of microembolic disease and circulating-antigen/antibody-complex-mediated vascular damage.

Embolic complications

The friable nature of the vegetations, their constant exposure to high pressure flow and the movement of the valve cusps are collectively responsible for the frequency with which fragments are thrown off into the systemic or pulmonary circulation. When the organism is pyogenic and of high virulence such infected emboli are capable of creating metastatic abscesses wherever they come to rest. Such abscesses are very characteristic of staphylococcal endocarditis and, as would be anticipated, occur in the lungs of drug addicts with tricuspid or pulmonary valve vegetations. Less virulent organisms tend either to be present in small numbers or not present in the emboli. Consequently impaction at the same peripheral site merely leads to a bland infarct without infection of the dead tissue. While such emboli may be carried out into any terminal branch of the systemic circulation those that pass to the brain are responsible for a significant proportion of the morbidity and mortality in cases of infective endocarditis. In 253 cases of bacterial endocarditis 52 (20%) developed cerebral emboli of whom 19 died.[25] Splenic emboli and the reaction to infection are responsible for producing the clinical signs of an enlarged and tender spleen. Renal emboli are one cause of overt haematuria. While microemboli are a common feature of bacterial endocarditis, major coronary emboli occur but are relatively rare. An important exception occurs in infective endocarditis of an aortic valve prosthesis, particularly in those types that have a central ball with peripheral flow of blood into the sinuses of Valsalva. The diversion of blood flow into the aortic sinuses by such prostheses directly channels emboli into the coronary artery orifices.

Circulating immune complexes

The prolonged bacteraemia that is so typical of infective endocarditis is commonly accompanied by circulating antigen/antibody complexes. The frequency with which circulating complexes are found varies with the method of their demonstration and ranges from 78% to 100% when using the ^{125}I–CIq/ binding assay.[26] In the acute phase of bacterial endocarditis there is an association of the presence of circulating immune complexes with the incidence of arthritis, subungual splinter haemorrhages, Osler's nodes, purpuric skin haemorrhages and glomerulonephritis. Biopsy of purpuric skin lesions has shown a vasculitis to be present and granular deposits of immunoglobulin can be demonstrated in the vessel wall;[27] in contrast, biopsy of the small red tender subcutaneous Osler's nodes suggests that they are purely embolic in origin with no immunologically determined vascular damage.[28] In contrast to the rising levels of immune complexes the serum complement falls. Bacterial antigens can be demonstrated both in the circulating complexes and in those deposited in the tissues.[29]

Immune-mediated mechanisms thus account for many of the clinical manifestations of bacterial endocarditis. In addition, the renal glomerular damage makes an important contribution to the morbidity and mortality. Studies in the pre-antibiotic era showed that 80% of patients dying from infective endocarditis had glomerular lesions identified by histology and that 15% of the mortality was due to renal failure.[30] Impairment of renal function, defined as haematuria or proteinuria greater than 150 mg per 24 hours, occurs in 50% of patients with infective endocarditis and, when present, indicates a worse prognosis. Renal biopsies studied by immunofluorescence suggest that virtually all cases of bacterial endocarditis have immune complexes within the glomeruli.[30] Complexes formed early

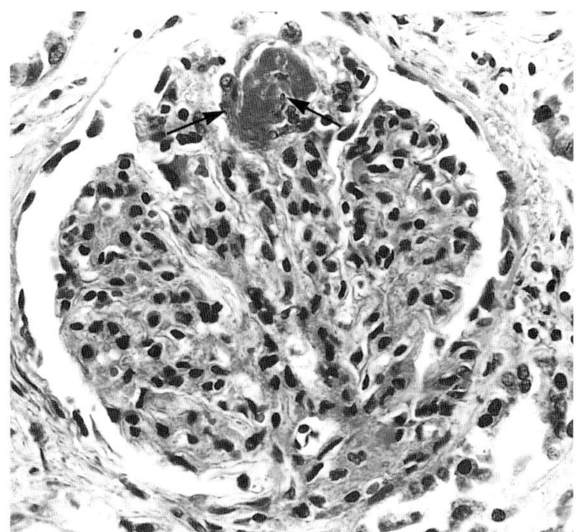

Fig. 7.14 Renal glomerulus in bacterial endocarditis. The glomerulus shows a focal segment of glomerulonephritis with a red fibrinoid appearance (arrows) contrasting with the more normal segments of the glomerulus.
Haematoxylin–eosin × 150

in the disease with antigen excess are deposited subepithelially; later, complexes with an antibody excess are deposited in the subendothelial zone and mesangium. At a histological level the most typical glomerular lesion is a focal proliferative form of glomerulonephritis (Fig. 7.14) with all gradations of severity up to a diffuse endocapillary form. In staphylococcal endocarditis acute renal failure still accounts for about 15% of the mortality.

The myocardial damage found in bacterial endocarditis, in part, is probably also determined by immune-complex-mediated vascular damage.

In the brain so-called mycotic aneurysms may also represent immune damage to large arteries; the term is a misnomer since there is no relation to fungal infection. The aneurysms range in size from being similar to the berry aneurysms that occur on the arteries of the circle of Willis to microscopic aneurysms on small parenchymal arteries within the cerebral cortex. The affected artery may or may not contain a small embolus within which organisms can be seen. A segment of the arterial wall shows fibrinoid necrosis of the media with a florid adventitial inflammatory response, the appearances being very similar to those of polyarteritis nodosa. Rupture leads to intracerebral haemorrhage, often combined with an area of infarction due to the embolisation.

LESIONS SIMULATING INFECTIVE ENDOCARDITIS

Infection is not the only mechanism by which thrombi can be produced on cardiac valves. In acute rheumatic fever and systemic lupus the valve cusps are swollen and along the apposition lines a row of small platelet thrombi are seen. These thrombi rarely exceed 1–2 mm in thickness and should not usually be confused with infective endocarditis. Any abnormal valve may develop slightly larger masses of surface thrombus, consisting mainly of platelets. In chronic rheumatic valve disease, for example, small masses of thrombi on the valve cusps, particularly in relation to calcification at the commissures of the mitral valve, are quite common. In bicuspid, calcific aortic valve stenosis small masses of thrombus are once again a relatively common finding. The recent clinical recognition that small microemboli to the retina are relatively common in patients with calcific aortic stenosis and mitral valve prolapse is a manifestation of the predisposition to the formation of platelet thrombi on abnormal valves. In general, the bland thrombi that occur in association with abnormal valves never reach the size of those seen in infective endocarditis.

Non-bacterial thrombotic endocarditis (NBTE)

In non-bacterial thrombotic endocarditis (NBTE) relatively large masses of thrombus develop on both the aortic and mitral valves. These vegetations may be up to a centimetre across and are often strikingly symmetrical in distribution on the aortic valve, being attached to the central nodulus Arantii of each cusp (Fig. 7.15). On the mitral valve the vegetations are attached symmetrically along the closure lines of both cusps (Fig. 7.16). The very size of the vegetations does lead to real difficulty in distinguishing the condition from true infective endocarditis. Histologically the vegetations are composed of platelets and fibrin with a mild inflammatory infiltrate. The underlying valve shows a minimal reaction although some

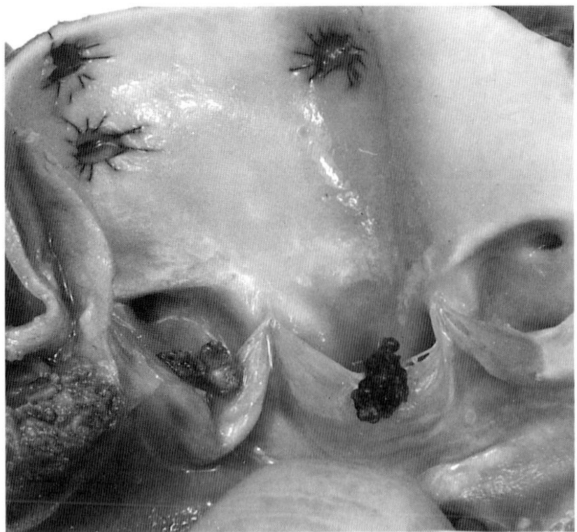

Fig. 7.15 Aortic valve NBTE. There are two vegetations, both of which are exactly at the central point of the cusp. The patient died within 2 weeks of cardiac surgery and the orifices of three vein grafts are shown.

organisation of the base of the vegetation may occur; no bacteria are present within the thrombus. While the condition is best known as non-bacterial thrombotic endocarditis (NBTE) the terms marantic endocarditis, endocarditis minima, endocarditis simplex and terminal endocardiosis are also used. Characteristically, non-bacterial thrombotic endocarditis occurs in patients who have died after weeks or months of a long debilitating illness. Particularly liable to develop NBTE are patients dying of carcinoma of the bronchus, stomach, pancreas and ovaries although no primary carcinoma is immune to association with the phenomenon. Occasional examples may be seen in terminal tuberculosis and in any chronic debilitating disease. A distinction between this condition and the formation of masses of thrombi occurring on grossly abnormal valves cannot easily be defined. This difficulty is responsible for much of the variation in published figures of the frequency of non-bacterial thrombotic endocarditis in the literature.

It is generally believed that the thrombi of non-bacterial thrombotic endocarditis develop on valves during the last few days of a terminal illness and hence are of little clinical significance. However, post-mortem studies in such cases demonstrate that quite a significant proportion of the thrombi on valves have given rise to systemic emboli.[31] Occasional clinical cases are described in which the embolic episodes occurred some weeks or months before death and were, in fact, the presenting feature of occult malignancy.

A post-mortem series is inevitably biased and the frequency of NBTE in patients with severe infectious diseases who recover may also be high.

The pathogenesis of the characteristic lesion of non-bacterial thrombotic endocarditis is thought to be a combination of underlying valve damage with an enhanced thrombotic tendency in these patients. The damage to the valve takes the form

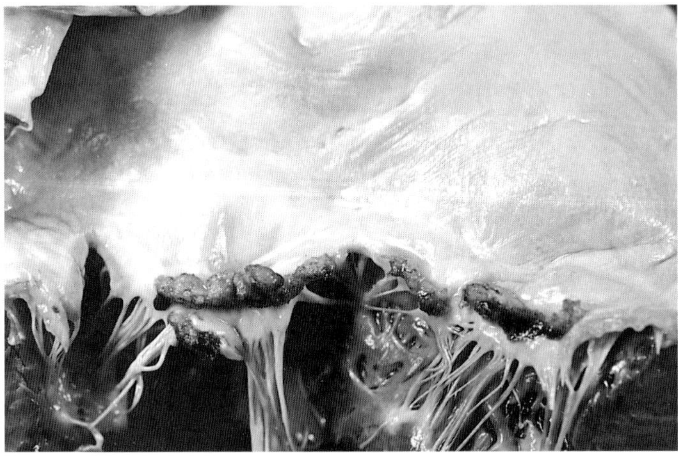

Fig. 7.16 Mitral valve NBTE. Vegetations are superimposed on the apposition lines of both cusps. The vegetations are relatively small, being 0.75 cm in thickness, but are quite exuberant and not unlike the appearances in Figure 7.3. Death from carcinoma of stomach.

of mild oedema and swelling of the subendothelial connective tissue of the valve and erosion of endothelium with exposure of the underlying collagen fibrils. This process has been postulated, largely on the basis of experimental work in animals, to be due to excess corticosteroid production as an accompaniment of stress. In patients with malignancy or severe infection increased platelet counts, increased plasma fibrinogen and activated factor VII levels and enhanced monocyte expression of Tissue Factor in the circulation are all postulated as factors in producing NBTE. Identical lesions may occur in any patient with acute disseminated intravascular coagulation,[32] quite apart from the presence of a debilitating disease. For the pathologist the issue with regard to non-bacterial endocarditis is how to avoid confusing the lesions with true infective endocarditis. In the final analysis it is the demonstration of organisms within the thrombus that distinguishes the two conditions. In some patients a terminal episode of non-bacterial thrombotic endocarditis becomes transformed into a true infective endocarditis through superimposed infection derived from the bacteraemia that is a not uncommon feature of the late stage of fatal illness.

REFERENCES

1. Freedman L, Valone J. Experimental infective endocarditis. Prog Cardiovasc Dis 1979; 22: 169–180.
2. Baddour LM, Christensen GD, Lowrance JH, Simpson WA. Pathogenesis of experimental endocarditis. Rev Infect Dis 1989; 11: 452–463.
3. Herzberg MC, MacFarlane GD, Gong K, Armstrong NN, Witt AR, Erickson PR, Meyer MW. The platelet interactivity phenotype of *Streptococcus sanguis* influences the course of experimental endocarditis. Infect Immunity 1992; 60: 4809–4818.
4. Homer KA, Whiley RA, Beighton D. Proteolytic activity of oral streptococci. FMS Microbiol Letters 1990; 67: 257–260.
5. Phair J, Clarke J. Immunology of infective endocarditis. Prog Cardiovasc Dis 1979; 22: 137–144.
6. McGowen D, Gillett R. Scanning electron microscopic observations of the surface of the initial lesions in experimental streptococcal endocarditis in the rabbit. Br J Exp Pathol 1980; 61: 164–171.
7. MacMahon S, Hickey A, Wilcken D, Wittes J, Feneley M, Hickie J. Risk of infective endocarditis in mitral valve prolapse with and without precordial systolic murmurs. Am J Cardiol 1986; 58: 105–108.
8. Bayliss R, Clarke C, Oakley C, Sommerville W, Whitefield A, Young S. The microbiology and pathogenesis of infective endocarditis. Br Heart J 1983; 50: 513–519.
9. Skehan J, Murray M, Mills P. Infective endocarditis: incidence and mortality in the North East Thames region. Br Heart J 1988; 59: 62–68.
10. Dressler F, Roberts W, Infective endocarditis in opiate addicts: analysis of 80 cases studied at necropsy. Am J Cardiol 1989; 63: 1240–1257.
11. Nahass RG, Weinstein MP, Bartels J, Gocke DJ. Infective endocarditis in intravenous drug users: a comparison of human immunodeficiency virus type 1-negative and -positive patients. J Infect Dis 1990; 162: 967–970.
12. Reisberg BE. Infective endocarditis in the narcotic addict. Prog Cardiovasc Dis 1979; 22: 193–204.
13. Watanakunakorn C. Prosthetic valve endocarditis. Prog Cardiovasc Dis 1979; 22: 181–192.
14. Bouvet A, Acar J. New bacteriological aspects of infective endocarditis. Eur Heart J 1984; 5: 45–48.
15. Cohen P, Maguire J, Weinstein L. Infective endocarditis caused by Gram-negative bacteria: a review of the literature 1945–1977. Prog Cardiovasc Dis 1980; 22: 205–242.
16. Sullivan N, Sutter V, Mims M, March V, Finegold S. Clinical aspects of bacteraemia after manipulation of the genitourinary tract. J Infect Dis 1973; 127: 49–55.
17. Wolff M, Regnier B, Witchitz S, Gibert C, Amoudry C, Vachon F. Pneumococcal endocarditis. Eur Heart J 1984; 5: 77–80.
18. Wall TC, Peyton RB, Corey GR. Gonococcal endocarditis: a new look at an old disease. Medicine (Baltimore) 1989; 68: 375–380.
19. Walsh T, Hutchins G, Bulkley B, Mendelsohn G. Fungal infections of the heart: analysis of 51 autopsy cases. Am J Cardiol 1980; 45: 357–366.
20. Baca OG. Pathogenesis of rickettsial infections — emphasis on Q fever. Eur J Epidemiol 1991; 7: 222–228.
21. Palmer S, Young S. Q-fever endocarditis in England and Wales 1975–81. Lancet 1982; ii: 1448–1449.
22. Tunkel AR, Kaye D. Endocarditis with negative blood cultures. N Engl J Med 1992; 326: 1215–1217.
23. Arnett E, Roberts W. Valve ring abscess in acute infective endocarditis. Frequency, location and clues to clinical diagnosis from a study of 95 necropsy patients. Circulation 1976; 54: 140–145.
24. Durack D, Beeson P. Experimental bacterial endocarditis I. Colonisation of a sterile vegetation. Survival of bacteria in endocardial vegetations. Br J Exp Pathol 1972; 53: 44–53.
25. Malquarti V, Saradarian W, Etienne J, Milon H, Delahaye J. Prognosis of native valve infective endocarditis: a review of 253 cases. Eur Heart J 1984; 5: 11–20.
26. Garnier J, Touraine J, Colon S. Immunology of infective endocarditis. Eur Heart J 1984; 5: 3–10.
27. Kauffman R, Thompson J, Valentin R, Daha M, van Es L. The clinical implications and pathogenic significance of circulating immune complexes in infective endocarditis. Am J Med 1981; 71: 17–25.
28. McKenzie P, Hawke D, Woodroffe A, Thompson A,

Seymour A, Clarkson A. Serum and tissue immune complexes in infective endocarditis. J Clin Lab Immunol 1980; 4: 125–132.
29. Inhan R, Redecha P, Knechtle S, Schnede S, van de Rijn I, Christian C. Identification of bacterial antigens in circulating immune complexes of infective endocarditis. J Clin Invest 1982; 70: 271–280.
30. Bayer AS, Theofilopoulos AN. Immunopathogenetic aspects of infective endocarditis. Chest 1990; 97: 204–212.
31. Olney B, Schattenberg T, Campbell J, Okazaki H, Lie J. The consequences of the inconsequential: marantic (non-bacterial thrombotic) endocarditis. Am Heart J 1979; 98: 513–522.
32. Kim H, Suzuki M, Lie J, Titus J. Non-bacterial thrombotic endocarditis (NBTE) and disseminated intravascular coagulation (DIC). Arch Pathol Lab Med 1977; 101: 65–68.

8

The pathology of cardiac transplantation

INTRODUCTION

Heart transplantation is now an accepted treatment for end-stage heart failure. Recent data from the Registry of the International Society for Heart Transplantation show a survival rate over 80% for the first year, reaching 75% at 5 years. More than 27 000 transplants have been registered worldwide, the vast majority in the last 7 or 8 years.

The most common indications for heart transplantation in adult populations are dilated cardiomyopathy and ischaemic heart disease. Other, less frequent indications are end-stage valvular heart disease, Chagas disease, hypertrophic cardiomyopathy, cardiac tumours and refractory arrhythmias.

Perioperative mortality rate related to heart transplantation can be divided into early (<30 days) and late (>30 days) mortality. The early mortality rate is up to 10% in adults and is related to complications such as poor preservation of the donor heart and prolonged ischaemic times during transport of the donor organ, or right-sided heart failure associated with high pulmonary vascular resistance during the early postoperative period. The late mortality rate, on the other hand, is closely related to both infection and acute rejection episodes during the first year post-transplant. Infection (23%)[1] and acute rejection (19%)[1] are major causes of death in the first 12 months after heart transplantation. Graft vascular disease — also called 'chronic rejection' — is the main cause of death after the first 12 months (30%).[1] Graft vascular disease remains the major unsolved problem of cardiac transplantation and is responsible for the loss of up to 10% of donor hearts per year after the first 2 years. The only available treatment is retransplantation, which poses an ethical problem because of the shortage of donors and the high mortality rate of a second cardiac transplant (up to 20%). The survival rate of retransplantation is significantly lower than that of primary transplant patients.[2] A recent assessment of 449 retransplanted patients showed that their survival rate at 1 year was 48%;[2] the frequency of both major postoperative complications and malignant neoplasms was also significantly increased when compared to first-time recipients.

The standard immunosuppressive treatment for heart transplantation includes azathioprine, corticosteroids and cyclosporin A. The last was added to the immunosuppressive schedule in the early 1980s and has allowed a significant decrease in the dosage of corticosteroids. There is, however, a considerable degree of renal toxicity with cyclosporin.

From the technical aspect, heart transplants can be divided into those in which the recipient's native heart is excised and replaced with a donor human heart (orthotopic) and those in which a donor human heart is inserted as an auxiliary pump ('piggyback' transplant). Since most cardiac transplants are performed in the orthotopic manner, this chapter will deal exclusively with the pathology findings in this form of heart transplantation.

EARLY PATHOLOGY

Hyperacute rejection

Hyperacute rejection is a rare event, becoming manifest in the operation theatre as soon as the donor heart is perfused. It results in a blue, hypercontracted 'stone heart'. The requirements for inotropic support are massive and the only therapeutic possibilities are either an artificial heart or immediate retransplantation with a second donor heart.

The mechanism underlying hyperacute rejection is not clear but it seems to be related to the presence of preformed HLA class I antibodies in the recipient, which would interact with the endothelial cells of the donor heart. A lymphocytotoxic antibody screen is used routinely to detect the presence of these antibodies and prevent hyperacute rejection. Another possible mechanism is based on the presence of preformed ABO blood group antibodies in the recipient, which would then react with the endothelial cells of the graft.

The clinical risk factors which have been related to hyperacute rejection are[3] a history of multiple blood transfusions, multiparity, and previous cardiac surgery and/or heart transplantation.

The hearts of patients dying of hyperacute rejection show severe dilatation of both ventricular cavities. The myocardium is flabby, with numerous minute petechial haemorrhages, mainly in the subendocardial area. Histological examination of the myocardium shows myocyte necrosis, interstitial oedema and haemorrhage. Fibrin and platelet thrombi are present occluding small vessels; the number of acute inflammatory cells is very variable.[4]

Unfortunately, this histological picture is quite similar to that of severe ischaemic damage to the graft. In donors who have been on inotropic support with catecholamines for long periods, the myocardial damage induced by the preservation procedure and prolonged ischaemic times during transport may combine to produce a similar histological picture.

Acute rejection

Acute rejection in the first postoperative year is the main complication and cause of death in patients who have undergone cardiac transplant. Rejection is diagnosed by means of endomyocardial biopsies, which are taken at regular intervals after transplantation. In general, they are obtained weekly during the first postoperative month and then every 2 weeks until the patient returns home. Most of the centres perform routine biopsies at 3, 6 and 12 months after transplantation and after that on a yearly basis unless there is a clinical suspicion of rejection. The diagnosis of rejection is still based exclusively on the biopsy findings. Numerous methods of diagnosing rejection by non-invasive methods including echocardiography, serial levels of cardiac enzyme or myocyte proteins such as troponin T and serial plasma levels of immune activation such as circulating soluble receptors have been tried but have not proved predictive.[5] Clinically, rejection is detected by the presence of signs and symptoms of left ventricular dysfunction, but these are not always present. Thus, the endomyocardial biopsy remains the 'gold standard' for the diagnosis and treatment of acute rejection. The Caves bioptome — used for right ventricular biopsies — has been available since 1973,[6] and serial right ventricular biopsies can be obtained from the patient with minimal risk.

One of the problems confronting histopathologists dealing with endomyocardial biopsies for the management of cardiac transplantation is the grading system. Many of the major cardiac transplant units over the world have developed — and use — their own grading system, which includes up to 10 subgroups.[7] This has made the comparison of different treatments and the assessment of survival related to the severity of rejection between different units very difficult. Most of the grading systems used were variations based on the Billingham system,[8] which was instituted at Stanford University in 1981. The Billingham grading system includes mild, moderate, severe and resolving or resolved rejection. Both mild and moderate rejection can be reversible, modifying the immunosuppressive schedule, whereas severe rejection is much more difficult to reverse.

In 1990 the International Society of Heart Transplantation set up a committee which devised a working formulation for the grading of acute rejection on endomyocardial biopsies.[9] This is the classification that has been adopted in order to make comparisons between different centres possible. This working formulation has a five-group system (Figs 8.1–8.4). Grade 0 does not show rejection. Grade 1 has a perivascular or interstitial lymphocytic infiltrate which can be focal (1A) or diffuse (1B), but the myocytes are intact. Grade 2 shows a single focus of inflammatory cells, with myocyte necrosis (myocytolysis) restricted to the area of the inflammatory infiltrate. Grade 3 is either a multifocal (3A) or a diffuse (3B) inflammatory infiltrate, with myocyte necrosis. Grade 4 is an 'aggressive' inflammatory cell infiltrate with lymphocytes, polymorphs and eosinophils; there is always myocyte necrosis, together with interstitial oedema, haemorrhage and variable degrees of vasculitis. 'Resolving rejection' should now be graded one grade less than in the

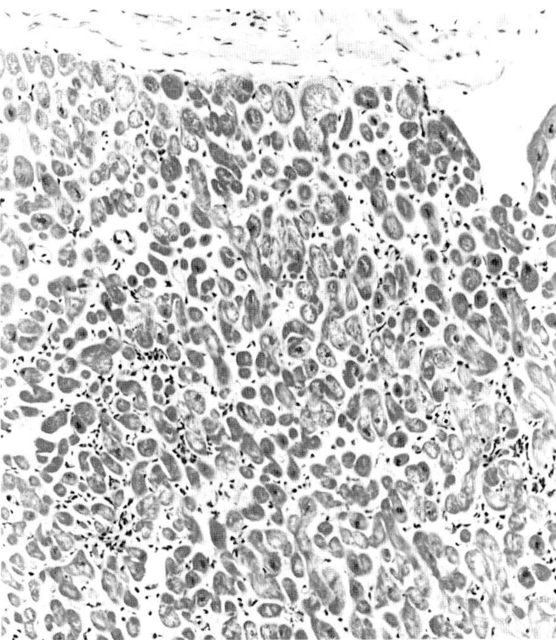

Fig. 8.1 Cardiac rejection grade 1B. There is a diffuse but sparse infiltrate of the interstitial tissues with lymphocytes but no myocyte damage.
Haematoxylin–eosin × 17.5

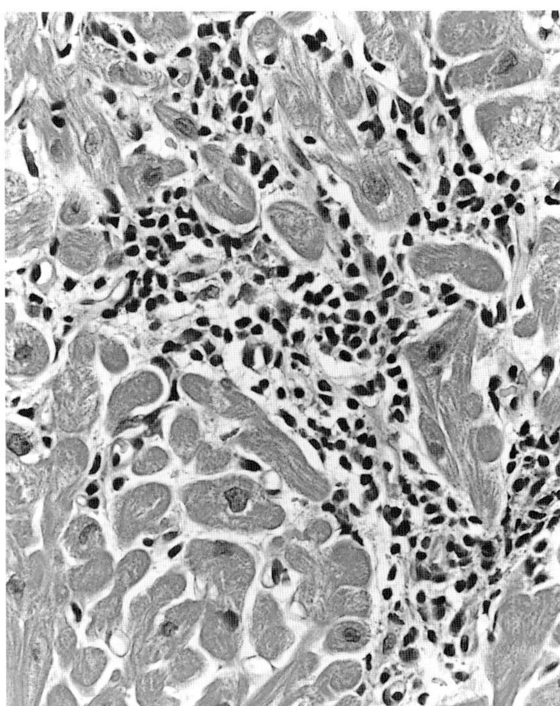

Fig. 8.2 Cardiac rejection grade 1A. There is a focus of interstitial inflammatory cells but no evidence of active myocyte damage.
Haematoxylin–eosin × 110

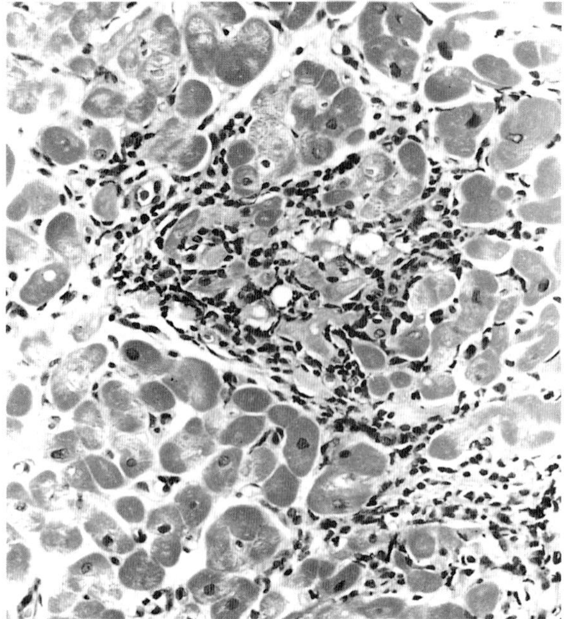

Fig. 8.3 Cardiac rejection grade 2. There is a single focus of interstitial inflammatory cells which surrounds individual myocytes. Within the focus the myocytes appear small with large vesicular nuclei. This focus would be graded 2 on the basis of evidence of myocyte damage.
Haematoxylin–eosin × 110

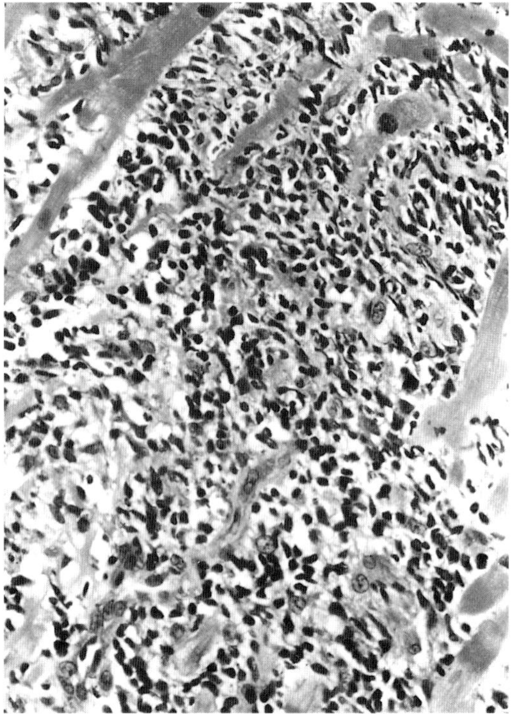

Fig. 8.4 Cardiac rejection grade 3A. There is both a focal and a diffuse severe interstitial inflammatory infiltrate with many large pironinophilic mononuclear cells. Active destruction of myocytes can be inferred by many spaces containing inflammatory cells without recognisable myocytes. In the infiltrate isolated surviving myocytes which are shrunken or have large hyperchromatic nuclei as evidence of damage can be seen.
Haematoxylin–eosin × 160

previous biopsy and 'resolved rejection' should be replaced by Grade 0.

Personal experience and that of others[10] shows the ISHT grading system to have some drawbacks and not to be entirely reproducible even among experienced pathologists. The major difficulties are that the grade is crucially dependent on recognising myocytolysis. This is very subjective. It is also dependent on recognising 'aggressive' lymphocytes, with the implication that there is cell-based myocyte destruction. While the international grading system has to be used to obtain publication of data its shortcomings are becoming apparent and revision is likely to occur.

Screening studies have determined that each endomyocardial biopsy should consist of three to five pieces of right ventricular myocardium, since this number reduces the degree of sampling error.[7] The matter of representative sampling increases in importance when applied to patients who have had a transplant for more than 1 year, since the odds of including an old biopsy site (Fig. 8.5) are increased. A recently published series[10] comparing the biopsy with autopsy findings has shown that the middle grades of rejection are often underestimated in a routine biopsy. Out of the analysis of 440 biopsies, the sensitivity for the middle grades was below 50%.[11]

Once obtained, the endomyocardial biopsies are fixed in formalin, processed routinely through paraffin and stained with haematoxylin–eosin and a trichrome stain in order to evaluate the degree of fibrosis. Other stains, such as methyl-green pyronine for lymphocytes, are sometimes used. Three deep levels should be cut out of the block.[12] Electron microscopy is not used routinely, since the processing takes too long in the clinical setting of acute rejection. Not only should the degree/severity of the rejection episode be evaluated on the biopsy, but also the presence/absence of infectious agents such as Cytomegalovirus (CMV), *Toxoplasma* and fungi.

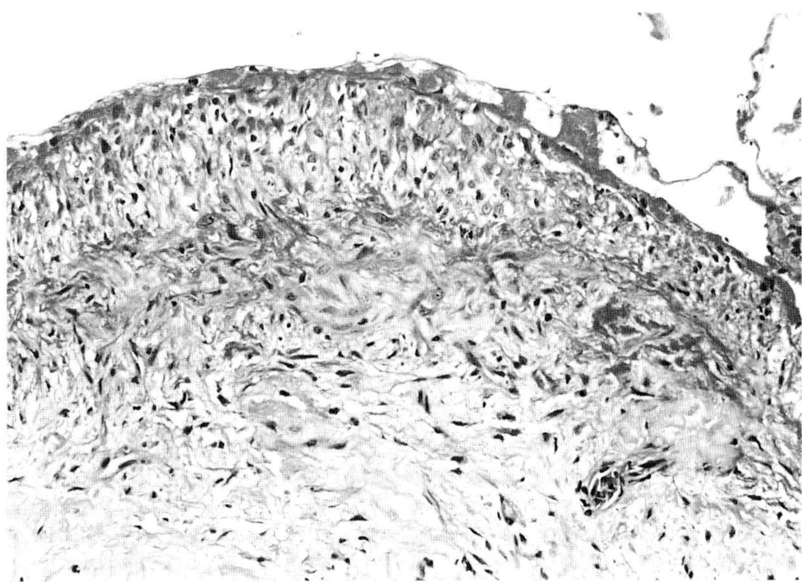

Fig. 8.5 Old biopsy site. There is a superficial zone of fibrin beneath which there are actively dividing fibroblasts. The developing fibrosis contains inflammatory cells and a considerable degree of disorganisation of the adjacent myocytes occurs. Fragments which contain an old biopsy site are excluded from analysis.
Haematoxylin–eosin × 45

Several attempts have been made to refine the histological diagnosis of rejection and to understand its pathophysiology better. It has been confirmed that the inflammatory cells present during an acute rejection episode adhere to the vascular endothelium[13,14,15] by means of adhesion molecules. This increases the likelihood of binding between the HLA system and the T cell receptors. ICAM-1 is an adhesion molecule expressed constitutively by endothelial cells and its expression increases after pretreatment with cytokines. VCAM-1 is an endothelial adhesion molecule, which is expressed by the endothelium only after induction by tumour necrosis alpha and interleukin-1. The presence of VCAM-1 has been shown to have a strong correlation with rejection of at least a moderate degree.[14] Thus there is no VCAM-1 expression on the endothelial cells if there is no active inflammation. Recently, it has also been shown that active inflammatory cells secrete tumour necrosis factor alpha during an acute rejection episode.[16] Further studies trying to identify subsets of T lymphocytes[17] showed an association between histological rejection and activation marker expression for CD25 (inflammatory cells expressing interleukin-2).

Hengstenberg[13] showed that myocytes express MHC class I antibodies after an episode of rejection in 68% of his cases, but they never express MHC class II antibodies. The expression of MHC I makes the myocytes susceptible to myocytolysis induced by cytotoxic T cells (T8). On the other hand, the interstitial cells, i.e. fibroblasts, leucocytes and endothelial cells, have been shown to express HLA, mainly DR and DP.

Other authors have investigated the relationship between acute rejection and viral infection[18] and have found that nucleic acids from herpesviruses were significantly more frequently retrieved from those biopsies showing rejection than from biopsies without rejection. They postulated that this finding could be relevant regarding the late development of graft vascular disease, since the viral infection could act as a trigger for smooth muscle cell proliferation. There are more proliferating cells (marked with Ki67) in those patients with moderate rejection.[18] Using a similar proliferative marker (PCNA), the increase in PCNA-positive cells with increasing degrees of rejection has been confirmed,[19] but the overlap between different categories of rejection is too large to allow its clinical use in the individual patient.

Other changes on the endomyocardial biopsy

Quilty effect

Quilty effect has been defined as a sharply demarcated band of lymphocytes present in the endocardium (Figs 8.6, 8.7) which may or not extend into the underlying myocardium but never 'damages' the myocytes. It has been named after the first patient to present with it. The Quilty effect is not related to rejection, but to high plasma levels of cyclosporin (>400 ng/ml).[20] No relationship has been shown between the presence of Quilty effect and that of graft vascular disease.

Cyclosporin-dependent fibrosis

This effect started to be reported in the early 1980s, when cyclosporin A was incorporated into the treatment of heart transplant patients.[8] It consists of a very fine network of fibrous tissue that encircles each myocyte individually.

Previous biopsy sites

There is a tendency for the bioptome used to obtain myocardial tissue to be passed into the same area at each procedure. It is therefore common to find that one or more of the biopsy fragments has been taken from the site of a previous biopsy. The frequency increases with the length of time after transplantation. Healed biopsy sites are recognised as areas of myocyte disorganisation, interspersed with foci of fibrosis. More recent biopsy sites show residual thrombosis and a florid fibroblastic proliferation (Fig. 8.8). It is not unusual for old biopsy sites to contain small giant cells with refractile material which is either starch or fibre introduced by the operator on to the bioptome itself during repeated biopsies.

Adipose tissue

The presence of adipose tissue in the endomyocardial biopsy taken from the right ventricle is common. The presence of mesothelial cells or nerve tissue is required for the diagnosis of perforation and should be reported to the clinician. Clinical sequelae are very rare, however, because the pericardium is usually obliterated by adhesions as a result of transplantation. Biopsies which contain subepicardial fat are easy to overinterpret because inflammatory cells extend into the superficial layers of the myocardium from the inflamed pericardium.

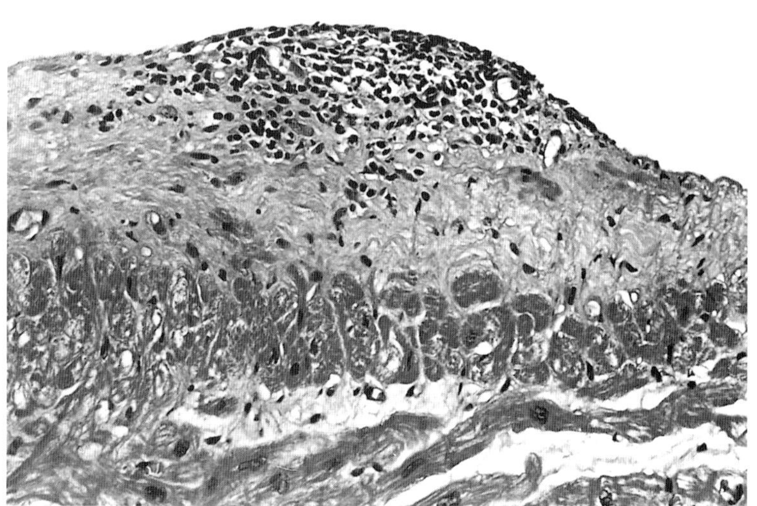

Fig. 8.6 Quilty effect. A small subendocardial focus of lymphocytes is well delineated from the underlying myocardium.
Haematoxylin–eosin × 110

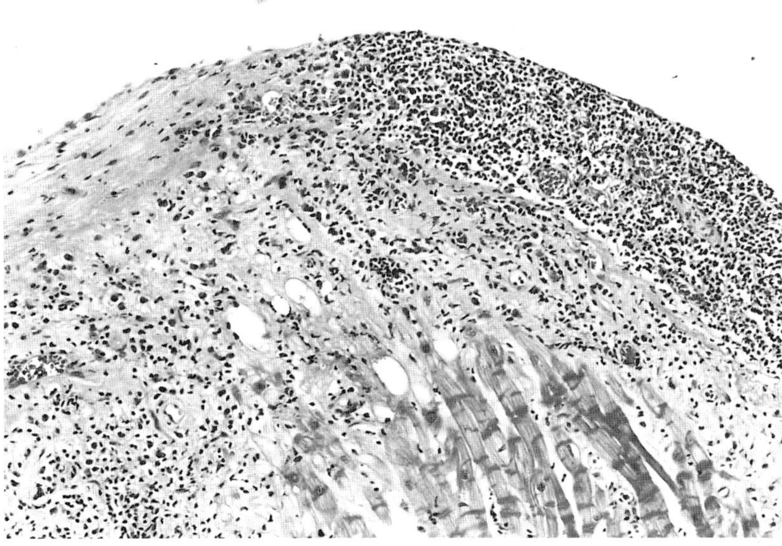

Fig. 8.7 Aggressive or expanding Quilty effect. A subendocardial focus of lymphocytes from which mononuclear cells extend into the underlying myocardium. Haematoxylin–eosin × 70

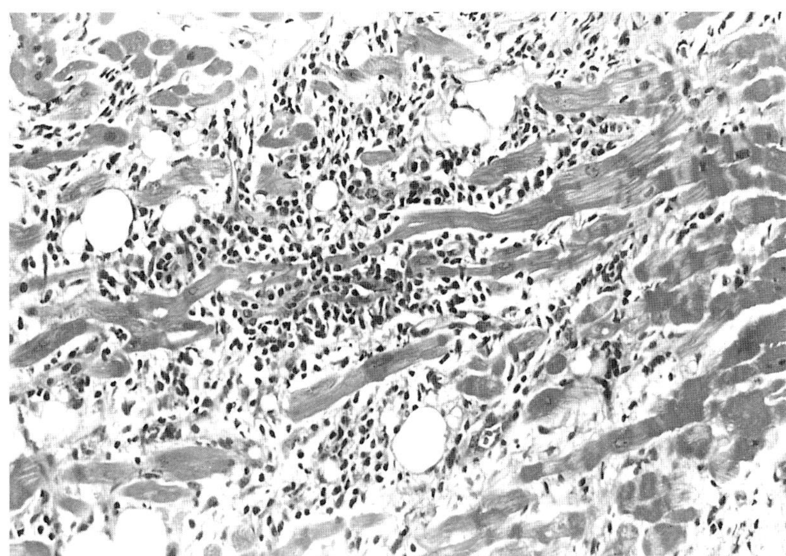

Fig. 8.8 Fat in biopsies for rejection. The biopsy contains a diffuse inflammatory infiltrate and a number of adipose cells. None of the other samples taken at the same time showed this appearance. This was interpreted as subpericardial non-specific inflammation.
Haematoxylin–eosin × 70

Vascular rejection

The majority of patients undergoing a rejection episode have a cellular response, with T lymphocytes predominantly involved. The myocyte is the target for cytotoxicity. However, a small percentage of transplanted patients will have vascular rejection. The diagnosis of vascular rejection is based on the presence of endothelial swelling and/or vasculitis, together with the presence of deposits of immunoglobulin (mostly IgG)[21] and complement in the vessels.[22] There is no simultaneous lymphocytic infiltrate and this type of rejection tends to occur mostly in the first 6 weeks after the transplant. In recent follow-up studies[22] the presence of vascular rejection has been associated both with acute decline in myocardial function and with a shorter time to development of chronic graft vascular disease,[23] although the numbers did not reach statistical significance. Acute vascular rejection has been seen relatively more frequently in the setting of Cytomegalovirus disease,[24] and this could be a relevant factor in the development of graft vascular disease, since the latter has also — at least in some of the transplant centres — been linked to the presence of Cytomegalovirus. Detailed histological studies using different immunohistochemical markers have shown[25] that most of the vacuolated cells that appear in the epicardial arteries during an episode of vascular rejection are modified smooth muscle cells, which would enter the intima through gaps in the internal elastic lamina. These cells have an extensively vacuolated cytoplasm, which stains negative for glycogen and only occasionally positive for lipids. Electronmicroscopy studies showed lack of concentric membranous lamellae and the presence of myofibrils in the periphery of the cell.

LATE PATHOLOGY

Cardiac allografts implanted longer than 12 months tend to show consistent findings. The grafts are increased in weight because of left ventricular hypertrophy. The development of cardiac hypertrophy has been considered as a risk factor for deterioration of left ventricular function. A recent study[26] has shown that myocyte hypertrophy appears relatively early after heart transplant and remains stable for up to 7 years.

Other late pathological findings are the presence of scarring due to old myocardial infarctions, with or without left ventricular dilatation and/or thrombi. At 1 year after transplantation the suture lines between the donor and recipient's atria will barely be visible as areas of fibrosis.

Histological examination of the myocardium will show established areas of scarring with a regional pattern, due to old myocardial infarction, or focal areas of fibrosis due to either previous rejection episodes or to graft vascular disease.

The main long-term complication in cardiac transplant recipients is graft vascular disease, which has also been called chronic rejection, accelerated arteriosclerosis, graft coronary disease, etc. The accepted nomenclature is now transplant-accelerated coronary artery disease (TACAD). The angiographic frequency of graft vascular disease has been reported as high as 50% at 5 years, for both the adult and the paediatric populations. It can be characterised as a 'silent' disease, since most of the patients will not feel any anginal pain, their hearts having been denervated during the surgical procedure. Graft vascular disease involves mainly the smaller epicardial vessels and the intramyocardial vessels and its characteristic angiographic appearance has been well described and classified.[27] There is pruning of the small branches and lack of collateral circulation. The diffuseness of graft vascular disease makes it difficult to diagnose in coronary angiograms, even when using digital angiography. Clinico-pathological studies[28] have shown that up to 100% of the normal-looking segments on coronary angiography were diseased when looked at histologically, with a severity ranging between mild and moderate. Unfortunately, the diffuse nature of the disease also makes it very difficult to treat, since neither coronary artery bypass grafting nor percutaneous transluminal angioplasty have been used successfully. The only available treatment remains retransplantation.

Risk factors for graft vascular disease

Most cardiac transplant units have analysed the risk factors in their patients developing graft vascular disease in an attempt to decrease the frequency of this complication. However, most — if not all — of these epidemiological studies have assessed the same risk factors as for native coronary artery disease, and graft vascular disease seems to be quite a different process.

Among the risk factors investigated for graft vascular disease have been hyperlipidaemia, hypertension, smoking and diabetes mellitus, but none of these have consistently shown a positive association. It was thought at one time that those patients with ischaemic heart disease would be at a higher risk of developing graft vascular disease postoperatively. This has proved to be a false assumption. The addition of cyclosporin A to the immunosuppressive protocol has not changed the frequency of graft vascular disease. The importance of the age of the donor has also been studied, under the assumption that elderly (> 35–40 years of age) donors would be at a higher risk. Most of the studies, however, do not confirm this theory. Hyperlipidaemia has been one of the few risk factors to come up as a strong predictor for graft vascular disease[29] in most of the studies. The reason for post-transplant hyperlipidaemia is still undetermined, although the use of corticosteroids and cyclosporin may play a role in it, steroids by increasing the production of apolipoprotein B by the liver and cyclosporin A by decreasing the clearance of steroids. Other authors have found that a high total cholesterol at 6 months after transplant[30] is a strong predictor for the development of graft vascular disease.

Serial angiographic studies up to 8 years after cardiac transplantation have shown that, although the coronary angiogram tends to underestimate the degree of involvement by graft vascular disease, there is an increase in the angiographic diagnosis of this entity, from 21% at 2 years to 43% at 5 years.[31] These authors split the population into 'slow' and 'fast' disease and found that the only significant difference between both groups was the high density lipoprotein plasma level. Long-term follow-up studies (> 2 years) have also shown that the presence of angiographic graft vascular disease identifies a subset of patients at high risk for cardiac events, i.e. acute myocardial infarction and sudden coronary death.[32]

Recently, a viral aetiology has been implicated in the development of graft vascular disease. It has been shown that Cytomegalovirus infection stimulates the expression of IgG Fc receptors on infected endothelial cells and that these activated endothelial cells could interact with granulocytes, resulting in endothelial damage. On the other hand, CMV has a glycoprotein similar to the heavy chain of the MHC class I molecule and can also bind to the light chain of the MHC class I molecule. CMV infection leads to an increased release of interferon gamma by activated T cells and this results in an upregulation of MHC class I expression on endothelial cells, which has been lately associated with the development of graft vascular disease.[33] Other clinical studies have found an increased frequency of Cytomegalovirus infection in patients with graft vascular disease when compared to transplanted patients without graft vascular disease,[34] and it has been postulated that the virus stays in a latent form within the vessel wall and may be 'activated' later on, resulting in an immunological reaction. In situ hybridisation techniques have confirmed the presence of Cytomegalovirus nucleic acids within endothelial cells, lymphocytes and smooth muscle cells of the vessels.[35] The mechanism by which CMV induces graft vascular disease, however, is still unknown.

Several institutions have assessed the effect of acute cellular rejection as a predictor of development of graft vascular disease.[36] It seems that the presence of moderate rejection early (during the first 3 months) after transplant is a predictor of angiographic graft vascular disease; others[37] have found that, on a long-term basis, the presence of more than one episode of severe rejection is also a predictor of graft vascular disease.

HLA matching has not been considered crucial in the setting of heart transplantation. However, recent studies[37] have shown preliminary results regarding a better outcome of those transplants in which there are no HLA mismatches. The presence of anti-HLA lymphocytotoxic antibodies has also been shown to be a predictor[38] of relatively poor outcome.

Histopathology of graft vascular disease

Examination of the arteries of transplanted hearts from subjects who died within 3 months shows that there is a diffuse infiltration of the intima by T lymphocytes. This 'endothelialitis' or 'intimitis' is postulated to be followed by smooth muscle cell proliferation in the intima.[39,40] Immunohistochemistry showed that the lymphocytes involved were T cells and amongst these most were T8 or cytotoxic T cells. Others[41] have found an approximately equal proportion of both CD4 and CD8 T lymphocytes beneath the endothelium, together with HLA-DR^{+} macrophages. They postulated that the endothelial cells of the graft stimulate CD4 T lymphocytes which, once activated, would release both cytokines and/or growth factors that would result in the proliferation of smooth muscle cells. Experimental studies have assessed the variations in time regarding lymphocytes and macrophages, and their relationship with graft vascular disease,[42] and found that the number of inflammatory cells increases with time, probably resulting in a sustained immunological injury that would result in a continuous stimulus for smooth muscle cell proliferation.

In the later and symptomatic stage of the disease concentric intimal thickening with a severe reduction in lumen diameter and an increase in wall thickness is present in the smaller epicardial arteries (Fig. 8.9) and first generation intramyocardial arteries.[43,44] The thickening is collagenous, with a high density of smooth muscle cells (Fig. 8.10). A distinct zone of lymphocytes and a few macrophages may be present close to the intimal medial border (Fig. 8.11). Lipid is inconstant and many foam cells are smooth muscle in origin. The histological picture is more complex in the larger epicardial arteries and focal plaques with lipid cores may occur. In these larger arteries the process is probably one of native plaques in the donor heart accelerated by graft disease. In the larger arteries superficial thrombosis occurs and its deposition into the intima leads to further intimal fibrosis. While graft vascular disease and native vessel atherosclerosis share common processes the balance between these is very different and the two diseases are morphologically easily distinguished (Table 8.1).

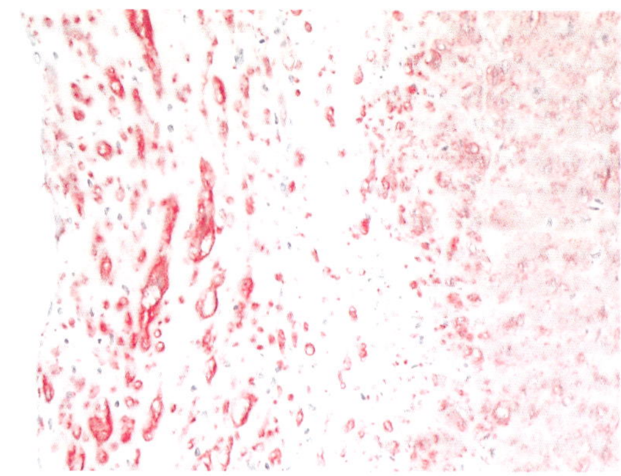

Fig. 8.10 Graft vascular disease — cell type. The section is stained by the alkaline phosphatase immunohistochemical method to show smooth muscle actin. The vast majority of the cells stain red in the intima and are therefore identified as smooth muscle in type.

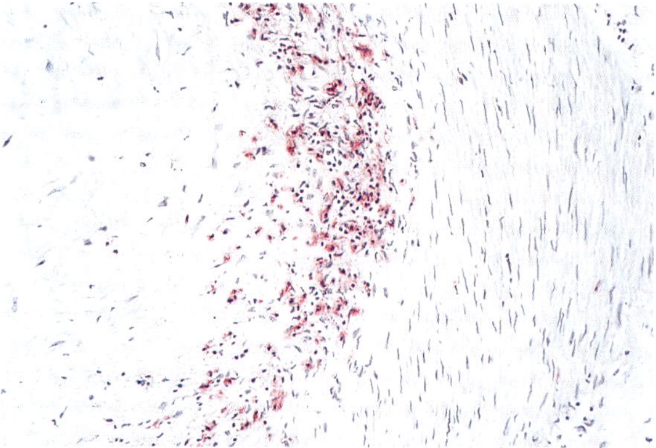

Fig. 8.11 Graft vascular disease — cell type. The section is stained by an antibody to T cells. At the intimal medial boundary there is a layer of T cells.

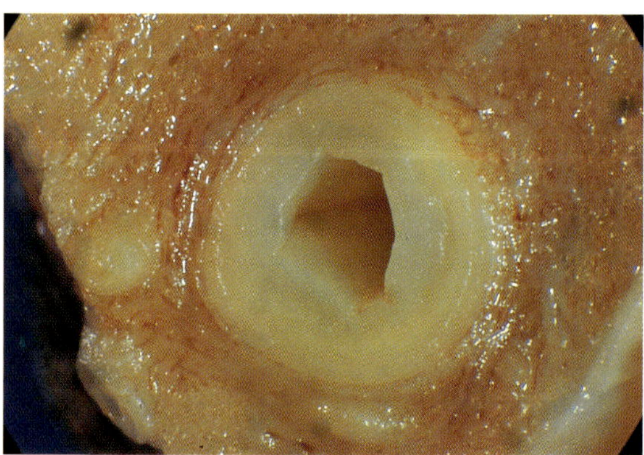

Fig. 8.9 Graft vascular disease. A small epicardial artery shows concentric thickening of the intima, narrowing the lumen.

Infections

Infection is another major cause of death during the first postoperative year. The reported frequency of infection ranges from 11%[45] to 20%. During the first postoperative month, most of the infections are liable to be nosocomial, including mainly staphylococci and Gram-negative microorganisms. Late postoperative infections are characterised by the

Table 8.1 Differences between graft vascular disease and atherosclerosis

	Graft vascular disease	Atherosclerosis
Focal or diffuse	Diffuse	Focal
Large epicardial	+	+++
Small epicardial	+++	+
Intramyocardial	+++	0
T lymphocytes	+++	+
Macrophage		
Early	0	+++
Late	+	+++
Lipid insudation	+	+++
Smooth muscle proliferation	+++	++

predominance of opportunistic infections such as *Pneumocystis carinii*, Cytomegalovirus and fungi.

A recent study[45] assessing the frequency of infection after the first postoperative year showed that the late risk of infections was around 13% at 2 years. Most of the infections (60%) were of bacterial origin. A review from Papworth including 323 patients did not show any difference regarding the frequency of infection when comparing patients treated with and without cyclosporin A.[46]

The diagnosis of Cytomegalovirus requires a fourfold increase in serological titres. Most of the Cytomegalovirus infections are reactivation of a prior infective episode. They tend to appear in the late postoperative period (>60 days) or whenever there is an increase in the immunosuppressive treatment, in order to treat a rejection episode. The frequency of Cytomegalovirus infection increases with donor–recipient mismatch. It is the main cause of pulmonary morbidity and it has also been involved in the pathogenesis of graft vascular disease. The typical 'bird's eye' intracytoplasmic inclusions are diagnostic, either in the myocytes — rarely — or in the pulmonary epithelium.

Lymphoproliferative disorders

Immunosuppressed patients have a higher than usual frequency of neoplasms overall. It has been estimated that the frequency of lymphoproliferative disorders in a transplant population is around 100 times more than that of the non-transplanted population. The most commonly encountered neoplasm in patients treated with cyclosporin is B-cell lymphoma, although other malignancies such as squamous cell carcinomas of the skin and gastrointestinal tract have also been reported.[47] The global frequency of post-transplant lymphoma has been reported as 3.4%[48] for those patients surviving the first postoperative month. It appears that the development of lymphoma after the first postoperative year carries a much higher morbidity and mortality rate (71% versus 38%) and that the late type tends to disseminate faster and to be more aggressive. The early type is generally nodal and responds well to a decrease in immunosuppression. Unfortunately, the risk is always present after transplant, remaining as high as 5% per year. B cell lymphomas can be either monoclonal or polyclonal; clonal analysis has shown that only the polyclonal subtype responds to immunosuppression. In most of the patients, Epstein–Barr virus DNA can be recovered from the B cells, implying a possible pathogenetic role for this infectious agent. It has been postulated that the lymphoproliferative disorder appears as a result of inadequate control by T cells of B cells infected with EBV. B-cell lymphomas in transplanted patients tend to involve more commonly the small bowel and rarely the central nervous system. However, the prognosis is still poor and lymphoproliferative disorders account for around 5–10% of late postoperative deaths. Recent surveys[49] of risk factors for the development of lymphoproliferative disorders have shown that one of them is the use of OKT3, which is a monoclonal antibody against $CD3^+$ T lymphocytes.

REFERENCES

1. Rose AG, Viviers L, Odell JA. Autopsy-determined causes of death following cardiac transplantation. Arch Pathol Lab Med 1992; 116: 1137–1141.
2. Ensley RD, Hunt S, Taylor DO, Renlund DG, Menlove RL, Karwande SV, O'Connell JB, Barr ML, Michler RE, Copeland JG, Miller LW. Predictors of survival after repeat heart transplantation. J Heart Lung Transplant 1992; 11: S142–S158.
3. Kemnitz J, Cremer J, Restrepo-Specht I, Haverich A, Ziemer G, Heublein B, Borst H-G, Uysal A, Georgii A. Hyperacute rejection in heart allografts. Path Res Pract 1991; 187: 23–29.
4. Rose AG, Cooper DKC, Human PA, Reichenspurner H, Reichart B. Histopathology of hyperacute rejection of the heart: experimental and clinical observations in allografts and xenografts. J Heart Lung Transplant 1991; 10: 223–234.
5. Laurent F, Benvenuti C, Mourtada A, Duval AM, Tavolaro O, Brun P, Rauss A, Loisance D, Cachera JP. Interêt de determiner la variation d'un indice de masse myocardique dans le diagnostic du rejet aigu d'une greffe cardiaque allogenique. Arch Mal Coeur 1990; 83: 1531–1537.
6. Caves PK. Percutaneous transvenous endomyocardial biopsy in human heart recipients. Experience with a new technique. Ann Thorac Surg 1973; 16: 325–326.
7. McAllister HA. Histologic grading of cardiac allograft rejection: a quantitative approach. J Heart Transplant 1990; 9: 277–282.
8. Billingham ME. Diagnosis of cardiac rejection by endomyocardial biopsy. Heart Transplant 1981; 1: 25–30.
9. Billingham ME, Cary NRB, Hammond ME, Kemnitz J, Marboe C, McAllister HA, Snovar DC, Winters GL, Zerbe A. A working formulation for the standardization of nomenclature in the diagnosis of heart and lung rejection: Heart rejection study group. J Heart Transplant 1990; 9: 587–593.
10. Nielsen H, Sorensen FB, Nielsen B, Bagger JP, Thayssen P, Baandrup U. Reproducibility of the acute rejection diagnosis in human cardiac allografts. The Stanford Classification and the International Grading system. J Heart Lung Transplant 1993; 12: 239–243.
11. Nakhleh RE, Jones J, Goswitz JJ, Anderson EA, Titus J. Correlation of endomyocardial biopsy findings with autopsy findings in human cardiac allografts. J Heart Lung Transplant 1992; 11: 479–485.
12. Billingham ME. The pathology of transplanted hearts. Sem Thorac Cardiovasc Surg 1990; 2: 233–240.
13. Hengstenberg C, Hufnagel G, Haverich A, Olsen EGJ, Maisch B. De novo expression of MHC class I and class II antigens on endomyocardial biopsies from patients with inflammatory heart disease and rejection following heart transplantation. Eur Heart J 1993; 14: 758–763.
14. Carlos T, Gordon D, Fishbein D, Himes VE, Coday A, Ross R, Allen MD. Vascular cell adhesion molecule-1 is induced on endothelium during acute rejection in human cardiac allografts. J Heart Lung Transplant 1992; 11: 1103–1109.
15. Allen MD, McDonald TO, Carlos T, Himes V, Fishbein D, Aziz S, Gordon D. Endothelial adhesion molecules in heart transplantation. J Heart Lung Transplant 1992; 11: S8–S13.
16. Arbustini A, Grasso M, Diegoli M, Bramerio M, Scotti Foglieni A, Albertario M, Martinelli L, Gavazzi A, Goggi C, Campana C, Vigano M. Expression of tumor necrosis factor in human acute cardiac rejection. Am J Pathol 1991; 139: 709–715.
17. Wijngaard PLJ, Tuijnman WB, Gmelig Meyling FHJ, van der Meulen A, Huytink M, Jambroes G, Schuurman H-J. Endomyocardial biopsies after heart transplantation. Transplantation 1993; 55: 103–110.
18. Jakel KT, Loning T, Arndt R, Rodiger W. Rejection, herpes virus infection, and Ki-67 expression in endomyocardial biopsy specimens from heart transplant recipients. Path Res Pract 1992; 188: 27–36.
19. Mann JM, Jennison SH, Moss E, Davies MJ. Assessment of rejection in orthotopic human heart transplantation using proliferating cell nuclear antigen (PCNA) as an index of cell proliferation. J Path 1992; 167: 385–389.
20. Pomerance A, Stovin PGI. Heart transplant pathology: the British experience. J Clin Pathol 1985; 38: 146–159.
21. Foerster A. Vascular rejection in cardiac transplantation. APMIS 1992; 100: 367–376.
22. Hammond EH, Ensley RD, Yowell RL, Craven CM, Bristow MR, Renlund DG, O'Connell JB. Vascular rejection of human cardiac allografts and the role of humoral immunity in chronic allograft rejection. Transplant Proc 1991; 23(Supp2): 26–30.
23. Hammond EH, Yowell RL, Price GD, Menlove RL, Olsen SL, O'Connell JB, Bristow MR, Doty DB, Millar RC, Karwande SV, Jones KW, Gay WA, Renlund DG. Vascular rejection and its relationship to allograft coronary artery disease. J Heart Lung Transplant 1992; 11: S111–S119.
24. Normann SJ, Salomon DR, Leelachaikul P, Khan SR, Staples ED, Alexander JA, Mayfield WR, Knauf DG, Sadler LA, Selman SS. Acute vascular rejection of the coronary arteries in human heart transplantation: Pathology and correlations with immunosuppression and cytomegalovirus infection. J Heart Lung Transplant 1991; 10: 674–687.
25. Normann SJ, Khan SR, Leelachaikul P, Salomon DR. Origin of cells in the coronary intima during acute vascular rejection of the transplanted human heart. J Heart Lung Transplant 1992; 11: 492–499.
26. Rowan RA, Billingham ME. Sustained myocardial hypertrophy seven years or more after heart transplantation: a morphometric study of endomyocardial specimens. J Heart Lung Transplant 1992; 11: 350–352.
27. Gao SZ, Alderman EL, Schroeder JS, Silverman JF, Hunt SA. Accelerated coronary vascular disease in the heart transplant patient: coronary arteriographic findings. J Am Coll Cardiol 1988; 12: 334–340.
28. Johnson DE, Alderman EL, Schroeder JS, Gao S-Z, Hunt S, DeCampli WM, Stinson E, Billingham ME. Transplant coronary artery disease: histopathologic correlations with angiographic morphology. J Am Coll Cardiol 1991; 17: 449–457.
29. Johnson MR. Transplant coronary disease: nonimmunologic risk factors. J Heart Lung Transplant 1992; 11: S124–S132.
30. Eich D, Thompson JA, Ko D, Hastillo A, Lower R, Katz S, Katz M, Hess ML. Hypercholesterolemia in long-term survivors of heart transplantation: an early marker of accelerated coronary artery disease. J Heart Lung Transplant 1991; 10: 45–49.
31. Davies H, Verney G, English T. The coronary arteries of

the transplanted human heart: studies of the development of disease based on serial angiography. Int J Cardiol 1991; 32: 35–50.
32. Uretsky BF, Kormos RL, Zerbe TR, Lee A, Tokarczyk TR, Murali S, Reddy PS, Denys BG, Griffith BP, Hardesty RL, Armitage JM, Arena VC. Cardiac events after heart transplantation: incidence and predictive value of coronary arteriography. J Heart Lung Transplant 1992; 11: S45–S51.
33. Kendall TJ, Wilson JE, Radio SJ, Kandolf R, Gulizia JM, Winters GL, Costanzo-Nordin MR, Malcom GT, Thieszen SL, Miller LW, McManus BM. Cytomegalovirus and other herpesviruses: do they have a role in the development of accelerated coronary arterial disease in human heart allografts? J Heart Lung Transplant 1992; 11: S14–S20.
34. Loebe M, Schuler S, Zais O, Warnecke H, Fleck E, Hetzer R. Role of cytomegalovirus infection in the development of coronary artery disease in the transplanted heart. J Heart Transplant 1990; 9: 707–711.
35. Wu T-C, Hruban RH, Ambinder RF, Pizzorno M, Cameron DE, Baumgartner WA, Reitz BA, Hayward GS, Hutchins GM. Demonstration of cytomegalovirus nucleic acids in the coronary arteries of transplanted hearts. Am J Pathol 1992; 140: 739–747.
36. Zerbe T, Uretsky B, Kormos R, Armitage J, Wolyn T, Griffith B, Hardesty R, Duquesnoy R. Graft atherosclerosis: effects of cellular rejection and human lymphocyte antigen. J Heart Lung Transplant 1992; 11: S104–S110.
37. Costanzo-Nordin MR. Cardiac allograft vasculopathy: Relationship with acute cellular rejection and histocompatibility. J Heart Lung Transplant 1992; 11: S90–S103.
38. Rose EA, Pepino P, Barr ML, Smith CR, Ratner AJ, Ho E, Berger C. Relation of HLA antibodies and graft atherosclerosis in human cardiac allograft recipients. J Heart Lung Transplant 1992; 11: S120–S123.
39. Hruban RH, Beschorner WE, Baumgartner WA, Augustine SM, Reitz BA, Hutchins GM. Accelerated arteriosclerosis in heart transplant recipients: an immunopathology study of 22 transplanted hearts. Transplant Proc 1991; 23: 1230–1232.
40. Paavonen T, Mennander A, Lautenschlager I, Hayry P. Endothelialitis in accelerated allograft arteriosclerosis in human cardiac transplant recipients. Transplant Proc 1992; 24: 342–343.
41. Salomon RN, Hughes CCW, Schoen FJ, Payne DD, Pober JS, Libby P. Human coronary transplantation-associated arteriosclerosis. Am J Pathol 1991; 138: 791–798.
42. Cramer DV, Wu GD, Chapman FA, Cajulis E, Wang HK, Makowka L. Lymphocytic subsets and histopathologic changes associated with the development of heart transplant arteriosclerosis. J Heart Lung Transplant 1992; 11: 458–466.
43. Billingham ME. Histopathology of graft coronary disease. J Heart Lung Transplant 1992; 11: S38–S44.
44. Liu G, Butany J. Morphology of graft arteriosclerosis in cardiac transplant recipients. Human Pathology 1992; 23: 768–773.
45. Hosenpud JD, Hershberger RE, Pantely G, Norman DJ, Hovaguimian H, Cobanoglu A, Starr A. Late infection in cardiac allograft recipients: profiles, incidence and outcome. J Heart Lung Transplant 1991; 10: 380–386.
46. Sharples LD, Caine N, Mullins P, Scott JP, Solis E, English TAH, Large SR, Schofield PM, Wallwork J. Risk factor analysis for the major hazards following heart transplantation — rejection, infection and coronary occlusive disease. Transplantation 1991; 52: 244–252.
47. Couetil JP, McGoldrick JP, Wallwork J, English TAH. Malignant tumors after heart transplantation. J Heart Transplant 1990; 9: 622–626.
48. Armitage JM, Kormos RL, Stuart RS, Fricker FJ, Griffith BP, Nalesnik M, Hardesty RL, Dummer JS. Post transplant lymphoproliferative disease in thoracic organ transplant patients: ten years of cyclosporine-based immunosuppression. J Heart Lung Transplant 1991; 10: 877–887
49. Swinnen LJ, Costanzo-Nordin MR, Fisher SG, O'Sullivan EJ, Johnson MR, Heroux AL, Dizikes GJ, Pifarre R, Fisher RI. Increased incidence of lymphoproliferative disorders after immunosuppression with the monoclonal antibody OKT3 in cardiac transplant recipients. New Engl J Med 1990; 323: 1723–1728.

9

The pericardium

THE NORMAL PERICARDIUM

The pericardium is a fibrous sac which surrounds the heart and the root of the great vessels. It consists of two layers: the epicardium, which is a single layer of mesothelial cells, covering the heart and continuous with the lining of the inner surface of the second pericardial layer, the fibrosa. The latter is 1–2 mm thick. The fibrosa is firmly attached to the sternum and to the left side of the diaphragm by ligaments and, in a more loose way, to the pleura. The pericardial cavity has two recesses: the transverse sinus, which lies between the great vessels and the atria, and the oblique sinus, which is between the venae cavae and the pulmonary veins. The latter accommodates any increase in the amount of fluid in the pericardial sac.[1]

Histologically, the pericardial lining consists of a single layer of mesothelial cells, which have microvilli. The fibrosa consists of collagen tissue arranged in thick wavy bands, and some elastic fibres.

Physiologically, the pericardium is a significant contributor to cardiac function and chamber filling, and contains mechanoreceptors and neuroreceptors located in the pericardium itself. Any increase in volume of the pericardial fluid does not immediately lead to a rise in pressure within the pericardial cavity; the mechanism responsible for this lag is the straightening of the collagen bundles that constitute the fibrosa layer.[2] In effect, considerable fluid can be accommodated before pressure rises. Distending the pericardial cavity at post mortem requires around 150 ml of fluid; in a living human subject, however, acute increases of smaller amounts of fluid may result in haemodynamic changes. The normal amount of fluid in the pericardial sac is around 20 ml. The pericardial fluid has a similar composition to plasma, with a slightly lower protein concentration and a relatively higher albumin level. It is always difficult at post mortem to judge the possible clinical effect of increased pericardial fluid since the actual volume does not bear a direct relation to the pressure on the heart and thus the impediment of filling. Some indication can be obtained by feeling the tension of the pericardial sac before it is opened. If fluid spurts out through a small incision it indicates clinically significant effusions.

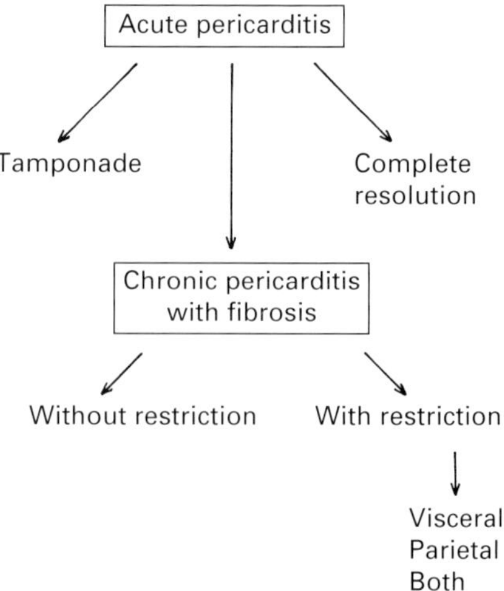

Fig. 9.1 Potential outcome of pericarditis

ACUTE AND CHRONIC PERICARDITIS

In the vast majority of cases, acute pericarditis is inflammatory in origin and has a significant fibrinous component. The amount of fluid in the pericardial sac increases only slightly and tamponade is very rarely seen. Chest pain is the dominant symptom.

The aetiology of acute pericarditis is varied, including viral pericarditis, tuberculous pericarditis, metabolic alterations such as uraemia, postinfarction pericarditis and postoperative pericarditis after cardiac surgery. Acute pericarditis may be a self-limiting short-term condition (Fig. 9.1) or pass into chronic forms which develop fibrosis with constriction over some years depending on the aetiology. Most of the idiopathic recurrent acute forms are probably related to viral infection, particularly with the Coxsackie group.

The term chronic pericarditis may be applied to infections such as tuberculosis or to the later effects of resolution of acute pericarditis by fibrosis of the exudate. Restriction with improvement of atrial and ventricular filling may or may not be present due to fibrosis in the visceral layer of the pericardium over the atria and ventricles or of the parietal pericardium or to a dense fibrous coat formed by fusion of the visceral and parietal layers. In this later stage foci of chronic inflammation (plasma cells and lymphocytes) still persist in the fibrous tissue and calcification is common. While common in tuberculous pericarditis calcification is by no means pathognomonic of this aetiology. Chronic pericarditis which does not produce constriction is unlikely to be diagnosed in life and is an incidental autopsy diagnosis. The diagnosis of constriction in life is, however, not always easy and the pathologist who finds severe fibrosis and calcification at autopsy is justified in asking the clinician to consider if, in retrospect, constriction was present. There are many causes of chronic restrictive pericarditis.[3] Some are relatively common; others very rare (Table 9.1).

Table 9.1 Causes of chronic pericardial constriction

Common
Infective
Post- and persistent viral infection (Coxsackie)
Tuberculosis
Connective tissue disorders
Scleroderma
Systemic lupus
Rheumatoid
Post-radiotherapy
Post cardiac surgery
Rare
Uraemia, sarcoidosis, asbestosis, histoplasmosis

Tuberculous pericarditis

Tuberculous pericarditis (Fig. 9.2) accounts for 4% of all cases of acute pericarditis and, in some of the older series, for approximately 6% of

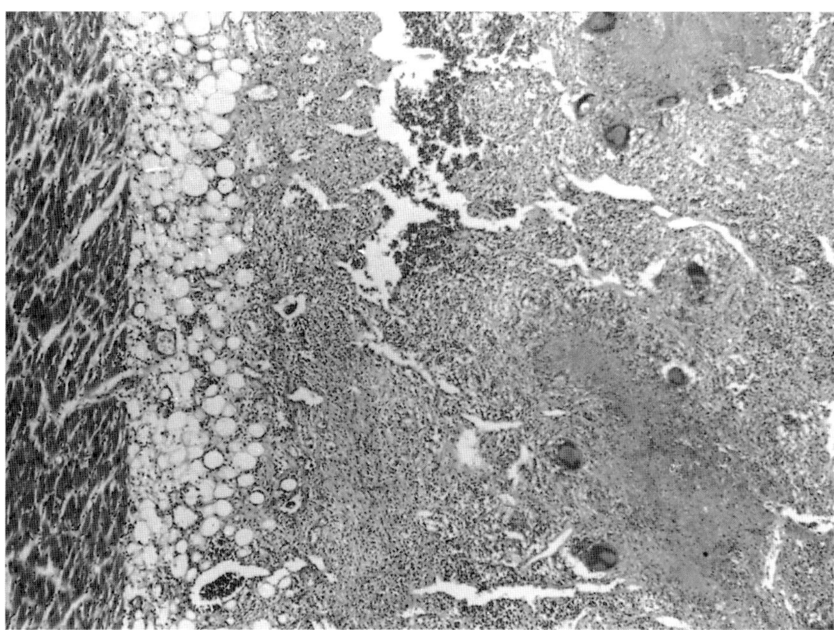

Fig. 9.2 Acute tuberculous pericarditis. The visceral pericardium is replaced by a thick layer of granulation tissue containing many caseating granulomas with giant cells. There is no invasion of the underlying myocardium.
Haemotoxylin–eosin × 18

all cases of cardiac tamponade. Although the frequency of tuberculosis has been progressively decreasing since the mid-1950s (due to the appearance on the market of anti-tuberculous drugs), in the last few years this decrease has come to a halt. This fact has been linked to the appearance of the acquired immunodeficiency syndrome (AIDS). The frequency of tuberculosis has been reported as significantly higher in Third World countries than in 'developed' Western countries. Tuberculous pericarditis is thought to occur in approximately 2% of cases of lung tuberculosis.[4]

Tuberculous pericarditis always appears in association with foci of tuberculosis somewhere else in the body. Pericardial involvement is due either to haematogenous spread from the lung or the genitourinary tract or to direct extension from the trachea, bronchi and mediastinal lymph nodes. In all cases, the histological findings are similar: during the first 2 weeks there is an increasing amount of fibrin deposited on the pericardium, as well as a mild degree of pericardial effusion. The pericardial fluid is mildly haemorrhagic and has a high concentration of proteins, together with a high white blood cell count consisting mainly of neutrophils. After the first 2 weeks the inflammatory cell population consists mostly of mononuclear cells, mainly lymphocytes. Later, in what some authors call the 'subacute stage',[4] typical tuberculous granulomas are seen, with formation of epithelioid cells, Langhans-type giant cells, caseous necrosis and a very small number of tubercle bacilli present in the lesions. In the more advanced stage there is a striking increase in the thickness of the pericardium, with fusion of both layers and the development of dense fibrosis resulting in constrictive pericarditis.

In areas of the tropics where endomyocardial fibrosis is endemic its clinical distinction in life from chronic constrictive pericarditis secondary to tuberculosis is not always easy.[5] Endomyocardial biopsies from patients with tuberculous constrictive pericarditis often show increased myocardial interstitial fibrosis and a mixed inflammatory cell infiltrate consisting mainly of lymphocytes and histiocytes. Occasional giant cells are present. Approximately half of the patients will show thickening of the endocardium, and on occasions tuberculous granulomas can be seen in the endocardium. On the other hand, endomyocardial biopsies obtained in patients with endomyocardial fibrosis also show increased interstitial fibrosis and a thickened endocardium, which does not always contain thrombus, either recent or organising. At the time the patient has his biopsy done, the eosinophils have already disappeared from the myocardium. Thus, the clinical findings have to be taken into account in order to help to make the correct diagnosis.

Most patients with pericardial tuberculosis will be in their third to fifth decade; they will give a history of typical symptoms such as shortness of breath, coughing and weight loss. The majority will have a positive PPD test, except if they have skin test anergy.

Cytological examination of the pericardial fluid shows an exudate, with high protein content, and an increase in mononuclear inflammatory cells. Acid-fast bacilli are seen, using special staining techniques, in approximately half the cases, but the results improve if culture techniques are used. However, since the culture of pericardial fluid takes a long time, between 4 and 6 weeks, pericardial biopsy has become the method of choice. Using polymerase chain reaction (PCR) techniques, the diagnosis of tuberculosis can be made much faster; the radiometric method allows testing for drug sensitivity in 2 weeks instead of the usual 5.

The reported mortality rate for pericardial tuberculosis is extremely variable, ranging from 3–40%, and is very much dependent on the type of treatment administered — with or without steroids, and medical versus surgical — and on the presence or absence of cardiac restriction. Recent reports[6] have shown that, provided there are no signs of cardiac compression, patients with tuberculous pericarditis do not require pericardiectomy and can be safely managed with medical treatment alone. On the other hand, however, surgical reviews on the indications for pericardiectomy[7] have shown that it can be performed with relatively low mortality rate (around 5%) and with a good late survival rate (72% at 5 years).

Tuberculous pericarditis has been reported lately in AIDS patients.[8–11] In general, tuberculosis appears as a disseminated disease in AIDS patients, but there are a few reports in which pericarditis was the presenting symptom. The amount of pericardial fluid present in the pericardial sac ranged from 600–1500 ml and all of the fluids grew *Mycobacterium tuberculosis* in culture. Multi-drug-resistant tuberculous pericarditis has also been reported in the setting of AIDS.[9]

Non-tuberculous pericarditis

Viral pericarditis

Many different viruses have been implicated in the aetiology of acute pericarditis. The most common are Coxsackie A and B, echoviruses and polioviruses. Diagnosis is made by a significant rise — generally fourfold — in viral titres in blood. Most of these patients are in their 20s and they generally give a history of a previous upper respiratory tract infection. Acute viral pericarditis is generally accompanied by pericardial effusions, which range from straw-coloured to haemorrhagic. The episode tends to be short-lived (1–2 weeks) in most cases.

Recurrent attacks may occur and it is this group which may progress to chronic constrictive pericarditis. Recurrent episodes have been particularly linked to Coxsackie infection.[12]

Other infectious pericarditis

Occasionally, a well-known venereal disease agent such as *Neisseria gonorrhoeae* is responsible for a bout of pericarditis.[13] This generally happens when the patient has articular involvement. In these cases, the pericardial effusion can be either purulent or fibrinous. Histoplasmosis may also cause a pericarditis which can progress to restriction.[14]

Pericarditis in connective tissue diseases

Acute pericarditis is virtually always present in acute rheumatic fever but resolves rapidly and does not progress to restriction.[15]

Pericarditis is a relatively common finding in patients with rheumatoid arthritis.[16] Autopsy data show that approximately 30–50%[17] of the patients have pericarditis and echocardiograms performed during life will show between 30% and 40% pericardial involvement. However, in life, patients with rheumatoid arthritis only rarely manifest any symptoms of pericarditis. In most of the studies reported, the mean age of the patients with pericarditis was 60 years and the average interval between the diagnosis of rheumatoid arthritis and the appearance of the symptoms of pericarditis was approximately 9 years. The male-to-female ratio was close to 1. In most of the patients, pericardial effusions were small; a few patients showed pericardial thickening. Analysis of the pericardial fluid shows leucocytosis, increased protein level (mainly gamma globulins), increased lactate dehydrogenase and cholesterol, and decreased complement and glucose levels. Sometimes, rheumatoid factor is present. Short- and intermediate-term follow-up studies have shown that, if the bout of acute pericarditis becomes complicated, i.e. results in constrictive pericarditis, the prognosis is bad, with the vast majority of patients dying within 2 years of the diagnosis. Constrictive pericarditis in the setting of rheumatoid arthritis tends to occur in older patients who have long-standing disease.[18] Extra-articular features appear in around 90% of patients, rheumatoid nodules being the most frequently reported. Histological examination of the pericardium discloses fibrous thickening, with variable numbers of chronic inflammatory cells. Occasionally, immunoglobulins and complement can be found both in the interstitium and the perivascular spaces when using immunofluorescence techniques, but this is not a constant finding. The presence of fibrinous strands results in adhesions between the parietal and the visceral pericardium and also in the formation of loculated spaces, which make a pericardiocentesis much more difficult — even impossible at times — and at the same time increase the morbidity of the procedure. The average amount of pericardial fluid present in the pericardial sac is around 600 ml. As in the other cases of rheumatoid arthritis with pericarditis, the liquid is slightly haemorrhagic, with high protein and lactic dehydrogenase levels, low glucose levels and leucocytosis.

In patients with systemic lupus erythematosus (SLE), pericarditis is the most common manifestation of cardiac involvement.[19,20] Up to a third of patients with SLE have symptoms of pericardial involvement and this figure increases to 80% when one includes autopsy cases. In general, cardiac tamponade is a rare event and the clinical signs of pericarditis disappear after treatment. In 2–3% of patients, however, cardiac tamponade appears as a life-threatening event. Cardiac tamponade is seen more frequently in patients with pleurisy, haemolysis and/or renal disease. Pericarditis is generally due to immunological involvement of the serosa in patients with lupus, but uraemia and sepsis have both to be ruled out before establishing the diagnosis of pericarditis. In general, uraemic pericarditis appears before starting haemodialysis and septic pericarditis has been seen after the patient has been on high-dose steroids.

Examination of pericardial tissue in patients with SLE shows, for those with constrictive pericarditis, pericardial thickening due to fibrosis, sometimes with fibrin deposition on the surface. A chronic inflammatory cell infiltrate is present, sometimes evenly distributed and at other times just in a perivascular location. Isolated case reports have shown immunoglobulin and complement deposition (IgA, IgG, IgM, C3c) both in a perivascular location and throughout the pericardium.[21] Antimyosin and antipericardial antibodies have also been reported, together with some more commonly seen antibodies such as anti-sarcolemmal and anti-subsarcolemmal.

The amount of pericardial fluid present varies from 300–1400 ml. The fluid has the characteristics of an exudate.

Pericardial involvement has occasionally been reported in the setting of mixed connective tissue disease.[22] This is a chronic inflammatory disease sharing clinical manifestations of systemic lupus erythematosus, scleroderma and polymyositis. The most common manifestations are Raynaud's syndrome, oesophageal involvement and lymphadenopathy. The cardiovascular spectrum includes acute pericarditis with or without pericardial effusion, and mitral valve prolapse.

Other causes

Acute pericarditis is a commonly seen complication in the setting of renal transplantation.[23] Recent reviews of nearly 1500 patients covering a 27-year period have shown an incidence of pericarditis of 2.4%. The aetiology of the pericarditis was uraemia in 40% of the cases, both uraemia and Cytomegalovirus in 12%, Cytomegalovirus in 9%, bacterial infections in 9% (*Bacteroides fragilis, Listeria monocytogenes, Staphylococcus epidermidis*) and tuberculosis and minoxidil in a single case each. A few cases remained without an aetiological diagnosis.

Acute pericarditis ranks among the most common complications seen in renal failure. The majority of patients have uraemic pericarditis, especially if they are having episodes of post-transplant acute renal failure. The use of high doses of steroids in the early post-transplant period can also be an adjuvant for the predominance of uraemic pericarditis in transplanted patients. Regarding tuberculosis, although it is a rare finding, the possibility of reactivating a latent focus in the post-transplant period is real and it does happen, occasionally. Tuberculous pericarditis can also be seen as one of the initial manifestations of the acquired immune deficiency syndrome, and points towards high-risk patients.

Pericarditis after cardiac surgery is quite common. During the first few days, there is a minor degree of haemorrhage together with fibrin deposition and an acute inflammatory cell infiltrate. With time, however, the fibrin becomes organised, the pericardium thickens and may result in constrictive pericarditis that, in time, will require surgical treatment.[24,25] Exposure to asbestos is associated with pericardial as well as pleural fibrosis, and constriction is reported.[26]

After mediastinal radiotherapy[27] dense fibrosis of either the visceral or parietal pericardium can lead to restriction (Fig. 9.3). Concomitant myocardial fibrosis, particularly in the right ventricle, as the result of the radiation may make clinical recognition of restriction difficult.

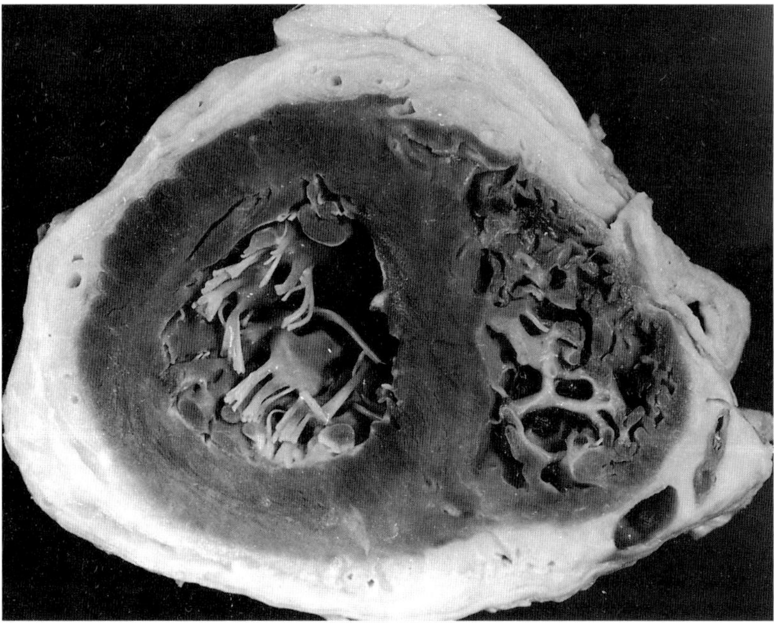

Fig. 9.3 Chronic constrictive pericarditis. The visceral pericardium is thickened and has calcified in areas. Fibrosis surrounds the epicardial coronary arteries. Previous radiotherapy to mediastinum; presented with constriction many years later.

The pericardium in AIDS

Cardiac disease can occur in approximately 7% of HIV-positive people. Cardiac involvement manifests itself as cardiac tamponade, dilated cardiomyopathy, refractory ventricular arrhythmias and infective endocarditis. Pericardial effusion results in cardiac tamponade in approximately a third of patients.[11] Both tuberculous and non-tuberculous pericarditis have been reported in AIDS patients; the most commonly retrieved microorganisms have been *Nocardia asteroides*, Herpes simplex virus and *Cryptococcus neoformans*. Sterile pericardial effusions have been reported in up to 15% of autopsies of AIDS patients.

Surgical excision in chronic constrictive pericarditis

In the relief of pericardial constriction the simplest procedure is the removal of a window of the anterior wall of the parietal pericardium. This may be followed by recurrence due to fibrosis in the visceral pericardium requiring stripping of the fibrous tissue of the myocardium itself.[28]

The material the pathologist receives from surgical excision of the pericardium should be examined in order to attempt a tissue diagnosis of the cause. Most of the material will be strips of fibrous tissue with calcification. It is advisable to examine a large proportion of the material looking for granulomas indicating tuberculosis or the palisaded granulomas of rheumatoid disease. The great majority of cases, however, will prove negative and the aetiology remain unknown.[29] In the developed world most are probably viral, whereas in areas where tuberculosis is still endemic this remains the most likely cause even if no granulomas are found.

PERICARDIAL TUMOURS

Approximately 10% of patients with terminal malignancy have cardiac involvement and, out of these, 85% have pericardial involvement. The presence of tumour cells in the pericardium may lead to a haemorrhagic pericarditis and cardiac tamponade, but this often goes unnoticed as its

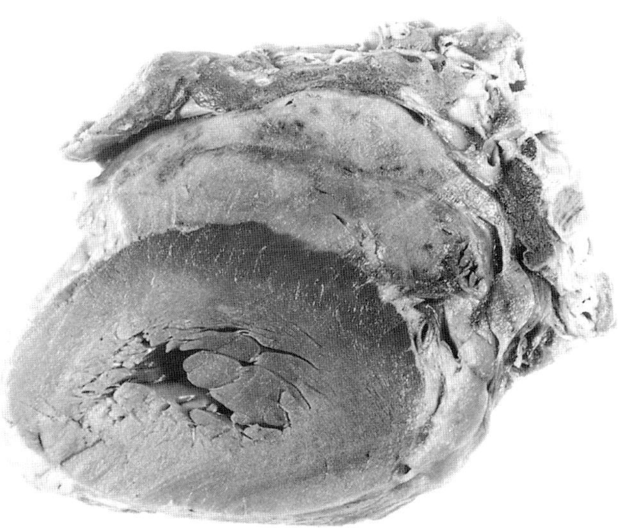

Fig. 9.4 Primary sarcoma of pericardium. There is a solid tumour applied to the visceral pericardium. Histology showed a malignant spindle cell sarcoma in which there were islands of mesothelial cells. This was interpreted as a mixed pattern mesothelioma but review suggested that the mesothelial element was benign pericardial proliferation in response to the tumour.

clinical signs are obscured by the presence of multiple metastases in other locations.

Secondary carcinoma is the most common cause of acute cardiac tamponade in clinical practice. Most of the patients with metastatic tumour in the pericardium have pericardial effusions, variable in size. Cytological examination of the pericardial fluid is mandatory.[30] The frequency of positive results is around 80%, with a false positive rate of around 3%. Cytologically positive pericardial effusions are treated with chemotherapy and/or radiotherapy, as long as the tumour is responsive.

The most common tumour to involve the pericardium is metastatic tumour from either a lung or breast carcinoma, or a lymphoma or leukaemia (80%). The tumours with the highest metastatic rate to the pericardium are melanoma and leukaemia (mainly by the haematogenous route), but lung and breast carcinomas occupy the first place in frequency because of their greater incidence. The average survival after diagnosis of pericardial involvement by tumour is short, ranging from 6–15 months in different series.[31]

Amongst the primary pericardial tumours, benign mesothelial/pericardial cysts are the most common and are diagnosed by being seen on chest radiograph as an incidental finding. They consist of a fibrous capsule lined by mesothelial-type cells and are usually unilocular although multiple cysts may occur. They do not cause symptoms but are often removed at a thoracotomy to see what they are. Haemangiosarcomas characteristically present as sudden tamponade due to haemorrhagic effusions but it is uncertain whether these tumours arise in the pericardium itself or in the atria (Chapter 11). Fibrosarcomas (Fig. 9.4) and liposarcomas, though very rare, are the most common primary malignant pericardial tumours.[32] Primary mesotheliomas of the pericardium are recorded but are too rare for it to be certain if there is a link with asbestosis.

REFERENCES

1. Spodick DH. Macrophysiology, microphysiology, and anatomy of the pericardium: A synopsis. Am Heart J 1992; 124; 1046–1051.
2. Watkins MW, LeWinter MM. Physiologic role of the normal pericardium. Annu Rev Med 1993; 44: 171–180.
3. Scully RE, Mark EJ, NcNeely WF, NcNeely BU. Case records of the Massachusetts General Hospital. Weekly clinicopathological exercises. N Engl J Med 1994; 330: 126–135.
4. Fowler NO. Tuberculous pericarditis. JAMA 1991; 266: 99–103.
5. Dave T, Narula JP, Chopra P. Myocardial and endocardial involvement in tuberculous constrictive pericarditis: difficulty in biopsy distinction from endomyocardial fibrosis as a cause of restrictive heart disease. Int J Cardiol 1990; 28: 245–251.
6. Long R, Younes M, Patton N, Hershfield E. Tuberculous pericarditis: long-term outcome in patients who received medical therapy alone. Am Heart J 1989; 117: 1133–1139.
7. DeValeria PA, Baumgartner WA, Casale AS, Greene PS, Cameron DE, Gardner TJ, Gott VL, Watkins L, Reitz BA. Current indications, risks, and outcome after pericardiectomy. Ann Thorac Surg 1991; 52: 219–224.
8. DeMiguel J, Pedreira JD, Campos V, Perez Gomez A, Porto JAL. Tuberculous pericarditis and AIDS. Chest 1990; 97: 1273.
9. Horn DL, Hewlett D, Alfalla C, Peterson S. Fatal hospital-acquired multi-drug resistant tuberculous pericarditis in two patients with AIDS. N Engl J Med 1992; 327: 1816–1817.
10. Supervia A, Campodarve I, Shaath M, Mellibovsky L, Cladellas M, Bruguera J. Pericarditis tuberculosa como primera manifestación de SIDA. Indicación de la pericardiocentesis diagnóstica. Rev Clin Esp 1993; 192: 150–151.
11. Anderson DW, Virmani R. Emerging patterns of heart disease in human immunodeficiency virus infection. Human Pathol 1990; 21: 253–259.
12. Muir P, Nicholson F, Tilzey AJ et al. Chronic relapsing pericarditis and dilated cardiomyopathy: serological evidence of persistent entero-virus infection. Lancet 1989; i: 804–807
13. Wilson J, Zaman AG, Simmons AV. Gonococcal arthritis complicated by acute pericarditis and pericardial effusion. Br Heart J 1990; 63: 134–135.
14. Picardi J, Kauffman C, Schwarz J, Holmes J, Phair J, Fowler N. Pericarditis caused by *Histoplasma capsulatum*. Am J Cardiol 1976; 37: 82–88.
15. Wood P. Chronic constrictive pericarditis. Am J Cardiol 1961; 7: 48–61.
16. Hara KS, Ballard DJ, Ilstrup DM, Connolly DC, Vollertsen RS. Rheumatoid pericarditis: clinical features and survival. Medicine (Baltimore) 1990; 69: 81–91.
17. Kahn M-F, Hayem G. Les pericardites rhumatoides. Ann Med Intern 1992; 143: 238–240.
18. Manji H, Raven P. Calcific constrictive pericarditis due to rheumatoid arthritis. Post Grad Med J 1990; 66: 57–58.
19. Kahl LE. The spectrum of pericardial tamponade in systemic lupus erythematosus. Arthritis and Rheum 1992; 35: 1343–1349.

20. Doherty NE, Siegel RJ. Cardiovascular manifestations of systemic lupus erythematosus. Am Heart J 1985; 110: 1257–1266.
21. Wolf RE, King JW, Brown TA. Antimyosin antibodies and constrictive pericarditis in lupus erythematosus. J Rheumatol 1988; 15: 1284–1287.
22. Beier JM, Nielsen HL, Nielsen D. Pleuritis-pericarditis — an unusual initial manifestation of mixed connective tissue disease. Eur Heart J 1992; 13: 859–861.
23. Sever MS, Steinmuller DR, Hayes JM, Streem SB, Novick AC. Pericarditis following renal transplantation. Transplantation 1991; 51: 1229–1232.
24. Cimino J, Kogan A. Constrictive pericarditis after cardiac surgery: report of three cases and review of the literature. Am Heart J 1989; 118: 1292–1301.
25. Kutcher M, King SI, Alimurung B, Craver J, Logue R. Constrictive pericarditis as a complication of cardiac surgery: recognition of an entity. Am J Cardiol 1982; 50: 742–748.
26. Davies D, Andrews M, Jones J. Asbestos induced pericardial effusion and constrictive pericarditis. Thorax 1991; 46: 429–432.
27. Cameron J, Oesterle SN, Baldwin JC, Hancock EW. The aetiologic spectrum of constrictive pericarditis. Am Heart J 1987; 113: 354–360.
28. Bashi V, John S, Ravikumar E, Jairaj P, Shyamsunder K, Krishnaswami S. Early and late results of pericardiectomy in 118 cases of constrictive pericarditis. Thorax 1988; 43: 637–641.
29. Blake S, Bonar S, O'Neill H, et al. Aetiology of chronic constrictive pericarditis. Br Heart J 1983; 50: 273–276.
30. Wiener HG, Kristensen IB, Haubek A, Kristensen B, Baandrup U. The diagnostic value of pericardial cytology. Acta Cytologica 1991; 35: 149–153.
31. Wilding G, Green HL, Longo DL, Urba WJ. Tumors of the heart and pericardium. Cancer Treat Rev 1988; 15: 165–181.
32. Butany J. The pericardium and its diseases. In Silver MD, ed. Cardiovascular pathology Churchill Livingstone 1991: p. 887.

10

The cardiac conduction system

INTRODUCTION

Dissociation of the cells of the early embryonic heart shows that there are two forms of myocyte. Most myocytes are totally quiescent but a minor subpopulation undergoes spontaneous regular contraction. The inert form is destined to produce the contractile (working) myocardium; the other form will produce the cells of the conduction system. The conduction system in the adult heart has two functions: first the initiation of a rhythmic impulse for contraction and second the rapid distribution of this stimulus for contraction to the cells of the working myocardium.

The generation of an impulse for contraction by conduction myocytes is a function of ion channels in the cell membrane, which allow a slow drift in electrical potential toward depolarisation in diastole. In contrast the cell membrane of contractile cells is electrically stable in diastole. Initiation of contraction and conduction are functions of myocytes and are independent of nerve impulses. Nervous control via release of chemical mediators from vagal and sympathetic nerves does, however, alter the rate of both the initiation of rhythm and speed of conduction.

In the adult heart within the cells of the conduction system (Table 10.1) there is further specialisation toward cells whose normal function is either the initiation of rhythm (nodal cells) or conduction (atrioventricular bundle and bundle branches). The normal conduction system is an integrated whole generating a regular impulse for contraction which is distributed in an orderly fashion to the ventricular myocardium. The normal sequence is:

Table 10.1 Function of myocytes in the adult heart

Type	Function		
	Initiation	Conduction	Contraction
Sinus node	+++(70)	Very slow	0
Atrio-ventricular node	++(40)	Very slow	0
Bundle of His	++(30)	Rapid	0
Bundle branches	+(25)	Rapid	0
Contractile myocardium	0	Slow	+++

1. Generation of an impulse at approximately 70 beats a minute by the sinus node. This rate can be altered by sympathetic (increased rate) or vagal (slowing) nerve impulses. The resting pulse rate of an individual is a reflection of the balance of vagal and sympathetic tone. The term sinus rhythm means the impulse generated in the sinus node is acting as the dominant pacemaker.

2. The impulse spreads diffusely to the atria initiating atrial contraction. While certain parts of the atrial muscle preferentially conduct the impulse by virtue of their anatomical site there is no specialisation in structure or function.

3. The impulse reaches the atrioventricular node and is held for an appreciable period of time. This allows atrial contraction to fill the ventricles.

4. The impulse leaves the atrioventricular node and is rapidly distributed to the ventricular myocardium via the atrioventricular bundle of His and the right and left bundle branches. The atrioventricular bundle of His is the only normal connection between the atria and ventricles.

It is an important facet of the conduction system that, while all its cells retain the function of automaticity, this is suppressed by being driven by the faster rhythm originating in the sinus node. The innate rhythm of the sinus node is the highest, with decreasing rates more distally in the conduction system. Rhythms initiated in the ventricles if the nodes are suppressed or destroyed are at rates of 30–40 beats a minute and tend to have intermittent pauses.

For the pathologist, the conduction system is a separate anatomical structure rather than a separate tissue and with a few exceptions it suffers the same pathological processes as the rest of the myocardium.

Pathological processes may delay or prevent conduction from one part of the heart to another or interfere with the generation of stimuli for contraction, leading to fast and/or irregular rhythms in atria or ventricles (tachycardia or fibrillation).

CONDUCTION DELAYS

Chronic long-term conduction disturbances usually involve an anatomical disruption of the atrioventricular bundle of His or bundle branches. Disruption of the bundle of His leads to atrioventricular heart block, in which the atria and ventricles are totally dissociated. The ventricular rate is unrelated to the atrial rate, and often slow — 30–40 a minute. Disruption of the bundle branches, if unilateral, leads to characteristic abnormalities in the electrocardiogram but not to symptoms because the ventricular myocardium is stimulated via the contralateral branch after a short delay. The delay is, however, sufficiently brief that contractile function of the ventricles and cardiac output are normal.

TACHYCARDIAS

The pathophysiology of tachycardias is a vast subject beyond the scope of this book. Nevertheless a basic knowledge of the ways in which tachycardias arise helps in understanding how morphological changes can contribute toward the generation of atrial tachycardias, atrial fibrillation and ventricular fibrillation or tachycardia. Tachycardias arise by three mechanisms.

Automaticity

Automaticity is a normal function of pacemaking cells but if the rate of discharge of a group of such cells becomes excessive tachycardia at rest occurs. Such arrhythmias arise from cells in the sinus node (sinus tachycardia) or in cells within the atrial muscle itself (atrial tachycardia) or in cells close to the atrioventricular node (junctional tachycardia). The lesions can be very focal and cured by ablation of very small areas of tissue. The pathophysiological basis, however, lies in abnormal function probably at cell membrane level rather than structural change visible by microscopy.

Re-entry tachycardia

This is by far the commonest mechanism generating tachycardias. A circular movement of an impulse round a central electrically inert area occurs. The stimulus arrives back at its starting point just at the moment when the tissue can be reactivated, and a self-perpetuating circuit of activation develops. The creation of the re-entry pathway may be pathophysiological (i.e. acute ischaemia) or structural (when fibrosis disturbs myocardial architecture) or a combination of the two. Examples of re-entrant tachycardias are chronic atrial fibrillation and episodic ventricular tachycardia. In normal cardiac muscle the wave of activation passes out from a central point in an orderly manner and then dies out. The conduction velocity in the long axis of the myocyte bundles is faster than that occurring in the transverse direction by a factor of approximately 3 but a symmetric wave front progression occurs in all directions. The different rates of conduction in the long and short axis reflect the orientation of tight junctions on the end of the myocyte.

In re-entry tachycardias there must be a central inert area of myocardial tissue caused, for example, by acute infarction or a focus of fibrosis. There must also be wave fronts proceeding at different rates and areas of tissue that block conduction in one direction but not the other. When such a circuit exists — and it may be single or multiple and large (many centimetres in length) or small — an extrasystolic beat can initiate a re-entrant tachycardia. The circuit may be in part made up of normal or anomalous conduction tissue or be entirely made up of working atrial or myocardial cells.

Triggered activity

After a myocyte has undergone depolarisation, conditions that include an increase in intracellular calcium and drugs such as digoxin may cause the membrane potential to oscillate and these swings may be of sufficient magnitude to trigger a further action potential. This is followed by a long train of additional contractions caused by the after-depolarisation variations in potential of the preceding impulse. The phenomenon is purely one of abnormal function, not structure. It is the possible mechanism for right ventricular outflow tachycardias and *torsades de pointe*, a particular form of ventricular tachycardia arising in the left ventricle.

THE ANATOMY AND STRUCTURES OF THE CONDUCTION SYSTEM

The sinus node

The sinus node, first described by Keith & Flack in 1907, lies at the junction of the superior vena cava and the right atrium close to the crest of the atrial appendage. The node (Figs 10.1, 10.2) consists of two types of myocyte. The central nodal cells are small and arranged in a complex interdigitating manner interspersed with connective tissue. Such central nodal cells contain very few myofilaments. The intracellular organised structures of myocytes (myofilaments, mitochondria, nuclei and sarcoplasmic reticulum tubules) occupy only 50% of the cell volume. In the contractile atrial myocytes these filaments and organelles comprise 90% of the total cell volume. The second type of myocyte is transitional in that it changes gradually from the morphology of the typical central type nodal cell to ordinary atrial myocytes. In some species, e.g. the rabbit, the zone of transitional cells is large; in others, e.g. the dog or the pig, it is narrow. Although the boundaries between the compact node and the transitional zone are usually distinct, the boundary between the transitional zone and the working right atrial myocardium is often poorly defined.

Dominant pacemaker cells — i.e. those that activate earliest, have the fastest rate of diastolic depolarization, the slowest rate of rise of the action potential upstroke and a gradual transition from diastolic to systolic depolarization — are gathered in a small area of about 0.3 mm^2 containing about 5000 cells that fire synchronously.[1] It is estimated that every cell in the pacemaker centre is coupled to other cells by at least 100

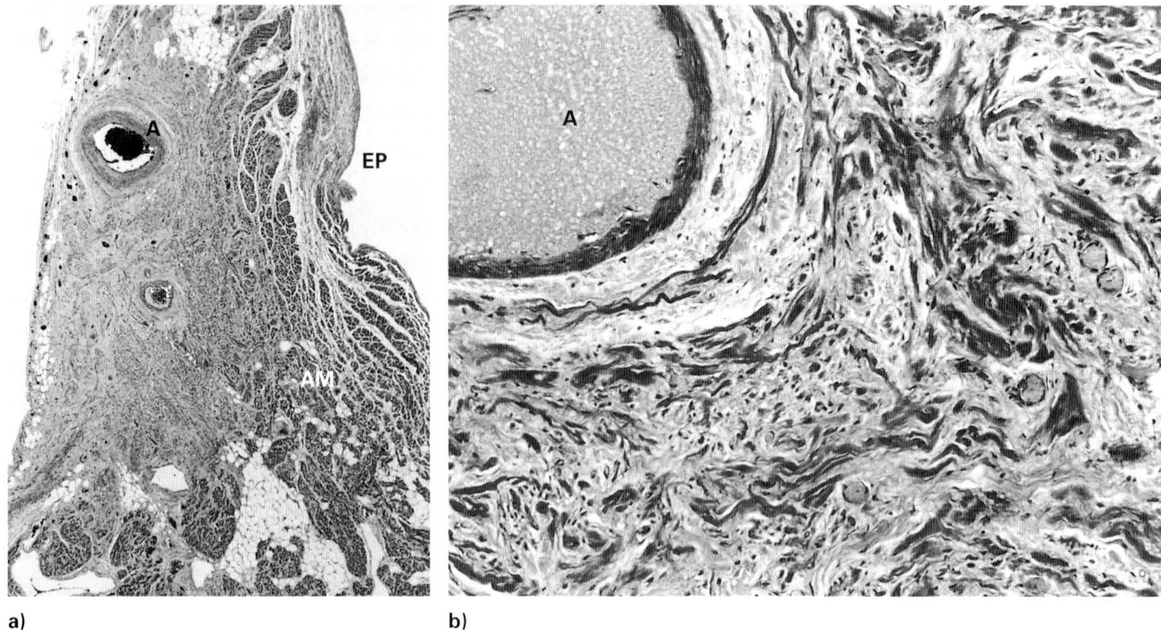

Fig. 10.1 a,b, Normal sinoatrial node. (**a**) At low power the node (arrows) lies around a central artery (A) just beneath the epicardium (EP). The node merges with adjacent atrial myocardium (AM). (**b**) At high power using trichrome stains which accentuate the staining of myocytes nodal cells are seen to be small and arranged in a complex network embedded in a connective tissue stroma.
(**a**) Haematoxylin–eosin × 7
(**b**) Picro–Mallory × 110

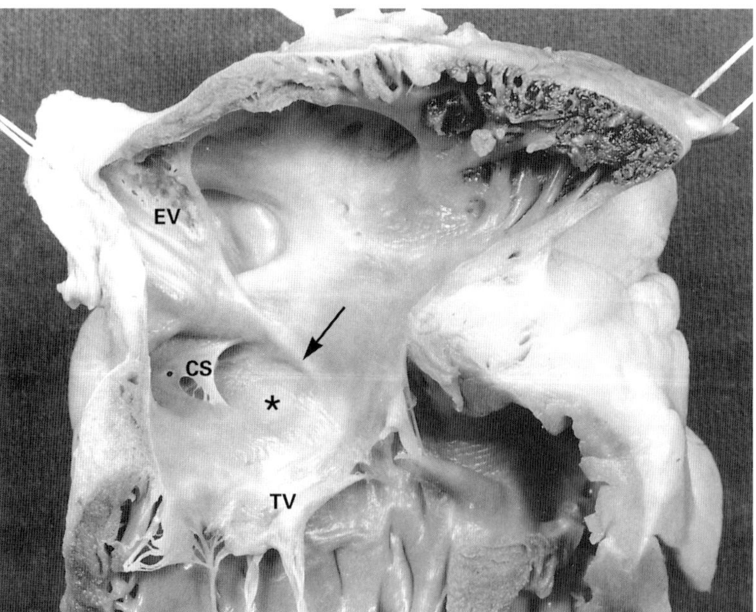

Fig. 10.2 Triangle of Koch. The atrial septum is viewed from the right. The triangle of Koch (*) is bounded by the coronary sinus (CS), the septal cusp of the tricuspid valve (TV) and the Tendon of Todaro (arrow). The tendon is the continuation of the valve of the inferior vena cava (Eustachian valve — EV).

gap junctions. The number of gap junctions, and thus the degree of electrical coupling between nodal cells, increases throughout the transitional zone towards the atrium.

A striking feature of the mammalian sinus node is the presence of abundant connective tissue surrounding individual myocytes.[2] Age-related changes in the sinus node are striking. In young individuals there are approximately equal proportions by volume of myocytes and collagen in the node. By 70 years of age in many individuals the proportion of the node occupied by nodal myocytes has fallen to 10%. There is nothing to suggest that the node increases in size with age and the data probably indicate an overall fall in the number of nodal myocytes. An increase in the amount of adipose tissue between the transitional nodal cells is also an age-related change.

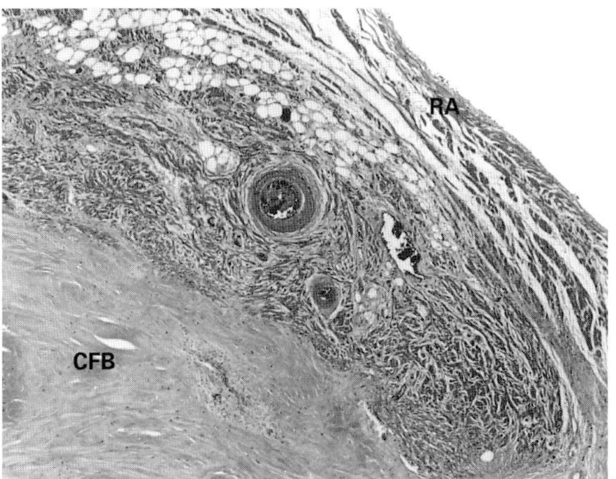

Fig. 10.3 Normal human AV node. The node is half oval with small myocytes applied closely to the central fibrous body (CFB). The node lies just beneath the right atrial endocardium (RA) and has a central artery. Haematoxylin–eosin × 16

The AV node and junctional tissues

The atrioventricular node lies just beneath the endocardium of the right atrium within the triangle of Koch. The triangle is bounded by the coronary sinus, the tendon of Todaro which attaches the eustachian valve to the central fibrous body, and the insertion of the septal cusp of the tricuspid valve (Fig. 10.2). The node lies closer to the apex of the triangle than to the base, which is formed by the ostium of the coronary sinus. The subepicardial fat invaginates into the posterior aspect of the atrial septum in the floor of the coronary sinus. Within this fat the nodal artery passes from its origin from the posterior descending coronary to reach the node.

The microanatomy of the human node is best appreciated in histological sections taken in the long axis of the atrial septum at right angles to the endocardium. The deep portion of the node is shaped like a half oval and applied closely to the central fibrous body (Fig. 10.3). The compact or deep portion of the node is made up of an interweaving mass of small myocytes embedded in a fibrous stroma (Fig. 10.4). This part of the atrioventricular node resembles the sinus node in structure and a proportion of the cells do not have transverse tubules and have very few myofibrils.[3]

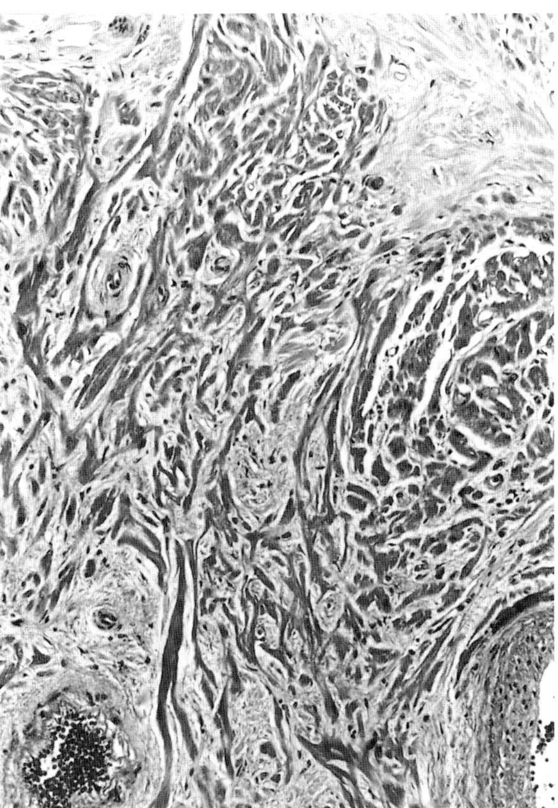

Fig. 10.4 Normal human AV node. The myocytes in the deep portion of the node have a characteristic interwoven arrangement.
Picro–Mallory × 70

Anteriorly the node begins to sink into the

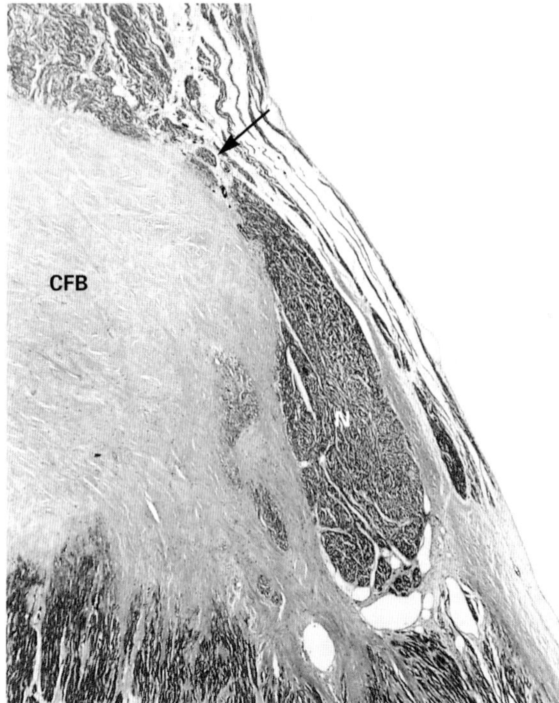

Fig. 10.5 Formation of AV bundle. The node (N) at this level has begun to penetrate the central fibrous body (CFB) but still retains some attachment to atrial muscle (arrow). Haematoxylin eosin × 18

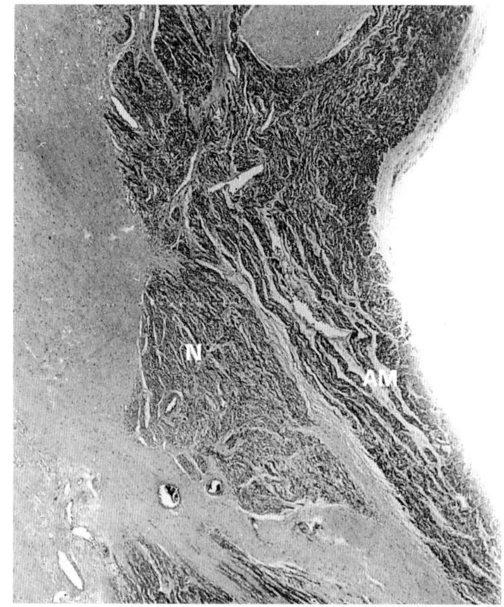

Fig. 10.6 Formation of AV bundle. The node (N) is now almost completely surrounded by fibrous tissue but still lies well over toward the right atrium from which it is separated by an overlay of atrial muscle (AM). Haematoxylin–eosin × 18

central fibrous body, finally entering and being completely encased by fibrous tissue. This is the morphological point at which the node is regarded as ending and the atrioventricular bundle of His begins (Figs 10.5, 10.6). Once within the tunnel of fibrous tissue all atrial input into the node ceases. The arrangement of myocytes within the penetrating bundle is in parallel regular arrays with the cells in end-to-end contact. The more irregular nodal type arrangement may, however, persist for some distance in the fibrous tunnel.

The deep portion of the node is covered by several superficial layers of transitional myocytes which form the contact between the deep node and the atrial myocardium. The node complex thus includes a deep portion and several superficial layers. Only the deep portion contains the characteristic small interweaving nodal myocytes. It is an unresolved semantic question whether the superficial layers of the node, composed of myocytes with properties transitional between deep nodal myocytes and the atrial myocytes, are strictly part of the node or form a paranodal structure.

Atrial input to the node

Considerable disagreement exists over the nomenclature and arrangement of the atrial input to the node and there is probably considerable individual variability in this regard.

On morphological criteria the major input enters the node posteriorly around the coronary sinus and via the superficial layers over the surface of the node in the mid-septal region. The deep portion of the node posteriorly bifurcates into two prongs. These are often very unequal in size and one or both may make connections to atrial myocytes. James[4] described an input which originated posteriorly around the Eustachian valve and passed forward beneath the septal endocardium to enter the node just before it penetrates the central fibrous body. It thus became a late input into the node, bypassing much of the deep node. In the experience of others the last nodal input is variable but usually derived from the superficial transitional layers of atrial muscle in the mid and anterior parts of the septum.[5]

Nodal structural variations

The deep portion of the node is closely applied to the central fibrous body but in many normal subjects, particularly in youth, apparently isolated islands of nodal-type tissue are embedded with the central fibrous body. Some at least of these archipelagos interconnect and form loops of tissue connecting to the deep node. In some otherwise normal hearts strands of myocardial tissue (Mahaim fibres) penetrate the central fibrous body to reach the ventricular septum and establish nodoventricular connections independent of the normal conduction system.

In the great majority of hearts the central fibrous body posterior to the node, where there is a pad of fat in the floor of the coronary sinus, is deficient and potentially atrial and ventricular myocardium abut. The gap is, however, usually closed by adipose tissue but occasional strands of myocytes are embedded in this tissue and may directly connect atria to ventricles.

In the ventricular free walls atrial and ventricular myocardium are usually regarded as totally separated and insulated by the connective tissue of the atrioventricular valve rings. The tricuspid valve ring is, however, only partially formed in many hearts and atria and ventricles are separated by adipose tissue only. A node-like mass of tissue exists as a remnant of the fetal ring of atrioventricular conduction tissue in up to 30% of normal hearts.[6] This remnant of nodal tissue, first recognised by Kent, does not usually establish atrioventricular continuity, running as it does in a circumferential plane.

Atrioventricular bundle of His

The penetrating portion of the atrioventricular bundle begins once the node has become completely enclosed within a tunnel in the central fibrous body (Fig. 10.7) and there is no potential for further atrial input. The atrioventricular bundle passes forward within the central fibrous body to emerge on the crest of the muscular interventricular septum where it joins the membranous septum.

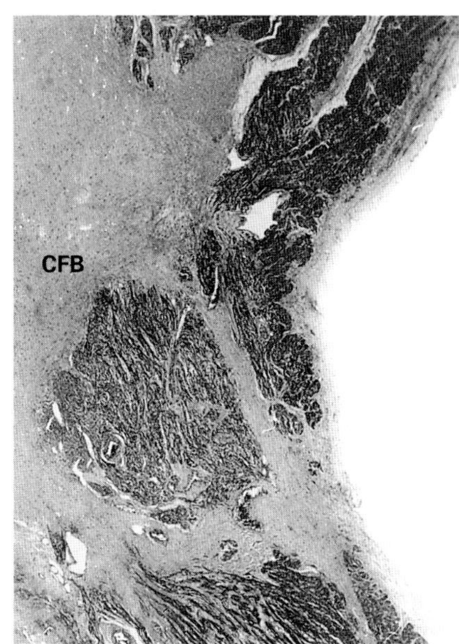

Fig. 10.7 Atrioventricular bundle of His. The AV bundle is now fully formed as a round muscle of regularly arranged conduction myocytes deeply embedded in the central fibrous body (CFB).

Within the tunnel the myocytes are arranged in a regular longitudinal fashion, a morphological indication that conduction is now rapid. The atrioventricular bundle is a slender structure no more than 2 mm in diameter. Within the fibrous body the atrioventricular bundle may be subdivided by fine fibrous trabeculae and there is some evidence that impulses destined for the right and left ventricles are already separate.

Bifurcating atrioventricular bundle and bundle branches

On the crest of the muscular septum the bifurcating portion of the atrioventricular bundle begins to give rise to the multiple slender fascicles of the left bundle branch (Fig. 10.8). These pass down the left side of the muscular septum just beneath the endocardium and ultimately form a network throughout the whole of the left ventricular endocardial surface. Each individual fascicle is very slender and passes at its origin between the endocardium of the left ventricular outflow and fibrous tissue in the upper septum. Loss of the

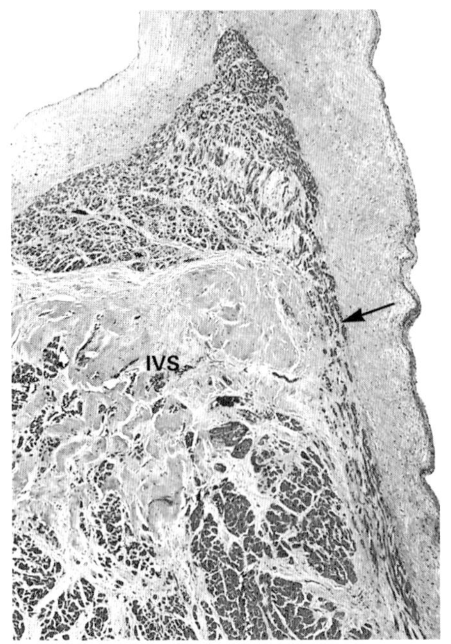

Fig. 10.8 Bifurcating atrioventricular bundle. The AV bundle is still encased in fibrous tissue and lies on the crest of the muscular interventricular septum (IVS). The upper septum at this site normally contains a lot of fibrous trabeculae. From the left side of the bundle one of the many slender fascicles (arrow) of the left bundle branch passes down beneath the endocardium of the septum.

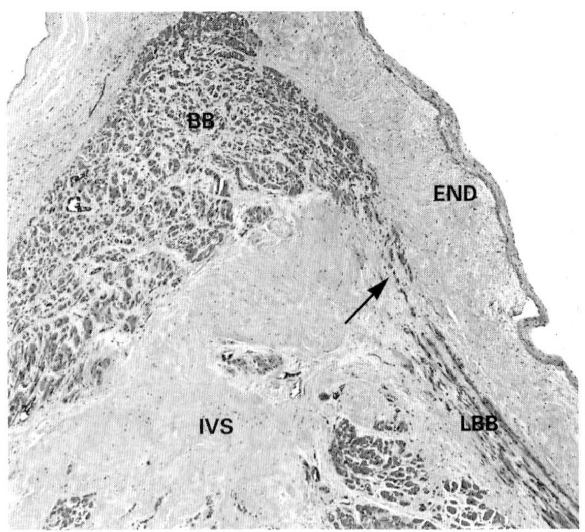

Fig. 10.9 Bifurcating AV bundle — origin of left bundle branch. A slender left branch fascicle (LBB) is present. At its origin from the bifurcating bundle (BB) it passes between the collagen tissue of the interventricular septum (IVS) and fibrosis beneath the endocardium (END) of the left ventricular outflow. Discontinuity of at least some fascicles with the bundle (arrow) is common with increasing age. Haematoxylin–eosin × 18

origin of some of the left branch fascicles is a common age-related change (Fig. 10.9). The pattern of left bundle branch fascicles in the septum is very variable. Many hearts have a preponderance of fascicles in the anterior and posterior portions, forming two streams, other hearts have a continuous fan or three main streams. These patterns can be discerned only by histological reconstruction. Although there have been gross dissections of the left branch it is not a structure easily visible to naked eye examination. In human hearts the individual myocytes within the left bundle branch fascicles are somewhat larger than the adjacent contractile myocytes and appear somewhat vacuolated because of a relative reduction in myofibrils compared with contractile myocytes (Fig. 10.10). The very large conduction myocytes with virtually no myofibrils described by Purkinje (Fig. 10.11) occur only in larger mammalian hearts such as the cow. This leads to a rather sterile semantic argument about the left bundle branch myocytes in human hearts. They are called by some Purkinje cells because their function is identical to those in larger mammalian hearts; others deny the use of the word because the strict morphological features described by Purkinje are absent in human hearts.

The right bundle branch is a single discrete muscle bundle formed as the continuation of the bifurcating bundle (Fig. 10.12). It may run immediately beneath the endocardium in the upper septum or pass through the muscular septum (Fig. 10.13) emerging beneath the endocardium lower down. Low in the septum it crosses the cavity of the right ventricle in what is called the moderator band in mammalian hearts. In human hearts the moderator band is less well formed and is just one of the trabeculae joining the septum to the base of the papillary muscles. From the free wall of the apex of the right ventricle a diffuse subendocardial network of conduction myocytes spreads throughout the ventricle.

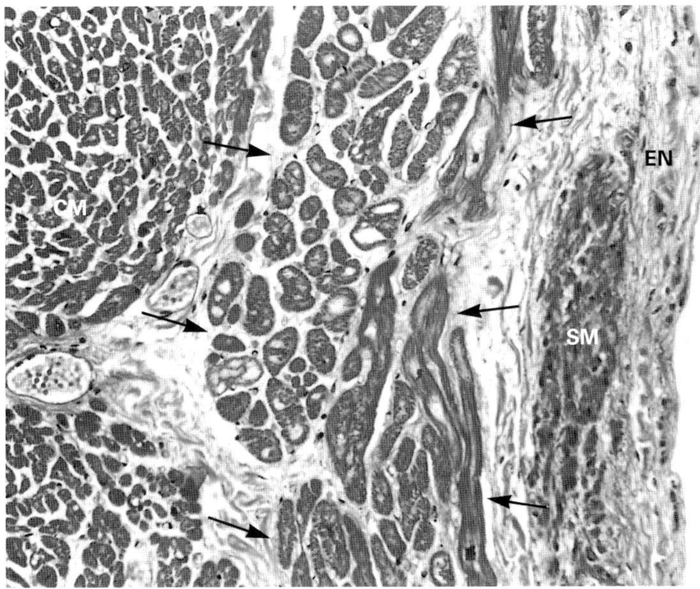

Fig. 10.10 Left bundle branch. The left bundle branch has been cut transversely in the mid-septal region. The endocardium (EN) contains some smooth muscle cells (SM). Beneath the endocardium there is a zone (arrows) of conduction tissue. Within this zone the myocytes are appreciably larger and more vacuolated than those of the underlying contractile myocardium (CM).
Haematoxylin–eosin × 110

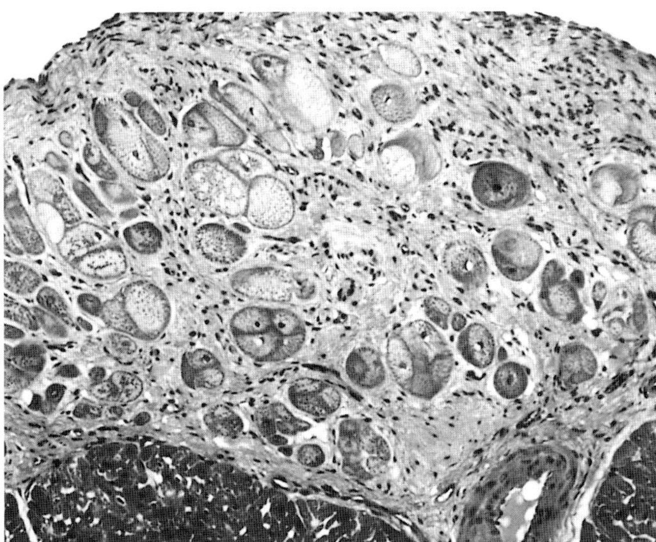

Fig. 10.11 Porcine Purkinje cells. The cells of the left bundle branch are very large and aggregates of two or three cells appear fused together and insulated by connective tissue from adjacent bundles.
Haematoxylin–eosin × 32

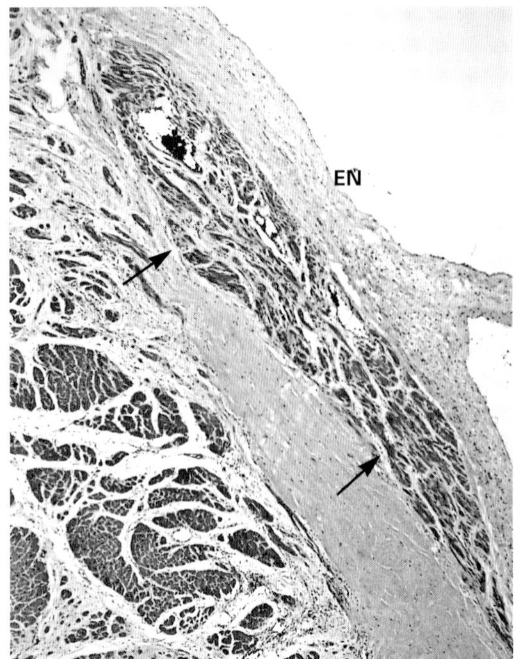

Fig. 10.12 Human right bundle branch. The right branch (arrows) is a single large bundle which runs down the septum just beneath the endocardium (EN). Haematoxylin–eosin × 28

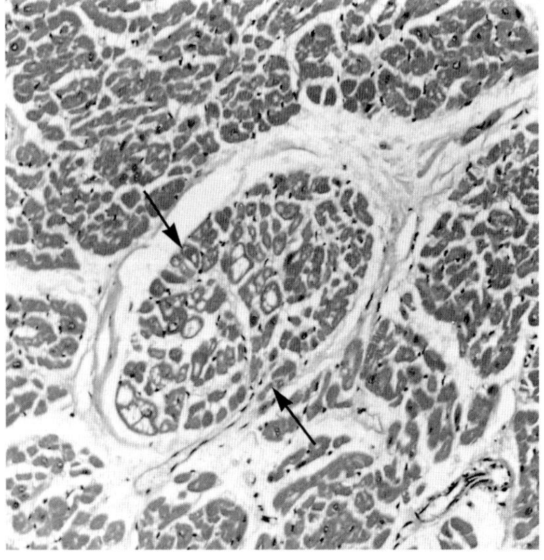

Fig. 10.13 Human right bundle branch. This example runs deep in the muscular septum and is recognisable because it is a discrete bundle (arrows) encased in connective tissue and because of the slightly larger more vacuolated appearance of the myocytes compared to the adjacent myocardium. Haematoxylin–eosin × 28

Accessory conduction pathways

In normal hearts the only electrical connection of the atria and ventricles is via the atrioventricular bundle of His. Accessory conduction paths however can exist and are divided[5] into those that lie in the left or right atrioventricular valve rings (parietal) and those that lie within the septum. Posterior septal pathways may activate either the right or the left side.

Parietal pathways

The majority of parietal anomalous conduction pathways consist of slender strands of normal working atrial myocytes embedded in connective tissue crossing the atrioventricular ring. Multiple slender strands and arborization of the ventricular end of the pathway over an area of a centimetre or more are common.[6] There are rare examples of paths that arise in persistent nodal-type tissue in the anterior tricuspid ring area, which should be appropriately regarded as Kent bundles,[7] but in general there is no morphological evidence of a delay-producing area in the vast majority of parietal accessory paths. On the left side, parietal anomalous bundles run in epicardial fat closely applied to the fibrous annulus of the mitral valve. On the right side, pathways simply run through the fat pad separating atrial and ventricular muscle.

Septal pathways

In the area immediately posterior to the atrioventricular node in the floor of the ostium of the coronary sinus, strands of normal atrial muscle may pass through the defect filled with fatty tissue which exists in the central fibrous body at this site. Access to this area can be achieved surgically by burrowing into the fat from the posterior interventricular sulcus because the pericardium is invaginated almost as far anteriorly as the atrioventricular node.[7]

Connections may also be present between the superficial atrial overlay myocytes beneath the endocardium of the right atrium and the ventricular septum through defects between the base of the septal cusp of the tricuspid valve and the central fibrous body. All these paths are composed of normal atrial myocytes.

MORPHOLOGICAL STUDIES IN ARRYTHMIAS AND CONDUCTION DISTURBANCE

Chronic sinoatrial disease

In the sick sinus syndrome the sinus node intermittently drops its rate, or even stops, for short periods. Escape rhythms take over from pacing cells in the atrioventricular nodal region if the pause continues long enough.

A consistent pattern can be observed in morphological studies of the sinus node.[8–11] Amyloid deposition within the node and adjacent atrial myocardium is one cause of sinoatrial block. A second cause is a loss of nodal myocytes in excess of the degree of loss normal for the age of the patient (Fig. 10.14). In many cases nodal myocytes are virtually absent, although the fibrous stroma of the node remains intact. The reason for the accentuated loss is unknown. Previous diphtheria, myocarditis, autoimmunity, rheumatic disease and large- or small-vessel disease have all been postulated but never proved to have a causal role. The third morphological pattern responsible for chronic sinoatrial disease is an aplastic or hypoplastic node in which even the basic collagenous structure of the node is absent. This form is found in younger subjects and may be the basis of familial cases.[12] Finally, cases are described in which the sinus node is morphologically normal.

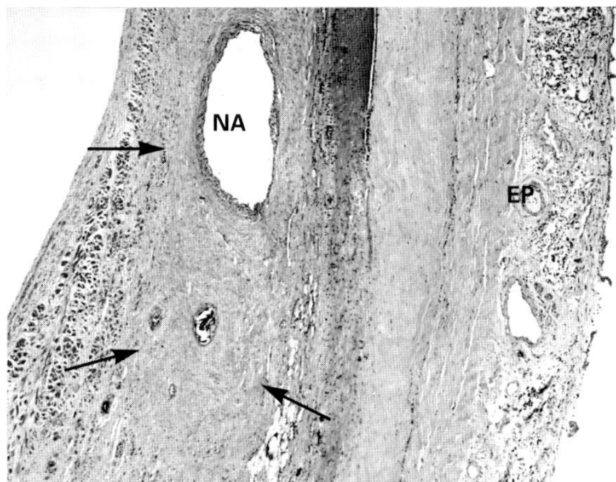

Fig. 10.14 Sino-atrial disease. In this patient with atrial fibrillation due to chronic rheumatic heart disease the SA node is recognisable as the collagenous structure (arrows) surrounding the nodal artery (NA). The node contains virtually no muscle cells. The epicardium is fibrotic and inflamed (EP).
Haematoxylin–eosin × 15

Atrial tachycardia and fibrillation

Atrial tachycardias in which a single focus is discharging at a regular high rate are the best examples of automaticity and are physiological rather than structural in origin. Atrial fibrillation represents multiple re-entry pathways in atrial myocardium associated in many cases with a decline in the dominance of the sinus node. The morphological basis for the non-uniform conduction in atrial muscle responsible for chronic atrial fibrillation is disruption by fibrosis. The fibrosis that develops with increasing age, or following chronic atrial dilatation, is often distributed in the long axis of muscle bundles and reduces the transverse spread of an impulse while still allowing longitudinal spread. It may also transect some muscle bundles, meaning that any impulse has to progress via a zigzag course. This disruption is the substrate for multiple re-entry pathways. Because it is a reflection of atrial fibrosis atrial fibrillation complicates any disease which leads to atrial dilatation and scarring and thus is common in all forms of cardiomyopathy, mitral valve disease and ischaemic heart disease. Deposition of amyloid material in atrial muscle also creates multiple re-entry pathways. The striking age-related frequency of atrial fibrillation is due to the increase in atrial fibrous and adipose tissue with age.

Junctional tachycardias

Junctional tachycardias arise in the conduction tissues of the atrioventricular rings that comprise the atrioventricular node, the penetrating atrioventricular bundle of His and accessory or anomalous atrioventricular connections.[13]

The term junctional tachycardias includes:

1. Re-entry tachycardia using an anomalous atrial ventricular conduction pathway situated

either in the septum or the lateral atrioventricular rings.
2. Intranodal reentrant tachycardia.
3. Tachycardia associated with nodoventricular connections.

Pre-excitation and re-entrant tachycardia involving anomalous atrioventricular pathways

Anomalous atrioventricular pathways (Figs 10.15, 10.16) lead to the early activation of a segment of ventricular myocardium through avoidance of the delay normally imposed by the deep portion of the atrioventricular node. The anomalous pathways may conduct in either one or both directions and can act as the afferent or the efferent limb of a re-entry circuit, using the conventional conduction system as the other limb. In pathological studies, all types of anomalous parietal and septal pathways have been shown to be associated with pre-excitation and tachycardia. Evidence of the function of these pathways is best shown by the success of surgical division and ablation in abolishing both pre-excitation and tachycardia. All these pathways are thought to represent persistence of atrioventricular connec-

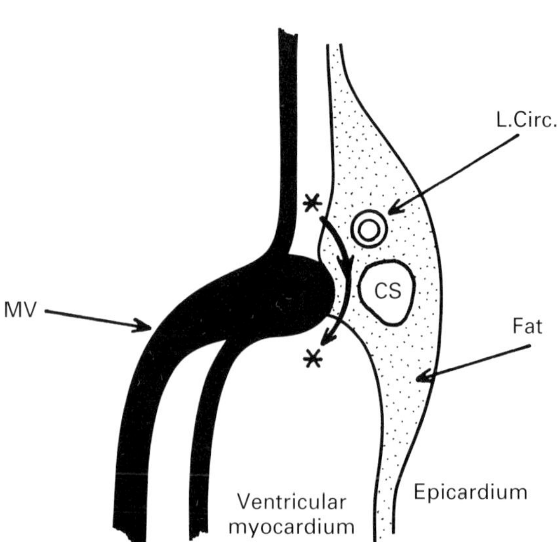

Fig. 10.15 Parietal anomalous conduction. The anomalous pathway (*) runs in the fat of the atrioventricular groove closely applied to the mitral valve (MV) annulus. In the left atrioventricular groove both the coronary sinus (CS) and the left circumflex artery lie close by in the fat.

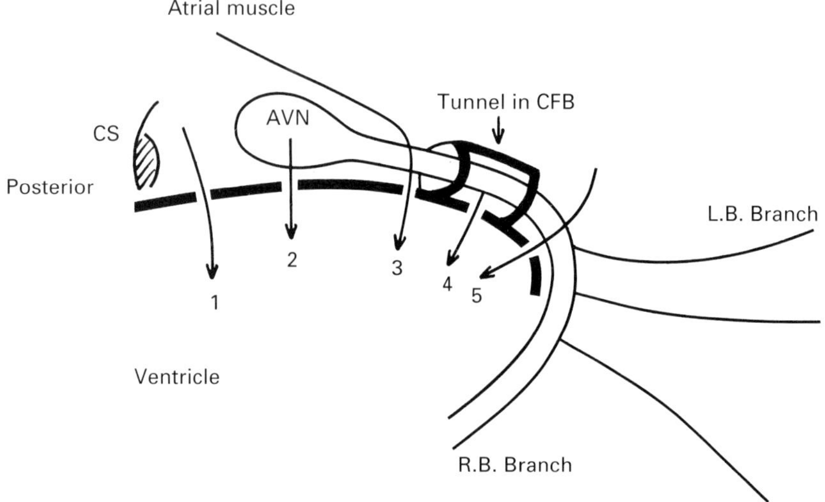

Fig. 10.16 Septal anomalous conduction. 1. Posteroseptal. 2. Nodo-ventricular (Mahaim). 3. Atrial overlay–ventricular (James). 4. AV bundle–ventricle (Mahaim). 5. Antero-septal. All these types of anomalous conduction join atria to ventricles outside the normal conduction system. All can be activated in both directions. 1, 3 and 5 shorten the PR interval by bypassing the delay at the AV node, 2 and 4 shorten it by lesser degrees merely bypassing the distal conduction system. CS = coronary sinus, AVN = atrioventricular node, CFB = central fibrous body

tions that exist in all developing mammalian hearts. There is a significant familial trend, with an autosomal dominant inheritance for persistence of these pathways.[14] Multiple accessory pathways have been reported[15] in up to 13% of patients with pre-excitation and are more common in the right parietal and postero-septal position.

Virtually all the anomalous pathways described either have a higher content of connective tissue than ordinary working myocardium or run within tunnels in collagenous tissue (Fig. 10.17). In general, fibrosis increases with age and if the same applies to conduction paths their electrophysiological properties may alter or they may cease to function. Fibrous proliferation is particularly striking around the central fibrous body and the concept that active remodelling of the margins of the node may contribute to sudden death or arrhythmias in infants has been put forward.[16] The prevalence of nodoventricular and fasciculoventricular Mahaim pathways does fall with age, being lower in adult than in infant hearts. Small strands of nerve tissue often accompany anomalous pathways and might be responsible for alterations in electrophysiological behaviour.

Conditions associated with pre-excitation

Patients with anomalous conduction paths are not immune to other diseases and cases of ischaemic heart disease or cardiomyopathy with pre-excitation probably reflect no more than coincidence. The myocardium of patients with uncomplicated preexcitation is not morphologically abnormal. A pre-excitation pattern is found in a high proportion of patients with Ebstein's anomaly,[17] and the anomalous connections are usually septal and/or right parietal. Two factors militate for the presence of anomalous pathways: the downward displacement of the septal cusp, increasing the chance of the atrial overlay fibres connecting with the septum, and connections via the dysplastic valve cusps often extensively covered by a layer of atrial muscle. In one case, the anomalous pathway originated in persistent nodal tissue in the anterior tricuspid ring.[5] Multiple pathways are common in Ebstein's anomaly.[15]

Hypertrophic cardiomyopathy has been shown to have an undue association with pre-excitation and in some families a single gene locus on chromosome 7 is responsible.[18] The pathways

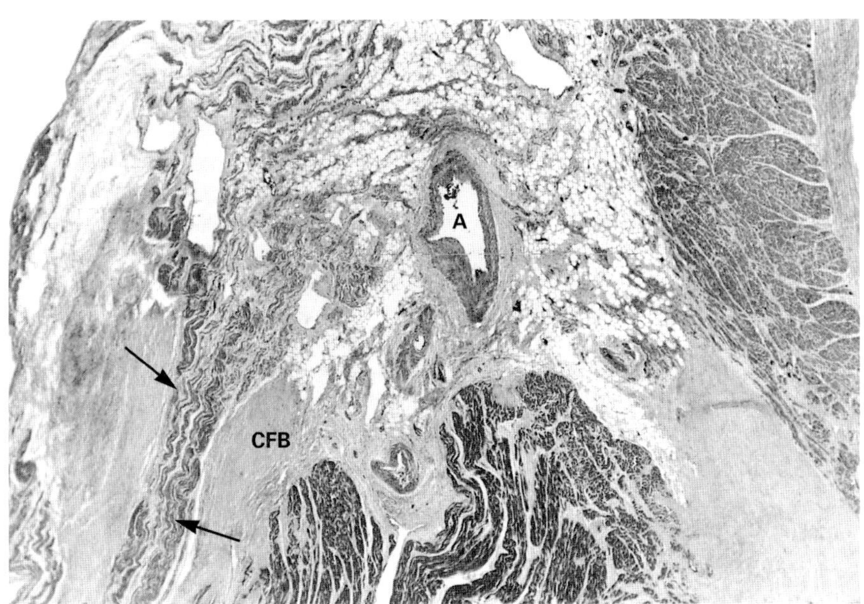

Fig. 10.17 Septal anomalous conduction. The central fibrous body (CFB) posterior to the node itself is penetrated by a discrete muscle bundle (arrows) joining atrial and ventricular myocardium. The nodal artery (A) is embedded in a pad of adipose tissue at this point. Haematoxylin–eosin × 18

present have been both parietal and septal, and usually they are inserted into areas of abnormally arranged ventricular muscle. It is not known whether there is a chance association with anomalous pathways or whether the abnormal growth of the ventricular myocardium actually establishes atrioventricular connections through areas where deficits in the fibrous body or annuli existed. Other abnormal myocyte configurations such as the rhabdomyomatous transformation of tuberous sclerosis[19] and infantile histiocytoid cardiomyopathy[20,21] are also associated with pre-excitation in infancy. In infantile histiocytoid cardiomyopathy, nodules of lipid-containing clear vacuolated cells develop within both the atrial and the ventricular myocardium. The condition has been given many names, reflecting a belief that either these cells are of histiocytic origin or that they represent transformed myocytes. The latter belief is more in accord with the consistent association of the condition with pre-excitation[20] and atrial and ventricular tachycardia.[21] The current view is that these nodules are myocardial hamartomas which possibly have Purkinje cell elements. The mortality of the condition is very high, but excision of nodules producing symptoms has now been reported.[21]

Pre-excitation has also been linked to mitral valve prolapse. There is no inherent reason why myxomatous changes in the floppy mitral cusp should invoke anomalous conduction because the paths are alongside the annulus rather than passing through it. An alternative view[22] is that the anomalous pathway itself causes asynchronous contraction of the posterior wall of the left ventricle, leading to prolapse of a cusp that is anatomically normal.

There is also a rare association of posterior left parietal paths with aneurysmal dilatation of the coronary sinus (Fig. 10.18), regarded as abnormal persistence of a cuff of atrial muscle associated with the sinus venosus.[23]

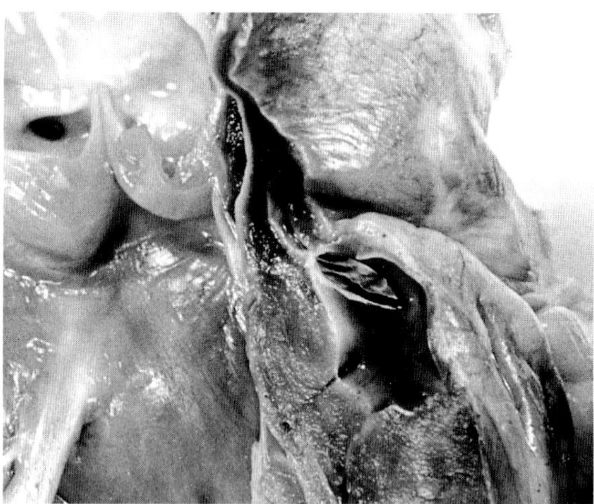

Fig. 10.18 Venous malformation with pre-excitation. The coronary venous sinus viewed in a cross section of the wall of the left ventricle is widely dilated and opens into the right atrium by a small orifice. Along with Ebstein's anomaly this is one of the few causes of pre-excitation which can be recognised macroscopically.

Intranodal re-entry tachycardia

Atrioventricular nodal re-entrant tachycardias are common and arise from dual conduction pathways within or close to the atrioventricular nodal area itself. Electrophysiological studies have shown a slowly conducting anterograde and a rapidly conducting retrograde limb within the node, beginning and ending in nodal tissue.[24] Surgical dissection around the nodal area has been described as highly successful in abolishing atrioventricular nodal re-entry tachycardia, a result that indicates that one limb of the circuit is paranodal. Such conflicting views presuppose that the limits of the atrioventricular node are being defined in an identical manner. The node contains a deep central portion, easily recognisable by its interweaving small myocytes, but the superficial node is made up of successive layers of myocytes which become progressively more like those of atrial muscle. The complexity of these layers makes histological demonstration of two conduction pathways and the limits of the node difficult. Arguments, however, are likely to continue over whether the intranodal tachycardias use atrial muscle immediately adjacent to the node as one pathway. In one autopsy study in which intranodal tachycardia had been demonstrated prior to death, no atrial connections to the node were found, suggesting a pure intranodal origin for the re-entry pathway.[25] A further possibility is that dual pathways are associated with the interconnecting islands of nodal tissue interspersed in the central fibrous body. This appearance, often known as fetal dispersion of the node, is found in a proportion of normal adult hearts. In three cases of junctional tachycardia complex malformations of the AV node, including reduplication with a right- and left-sided node have been found.[26] Incessant tachycardia associated with atrioventricular nodal re-entry and a long PR interval have also been postulated to represent accessory atrioventricular nodal tissue close to the normal conduction axis,[27] a role for which nodal tissue in the central fibrous body is an obvious candidate. However, one autopsy study revealed a long and tortuous septal anomalous connection between atrial and ventricular muscle made up of normal atrial myocytes.[28]

Tachycardia associated with nodo- and fasciculoventricular pathways

The nodo- and fasciculoventricular pathways described by Mahaim have been associated with both pre-excitation and tachycardia in clinicopathological studies.[29] However, there is continuing clinical debate over whether these anomalous connections play a part in maintaining tachycardia. Some evidence shows that this group of connections may coexist with intranodal re-entry, which may be the active cause of the tachycardia.[13] It is becoming increasingly clear to morphologists working in this field that nodoventricular and fasciculoventricular connections are very common in otherwise normal hearts taken from subjects not known to have any arrhythmias. If these pathways are important in initiating tachycardias, the question is why do they become functional in only a minority of subjects who possess these paths?

The short PR interval/normal QRS complex

The Lown–Ganong–Levine syndrome, with its short PR interval and normal QRS complex, is as yet not firmly based on an anatomical substrate. Paths that join the atria either to the distal atrioventricular node or to the penetrating atrioventricular bundle itself are reported but lack electrophysiological data which would exclude the presence of fast intranodal pathways.[30] Another postulated mechanism is hypoplasia of the node itself.

Ventricular arrhythmias

Chronic ischaemic heart disease

The margins of the fibrous scars that result from myocardial infarction are never sharply defined and, at the lateral borders, clumps and strands of surviving myocardium are embedded in collagen. In the great majority of infarcts, a thin layer of myocardium survives just beneath the endocardium, forming ribbon-like anastomosing strands of muscle (Fig. 10.19). This sheet of muscle, up to 1 mm and 10 cells in thickness,[31] owes its survival to diffusion of oxygen across the endocardium from the cavity of the left ventricle and contains inevitably a number of conduction myocytes (Purkinje cells). This muscle sheet joins with more normal myocardium at the lateral margins of the infarct. Total transmural infarction is rare and a thin sheet of subpericardial surviving muscle is also common in ischaemic scars. Therefore, a potential substrate for a re-entry circuit, either around the complete circumference of the infarct or confined to the subendocardial zone, exists in many ischaemic scars.[31]

Only a minority of patients who have ischaemic scars, however, are troubled by ventricular arrhythmias; the results of autopsy studies and examination of the material resected during successful eradication of tachycardia have shown the importance of several additional factors. Clinical studies in which the origin of the tachycardia is mapped show that, over the ischaemic scar, potentials are fractionated and early endocardial activation relative to the epicardium occurs.[32] The area of endocardium over which a re-entry circuit can be located is recorded as anything from small (2–3 cm^2) to very large (10–12 cm^2) in size. Resection, particularly of the margins of an aneurysmal scar, is often successful in abolishing tachycardia. Histological examination of resected material from successful ablations shows the endocardium to be thickened by elastic tissue and collagen, beneath which there is a

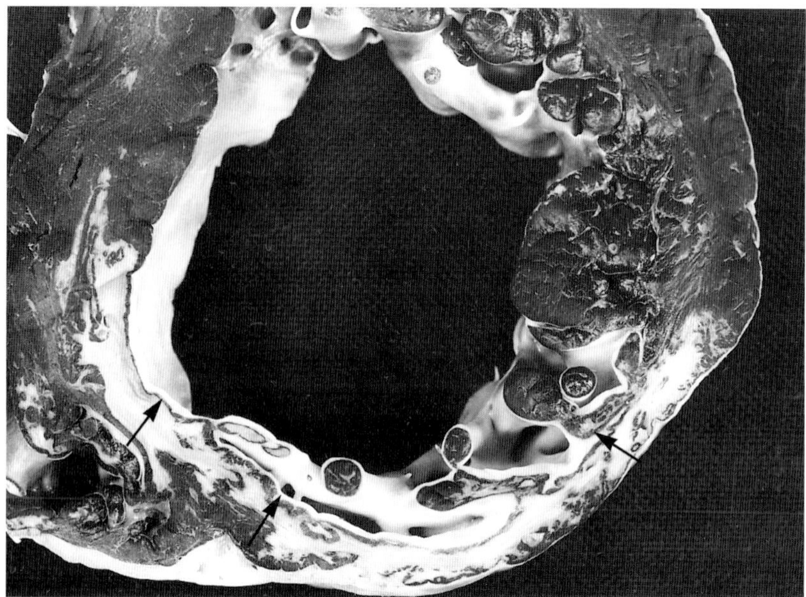

Fig. 10.19 Ischaemic scar related ventricular tachycardia. This postero-septal healed infarct was associated with fatal ventricular tachycardia. Embedded in the dense white fibrous scar tissue there is a subendocardial ribbon of surviving myocytes (arrows). There are also clumps and strands of residual myocardium in the subepicardial area and throughout the scar. There is marked endocardial thickening in the region of the scar.

layer of collagenous tissue in which there are embedded strands of myocardial muscle cells comprising 10–50% of the tissue.[33] Ultrastructural studies[34] show that the myocytes comprise both contractile and conduction (Purkinje) cells. The contractile myocytes show marked myocytolysis, i.e. a loss of myofibrillary content thought to represent a chronic hypoxic state (Fig. 10.20), whereas the Purkinje cells are normal in structure. Following a successful subendocardial resection, the endocardium once again undergoes fibro-elastic thickening but the arrhythmia does not recur in the absence of surviving subendocardial myocytes. It is not possible in morphological studies to establish the mechanism by which the tachycardia is initiated but such studies do indicate the importance of a particular geometric configuration, with anastomosing ribbons of sub-endocardial myocytes embedded in collagen. An important additional factor is chronic hypoxia, perhaps related to increasing endocardial fibro-elastosis.

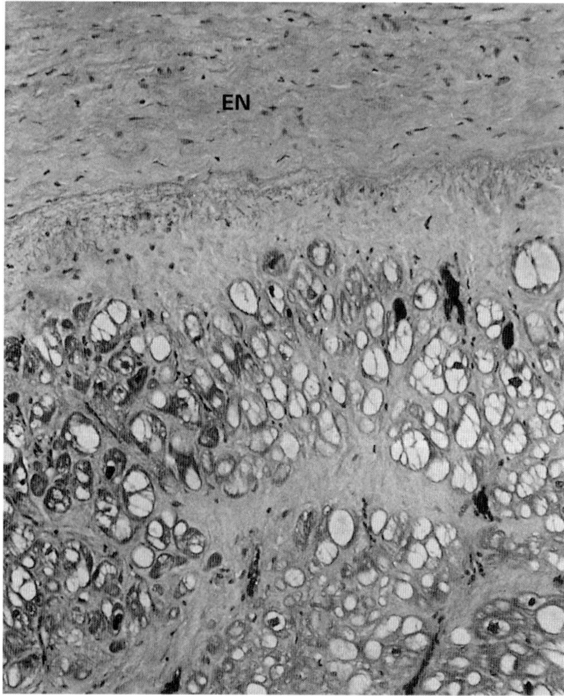

Fig. 10.20 Scar-related ventricular tachycardia. Beneath the thickened endocardium (EN) there is a zone of myocytes which show extreme vacuolation due to the loss of myofibrils. Resected scar to control ventricular tachycardia. Haematoxylin–eosin × 110

Non-ischaemic arrhythmogenic ventricular disease

The concept of fibrosis breaking the mass of myocardial cells into smaller interconnecting units, thereby providing a basis for re-entry, is also relevant to non-ischaemic disease. Hypertrophic cardiomyopathy is associated with a high incidence of ventricular tachycardia and the configuration of whorls of myocytes arranged around foci of connective tissue seems an ideal substrate for re-entry. The end-stage of a dilated cardiomyopathy is also associated with considerable interstitial fibrosis and tachycardias and sudden death are common. Ventricular arrhythmias are also strongly associated with myocardial sarcoidosis in both the acute phase, when granulomas are present, and the burnt-out phase, when granulomas are absent. The scars resulting from healed sarcoidosis are irregular in outline and often become aneurysmal, suggesting that similar mechanisms to those in ischaemic scars will operate.

Any ventricle in which there is severe hypertrophy will undergo a marked increase in interstitial fibrosis and focal myocyte damage, thereby providing a substrate for arrhythmias and, as would be anticipated, the incidence rises as ventricular function fails. This is particularly likely to occur in the infundibular portion and leads to both outflow obstruction and arrhythmias or sudden death in, for example, Fallot's tetralogy.[35]

Ventricular arrhythmias arising in the right ventricle

Gross right ventricular hypertrophy is associated with considerable interstitial fibrosis which occurs in a coarser pattern than is found in left ventricular hypertrophy. The formation of trabeculae of muscle divided by broad bands of connective tissue is particularly characteristic of the outflow tract in Fallot's tetralogy and may explain the occurrence of arrhythmias even after surgical correction.[35]

There is a spectrum of morphological changes in non-hypertrophied right ventricles associated with recurrent ventricular tachycardias which arise on the right side. These changes range from, at one extreme, an apparently normal right ventricle through right ventricular dysplasia and isolated right ventricular cardiomyopathy to, at the other extreme, Uhl's anomaly. The morphological features to which these names have been applied merge and overlap to such an extent that it is not certain whether they do represent different conditions.[36]

In Uhl's anomaly, the whole of the right ventricle is paper-thin and dilated. Histology shows virtually no myocardial muscle with close apposition of the endocardium and epicardium and islands of fibrous tissue mixed with adipose tissue. In right ventricular dysplasia[37] a segment of the right ventricular wall is thinned and replaced by adipose and fibrous tissue intermingled with myocytes (Chapter 5). The area involved is often the anterior free wall related to the outflow tract but it may also be lateral or posterior. In what is described as right ventricular isolated cardiomyopathy, the histological changes are similar but more diffuse in distribution.[38,39] Adipose tissue is normally present in the right ventricular free wall and therefore its presence in an abnormal ventricle cannot be regarded as specific for right ventricular dysplasia. A set of clinical and pathological criteria have now been established[40] to try and unify the diagnosis of what is now known as arrhythmogenic right ventricular dysplasia. Concomitant milder left ventricular involvement is common.[41]

Patients with right ventricular tachycardia but without clinical evidence of any contractile abnormality are often regarded as idiopathic or 'innocent'. A high incidence of morphological abnormalities detected by right ventricular biopsy is reported.[42] A small proportion of patients do have an occult myocarditis; the majority of the remainder show a mild increase in the amount of interstitial fibrosis but overall one-third of patients have a normal biopsy.

Atrioventricular conduction defects

One aspect of histopathological studies of the conduction system is confirmation of the anatomical site at which atrioventricular block has occurred. In this respect, excellent correlation with electrophysiological studies can be found, and confirms that the site of chronic atrioventricular block is usually distal to the atrioventricular node.

A second aspect lies in determining the nature of the destructive process. In this respect, distinction must be made between patients in whom atrioventricular block is the sole manifestation and patients who have any of the many known systemic or cardiac diseases that can be complicated by atrioventricular block. The relative proportions of the causes of chronic atrioventricular block in any clinical series will be influenced by the selection of patients from the two groups.

In large series of patients referred for long-term pacing who do not have other overt systemic disease, the commonest cause of chronic atrioventricular block is the entity known as idiopathic bilateral bundle branch fibrosis. Although this term is clumsy, it is an accurate description of a process in which conduction fibres vanish from the bifurcating atrioventricular bundle and proximal bundle branches. The disease was known to the pathologists who made the first morphological studies of atrioventricular block in the late 19th century but two somewhat different forms of the disease have been stressed subsequently by Lev[43] and Lenègre.[44] Both authors emphasise that the disease is most common in subjects over 65 years of age and is the culmination of a process which may evolve over 10 years or more. Lev stresses a form of the disease in which the initial loss of conduction tissue takes place in the proximal left bundle branch. The left bundle branch has numerous fine fascicles arising independently from the bifurcating bundle; each runs between the endocardium of the ventricular outflow and the connective tissue of the upper ventricular septum. Lev postulates that the fascicles are compressed between the two masses of collagen each time the ventricle contracts. The conduction fibres ultimately vanish, leaving open spaces which still outline the original site of the bundle branch in the connective tissue (Fig. 10.21). The process is ubiquitous in old age and appears to be accelerated by hypertension; it is only in extreme cases that the loss of conduction tissue extends into the bifurcating bundle and atrioventricular block develops, usually after a long period of left bundle branch block. Lev envisages the process as a combination of age and 'wear and tear'. In many cases, there is some associated fibrosis and microscopic foci of calcification in the upper interventricular septum. In a proportion of cases there is also hyaline thickening of the small arteries within the penetrating atrioventricular bundle. There is no evidence to suggest that

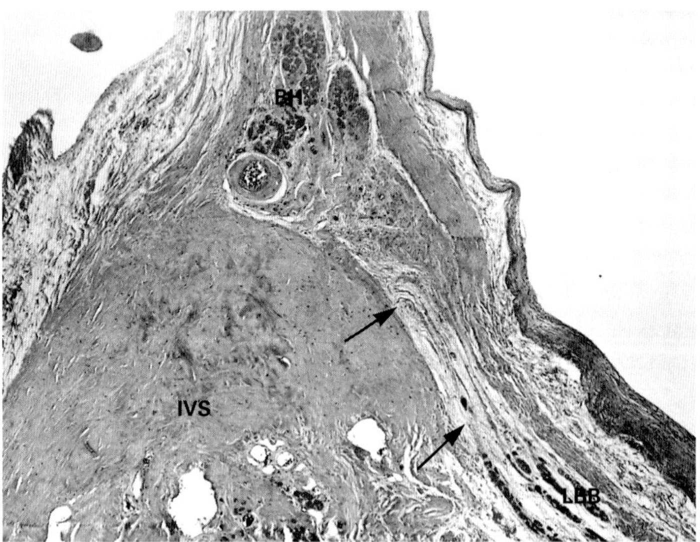

Fig. 10.21 Idiopathic bundle branch fibrosis. In this Lev form of the disease there is discontinuity (arrows) between the left bundle branch (LBB) and the bifurcating bundle of His (BH). At the site of conduction tissue loss there are open spaces in the tissue. There is also extensive replacement of conduction tissue in the bifurcating bundle by fibrosis. The upper septum (IVS) is also fibrotic. The wall of a small artery in the bundle is thickened. Haematoxylin–eosin × 18

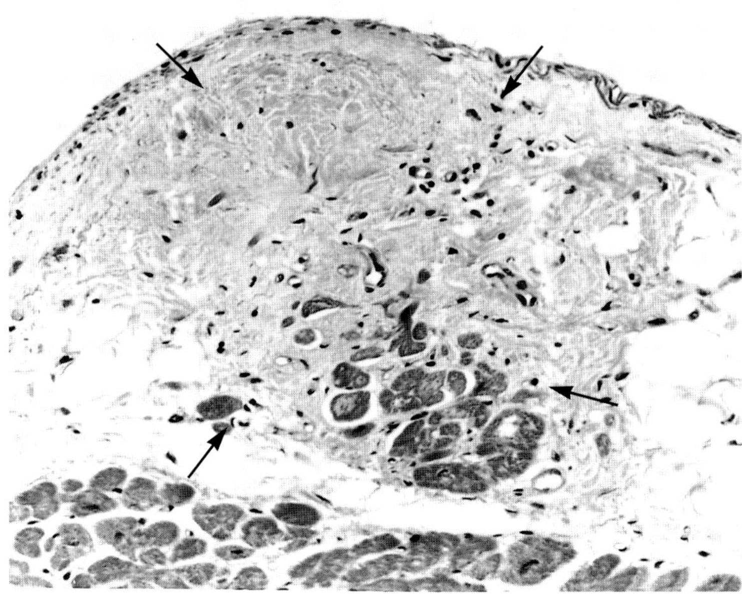

Fig. 10.22 Idiopathic bundle branch fibrosis. In this Lenègre form of the disease the right bundle branch (arrows) is seen in its subendocardial portion at mid-septal level. The branch (arrows) is cut transversely and the number of myocytes is approximately one third of normal. In areas where conduction cells have vanished there is fibrous replacement of the tissue. Haematoxylin–eosin × 45

atheroma of epicardial coronary arteries is implicated directly in Lev's disease.

Lenègre described cases of idiopathic bundle branch fibrosis in which either diffuse or focal segments of both the right (Fig. 10.22) and left bundle branches (Fig. 10.23) showed a progressive loss of conduction fibres with replacement fibrosis, but the spaces so characteristic of Lev's disease were absent. In these areas of fibrosis, occasional degenerate conduction cells survive, associated with small foci of chronic inflammatory cells, but in general there is no evidence of an acute myocarditis. The myocardium immediately adjacent to the bundle branches is normal. Loss of conduction fibres also extends into the more distal portions of the right and left branches. In extreme cases, conduction fibres are lost throughout the Purkinje network of the left ventricle.

Speculation with regard to the aetiology of Lenègre's disease includes previous acute myocarditis and a 'myopathic' process selective for conduction fibres. The latter is supported by the similarity of the morphological changes to those

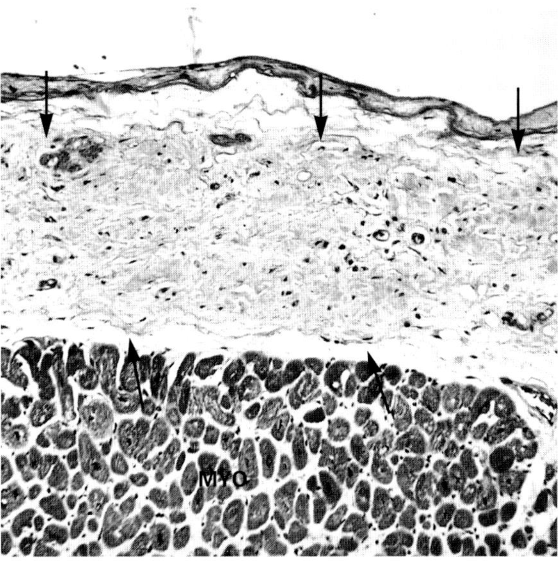

Fig. 10.23 Idiopathic bundle branch fibrosis. The left bundle branch is cut transversely at mid septal level. In the subendocardial zone fibrous tissue (arrows) replaces the broad band of conduction cells (cf Fig. 10.10). The adjacent contractile myocardium (MYO) is normal.

found in the conduction system in patients with some familial conduction disturbances or dilated cardiomyopathies, the association of Lenègre's disease with an increase in left ventricular mass with mild diffuse interstitial fibrosis and the occasional occurrence of the disease in relatively young individuals. Although autoantibodies specific for Purkinje cells have been demonstrated, immune-based destruction of the conduction system has not been established as a contributory factor in bundle branch fibrosis.

Within the spectrum of idiopathic bundle branch fibrosis overall, more cases conform to the Lev than the Lenègre type, but many cases have features of both diseases. It is therefore impossible to determine from a morphological study of autopsy cases whether idiopathic bundle branch fibrosis represents the end-stage of one, two or several disease processes.

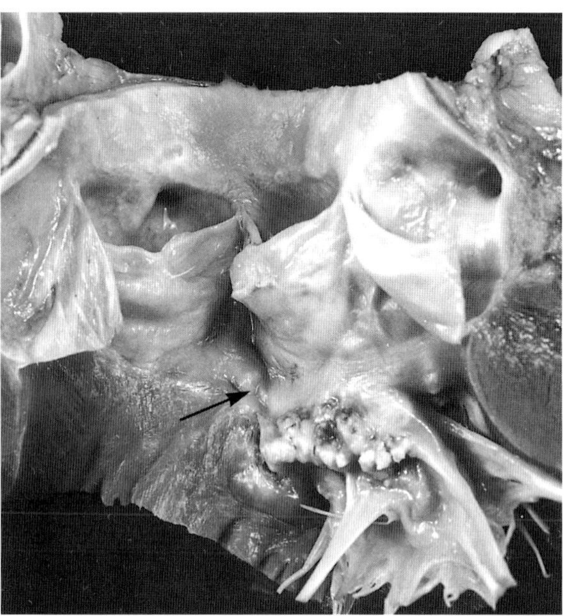

Fig. 10.24 Calcific AV block. Mitral ring calcification has extended into the base of the membranous septum (arrow) and caused permanent AV block.

Ischaemic heart disease and chronic atrioventricular block

Coronary atheroma is responsible for chronic atrioventricular block when acute infarction destroys totally a segment of the conduction system and the patient survives. The most common pattern encountered is destruction of both bundle branches within one or more episodes of septal infarction due to occlusion of the left anterior descending artery. An occlusion of the right coronary artery that has extended into the nodal artery itself with subsequent destruction of the node is more rare. In one study of 13 patients with ischaemic chronic atrioventricular block, 10 were found to have intrahisian block with left anterior descending disease and three to have nodal block with right coronary artery disease.[45]

Calcific atrioventricular block

The term calcific atrioventricular block is usually applied to transection of the conduction system by a mass of calcium large enough to be visible on X-ray or echocardiography in life and by naked eye examination at autopsy.[46,47] The penetrating atrioventricular bundle is anatomically very close to the medial aspect of the mitral valve ring, to the membranous interventricular septum and to the aortic valve. Nodular calcification at

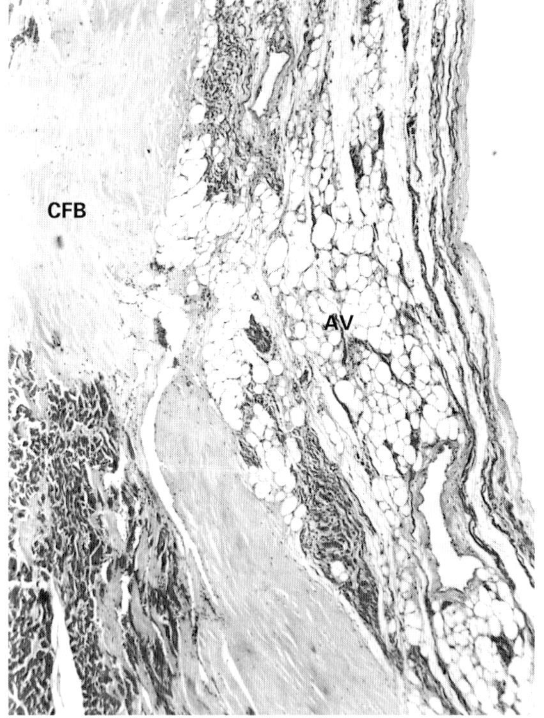

Fig. 10.25 Conduction system in dystrophia myotonica. The AV nodal area (AV) shows extensive loss of conduction tissue with replacement by adipose tissue (CFB — central fibrous body).
Haematoxylin–eosin × 18

any of these sites, due to any cause, may extend outward sufficiently to disrupt the conduction system (Fig. 10.24). Extension of calcium from the valve into the upper septum may complicate any form of aortic stenosis, whether in a tricuspid or bicuspid valve. The clinical association of atrioventricular block with massive mitral ring calcification in old age is often known as Rytand's syndrome. Accelerated soft-tissue calcification in Paget's disease of bone or renal failure may lead to similar mitral ring calcification and atrioventricular block.

Cardiomyopathy and atrioventricular block

Patients with idiopathic dilated cardiomyopathy have diffuse loss of conduction fibres with replacement fibrosis, particularly in the distal bundle branches, which is manifest clinically as a high incidence of left bundle branch block. Complete atrioventricular block is rare because of the short clinical course. In comparison, subjects with familial cardiomyopathies have a tenfold incidence of atrioventricular block and those with inherited neuromyopathies have an even higher incidence of cardiac involvement characterised by conduction rather than contraction abnormalities. Conduction abnormalities may precede the manifestation of skeletal muscle disease. In dystrophia myotonica, conduction fibres are replaced by fat rather than fibrous tissue (Fig. 10.25); the results of electrophysiological studies suggest that the loss is at all levels in the conduction system. Detailed pathological studies of isolated examples of any of the rarer forms of neuromyopathies indicate a non-specific loss of conduction tissue at all levels.[48] The results of clinical studies of patients with progressive external ophthalmoplegia (Kearns–Saye syndrome) suggest that the Purkinje cells of the more distal bundle branches are involved selectively.[49] In Duchenne and Becker's muscular dystrophy dystrophin is abnormal in conduction tissue and in part the loss of specialised conduction myocytes is by mechanisms identical to those in skeletal muscle. The conduction tissue contains a splice form of dystrophin more usually associated with brain tissue and its absence from the cell membrane may lead to electrophysiological dysfunction rather than cell death.[50]

Familial conduction defects are a heterogeneous group.[51] The simplest form is absence of a segment of a bundle branch, usually the right, not associated with progression of the conduction defect. Another form is a slowly progressive loss of conduction fibres throughout both bundle branches and both nodes, culminating in complete atrioventricular block later in life. One family with this form of the disease has been described in whom there is a genetic defect in connexin 40 which is present in large amounts in conduction tissue. Connexins are concerned with the gap junctions, which control cell to cell

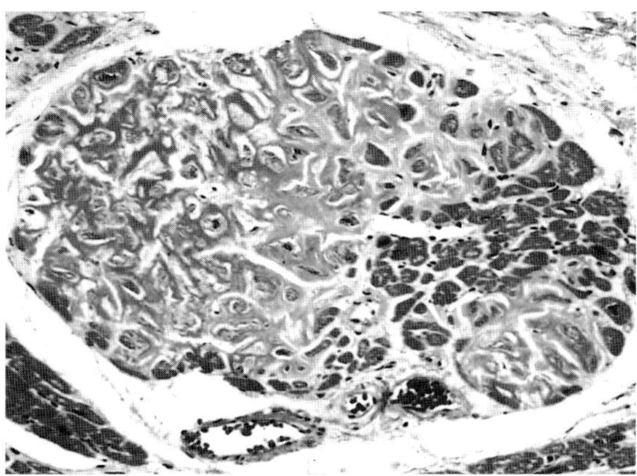

Fig. 10.26 Amyloid in conduction system. Within the right bundle branch there is a lattice of amyloid and considerable loss of conduction tissue.
Haematoxylin–eosin × 38

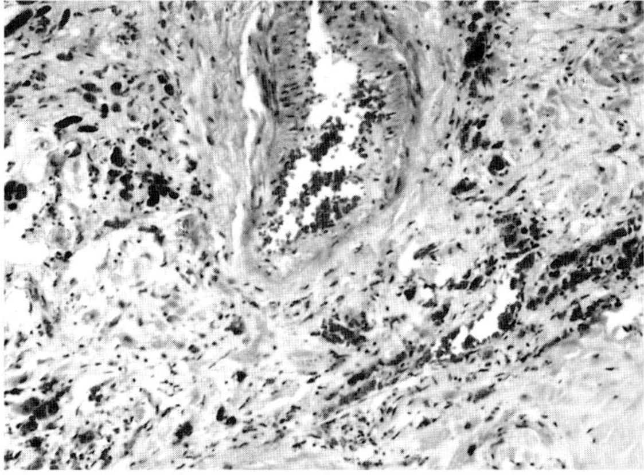

Fig. 10.27 AV node in haemachromatosis. The node can be recognised by the central artery. There is virtual total loss of nodal myocytes and heavy deposition of iron pigment in the interstitial tissues.
Haematoxylin–eosin × 38

contact and thus the electrical impulse spread. In affected families, sudden death seems to be more common than would be anticipated from the severity of the conduction defect.

Amyloid heart disease is strongly associated with sinoatrial disease and atrial fibrillation, reflecting the high degree of atrial involvement. Amyloid is, however, also deposited in the distal conduction system, causing bundle branch block which may proceed to complete AV block (Fig. 10.26). In haemochromatosis iron deposition in the AV node is a feature of the late stage and may cause AV block (Fig. 10.27).

Congenital complete atrioventricular block

Congenital heart block which is not associated with other complex congenital cardiac malformations has been shown to have two morphological varieties.[52] In the most common form, the inferior limbus of the atrial septum inferior to the foramen ovale is deficient in atrial myocytes and is formed predominantly of adipose tissue. Buried within the central fibrous body is tissue representing the deep portion of the atrioventricular node but, in the absence of an atrial nodal component, no connection is established between atrial muscle in the upper septum and the atrioventricular conduction axis. The more distal penetrating and bifurcating atrioventricular bundles are normal. This form of atrioventricular block has been specifically linked with maternal connective tissue disorders, predominantly systemic lupus erythematosus but also rheumatoid arthritis and dermatomyositis.[53] The mothers are characterised by possession of anti-RO and anti-La antibodies to soluble tissue ribonucleoprotein antigens. These antibodies cross the placenta and will bind fetal cardiac tissue, but specificity for conduction tissue has not been well established. Maternal lupus is thus an example of passively acquired autoimmune injury, but it is uncertain why the antigen is expressed only in the fetus and not in the adult heart of the mother herself. Systemic lupus in the adult produces a very different cardiac involvement with valvulitis and vasculitis. Conduction defects are rare. Subclinical maternal lupus is one cause of several siblings having congenital atrioventricular block and may be confused with a genetic familial conduction tissue defect.

The second form of congenital heart block has a well formed node with a deep and a superficial portion but no continuity is made with the ventricular conduction axis (nodoventricular dissociation). This rarer form of congenital block is not related to maternal connective tissue disorder. It may be related to some of the familial bundle branch defects. The rare primary 'tumour' of the atrioventricular node (mesothelioma) (Chapter 11) is due to growth of rests of pericardial tissue persisting within the node and reflecting its original histogenesis on the posterior interventricular sulcus.

THE CONDUCTION SYSTEM IN CONNECTIVE TISSUE DISEASES

An inflammatory aortitis is found in association with the HLA-B27-related diseases, including ankylosing spondylitis and Reiter's syndrome.[54] The distortion of the aortic root leads to aortic regurgitation while extension of the inflammatory process outside the aorta may involve the immediately adjacent atrioventricular node. Conduction disturbances and aortic regurgitation are therefore closely linked. Heart block is predominantly suprahisian in HLA-B27-related disease. A different mechanism is responsible for complete atrioventricular block in rheumatoid arthritis, where a granuloma in the upper septum or mitral/aortic rings transects the conduction system, usually at the level of the bifurcating atrioventricular bundle. In systemic sclerosis, connective tissue within the atrioventricular node proliferates and, in association with small vessel obliteration, leads to nodal destruction.[55,56] Bundle branch destruction also occurs in association with the widespread myocardial scarring. A virtually identical histological picture can be produced by irradiation to the heart.[57] In adult systemic lupus, focal necrosis and fibrosis associated with an arteritis in the node have been described.[58] About 70% of cases of dermatomyositis have evidence of cardiac involvement with conduction defects being common and one of the leading causes of death.[59] The cardiac damage which principally affects the bundle branches has been linked to antibodies to ribonucleoproteins, although it is not known why there are similar antibodies in systemic lupus erythematosus that affect only the fetus and not the mother.

MYOCARDITIS AND ATRIOVENTRICULAR BLOCK

All forms of myocarditis may involve the conduction system, the bundle branches being particularly vulnerable. Mild cases are usually detected by electrocardiography in patients with systemic viral infections. Complete atrioventricular block identifies the rare examples of more severe involvement, but even so ultimate reversion to sinus rhythm is usual. In one series of 10 patients with myocarditis and complete atrioventricular block, only two had permanent conduction defects.[60] Histological confirmation of an inflammatory infiltrate in the conduction system exists largely in case-reports. Most cases of atrioventricular block in the acute phase of diphtheria are due to the direct effect of the exotoxin on conduction myocytes, causing cell death. Long-term conduction defects are an appreciable risk. Chagas disease (South American trypanosomiasis) carries a high risk of bundle branch block and atrioventricular block in the initial acute myocarditic phase, and in the later chronic stage. In the latter, bundle branch destruction occurs as part of a generalised myocardial scarring; arrhythmias may be enhanced by the neuronal damage that occurs within the heart in Chagas disease. Worldwide, Chagas disease may be the commonest cause of chronic atrioventricular block. Septal gummata in syphilis used to be a classic cause of complete atrioventricular block and they are still reported sporadically, as are tuberculomas destroying the conduction system.[61] Myocarditis due to Lyme borreliosis has a particular predilection for the conduction system and permanent AV block may occur.[62] Sarcoidosis, when involving the heart, may produce a large granulomatous mass most frequently occurring in the upper interventricular septum and the atrial muscle in the vicinity of the aortic root. Destruction of the conduction system leads to sudden death and atrioventricular block.[63] Sudden death may reflect either conduction defects or the high frequency of ventricular arrhythmias with myocardial scarring and aneurysm formation. Involvement of the sinus node by giant cell granulomas in sarcoid is also recorded.[64]

BUNDLE BRANCH BLOCK

Many myocardial diseases are associated with bundle branch block; conversely, mass electrocardiographic surveys have revealed that many apparently healthy individuals have bundle branch block. The prognosis of bundle branch block reflects that of the underlying myocardial disease and is therefore very variable.

Left bundle branch block

Common to all descriptions of the anatomy of the left bundle branch is that a series of slender fascicles arise from a considerable length of the bifurcating atrioventricular bundle as it lies at the crest of the muscular interventricular septum. Some individuals possess anterior and posterior streams of fascicles of equal size, some have a preponderance of one and others have an additional middle stream in the upper third of the septum. In all individuals, however, by the time the fascicles reach the lower third of the septum there is a contiguous sheet of conduction tissue in the subendocardium. There is general agreement that complete left bundle branch block is associated with severe loss of conduction tissue. This may be proximal and focal, as in old age, hypertension, aortic valve disease and some patients with ischaemic heart disease, or diffuse and distal, as in the myopathies and severe ischaemic damage. The electrocardiographic patterns described as indicating partial bundle branch block, hemiblock or left-axis deviation are now agreed to be due to lesser degrees of fascicular loss than that of complete bundle branch block.[65] Left anterior hemiblock has not been found to be specifically associated with damage confined to the anterior portion of the bundle branch but to more diffuse loss.[66] In contrast, left posterior hemiblock, particularly in association with inferior infarction, is associated with damage concentrated on the posterior division of the left branch.[67] The age-related sclerosis of the upper interventricular septum described by Lev is potentiated by any disease causing left ventricular hypertrophy[68] and is the non-specific factor unifying many causes of left bundle branch block.

Right bundle branch block

The right bundle branch is the continuation of the penetrating atrioventricular bundle and runs as a single discrete bundle beneath the endocardium of the ventricular septum to reach the base of the anterior papillary muscle; from here it runs in the moderator band to form a rich anastomosing network of conduction fibres throughout the right ventricle.

The discrete nature and subepicardial position of the bundle branch at the rim of the right ventricular outflow make it liable to mechanical trauma from catheters (a situation that has no analogue on the left side of the heart). The main stem of the right branch is very variable in size and in the number of myocytes it contains as viewed in cross-section. Focal hypoplasia is one cause of congenital right bundle branch block. The discrete nature of the right bundle branch also means that destruction with an area of infarction, particularly anteroseptal in distribution, is common. Severe right ventricular hypertrophy is associated with diffuse subendocardial fibrosis within the outflow tract, a process that may also involve the right bundle branch.[69]

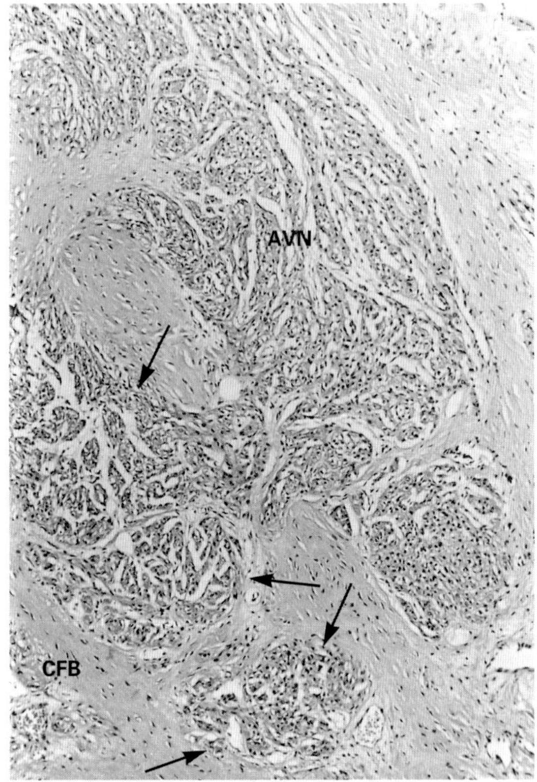

Fig. 10.28 Infant AV node. The main body of the node (AVN) is shown just prior to its forming the penetrating bundle. Within the central fibrous body (CFB) are islands of nodal tissue (arrows) which join with the main node. With age these separate portions vanish to leave the nodal structure seen in adults. This process of 'remodelling' is a normal phenomenon but is regarded by some authorities as being accompanied by electrical instability. Haematoxylin–eosin × 105

STRUCTURAL ABNORMALITIES OF THE CONDUCTION SYSTEM IN SUDDEN UNEXPLAINED DEATH

Numerous case-reports suggest that an examination of the conduction system for structural abnormalities may elucidate the cause of sudden unexplained death, particularly in young subjects. Abnormalities of the atrioventricular node (Fig. 10.28), nodo-ventricular (Fig. 10.29) and fasciculo-ventricular connections (Fig. 10.30), an intramyocardial course for the right bundle

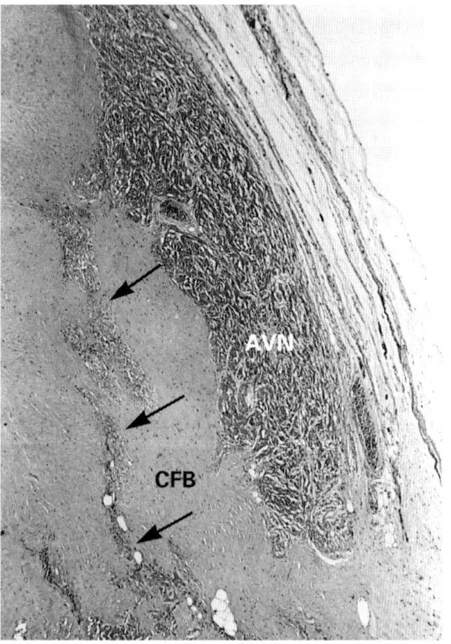

Fig. 10.29 AV nodal loops. The main portion of the node (AVN) is normally applied to the edge of the central fibrous body. A separate mass of nodal tissue (arrows) forms a loop from the node itself in the central fibrous body (CFB) and continues down to the upper interventricular septum. Serial sections showed a portion to also enter the node distally. Haematoxylin–eosin × 6.5

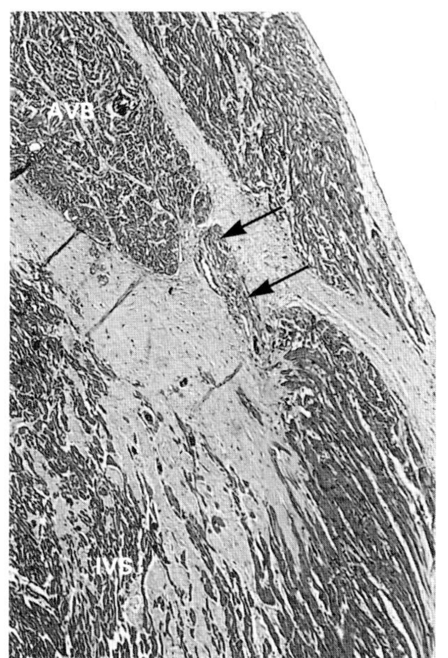

Fig. 10.30 Fasciculo-ventricular connection. A muscle bundle (arrow) joins the AV bundle (AVB) to the upper interventricular septum (IVS), bypassing the bundle branches.
Haematoxylin–eosin × 16

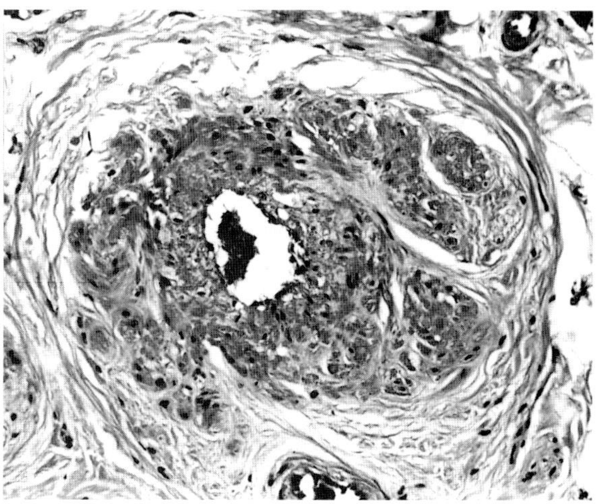

Fig. 10.31 Nodal artery dysplasia. The artery shows bizarre proliferation and disorganisation of the medial smooth muscle, producing a thick-walled vessel.
Haematoxylin–eosin × 95

branch, undue sclerosis or fatty infiltration of the conduction system for the age of the subject, and small vessel disease have all postulated to be causes of sudden death in apparently fit young individuals.[70,71] Sudden death has been documented in patients with pre-excitation who have not had previous episodes of significant tachycardia and no other abnormality at autopsy apart from an anomalous conduction pathway.[72] It is therefore not impossible that sudden death in a young subject who was previously asymptomatic could be due to pre-excitation or a re-entry arrhythmia.

In a study[73] of the conduction system in 18 cases of unexplained sudden death in South East Asian immigrants, it was found that 14 had fetal dispersion of the atrioventricular node and 13 had accessory conduction pathways (72%), of which three were atrio-fascicular, eight nodo-ventricular and five fasciculo-ventricular. In a control group of 124 hearts taken from subjects in whom death was accidental, 35 (28%) were found to have similar perinodal anatomical abnormalities. In another case control study[74] of the AV nodal artery in cases of unexplained sudden death 12 of 27 (44%) were found to have nodal arterial dysplasia (Fig. 10.31) while in the 17 control accidental deaths one case was found (6%). Our own work suggests that when serial sectioning is carried out focal areas of medial disorganisation in control hearts are found in the nodal artery with a high frequency. It seems that anatomical abnormalities of the conduction system or its vasculature are not uncommon in normal hearts, but that such abnormalities may be more common in hearts of subjects who suffer sudden unexpected death. It is, however, very important to bear in mind that the vast majority of reports linking sudden unexplained death to a wide range of isolated, and often minor, morphological abnormalities of the conduction system are case-reports and therefore uncontrolled. They are also highly selected cases and do not represent a consecutive series of sudden unexplained deaths in young individuals.

THE PATHOLOGY OF PACING

Complete heart block is now treated by placing permanent electrodes in the right side of the heart via the superior vena cava. The catheter tip is impacted on to the endocardium of the right

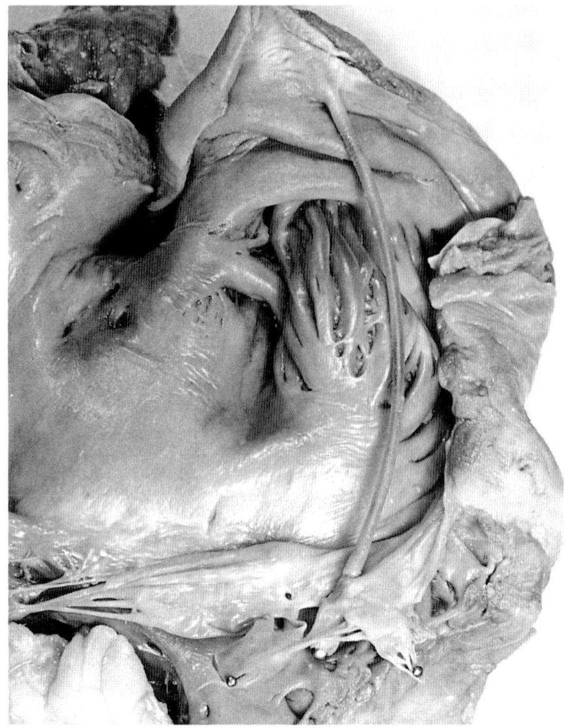

Fig. 10.32 Pacing catheter. A long-term pacing catheter is firmly attached by a fibrous sheath to the atrial wall and the tricuspid valve.

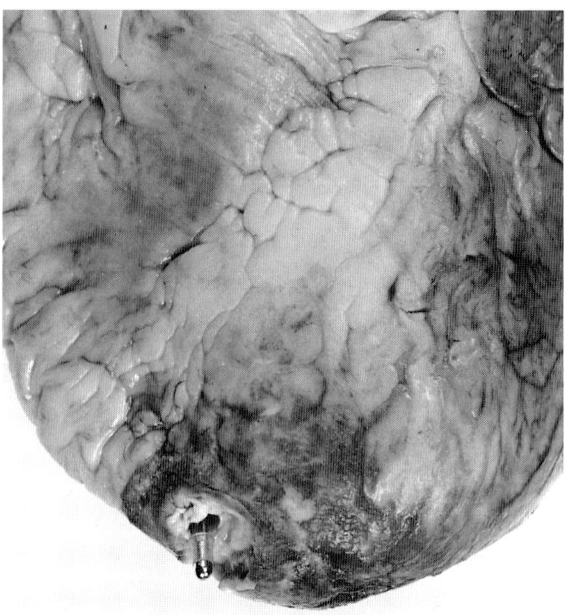

Fig. 10.33 Pacing catheter displacement. The catheter tip has worked through into the pericardium. Failure to pace occurred after a long period of successful stimulation at low threshold.

ventricle and a subcutaneous unit is placed in the axilla. The catheter becomes very firmly adherent to the endocardium through the formation of a sheath of tissue containing smooth muscle cells and ultimately collagen. This probably arises by organisation of thrombus. A similar sheath often attaches the catheter to the tricuspid valve and to the opening of the vena cava into the atrium (Fig. 10.32). Pacing failure after a long period of successful function may be due to a number of conditions. The unit itself may fail. Units are always removed at autopsy and can be returned for testing. Breaks or cracks in the catheter are virtually impossible to detect after death unless they are gross. The removal of a densely-adherent catheter intact is well nigh impossible at autopsy. The catheter tip may have become displaced. At times this may be very obvious when perforation of the myocardium occurs (Fig. 10.33) but is more often due to fibrosis around the tip at its site of impaction. Pacing catheters may also become mobile within a fibrous sheath and this can be tested by gently pulling the catheter to see if there is movement. The detection of these various forms of pacing failure at autopsy is, however, often impossible unless the reason is gross displacement of the catheter.

REFERENCES

1. Bouman LN, Jongsma HJ. Structure and function of the SA node: a review. Eur Heart J 1986; 7: 94–104.
2. Davies MJ. Pathology of atrial arrhythmias. In: Davies MJ, Anderson RH, Becker AE eds. The conduction system of the heart. London: Butterworths, 1983: 203.
3. Vassal-Adams PR. Ultrastructure of the human AV conduction tissue. Eur Heart J 1983; 4: 449–460.
4. James TN. Anatomy of the heart A-V node with remarks pertinent to its electrophysiology. Am Heart J 1961; 62: 756–771.
5. Becker AE. Morphological basis of pre-excitation. In: Davies MJ, Anderson RH, Becker AE eds. The conduction system of the heart. London: Butterworths, 1983: 183.
6. Anderson RH, Davies MJ, Becker AE. Atrioventricular ring specialised tissue in the normal heart. Eur J Cardiol 1974; 2: 19–27.
7. Sealy WC, Gallagher JJ. The surgical approach to the septal area of the heart based on experience with 45 patients with Kent bundles. J Thorac Cardiovasc Surg 1980; 79: 542–551.
8. Thery C, Gosselin B, Lekieffre J, Warembourg H. Pathology of sinoatrial node. Correlations with electrocardiographic findings in 111 patients. Am Heart J 1977; 93: 735–740.
9. Evans R, Shaw DB. Pathological studies in sinoatrial disorder (Sick Sinus Syndrome). Br Heart J 1977; 39: 778–786.
10. Demoulin JC, Kulbertus AE. Pathological correlates of atrial arrhythmias. In: Kulbertus HE ed. Reentrant arrhythmias mechanisms and treatments. Lancaster: MTP, 1977: 99.
11. Sugiura M, Ohkawa A. A clinicopathological study on sick sinus syndrome with histological appearances of the sinoatrial node. Jap Circ J 1980; 44: 497–504.
12. Bharati S, Nordenberg A, Bauerfiend R et al. The anatomic substrate for the sick sinus syndrome in adolescence. Am J Cardiol 1980; 46: 163–172.
13. Ward DE, Camm AJ. Clinical Electrophysiology of the Heart. London: Edward Arnold, 1987: 173
14. Vidaillet HJ, Presley JC, Henke E, Harrel FE, Ferman LD. Familial occurrence of accessory atrioventricular pathway (pre-excitation syndrome) N Engl J Med 1987; 317: 65–69.
15. Colavita PG, Packer DL, Presley JC. et al. Frequency, diagnosis and clinical characteristics of patients with multiple accessory atrioventricular pathways. Am J Cardiol 1987; 59: 601–606.
16. Marino TA, Kane BM. Cardiac atrioventricular junctional tissues in hearts from infants who died suddenly. J Am Coll Cardiol 1985; 5: 1178–1184.
17. Smith WM, Gallagher JJ et al. The electrophysiological basis and management of symptomatic recurrent tachycardia in patients with Ebstein's anomaly of the tricuspid valve. Am J Cardiol 1982; 49: 1223–1234.
18. Hauser AM, Gordon S, Timmis GC. Familial hypertrophic cardiomyopathy and pre-excitation. Am Heart J 1984; 107: 176–178.
19. Jayakar PB, Stanwick RS, Seshia SS. Tuberous sclerosis of Wolff–Parkinson–White syndrome. J Pediatr 1986; 108: 259–260.
20. Gottlieb AV, Chan M, Palmer WH, Huang SN. Ventricular pre-excitation syndrome. Accessory left atrioventricular connection and rhabdomyomatous myocardial fibers. Arch Pathol Lab Med 1977; 101: 486–489.
21. Kearney DL, Titus JL, Hawkins EP, Ott DA, Garson A. Pathologic features of myocardial hamartomas causing childhood tachycardia. Circulation 1987; 75: 705–710.
22. Drake CE, Hodsden JE, Sridharan MR, Flowers NC. Evaluation of the association of mitral valve prolapse in patients with WPW type electrocardiogram and its relation to ventricular activation pattern. Am Heart J 1985; 109: 83–87.
23. Gerlis LM, Davies MJ, Boule R, Williams G, Scott H. Pre-excitation due to accessory sino-ventricular connections associated with coronary sinus aneurysms. A report of two cases. Br Heart J 1985; 53: 314–322.
24. Scheinman MM. Atrioventricular reentry. Lesions learned from radiofrequency modification of the node. Circulation 1992; 85: 1619–1620.
25. Scheinman MM, Gonzalez R, Thomas A, Ullyot D, Bjarati S, Lev M. Reentry confined to the AV node: electrophysiology and anatomic findings. Am J Cardiol 1983; 49: 1814–1818.
26. Bharati S, Moskowitz WB, Scheinman M et al. Junctional tachycardias: anatomic substrate and its significance in ablative procedures. J Am Coll Cardiol 1991; 18: 179–186
27. Ward DE, Camm AJ. Ventriculo-atrial conduction over accessory pathways exhibiting decremental properties. Eur Heart J 1982; 3: 267–275.
28. Critelli G, Gallagher JJ, Monda V, Coltorti F, Scherillo M, Ross L. Anatomic and electrophysiologic substrate of the permanent form of junctional reciprocating tachycardia. J Am Coll Cardiol 1984; 4: 601–610.
29. Gmenier R, Ng CK, Hammer L, Becker AE. Tachycardia caused by an accessory nodo-ventricular tract: a clinico-pathological correlation. Eur Heart J 1984; 5: 233–242.
30. Brechenmacher C. Atrio-His bundle tracts. Br Heart J 1975; 37: 853–859.
31. Bolik DR, Hackel DB, Reimer KA, Ideker RE. Quantitative analysis of myocardial infarct structure in patients with ventricular tachycardia. Circulation 1986; 74: 1266–1279.
32. Cox JL. Anatomic-electrophysiologic basis for the surgical treatment of refractory ischaemic ventricular tachycardia. Ann Surg 1983; 198: 119–129.
33. Fenoglio JJ, Pham TD, Harken AH, Horowitz LN, Josephson ME, Wit AL. Recurrent sustained ventricular tachycardia: structure and ultrastructure of subendocardial regions in which tachycardia originates. Circulation 1983; 68: 518–533.
34. Silver MA. Morphologic substrates of ventricular arrhythmias. Clin Prog Electrophys Pacing 1986; 4: 1
35. Sullivan ID, Presbitero P, Gooch VM, Aruta E, Deanfield JE. Is ventricular arrhythmia in repaired tetralogy of Fallot an effect of the operation or a consequence of the course of the disease? A prospective study. Br Heart J 1987; 58: 40–44.
36. Gerlis LM, Schmidt-Ott SC, Ho SY, Anderson RH. Dysplastic conditions of the right ventricular myocardium: Uhl's anomaly v arrhythmogenic right ventricular dysplasia. Br Heart J 1993; 69: 142–150.
37. Marcus FI, Fontaine GH, Guiraudon G, Frank R,

Laurenceau JL, Malergue C, Grosgogeat Y. Right ventricular dysplasia: a report of 24 adult cases. Circulation 1982; 65: 384–398.
38. Fitchett DH, Sugrue DD, Macarthur CG, Oakley CM. Right ventricular dilated cardiomyopathy. Br Heart J 1984; 51: 25–29.
39. Ibsen HHW, Baandrup U, Simonsen EE. Familial right ventricular dilated cardiomyopathy. Br Heart J 1985; 54: 156–159.
40. McKenna WJ, Thiene G, Nava A, Fontalian F, Blonistrom-Lundqvist C et al. Diagnosis of arrhythmogenic right ventricular dysplasia/cardiomyopathy. Br Heart J 1994; 71: 215–218.
41. Miani D, Pinamonti B, Bussani R et al. Right ventricular dysplasia: a clinical and pathological study of two families with left ventricular involvement. Br Heart J 1993; 69: 151–158.
42. Morgera T, Salvi AE, Silvestri F, Camerini F. Morphological findings in apparently idiopathic ventricular tachycardia. An echocardiographic haemodynamic and histological study. Eur Heart J 1985; 6: 323–334.
43. Lev M. The pathology of complete atrioventricular block. Prog Cardiovasc Dis 1964; 6: 317–336.
44. Lenègre J. Aetiology and pathology of bilateral bundle branch fibrosis in relation to complete heart block. Prog Cardiovasc Dis 1964; 6: 409–444.
45. Ginks W, Sutton R, Siddons H, Leatham A. Unsuspected coronary artery disease as a cause of chronic atrioventricular block in middle age. Br Heart J 1980; 44: 699–703.
46. Fulkerson PK, Beaver BM, Auseon JC, Graber HL. Calcification of the mitral annulus. Aetiology, clinical associations, complications and therapy. Am J Med 1979; 66: 967–977.
47. Takamoto T, Popp RL. Conduction disturbances related to the site and severity of mitral annular calcification. A 2 dimensional echo and electrocardiographic correlative study. Am J Cardiol 1983; 51: 1644–1649.
48. Dunnigan A, Pierpont ME, Smith SA et al. Cardiac and skeletal myopathy associated with cardiac dysrhythmias. Am J Cardiol 1984; 53: 731–737.
49. Roberts NK, Perloff JK, Kark RA. Cardiac conduction in the Kearns–Sayre syndrome. Am J Cardiol 1979; 44: 1396–1400.
50. Bies RD, Friedman D, Roberts R, Perryman MB, Caskey CT. Expression and localization of dystrophin in human cardiac Purkinje fibers. Circulation 1992; 86: 147–153.
51. Barak M, Herschkowitz S, Shapiro L, Roguin N. Familial combined sinus node with atrioventricular conduction dysfunctions. Int J Cardiol 1987; 15: 231–239.
52. Ho SY, Esscher E, Anderson RH, Mitchaelsson M. Anatomy of congenital complete heart block and relation to maternal RO antibodies. Am J Cardiol 1986; 58: 291–294.
53. Taylor PV, Scott JS, Gerlis LM, Esscher E, Scott O. Maternal antibodies against foetal cardiac antigens in congenital complete heart block. N Engl J Med 1986; 315: 667–672.
54. Peeters AJ, Wolde ten S, Sedney MI, Dijkmans BAC. Heart conduction disturbance: an HLA-B27 associated disease. Ann Rheum Dis 1991; 50: 348–350.
55. Bulkley BH, Ridolfi RL, Salyer WR, Hutchins GM. Myocardial lesions of progressive systemic sclerosis — a cause of cardiac dysfunction. Circulation 1976; 53: 483–490.
56. Roberts NK. The prevalence of conduction defects and cardiac arrhythmias in progressive systemic sclerosis. Ann Intern Med 1981; 94: 38–40.
57. Slama MS. Complete AV block following mediastinal irradiation. PACE 1991; 14: 1112–1118.
58. Bharati S, Fuente JM, Kallen RJ, Freij Y, Lev M. Conduction system in systemic lupus with AV block. Am J Cardiol 1975; 35: 299–304.
59. Askari AD, Huettner TL. Cardiac abnormalities in polymositis and dermatomyositis. Semin Arthritis Rheum 1982; 12: 208–219.
60. Karjalainen J, Vitasalo M, Kala R, Keikkila J. 24-hour electrocardiographic recordings in mild acute infectious myocarditis. Ann Clin Res 1984; 16: 34–39.
61. Stovin PG. Isolated interventricular septal tuberculoma causing complete heart block. Thorax 1982; 45: 49–50.
62. Van der Linde MR, Crijns JGM, de Koning J et al. Range of atrioventricular conduction disturbances in Lyme borreliosis: a report of four cases and review of other published reports. Br Heart J 1990; 63: 162–168.
63. Fleming HA. Sarcoid heart disease. Br Med J 1986; 292: 1095–1096.
64. Silverman KJ, Hutchins GM, Bulkley BH. Cardiac sarcoid: a clinicopathological study of 84 unselected patients with systemic sarcoidosis. Circulation 1978; 58: 1204–1211.
65. Kulbertus HE. The hemiblocks — ten years' experience. New York: Boehringer-Ingelheim, 1979.
66. Demoulin JC, Simar LJ, Kulbertus HE. Quantitative study of left bundle branch fibrosis in left anterior hemiblock. A stereological approach. Am J Cardiol 1975; 36: 751–756.
67. Rizzon P, Rossi L, Baissus C, Demoulin JC, Dibaise M. Left posterior hemiblock in acute myocardial infarction. Br Heart J 1975; 37: 711–720.
68. Lev M, Unger PN, Rosen KM, Bharati S. The anatomic base of the ECG abnormality of left bundle branch block. Adv Cardiol 1975; 14: 16–24.
69. Lev M, Unger PN, Lesser ME, Pick A. Pathology of the conduction system in acquired heart disease: complete right bundle branch block. Am Heart J 1961; 61: 593–614.
70. Bharati S, Lev M. Congenital abnormalities of the conduction system in sudden death in young adults. J Am Coll Cardiol 1986; 8: 1096–1104.
71. Cohle SD. Pathologic changes of the cardiac conduction system in sudden unexplained death — a review. Pathol Annu 1991; 26: 33–57.
72. Weidermann CJ, Becker AE, Hopferwieser T et al. Sudden death in a young competitive athlete with WPW syndrome. Eur Heart J 1987; 8: 651–655.
73. Kirschner RH, Echner FAO, Baron RC. The cardiac pathology of sudden unexplained nocturnal death in SE Asian refugees. JAMA 1987; 256: 2700–2705.
74. Burke AP, Subramanian R, Smialek J, Virmani R. Nonatherosclerotic narrowing of the atrioventricular node artery and sudden death. J Am Coll Cardiol 1993; 21: 117–122.

11

Cardiac tumours

INTRODUCTION

Primary cardiac tumours are rare. Reviews of large autopsy series, including one of 480 331 cases, show a frequency ranging from 0.0017–0.33%.[1] The majority of primary cardiac tumours are benign, most being atrial myxomas.[2] In contrast, secondary carcinoma involving the heart, from a wide range of primary sites, particularly breast, bronchus and stomach, is 20–40 times more common than primary tumours.

CLINICAL MANIFESTATIONS

The clinical manifestations of cardiac tumours, whether primary or secondary, depend on their location within the heart rather than on their histological type. Unfortunately, the symptoms are non-specific and this often results in delayed diagnosis.

Many cardiac tumours, whether primary or secondary, project into a cardiac cavity as a polypoid mass. Such masses may obstruct blood flow, examples being left atrial myxoma simulating mitral stenosis and tumours growing into the right ventricular outflow tract simulating pulmonary stenosis. All intracavity tumours have the potential to be the source of pulmonary or systemic emboli of fragments of tumour, or of thrombus from the surface of the tumour. Two-dimensional echocardiography is a very sensitive means of demonstrating intracavity masses in the heart and is the most widely used method of demonstrating cardiac tumours in vivo.

Intramyocardial tumours are often clinically silent but may cause ventricular or atrial arrhythmias. If strategically sited, complete heart block can be caused due to pressure on/or destruction of the atrioventricular node and the penetrating or bifurcating AV bundle.

Pericardial involvement by tumours leads to pericarditis, blood-stained effusions and often tamponade. Such clinical pictures are commonly due to secondary carcinoma involving the heart but are also pathognomonic of the presentation of the rare primary right atrial haemangiosarcoma. Cardiac tumours may cause a systemic upset including fever, weight loss, arthritis, high ESR, a polymorphonuclear leucocytosis and skin rashes. This picture is most commonly seen with left atrial myxomas but can occur with other cardiac tumours.

PRIMARY BENIGN CARDIAC TUMOURS

Benign cardiac tumours can be divided into two groups: those that are myxomas and those that are not. Myxomas are almost, but not completely, confined to the atria and develop in adult life. Other benign cardiac tumours tend to appear in a younger age group and to involve the ventricles more frequently than the atria: 12–50% of all primary benign cardiac tumours[3] reported in series are not myxomas. Such data are, however, highly selected and must not obscure the fact that by far and away the most common benign cardiac tumour is the atrial myxoma.

Rarely, in infants, benign cardiac tumours present simultaneously with another cardiac malformation[4] such as Ebstein's malformation of the tricuspid valve.

The majority of benign cardiac tumours occur without associated disease and are not familial; however, a few associations of cardiac tumours with hereditary syndromes have been reported.[5] 50% of the cardiac rhabdomyomas that occur in children are associated with tuberous sclerosis; in this instance the tumours are intramyocardial and often multiple instead of being intracavitary as in the spontaneous cases. Cardiac fibromas have been found in association with the naevoid basal-cell carcinoma syndrome, and cardiac myxomas have been described in association with pigmented skin lesions, peripheral nerve tumours and endocrine neoplasms.[6]

Myxomas

Atrial myxomas are the most common primary benign cardiac tumour, accounting for up to 83% of all cardiac tumours in some series.[3] Myxomas are slightly more common in women than in men and generally located (>90% of cases) in the left atrium. However, occasional right atrial myxomas and bilateral myxomas are reported.[1] Clinically, up to 50% of myxomas manifest general constitutional signs and symptoms such as fever, raised erythrocyte sedimentation rate, hypergammaglobulinaemia, arthralgia and weight loss. Symptoms due to obstruction of the mitral valve are also frequent (40–90%), often presenting with disproportionately high levels of pulmonary hypertension. Peripheral embolisation can be the presenting symptom in around 30% of cases; most of them are cerebral emboli. Recent reviews show that up to 8% of patients with an atrial myxoma die while awaiting surgery. The imaging method of choice to diagnose atrial myxomas is two-dimensional echocardiography, although computerised tomography and magnetic resonance imaging are useful for localising the tumour and determining its size.

The majority of myxomas are solitary. However, a familial myxoma syndrome has been described,[6] its features including: cardiac myxoma, widespread skin freckles, mainly on the face and trunk (68%), non-cardiac myxomatous tumours or neurofibromas (57%), endocrine neoplasms (adrenal, testicular and thyroid tumours, 30%) and a high family frequency (34% of the first-degree relatives of the affected population show at least one feature of the syndrome). In this familial syndrome the myxoma has a somewhat different biological behaviour from that of other non-familial myxomas: the frequency of recurrence is much higher (34%), the tumour may be in a ventricle, and it is multiple in up to 50% of cases. This genetic syndrome has been differentiated from the sporadic myxomas by the following acronyms: NAME (N = naevi, A = atrial myxoma, M = mucocutaneous myxoma, E = ephelides) or

LAMB (L = lentigines, A = atrial myxoma, M = mucocutaneous myxomas, B = blue naevi).

Macroscopic appearances of myxomas

Myxomas are soft masses, sessile or pedunculated, with a pedicle attached to the limbus of the fossa ovalis (Fig. 11.1). Although there is a great variability in weight and size, they may measure up to 6 cm in their biggest dimension, and weigh up to 120 g. They may be smooth (Fig. 11.2) or have a villous appearance (Figs 11.3, 11.4). They may be partially covered by thrombus. On section, there are usually translucent, gelatinous areas intercalated with haemorrhagic areas (Fig. 11.4).

Atrial myxomas arise from the endocardium and can relatively easily be separated from the underlying atrial myocardium at surgery (Fig. 11.4). However, the standard surgical procedure is to remove a cuff of adjacent endocardium and a segment of myocardium abutting on the base of the myxoma. The aim of this procedure is to reduce the risk of recurrence, which is high if the tumour is simply pulled away from the atrial wall. Recurrence of an atrial myxoma represents regrowth of the tumour from clumps of myxoma cells left behind in the adjacent endocardium. In examining excised myxomas histologically, adjacent endocardium should be checked for completeness of resection.

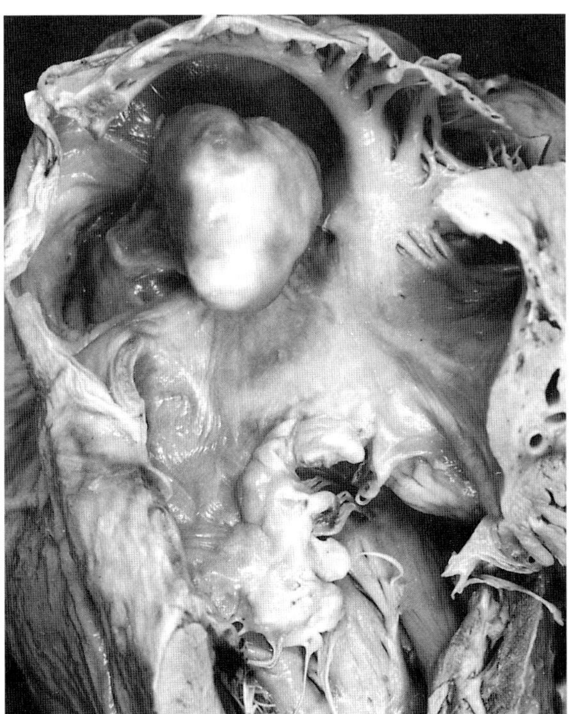

Fig. 11.1 Atrial myxoma. A smooth ovoid right atrial myxoma is attached to the fossa ovalis by a stalk.

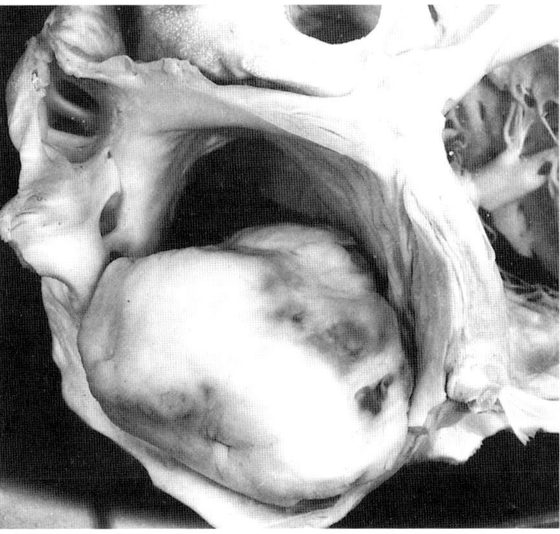

Fig. 11.2 Atrial myxoma. The left atrium is almost filled by a smooth atrial myxoma attached to the atrial septum. Reproduced from Pathology of Cardiac Valves (1980) with permission of M. J. Davies and publishers Butterworth–Heinemann Ltd.

Histological appearance of myxomas

The histogenesis of atrial myxomas has provoked much discussion. The issue remains unresolved. The histological pattern is very characteristic, but does not closely resemble any other tumour arising outside the heart.

The histological appearances are very variable, both between different myxomas and in different areas of a single myxoma (Figs 11.5, 11.6). The bulk of the tumour is made up of a myxoid stroma which is rich in glycosaminoglycans and stains positively with PAS and Alcian blue. Embedded in the stroma are the myxoma cells. The term 'lepidic' (scale-like) has been applied to these cells, drawing attention to their polygonal shape. Myxoma cells in fact vary widely in morphology. Isolated myxoma cells embedded in the stroma

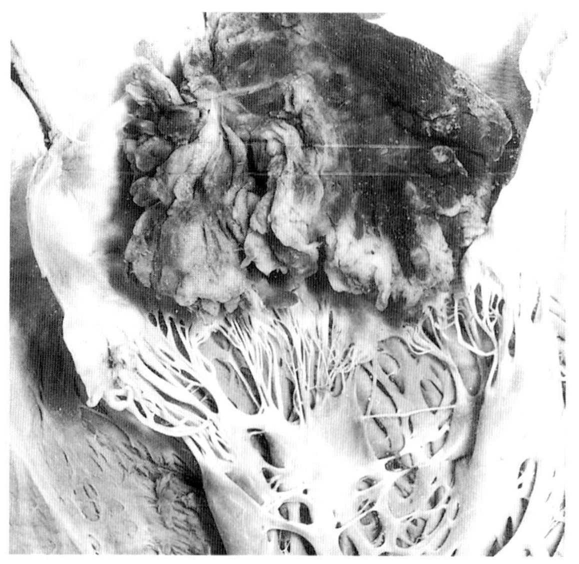

a)

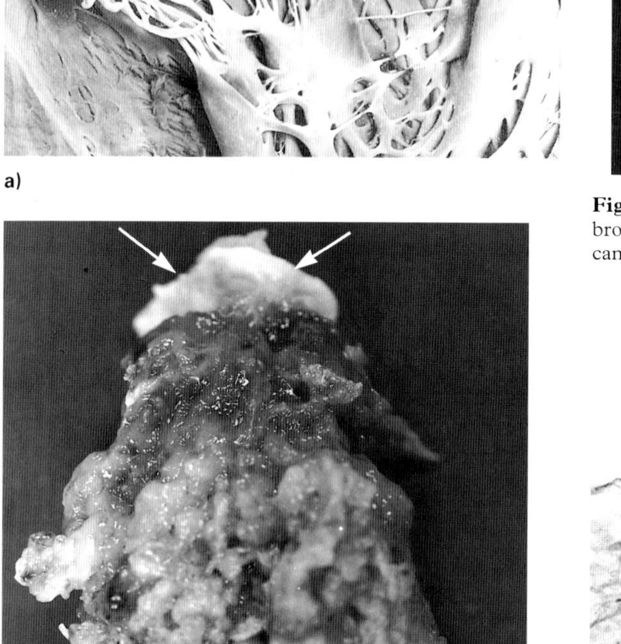

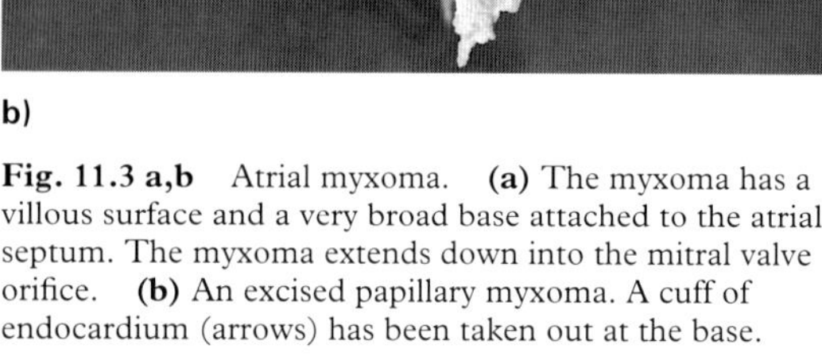

b)

Fig. 11.3 a,b Atrial myxoma. **(a)** The myxoma has a villous surface and a very broad base attached to the atrial septum. The myxoma extends down into the mitral valve orifice. **(b)** An excised papillary myxoma. A cuff of endocardium (arrows) has been taken out at the base.

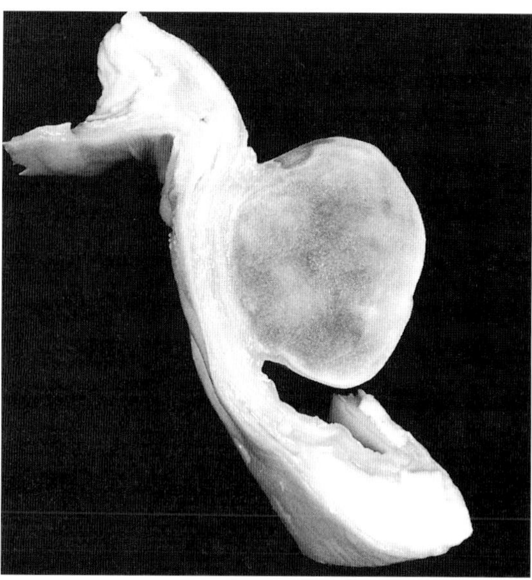

Fig. 11.4 Atrial myxoma. This myxoma is attached on a broad base to the atrial septum. The tumour is superficial and can be peeled away with the endocardium.

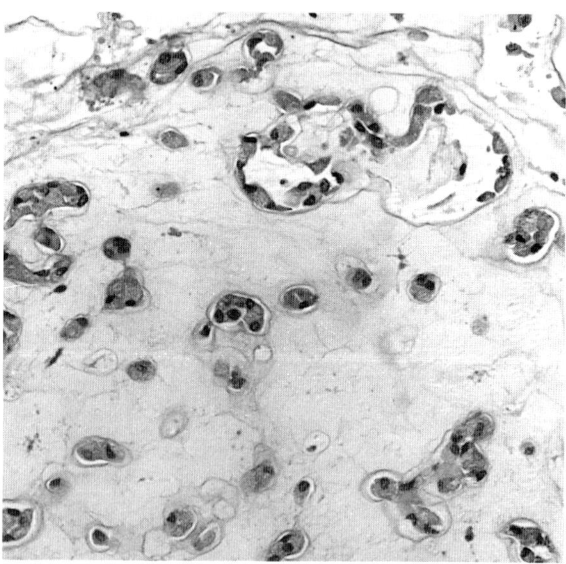

Fig. 11.5 Atrial myxoma — histology. The myxoma cells in this case conform to the classic description, being polygonal in shape and occurring in small clumps embedded in a mucinous stroma.
Haematoxylin–eosin × 105

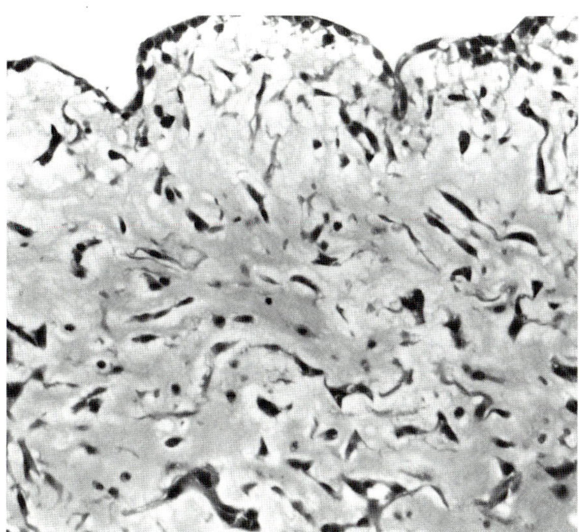

Fig. 11.6 Atrial myxoma — histology. In this field cells are stellate in shape and occurring single or in small clumps. The surface of the tumour is covered by myxoma cells. Haematoxylin–eosin × 105

are often spindle-shaped or stellate. A very characteristic appearance is of more stellate myxoma cells arranged in a cuff around a small central space. Use of immunohistochemical markers shows the space to be lined by endothelial cells to which the myxoma cells are loosely attached. Mitotic figures within myxoma cells are usually rare but an occasional tumour shows frequent mitotic figures. The most characteristic histological appearances of a myxoma may occur throughout the tumour or be confined to the area adjacent to the base. Myxomas in which the characteristic appearance is confined to small areas of the tumour are those which have undergone extensive degeneration. In rare cases myxomas contain gland-like structures with spaces lined by columnar or cuboidal epithelium.[7] The presence of typical myxoma cells elsewhere distinguishes such appearances from secondary adenocarcinoma.

Biochemical analysis of the myxoma matrix has shown that 65% of the stroma consists of proteoglycans, of which 85% is chondroitin sulphate. Recent studies with a cartilage-derived hyaluronic-acid-binding protein have shown that the stroma of the myxoma contains hyaluronic acid,[8] which would be responsible for the gelatinous appearance and consistency.

Other elements found in the matrix include old and recent haemorrhage; iron pigment contained within macrophages is very common. Calcium-encrusted elastic fibrils are also common and may invoke a giant-cell reaction. Close to the base of the tumour thick-walled arteries are common, with a local proliferation of smooth muscle cells that appears to spread out into the stroma from the artery.

Immunohistochemical studies of myxomas show the myxoma cell to stain fairly constantly with PGP 9.5 (Fig. 11.7) and less consistently with NSE and S100. Use of these stains demonstrates that the surface of myxomas may be partially covered by endothelial cells but also partially by myxoma cells.

The wide variation in appearances within atrial myxomas makes it necessary to study several tissue blocks from each case. Identification of an area with the most typical appearances (Figs 11.6, 11.8) is helpful in distinguishing between atrial myxomas and low-grade sarcomas. Some of the appearances of cellular myxomas (Fig. 11.6), particularly if mitotic figures are present, are not easy to distinguish from a myxosarcoma. We have never seen a myxosarcoma which has areas showing appearances like those in Figs 11.8–11.9.

Many myxomas contain large numbers of basophils and eosinophils within the stroma and

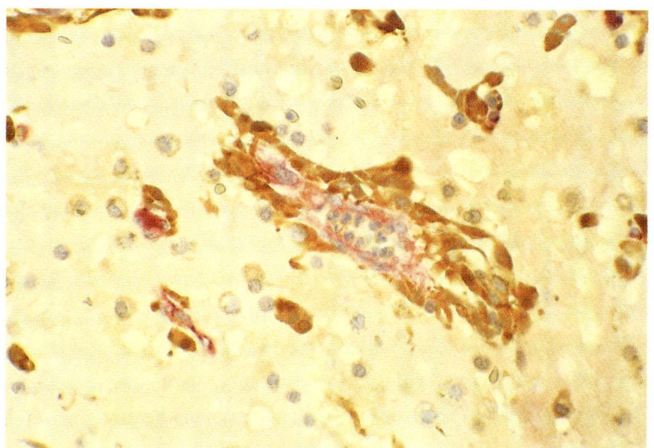

Fig. 11.7 Atrial myxoma — histology. Immunohistochemical staining of an atrial myxoma. The myxoma cells are positive for PGP 9.5 (brown) and occur both as isolated cells in the stroma and as a large clump. Within the centre of this clump are endothelial cells staining for EN4 (red).

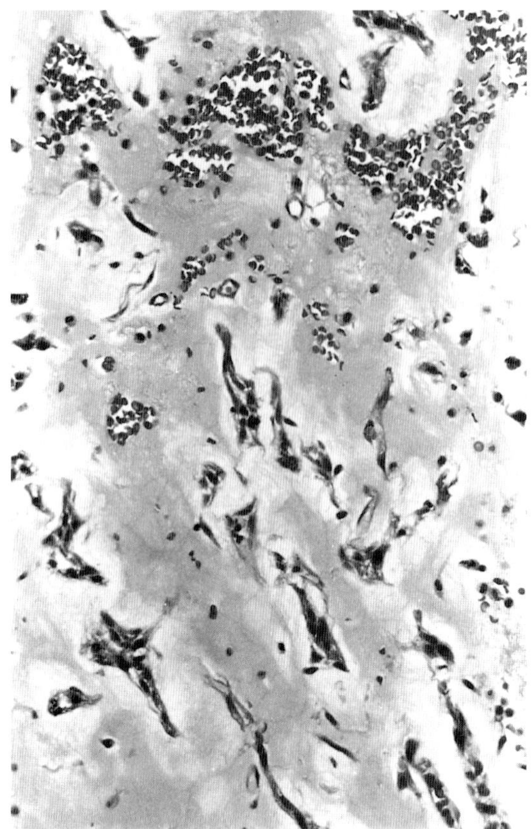

Fig. 11.8 Atrial myxoma — histology. In this field the clumps of myxoma cells are lying within a paler staining space within the stroma. Red cells are extravasated into the stroma in one area.
Haematoxylin–eosin × 105

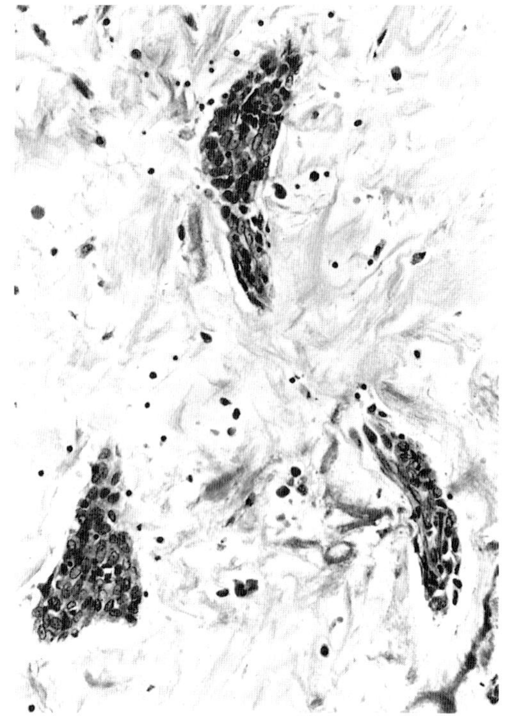

Fig. 11.9 Atrial myxoma — histology. In this field myxoma cells are arranged in large masses without individual cells loose in the stroma. The stroma contains numerous plasma cells.
Haematoxylin–eosin × 105

also plasma cells and lymphocytes. Chronic inflammatory cells are more common around the vascular structures and it has been postulated that this perivascular location could be the result of the release of interleukins by the inflammatory cells (mostly interleukin-6) inducing new vessel formation. Interleukin-6 is known to be a potent stimulus for the synthesis of immunoglobulins, and it also induces the release of acute phase proteins, which are seen in more than 50% of patients with an atrial myxoma. It has been postulated that the release of IL-6 is responsible for the immunological features seen in these patients.[9]

Biological behaviour of myxomas

Clinical studies show that some myxomas increase in size rapidly while others have apparently been present for years and are static in size. In accord with these observations some excised myxomas have numerous myxoma cells, often with mitosis present, while others show extensive degeneration and myxoma cells are sparse.

Fragments of myxomas do embolise to the arteries of other organs, particularly the brain (Fig. 11.10). The myxoma may persist at the local site[10] but there are no indubitable reports of genuine metastatic growth at the site. Recurrence at the site of excision in the heart represents regrowth following failure to totally excise the base. The NAME syndrome (see above) is an exception in that recurrence is common and often takes place at sites remote from the original excision: this appears to reflect a general tendency of the whole endocardium to produce myxomas in these patients.

Local recurrences have been divided into septal, which are probably due to incomplete resection of the tumour, and extraseptal. The

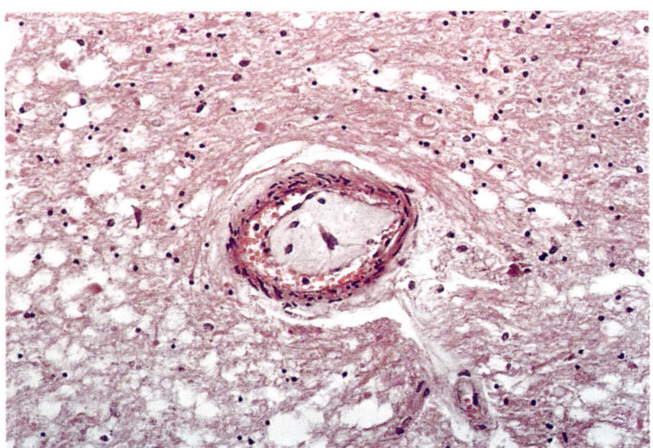

Fig. 11.10 Atrial myxoma — cerebral emboli. A small cerebral artery contains a fragment of an atrial myxoma. Haematoxylin–eosin × 345

reported frequency of recurrence varies from 5–14%;[11] such figures warrant serial echocardiographic follow-up of all patients who have had a cardiac myxoma surgically excised.[12] Other risk factors for recurrence are failure to identify more than one tumour at initial presentation, intracardiac seeding and embolisation. Patients with the 'myxoma syndrome' have a higher frequency of recurrence than patients with sporadic myxoma.[13]

It must be made clear that left atrial sarcomas can macroscopically exactly simulate myxomas and be diagnosed as such by clinicians. It is mandatory to examine all intracavitary tumours histologically to exclude a diagnosis of sarcoma. The histological appearance of sarcomas is very different from that of myxomas and we have never seen a tumour showing transitions between a true myxoma and a sarcoma.

Histogenesis of myxomas

Immunohistochemistry has been carried out in an attempt to determine the origin of the lepidic cells. A review of over 100 cases of myxoma studied by different authors[14–17] shows that myxoma cells nearly always stain for vimentin, actin and PGP 9.5; less frequently for S-100, factor VIII and desmin, NSE and synaptophysin. These immunohistochemical data point to a mesenchymal origin of the cells, possibly with some degree of neuroendocrine differentiation. A panepithelial marker for fetal mesenchymal cells, lu-5,[16] has also been shown to stain myxoma cells, and this has been taken as proof of the mixed (endodermal and mesenchymal) origin of the cells. In rare cases myxomas also contain glandular formations which stain for cytokeratins, epithelial membrane antigen (EMA) and carcinoembryonic antigen (CEA).

Electronmicroscopy studies[14] have described two different types of 'lepidic' cells: one has a stellate shape, with a round nucleus and variable amounts of rough endoplasmic reticulum in the cytoplasm, together with low-density material granules; cytoplasmic processes are also present, helping to connect with other similar cells. The other type of lepidic cell is round or fusiform, with a prominent nucleolus, Golgi areas in the cytoplasm, many mitochondria and intermediate filaments. These intermediate filaments have been taken as proof of the mesenchymal origin of the lepidic cells, which can be considered as being in different stages of differentiation and thus reacting differently to the immunohistochemical markers that have been used. Further electronmicroscopy studies confirmed that the myxoma cells are mesenchymal cells,[18] with abundant rough endoplasmic reticulum and intermediate filaments in the cytoplasm, and no Weibel–Palade bodies; scanning electronmicroscopy confirmed that the cells lining the surface of the tumour were all interconnected by interdigitating cellular processes. Analysis of the matrix of the tumour has shown it to consist of a network of reticulin fibres, together with collagen and a few capillaries. The basic matrix substance is mostly chondroitin sulphate with some hyaluronic acid. The ground substance is synthesised by the myxoma cells themselves within the tumour.

Although some authors do not accept these different cellular categories, the use of electron microscopy has at least solved the argument regarding the origin of the myxoma: it has been shown that it does not have a thrombotic origin. On the other hand, the morphological resemblance of the lepidic cells to those present in the limbus of the fossa ovalis has given rise to the theory that the myxoma arises from embryological remnants (multipotential mesenchymal cells) in the fossa ovalis area. It is difficult, however, to use the same theory to explain the presence of myxomas in other areas of the heart, although embryonic cells have been found in the subvalvular regions.

Recent reports of DNA analysis[19,20] of cardiac myxomas has shown that, out of 39 myxomas analysed, 34 (87%) were diploid and five (13%) were aneuploid. Out of the 34 diploid myxomas, however, eight (23%) had a high proliferative fraction, and in this subgroup four patients had either an embolic phenomenon or a recurrence and three had multiple myxomas. Among the patients with aneuploid tumours, one had a recurrence. It has been postulated that the presence of a high proliferative fraction could be an indicator of aggressive behaviour in these tumours. The data are, however, biased by inclusion of cases that are likely to be the familial syndrome and it is not clear whether the data apply to isolated non-familial myxomas.

Other benign cardiac tumours

Rhabdomyomas

These tumours are seen almost exclusively in the paediatric age group and are considered the second most common benign primary cardiac tumour.[21] Up to 50% of rhabdomyomas are associated with tuberous sclerosis. The remainder are sporadic.[22] The vast majority appear in children under 15, and over 50% are found in children under 1 year; there is a striking male predominance.[23] They are a well-recognised cause of arrhythmias in the paediatric age group. Rhabdomyomas tend to be multiple and if so they involve the left ventricle. Histologically, they consist of nodules of large cells with clear cytoplasm (Fig. 11.11). These cells have cross-striations and stain positive for myoglobin, desmin, vimentin and actin, but not for S-100.

In the paediatric age group, cardiac arrhythmias are the presenting feature of a condition which has been considered to be either multiple Purkinje cell hamartomas or a form of cardiomyopathy. Small, ill-defined grey-white myocardial nodules are present, each consisting of large cells with granular cytoplasm. Electronmicroscopy studies show disorganisation of the cristae of the mitochondria together with dense mitochondrial inclusions. The condition (oncocytic cardiomyopathy) is considered in Chapter 5.

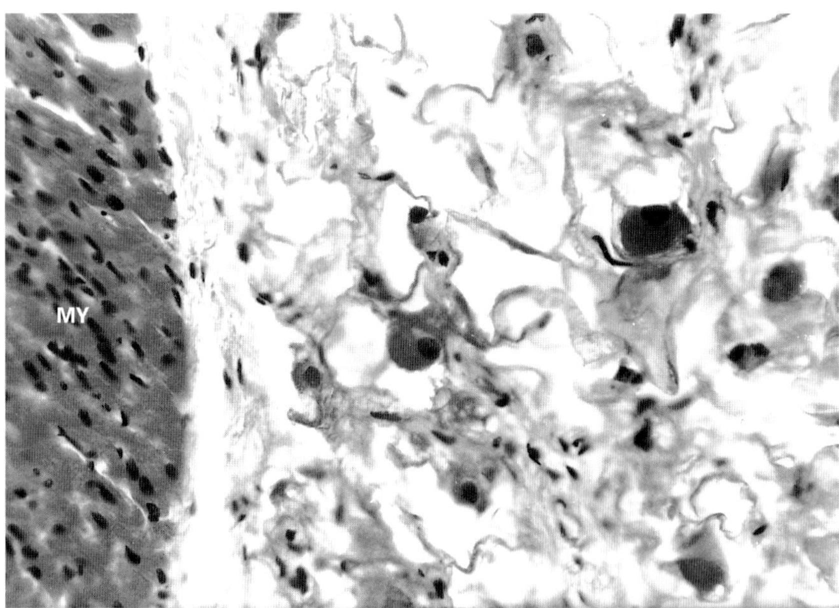

Fig. 11.11 Rhabdomyoma. The tumour cells are large and vacuolated and appear to have the nuclei suspended within an empty space. The cells also contain eosinophilic conglomerates of myofibrillary material which are often around the nuclei. There is an abrupt transition between normal myocardium (MY) and the cells of the rhabdomyoma. Haematoxylin–eosin × 160

Fibromas

Fibromas are seen most frequently in children under 10 years of age. They are single, well-defined nodules, located in the left ventricular myocardium, usually the septum, and may be massive, causing obstruction to blood flow and sudden death (Fig. 11.12). Sudden death has been reported when the tumour involves the ventricular septum.[24] Mitotic figures are not present; dystrophic calcification is quite common[25] and a helpful diagnostic feature.[26] In some series[21] cardiac fibromas have been described as small and multicentric. They may present with an infiltrative pattern[25] similar to that seen in the extra-abdominal desmoid tumours, but they do not recur. The tumours, although well defined, do not have a fibrous tissue capsule. Their centre can show cystic degeneration. Electronmicroscopy shows that the tumour consists of fibroblasts, elastic fibres, collagen and degenerating myocardial cells.

Lipomas

Lipomas can be located anywhere in the heart: some are subendocardial, some have been reported to extend from the epicardium through the myocardium into a cardiac cavity.[27] Some form lobulated masses attached externally to the pericardium (Fig. 11.13). Lipomas have to be differentiated from lipomatous hypertrophy of the atrial septum or adipose infiltration of the right ventricle. While true lipomas are said to consist of mature lipocytes and lipomatous hypertrophy of immature lipocytes, the distinction in practice is made on whether the mass of fat is discrete (lipoma) or merges diffusely with adjacent

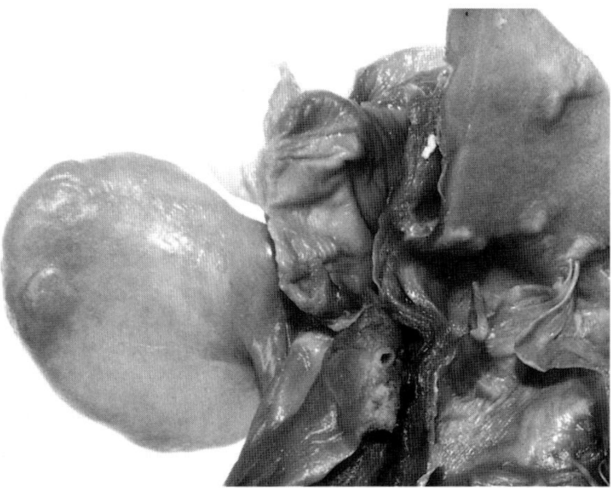

Fig. 11.13 Cardiac lipoma. A subepicardial lipoma projects out from the right border of the heart.

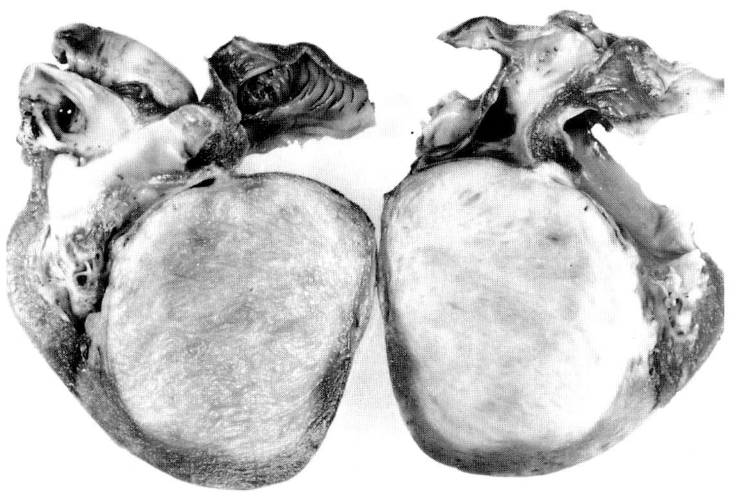

Fig. 11.12 Cardiac fibroma. A large solid tumour replaces the entire ventricular septum. The cut surface is uniform and white with a whorled appearance.

tissue (lipomatous hypertrophy). The vast majority of cardiac lipomas are asymptomatic and discovered as incidental autopsy findings. In size they range from 1 cm to over 15 cm across; it is only the largest which are discovered in life, either by being seen as a mass in a chest radiography or during echocardiography carried out for other purposes or because they project into a cardiac cavity. Projection into the right ventricular outflow is the most common. Lipomas involving the heart are rare but the exact frequency is impossible to determine because most are small and pass unrecorded at autopsy.

Mesotheliomas of the atrioventricular node

This tumour is very rare, but is a recognised cause of sudden cardiac death. The tumour is small, up to 2 cm in diameter, situated in the atrial septum at the site of the AV node, and cystic on cross section. The histological appearance is of glandular spaces containing PAS-positive material and lined by epithelioid cells (Figs 11.14, 11.15). The histological appearances mimic some tumours of the testes, ovaries and kidneys. They are seen more frequently in adult women and can result in complete heart block,[28,29] ventricular fibrillation and sudden death. To our knowledge, the condition has never been diagnosed in life; the diagnosis has always been made at post mortem in patients known to have complete heart block or who die suddenly. The lesion has been called 'the smallest tumour capable of causing sudden death'.[24] The origin of the tumour is still a matter of debate, since some authors believe it to be of mesothelial origin.[24] The AV node embryologically is formed on the posterior surface of the heart and is carried anteriorly into the septum in a folding process; it is postulated that the AV node can carry embryonic mesothelial cells in from the pericardial surface. Others[30] have found strong positive staining for epithelial markers such as CEA, keratin and EMA, a finding which supports the theory of an endodermal origin.

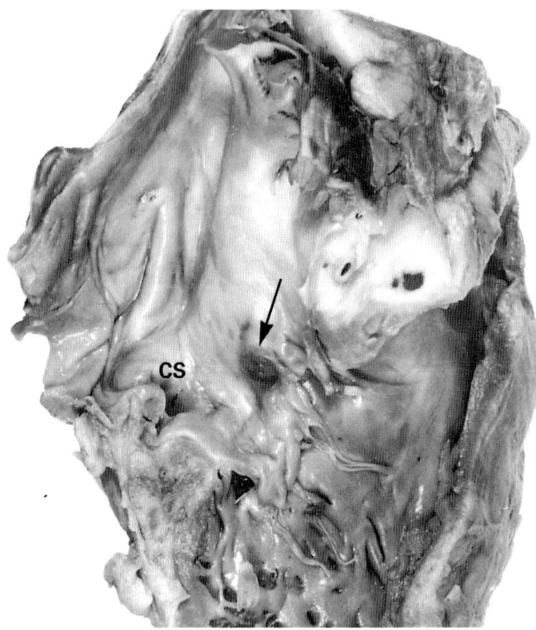

Fig. 11.14 Mesothelioma of AV node. A small nodule is visible (arrow) beneath the endocardium of the right atrium just anterior to the coronary sinus (CS).

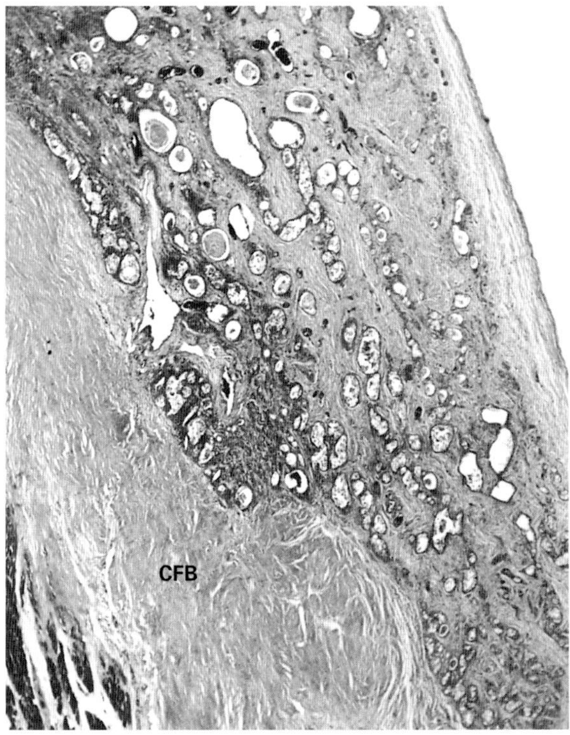

Fig. 11.15 Mesothelioma of AV node. A tumour with multiple cystic spaces replaces the AV node (CFB = central fibrous body).
Haematoxylin–eosin × 19

Papillary fibroelastomas

These are small papillary tumours which appear on cardiac valves or the endocardium (Figs 11.16, 11.17). They must be differentiated from Lambl's excrescences and from an atrial myxoma. Lambl's excrescences are multiple and appear on the apposition points of the valve cusps. Although papillary fibroelastomas are generally an incidental autopsy finding, there are a few reports in the literature of coronary occlusion (when a papillary fibroelastoma on an aortic valve cusp swings into a coronary orifice) or of transient ischaemic attacks from microemboli originating from tumours on the mitral[31,32] or the aortic valve. Papillary fibroelastomas tend to be located in the central area of the valve, on the atrial side if they are on an atrioventricular valve and on the ventricular surface of the aortic or pulmonary valves. They vary in size from a few millimetres to a few centimetres. They have a very characteristic appearance, particularly when examined under water. Histologically they consist of a central core of vascularised fibrous tissue, and innumerable fronds covered by endothelial-like cells. The actual demonstration that these cells are endothelial is difficult. In our experience they are sporadically positive only for Q Bend or EN4.

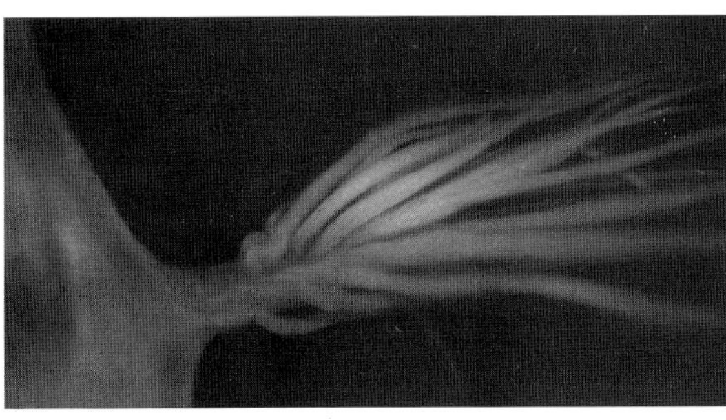

a)

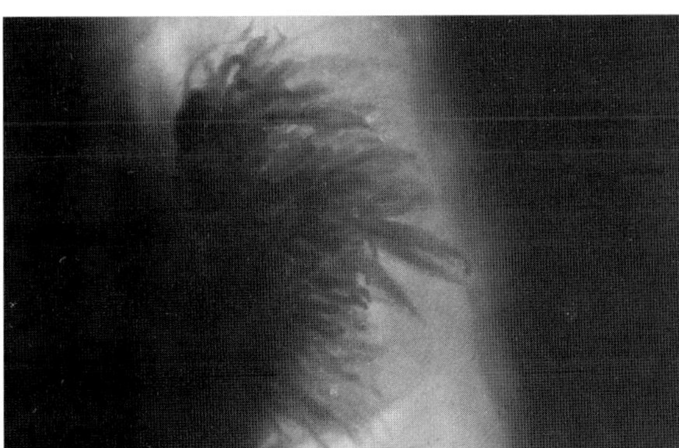

b)

Fig. 11.16 a,b Papillary fibroelastoma. Two examples are shown. One has a broad base and multiple fine fronds simulating the appearances of an open sea anemone. The other has a stalk to which are attached several thicker fronds.

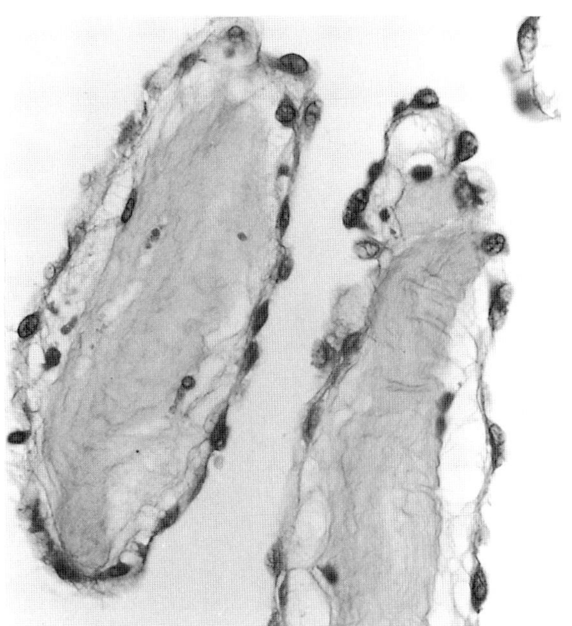

Fig. 11.17 Papillary fibroelastoma — histology. Each frond has a fine connective tissue stroma covered by plump cuboidal cells. These are presumably of endothelial origin. Haematoxylin–eosin × 280

Cardiac haemangiomas

Recent reports[33,34] show that these tumours are variable in size (up to 10 cm in diameter) and ill-defined, and that they can compress surrounding structures such as the left anterior descending coronary artery.[34] Approximately 50% are in the right-sided cavities.[33] They can result in sudden death and, if they rupture outward, can lead to cardiac tamponade. Many small examples, however, are found just beneath the visceral pericardium as incidental autopsy findings (Fig. 11.18). Haemangiomas may be capillary or cavernous.

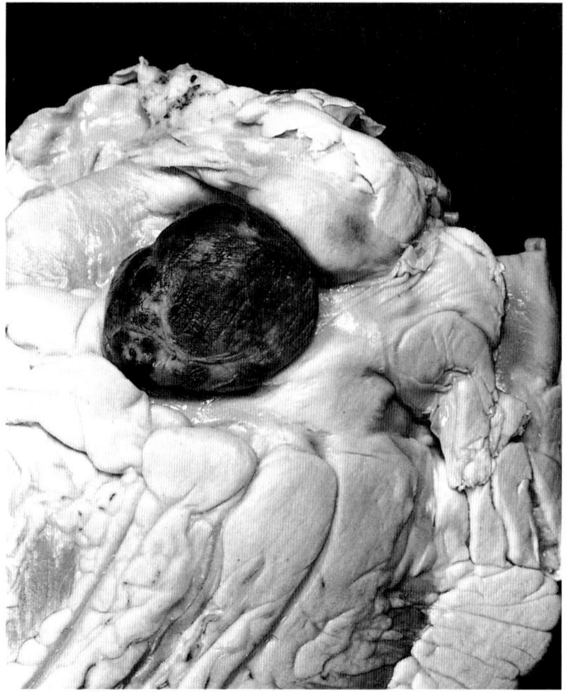

Fig. 11.18 Haemangioma. A dark red nodule 4 cm across is present over the pericardial surface of the posterior wall of the heart over the left atrioventricular region.

There is no mitotic activity or necrosis, this lack making the differential diagnosis from angiosarcoma. They all stain with endothelial immunohistochemical markers.

Other rare benign cardiac tumours

Other rare benign cardiac tumours which have been reported in recent review series include a glomangioma of the atrioventricular node and teratomas.[21] Teratomas usually occur in the atrial septum and form cystic masses distinguishable from mesotheliomas of the AV node by the presence of other mesodermal components such as cartilage. Benign leiomyomas may develop from the endocardium of any chamber but are most common in the right ventricular outflow (Fig. 11.19).

PRIMARY MALIGNANT CARDIAC TUMOURS

Primary malignant tumours of the heart are very rare. They form 20–25% of all primary cardiac tumours. Recent reviews of nearly 100 primary

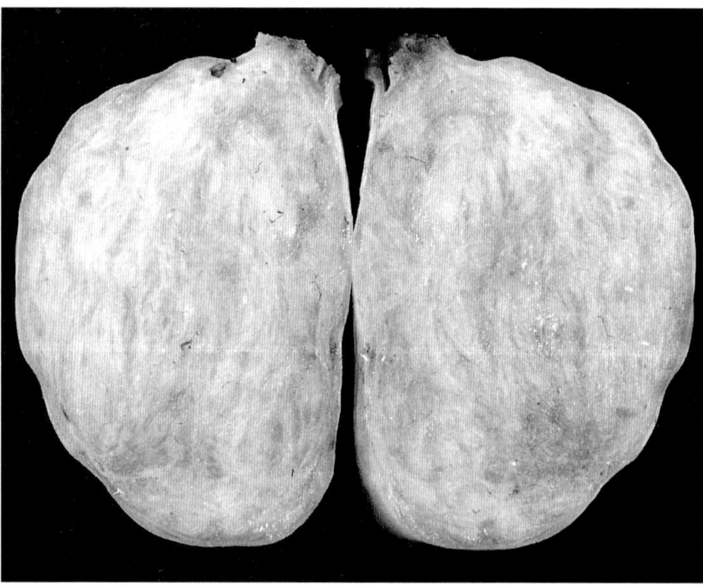

Fig. 11.19 Benign leiomyoma right ventricle. The tumour presented as a mass in the right ventricular outflow in a woman of 69. Exploration showed a pedunculated solid tumour attached to the endocardium in the outflow tract. It was easily excised — the cut surface is uniform, white and with a whorled appearance. This white solid appearance is totally unlike that of a myxoma.

cardiac sarcomas[35,36] show that angiosarcomas are the most frequent (33%), followed by undifferentiated sarcomas (19%). The majority of patients with cardiac sarcomas will have pulmonary and other systemic metastases at the time of diagnosis, which is one of the reasons for their poor survival rate (median less than 12 months).[36]

Angiosarcomas

Angiosarcomas have a strong predilection for the right atrium and metastasise early, by haematogenous spread. The most frequent sites for metastases are the lungs and the liver. Angiosarcomas can present as multiple or single nodules, variable in diameter and filling the cardiac cavity, with or without infiltration of the atrial wall. Angiosarcomas have a marked tendency to spread into the pericardium (Fig. 11.20) and presentation with recurrent blood-stained effusions is common. It is a moot point whether right atrial angiosarcomas actually arise within the pericardium or within the myocardium because by the time of autopsy or surgical exploration transmural atrial involvement is common. Histologically, the cells lining the vascular channels are anaplastic and mitoses are frequent (Fig. 11.21). It is characteristic of angiosarcomas arising in the heart that very well differentiated areas appearing 'benign' coexist with more anaplastic areas,

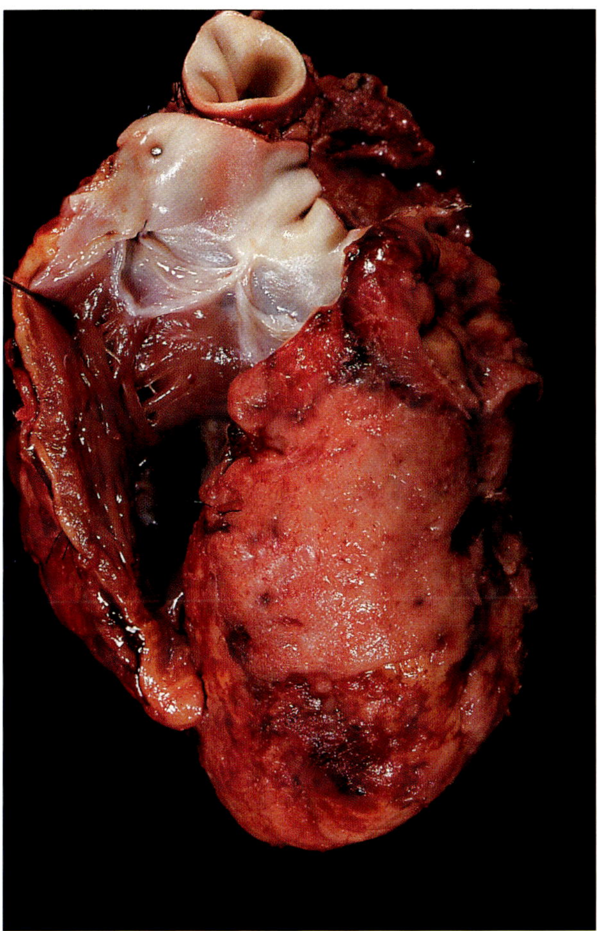

Fig. 11.20 Haemangiosarcoma. The visceral pericardium is covered by a sheet of haemorrhagic tumour which encases both ventricles.

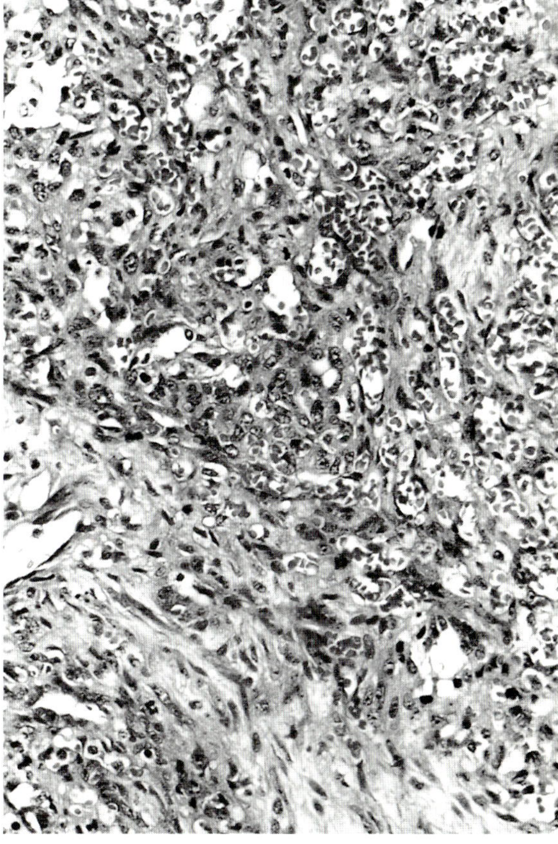

Fig. 11.21 Cardiac angiosarcoma. In part the tumour is made up of anaplastic spindle-shaped cells but in other areas there is formation of vascular channels containing red cells. Haematoxylin–eosin × 110

creating the possibility of a sampling error in diagnosis on biopsy material. It is unclear whether angiosarcomas arise in pre-existing benign angiomas because by the time of autopsy the tumour is too extensive for this to be ascertained.

Cardiac sarcomas

The left atrium is the preponderant site for connective tissue sarcomas, which protrude into the cavity (Fig. 11.22) and thus on echocardiographic grounds can be easily mistaken for atrial myxomas. Rapid growth and embolic phenomena are common to all atrial sarcomas.

The histological appearances can be that of any sarcoma, including fibrosarcoma, myxosarcoma and osteogenic sarcoma. While some sarcomas are histologically uniform many show a mixture

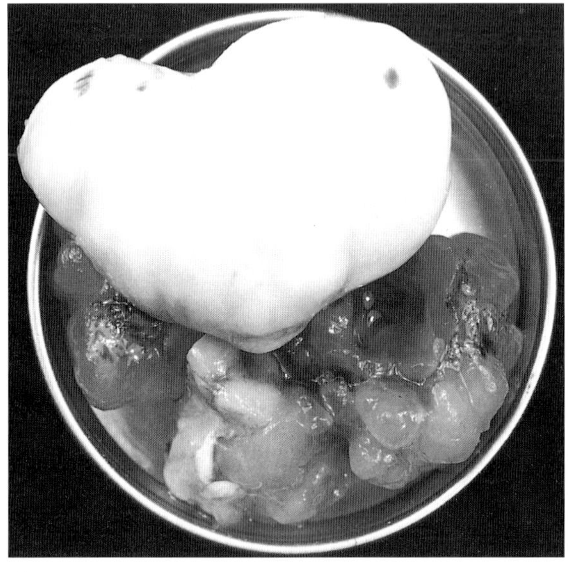

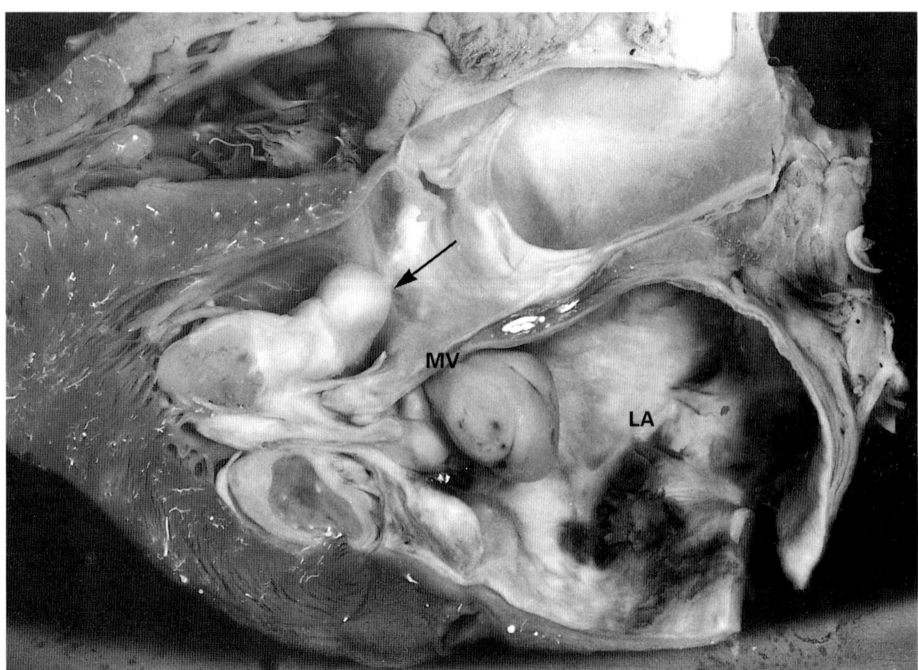

Fig. 11.22 a,b Cardiac sarcoma. **(a)** Specimen excised surgically as an atrial myxoma. The tumour is clearly biphasic with one solid white component and another papillary and myxoid. While either appearance individually is consistent with a myxoma, to have both is very rare and histology showed the tumour was a sarcoma. **(b)** At autopsy some months later the tumour has recurred in the left atrium (LA) and extends through the mitral valve (MV) to protrude up into the left ventricular outflow (arrow).

of differentiation patterns. More rarely, differentiation toward neural or synovial types of sarcoma occurs. The exact histogenesis and origin of these sarcomas is unclear. They do not necessarily arise in the atrial septum and are usually regarded as arising from undifferentiated mesenchymal cells in the endocardium. Semantic difficulties often arise over these sarcomas, which generate a plethora of individual reports of cases in which the differentiation pattern is uniform and unusual. When a monomorphic differentiation pattern exists it can be used to name the tumour, i.e. fibrosarcoma, leiomyosarcoma etc, but when a mixed pattern exists the general term mixed left atrial sarcoma is most appropriate. In practice most sarcomas consist of spindle-shaped cells with a high mitotic rate and show no particular differentiation pattern (Fig. 11.23). The most frequent semantic difficulty is over rhabdomyosarcomas. Some would use this term if these were areas showing strap-like tumour cells (Fig. 11.24) or if there were tumour cells containing myofibrils (Fig. 11.24), others only when this is the dominating pattern of differentiation. For all these reasons it is difficult to gain from the literature a clear impression of the prognosis of cardiac sarcoma in relation to tumour type. Better survival has been shown to be associated with absence of necrosis, low mitotic counts and left-sided situation. The last reflects early diagnosis rather than inherently different behaviour.

Sarcomas which have a predominant osteogenic differentiation are infiltrative and very aggressive; origin elsewhere in the body has to be excluded.[37] In all cases, a primary osteosarcoma has to be ruled out before making the diagnosis of primary cardiac osteosarcoma. Immunohistochemistry will show positive staining for vimentin, without staining for epithelial markers such as cytokeratin. Metastases are frequent and early, via the haematogenous route. The prognosis is bad, but a few patients[37] have survived up to 5 years after partial

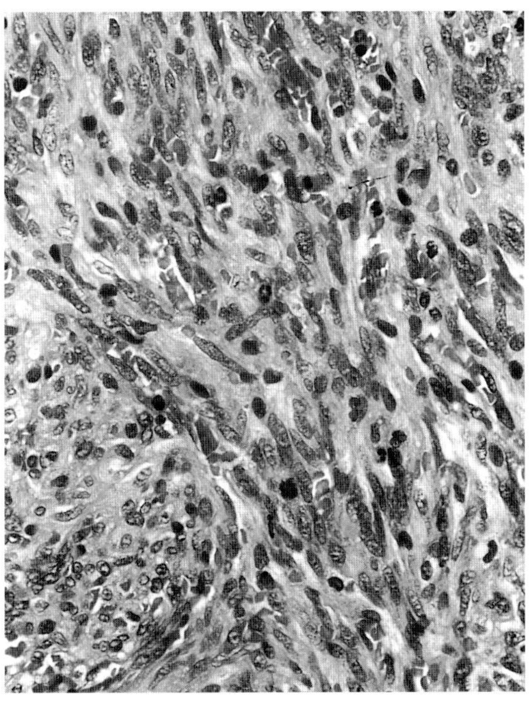

Fig. 11.23 Undifferentiated cardiac sarcoma. The tumour shows a uniform spindle-shaped cell morphology with a very high mitotic rate.
Haematoxylin–eosin × 110

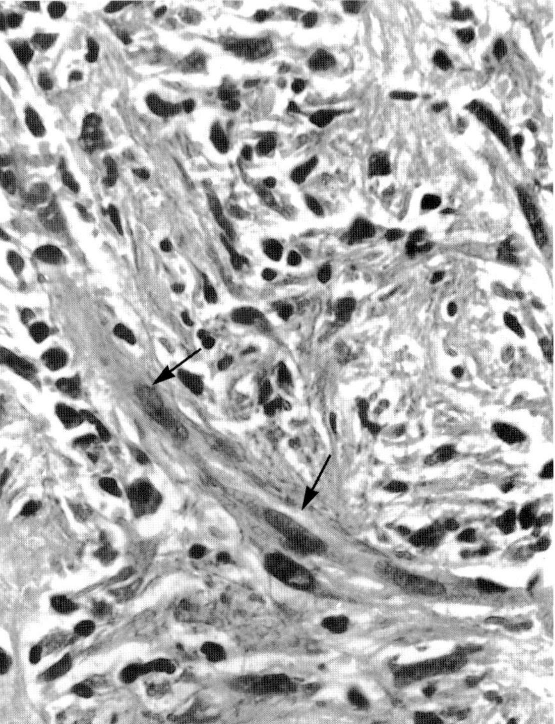

Fig. 11.24 Cardiac sarcoma — myogenic differentiation. Elongated, strap-like tumour cells are present in some areas (arrows).
Haematoxylin–eosin × 280

surgical resection. Pure fibrosarcomas of the heart are well defined nodules and histologically they consist of spindle cells with abnormal mitotic figures. They also metastasise early, through the blood, to the lungs and liver, and their prognosis is poor.

Malignant fibrous histiocytoma of the heart is a very rare tumour. It is relatively more common in women and tends to appear in the left atrium. It generally appears as a whitish-grey multilobulated invasive mass. As with the fibrosarcoma, prognosis is poor, but the occasional case of survival for 18 months after incomplete surgical excision has been reported.[38]

Sarcomas showing clear myogenic differentiation have two incidence peaks; one in childhood and one in later life, around the seventh decade. There is a slight male predominance, particularly in the paediatric age group. In contrast to primary cardiac rhabdomyomas no association with tuberous sclerosis has been reported. The tumour involves any part of the heart, although ventricular septal involvement has been described more frequently in children.[39] The tumour can result in sudden death by involvement of the atrioventricular node. Primary cardiac rhabdomyosarcomas may be multiple. They are generally infiltrative and extend into the pericardium and great vessels in over a third of cases. Death can occur from bleeding into the pericardial sac. Metastases are present in about 70% of patients at the time of diagnosis, generally to the lungs and mediastinal lymph nodes. Median survival is 6 months. The histological type does not seem to modify prognosis. The tumour cells show cross-striations, which are considered to be pathognomonic.

Primary liposarcoma of the heart[40,41] is another rare tumour. It is intracavitary and like all sarcomas has to be differentiated from an atrial myxoma. Although the number of reported cases is small, there seems to be no site of predilection. Pulmonary and osseous metastases were present in most of the reported cases and the mean survival was 8 months.

Other reportedly rare differentiation patterns in primary sarcomas of the heart are leiomyosarcoma, myxosarcoma, synovial sarcoma and neurofibrosarcoma. The cardiac sarcomas which show a single differentiation pattern are often reported in the literature while most undifferentiated sarcomas and myxosarcomas go unreported, creating a publication bias. Personal experience suggests that in practice single differentiation patterns are most unusual.

Primary cardiac lymphomas

These constitute 1.6% of the AFIP series of primary cardiac tumours,[24] and increasingly are in association with AIDS. They tend to involve the right side of the heart and spread through the cavity walls or protrude into the right ventricular outflow (Fig. 11.25) or atria. On macroscopic examination they look nodular and are relatively more common in the atrioventricular groove.[42] Histologically, they generally are B-cell, non-Hodgkin's lymphomas. There have been

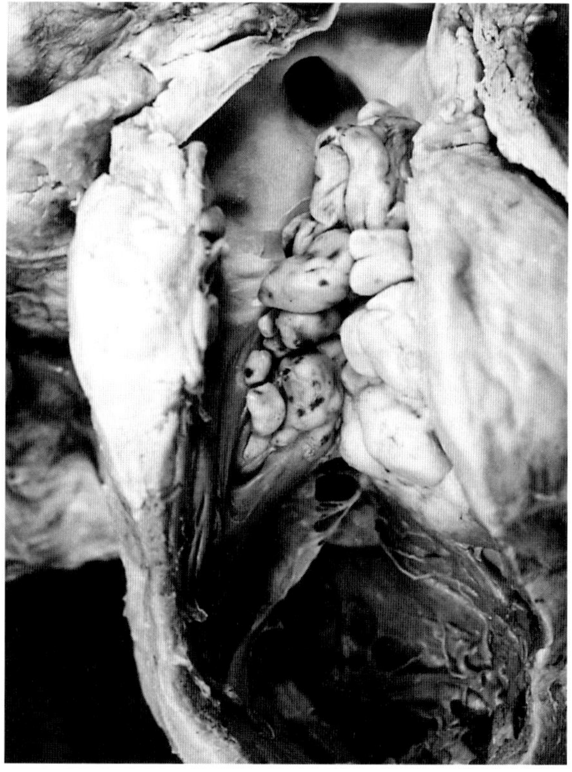

Fig. 11.25 Lymphoma of the heart. A polypoidal mass grows from the cavity of the right ventricle through the pulmonary valve into the pulmonary artery. This macroscopic spread is common to any malignant cardiac tumour, although this case was a B-cell lymphocytic lymphoma with extracardiac disease present.

occasional reports of coronary artery occlusion by lymphoma cells, and coronary artery aneurysm secondary to destruction of the vessel media by lymphoma cells.[43]

Patients with the acquired immunodeficiency syndrome may develop diffuse or nodular deposits of a lymphoma which is B cell in type or Kaposi's sarcoma involving the pericardium.[44,45]

Involvement of the myocardium and pericardium is seen in cases of widespread Kaposi's sarcoma, which has a special predilection for the pericardium. Although cardiac involvement is not uncommon, the mortality rate due to cardiac involvement is low.

Primary pericardial tumours

Tumours arising in the pericardium are exceedingly rare if the right atrial angiosarcoma is excluded.

Primary pericardial mesotheliomas encase the heart, producing a clinical picture similar to constrictive pericarditis. The tumour is so rare that a relation to asbestosis is neither proved nor disproved. Pleural mesotheliomas often directly invade the pericardium and the diagnosis of a primary pericardial tumour can only be sustained when both pleural cavities are clear of tumour. Fibrosarcomas have also been reported.

SECONDARY CARDIAC TUMOURS

The patterns of secondary involvement of the heart[46] include:

1. Direct invasion of pericardium or atrial walls
2. Pericardial nodular involvement
3. Intramyocardial deposits with or without protrusion into a cavity
4. Endocardial deposits

Most cardiac involvement goes clinically unnoticed and is discovered incidentally at autopsy. When secondary involvement is clinically diagnosed it is usually due to a haemorrhagic effusion and a pericarditis which may progress to tamponade. Echocardiography will detect secondary deposits which project into a cavity (Fig. 11.26). Systemic

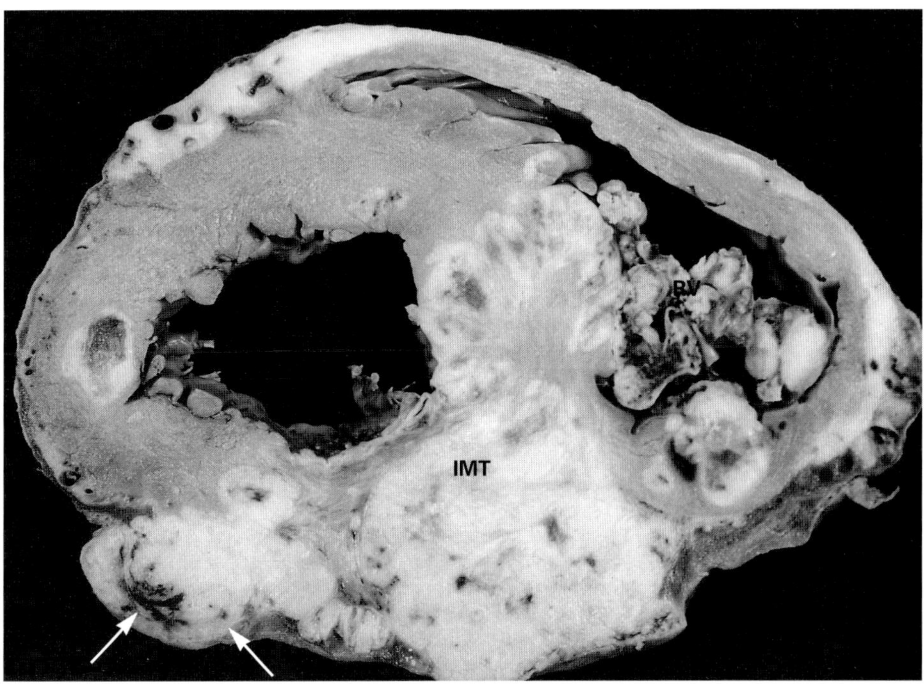

Fig. 11.26 Secondary carcinoma of the heart. The transverse slide of the ventricles shows three of the patterns of secondary carcinoma — intracavity masses in the right ventricle (RV), intramyocardial tumour (IMT) and nodules projecting into the pericardium (arrows).

emboli and rarely constitutional symptoms may lead to confusion with atrial myxomas. Intramyocardial deposits are usually silent although they occasionally act as a focus for atrial and ventricular arrhythmias. Tumour deposits on valves are a rare pathological curiosity.[46]

Myocardial involvement, when not associated with direct invasion from adjacent tissues, represents haematogenous spread and, given the high blood flow to the myocardium, is surprisingly rare when compared to the liver. Considerable philosophical thought has been published concerning the mechanism for the relative resistance of the myocardium to tumour growth.[47]

The frequency of secondary involvement of the heart in malignant tumours ranges at autopsy from 0.2–6.5%. Variation of this degree reflects many factors such as the care taken to examine the heart, whether microscopy was used and the extent of any bias introduced when series under study contain a high proportion of primary sites with marked predilection for the heart, e.g. bronchus. A recent study assessing the incidence of cardiac metastasis[47] has shown that squamous cell carcinoma of the lung and adenocarcinoma of the kidney have the highest reported frequency of metastasis to the heart. A 14-year study involving 3314 consecutive autopsies showed that out of 806 cases with a neoplasm 12% had cardiac involvement.[46,48] Myocardial involvement was twice as common as pericardial involvement, particularly in carcinoma of the lung. However, some studies[48] have shown that the pericardium is the structure most commonly involved, mainly with direct invasion by squamous cell carcinoma of the lung and carcinoma of the breast. Pericardial effusion seems to be a constant finding with these two tumours, whereas the myocardium shows metastatic deposits mainly with melanoma and lymphoma, probably due to a haematogenous spread.

Isolated pericardial involvement by tumour ranged from 8–16% in another series.[49] Pericardial involvement without simultaneous myocardial involvement was seen in the majority (75%) of cases. The diagnosis of pericardial involvement, made generally through the presence of a neoplastic pericardial effusion, has prognostic importance

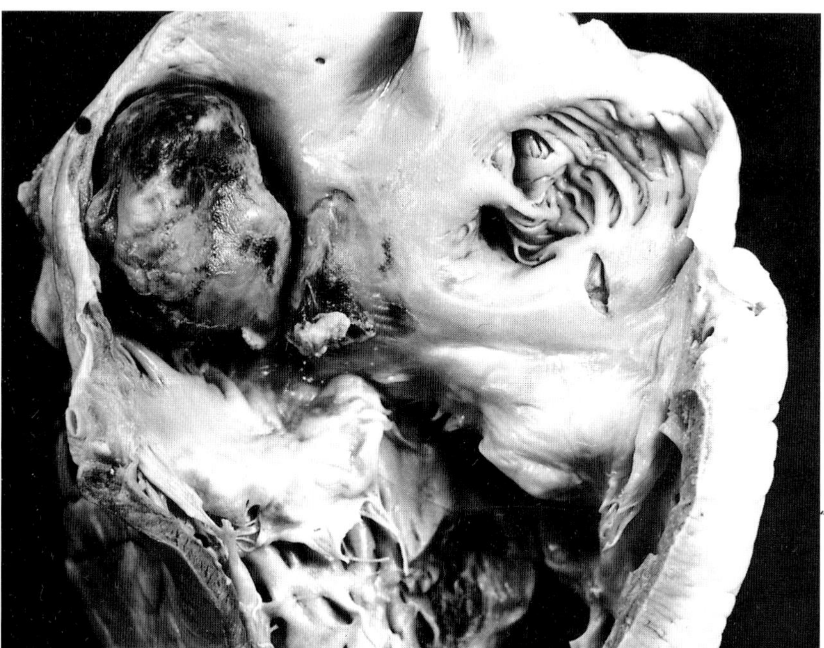

Fig. 11.27 Tumour spread via vena cava. A renal adenocarcinoma had spread up the inferior vena cava to protrude into the cavity of the right atrium.

since — in general — the median survival after its diagnosis is only 3 months. These pericardial effusions tend to recur, and cardiac tamponade is a frequent complication. Cytological analysis of the pericardial effusion yields variable results; however, if combined with a pericardial biopsy the results are significantly better. Squamous cell carcinoma of the lung is the most common metastatic tumour to be diagnosed in a pericardial effusion.

A further form of secondary involvement of the heart by malignant tumours is protrusion into the right atrium of tumour that has extended upward along the lumen of the inferior vena cava (Fig. 11.27). In these cases a lobulated mass is often detected by echocardiography within the atrial cavity; the component of tumour in the lumen of the inferior vena cava may not be recognised until surgical removal is attempted or autopsy is carried out. Certain tumours such as hepatomas, renal adenocarcinomas and ovarian stromal tumours have a particular affinity for this form of spread and the slow growth is associated with long survival and perplexing clinical signs. Carcinomas of the bronchus may spread in a like manner along a pulmonary vein into the left atrium but the more rapid growth of the bronchial tumour means that the clinical course is short and a diagnostic problem is not posed.

REFERENCES

1. Chitwood WR. Cardiac neoplasms: current diagnosis, pathology and therapy. J Card Surg 1988; 3: 119–154.
2. Lie JT. The identity and histogenesis of cardiac myxomas. Arch Pathol Lab Med 1989; 113: 724–726.
3. Blondeau Ph. Primary cardiac tumours — French studies of 533 cases. Thorac Cardiovasc Surgeon 1990; 38: 192–195.
4. Russell GA, Dhasmana JP, Berry PJ, Gilbert-Barness EF. Coexistent cardiac tumours and malformations of the heart. Int J Cardiol 1989; 22: 89–98.
5. Vidaillet HJ. Cardiac tumors associated with hereditary syndromes. Am J Cardiol 1988; 61: 1355.
6. Vidaillet HJ, Seward JB, Fyke FE, Su WPD, Tajik AJ. 'Syndrome myxoma': a subset of patients with cardiac myxoma associated with pigmented skin lesions and peripheral and endocrine neoplasms. Br Heart J 1987; 57: 247–255.
7. Goldman BI, Frydman C, Harpaz N, Ryan SF, Loiterman D. Glandular cardiac myxomas. Cancer 1987; 59: 1767–1775.
8. Hendin BN, Longaker MT, Finkbeiner WE, Roberts LJ, Stern R. Hyaluronic acid deposition in cardiac myxomas: localization using a hyaluronate-specific binding protein. Am J Cardiovasc Pathol 1990; 3: 209–215.
9. Jourdan M, Bataille R, Seguin J, Zhang XG, Chaptal PA, Klein B. Constitutive production of interleukin-6 and immunologic features in cardiac myxomas. Arthritis Rheum 1990; 33: 398–402.
10. Samaratunga H, Cominos D. Cerebral metastasis of an atrial myxoma mimicking an epithelioid hemangioendothelioma. Am J Surg Pathol 1994; 18: 107–111.
11. Markel ML, Waller BF, Armstrong WF. Cardiac myxoma. Medicine (Baltimore) 1987; 66: 114–125.
12. Attum AA, Johnson GS, Masri Z, Girardet R, Lansing AM. Malignant clinical behavior of cardiac myxomas and 'myxoid imitators'. Ann Thorac Surg 1987; 44: 217–222.
13. Warsinger ML, Wasserman AG, Goldstein H, Steinberg JS, Mills M, Katz RJ. Multiple cardiac myxomas with multiple recurrences: unusual presentation of a 'benign' tumor. Ann Thorac Surg 1987; 44: 77–78.
14. Govoni E, Severi B, Cenacchi G, Laschi R, Pileri S, Rivano MT, Alampi G, Branzi A. Ultrastructural and immunohistochemical contribution to the histogenesis of human cardiac myxoma. Ultrastruct Pathol 1988; 12: 221–233.
15. Krikler DM, Rode J, Davies MJ, Woolf N, Moss E. Atrial myxoma — a tumour in search of its origins. Br Heart J 1992; 67: 89–91.
16. Curschellas E, Toia D, Borner M, Mihatsch MJ, Gudat F. Cardiac myxomas: immunohistochemical study of benign and malignant variants. Virchows Archiv A Pathol Anat 1991; 418: 485–491.
17. Tanimura A, Kitazono M, Nagayama K, Tanaka S, Kosuga K. Cardiac myxoma: morphologic, histochemical and tissue culture studies. Hum Pathol 1988; 19: 316–322.
18. Zhang P, Jones JW, Anderson WR. Cardiac myxomas — correlative study by light, transmission and scanning electron microscopy. Am J Cardiovasc Pathol 1989; 2: 295–300.
19. Seidman JD, Berman JJ, Hitchcock CL, Becker RL, Merner W, Moore GW, Virmani R, Yetter RA. DNA analysis of cardiac myxomas. Hum Pathol 1991; 22: 494–500.
20. Kotylo PK, Kennedy JE, Waller BF, Sample RB. DNA analysis of cardiac myxomas. Chest 1991; 99: 1203–1207.
21. Molina JE, Edwards JE, Ward HB. Primary cardiac tumors: experience at the University of Minnesota. Thorac Cardiovasc Surgeon 1990; 38: 183–191.
22. Burke AP, Virmani R. Cardiac rhabdomyoma: a clinicopathologic study. Mod Pathol 1991; 4: 70–74.
23. Murphy MC, Sweeney MS, Putnam JB, Walker WE, Frazier OH, Ott DA, Cooley DA. Surgical treatment of cardiac tumors: a 25-year experience. Ann Thorac Surg 1990; 49: 612–618.
24. McAllister HA, Fenoglio JJ. Tumors of the cardiovascular system, in: Atlas of tumor pathology. Washington, DC: AFIP, 1978; fasc. 15.

25. Tazelaar HD, Locke TJ, McGregor CGA. Pathology of surgically excised primary cardiac tumors. Mayo Clin Proc 1992; 67: 957–965.
26. Parmley LF, Salley RK, Williams JP, Head GB. The clinical spectrum of cardiac fibroma with diagnostic and surgical considerations: noninvasive imaging enhances management. Ann Thorac Surg 1988; 45: 455–465.
27. Anderson DR, Gray MR. Mitral incompetence associated with lipoma infiltrating the mitral valve. Br Heart J 1988; 60: 169–171.
28. Evans DW, Stovin PGI. Fatal heart block due to mesothelioma of the atrioventricular node. Br Heart J 1986; 56: 572–574.
29. Subramanian R, Flygenring B. Mesothelioma of the atrioventricular node and congenital complete heart block. Clin Cardiol 1989; 12: 469–472.
30. Robertson AL. The origin of primary tumors of the atrioventricular node. Arch Pathol Lab Med 1990; 114: 1198.
31. McFadden PM, Lacy JR. Intracardiac papillary fibroelastoma: an occult cause of embolic neurologic deficit. Ann Thorac Surg 1987; 43: 667 669.
32. Mann J, Parker DJ. Papillary fibroelastoma of the mitral valve: a rare cause of transient neurological deficits. Br Heart J 1994; 71: 6.
33. Burke A, Johns JP, Virmani R. Hemangiomas of the heart. Am J Cardiovasc Pathol 1990; 3: 283–290.
34. Grenadier E, Margulis T, Palant A, Safadi T, Merin G. Huge cavernous hemangioma of the heart: a completely evaluated case report and review of the literature. Am Heart J 1989; 117: 479–481.
35. Burke AP, Cowan D, Virmani R. Primary sarcomas of the heart. Cancer 1992; 69: 387–395.
36. Putnam JB, Sweeney MS, Colon R, Lanza LA, Frazier OH, Cooley DA. Primary cardiac sarcomas. Ann Thorac Surg 1991; 51: 906–910.
37. Burke AP, Virmani R. Osteosarcomas of the heart. Am J Surg Pathol 1991; 15: 289–295.
38. Glock Y, Binon JP, Coca F, Rochiccioli JP, Duboucher C, Calazel J, Puel P, Bernadet P. Histiocytome fibreux malin ventriculaire droit et de l'artère pulmonaire. Ann Chir: Chir Thorac Cardio-vasc 1990; 44: 94–97.
39. Hui KS, Green LK, Schmidt WA. Primary cardiac rhabdomyosarcoma: definition of a rare entity. Am J Cardiovasc Pathol 1988; 2: 19–29.
40. Cafferty LL, Epstein JI. Primary liposarcoma of the right atrium. Hum Pathol 1987; 18: 408–410.
41. Paraf F, Bruneval P, Balaton A, Deloche A, Mikol J, Maitre F, Scholl JM, Prudhomme de Saint Maur P, Camilleri JP. Primary liposarcoma of the heart. Am J Cardiovasc Pathol 1990; 3: 175–180.
42. Allen DC, Alderdice JM, Morton P, Mollan RAB, Morris TCM. Pathology of the heart and conduction system in lymphoma and leukaemia. J Clin Pathol 1987; 40: 746–750.
43. Gardiner DS, Lindop GBM. Coronary artery aneurysm due to primary cardiac lymphoma. Histopathology 1989; 15: 537–552.
44. Kaul S, Fishbein MC, Siegel RJ. Cardiac manifestations of acquired immune deficiency syndrome: a 1991 update. Am Heart J 1991; 122: 535–544.
45. Goldfarb A, King CL, Rosenzweig BP, Feit F, Ramat BR, Rumancik WM, Kronzon I. Cardiac lymphoma in the acquired immunodeficiency syndrome. Am Heart J 1989; 118: 1340–1344.
46. Abraham KP, Reddy V, Gattuso P. Neoplasms metastatic to the heart: review of 3314 consecutive autopsies. Am J Cardiovasc Pathol 1990; 13: 195–198.
47. Weiss L. An analysis of the incidence of myocardial metastasis from solid cancers. Br Heart J 1992; 68: 501–504.
48. MacGee W. Metastatic and invasive tumour involving the heart in a geriatric population: a necropsy study. Virchows Archiv A Pathol Anat 1991; 419: 183–189.
49. Marek A, Rey JL, Jarry G, Hermida JS, Pleskof A, Kralstein J, Frishman W. Malignant pericardial diseases: diagnosis and treatment. Am Heart J 1987; 113: 785–790.

12

How to examine the heart and cardiac biopsies

AUTOPSY EXAMINATION

The technique used to examine the heart depends on the questions asked by those who requested the autopsy. There is no universally applicable technique. Most of those who carry out autopsies will have learnt the traditional method of opening the heart sequentially in the sequence of blood flow starting at the inferior vena cava.

In this technique the heart is removed from the lungs by placing a finger through the transverse sinus and then dividing the aorta and main pulmonary artery about 3 cm above the aortic valve. The pulmonary veins can then be identified and divided. Finally the superior vena cava is divided about 2 cm above where the crest of the right atrial appendage meets the vena cava, thus preserving the sinus node, and the inferior vena cava is divided close to the diaphragm. The prosecutor now has an isolated but intact heart in which the venous connections have been confirmed as normal.

From this point on there are many methods which can be used to examine the heart. The traditional method is to:

1. open the right atrium by a cut from the inferior vena cava into the right atrial appendage
2. open the tricuspid valve laterally down to the apex of the right ventricle
3. cut from the apex of the right ventricle through the pulmonary valve into the pulmonary artery
4. join two pulmonary veins across the roof of the left atrium to view the inside of the chamber

5. cut through the mitral valve orifice laterally down to the apex of the left ventricle
6. cut from the apex of the left ventricle up through its outflow tract into the aorta.

There are two variations in this final cut. It may be made through the anterior cusp of the mitral valve itself or pass anteriorly, leaving a flap of anterior wall of the ventricle hinged on an intact anterior cusp of the mitral valve.

This traditional method has the virtue of examining structure in detail. It has the disadvantages of destroying any understanding of the valve function, of poorly demonstrating the regional distribution of ischaemic myocardial damage and ventricular shape and of having no correlation with the echocardiographic planes used by clinicians.

For these reasons most professional cardiovascular pathologists have abandoned this technique and most of the illustrations in this book are made using other techniques. This chapter describes the variations in technique available for examining the heart. Perhaps the most important variation lies in routinely taking a transverse 1 cm thick slice across the ventricles before opening the rest of the heart. Such slices allow accurate recording of ventricular shape and of the distribution of ischaemic damage.

Assessment of hypertrophy and ventricular shape

Total heart weight

The measurements that can be made, and their limitations, must be understood. It is easy, and useful, to record total fixed or fresh heart weight but this must be accompanied by an indication of body weight. Normal values are published that allow the degree of heart weight increase to be calculated for a particular body size.

Practical difficulties, however, arise with the definition of normality. The heart sizes of normally active individuals dying suddenly outside hospital are very different from the heart sizes of those dying in hospital from non-cardiac disease. The hearts of athletic normal individuals are greater than normal but sedentary individuals.

One approach[1] is to use a formula based on the regression equation determined by plotting total heart weight against total body weight in a series of normal individuals dying suddenly of non-cardiac causes (Table 12.1). Using this approach the predicted normal total heart weight, left ventricular and right ventricular weights are shown in Table 12.2. Such prediction figures allow calculation of the percentage increase in total heart weight for an individual. That is, a male of 80 kg body weight with a total heart weight of 500 g has a percentage increase of total heart weight of (500 – 419)/419 or 19.3%. This approach does however hide the considerable individual variation that exists and to be 90% confident that cardiac enlargement existed an increase of over 30% is needed. The variation is largely due to physical activity: in a sedentary male a 20% increase is likely to indicate hypertrophy while in a male who runs regularly 30% would be needed.

Other figures and methods are quoted. Hudson[2] stated that the total heart weight for

Table 12.1 Prediction equations for fixed heart weight (FHW), isolated LV weight (LVW) and isolated right ventricular weight (RVW) for normal males and females in grams. (x = body weight in kg). Fixed total heart weight exceeds that of the fresh heart by approximately 5%. Isolated ventricular weights are always based on fixed material

	Males	Females
FHW	$3.44x + 144$	$4.45x + 85.4$
LVW	$1.80x + 43.5$	$1.18x + 64.3$
RVW	$0.64x + 12.8$	$0.39x + 19.9$

Table 12.2 Predicted total fixed heart weight, isolated left ventricular (LVW) and isolated right ventricular weight (RVW) for body weight in kg[1] in males and females

	Body weight	FHW	LVW	RVW
Females	30	219	99	32
	40	264	110	36
	50	308	122	39
	60	352	131	43
	70	396	145	47
Males	40	282	116	38
	50	316	134	45
	60	350	152	51
	70	385	170	58
	80	419	188	64
	90	454	206	70
	100	488	223	77

males was 0.45% and females 0.4% of total body weight. In the hypothetical example above an 80 kg male has a predicted heart weight of 360 g but no confidence limits are given. In a larger series of hearts from subjects dying in hospital[3] much lower figures are cited for normality. An 80 kg male is predicted to have a heart weight of 349 g with a 95% confidence limit for hypertrophy of 461 g (Table 12.3). The differences between these normal ranges are due to the source of the normal hearts. Pathologists should use the data that correspond most closely to the case they are considering. If that is of a fit person dying outside hospital the series that give a higher normal range are the most applicable.

Pathologists using words like mild, moderate and severe hypertrophy in autopsy reports that are going to be used for medical-legal purposes or audit should be prepared to discuss their usage in the light of the above figures. Without a body weight there is no discussion possible and a subjective opinion is not likely to be accepted readily.

Total heart weight is a useful measurement because it is directly related to left ventricular mass and therefore gives information on left ventricular hypertrophy. If the total heart weight is within the normal range for body size there cannot be significant left ventricular hypertrophy. Pathologists should avoid giving a subjective report that left ventricular hypertrophy was present while recording discordant objective data such as a normal total heart weight for body size. Total heart weight, however, gives no indication of the presence or absence of right ventricular hypertrophy.

All the other measurements of ventricular hypertrophy are either time-consuming and accurate or easy and inaccurate.

Table 12.3 Predicted total fixed heart weight for body weight in males and females (95% confidence upper limit in brackets)[3]

	Body weight	Fixed total heart weight
Female	30	196 (287)
	40	216 (317)
	50	243 (356)
	60	262 (385)
	70	280 (411)
Male	40	247 (325)
	50	276 (364)
	60	302 (399)
	70	327 (431)
	80	349 (461)
	90	371 (489)
	100	391 (416)

Isolated ventricular weights

Once the heart is fixed accurate measurements of ventricular hypertrophy can be made by dissecting the muscle of right and left ventricles free from the other constituents of the heart.[4] It is totally destructive of the specimen and takes 10–15 minutes. The epicardial fat is scraped away, following which the atria and valve tissue are cut off. The interventricular septum is functionally a component of the left ventricle, from which the right ventricular free wall can be separated (Fig. 12.1). The isolated weights of the two ventricular muscle masses can be compared to give relative degrees of hypertrophy.

The normal values for the Fulton technique are:

1. a combined ventricular weight of less than 250 g
2. an isolated right ventricular weight of less than 65 g
3. an isolated left ventricular weight (septum plus free wall) of 190 g.
4. a left-to-right isolated mass ratio between 2.3 and 3.3.

The Fulton technique is mandatory for any serious consideration of right ventricular hypertrophy.

Wall thickness

Wall thickness measurements taken in isolation are poor indicators of hypertrophy. In the left ventricle wall thickness must be related to cavity diameters. For example, if the LV cavity is very small the wall thickness can be 1.5–2.0 cm, yet with a normal isolated left ventricular weight. Some hearts with a normal LV mass appear either to arrest in systole or to go into rigor post mortem, producing high wall thickness measurements. The converse is also true, in that a dilated

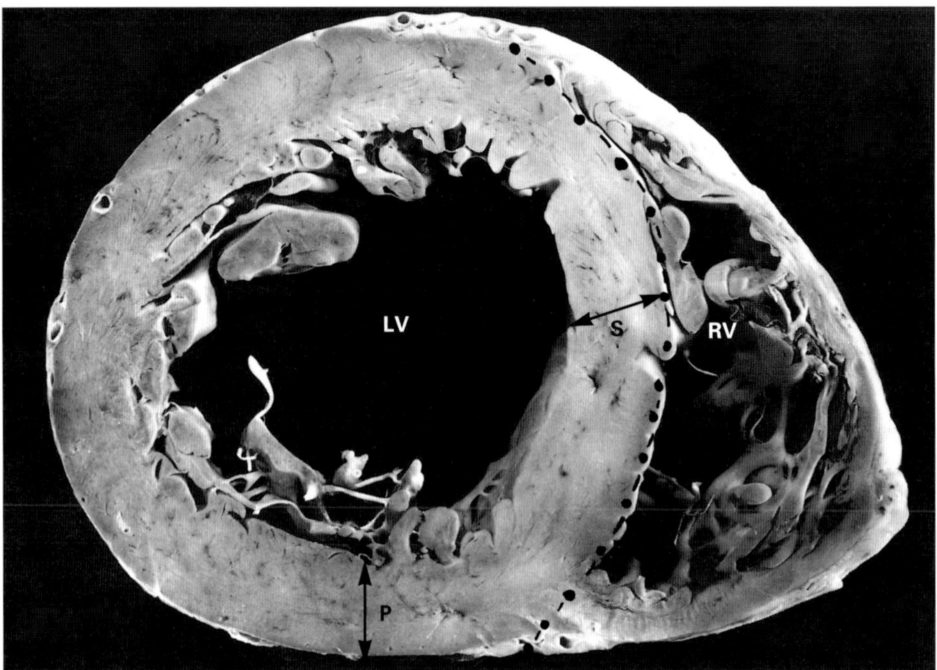

Fig. 12.1 Fulton technique. The left ventricular myocardium (LV) forms a circle and includes the septum (S). The right ventricle (RV) is a triangular structure attached to one side. The plane of the separation of right and left ventricle is shown.

left ventricle with a cavity diameter of over 8 cm can have a normal wall thickness yet an isolated muscle mass of more than twice normal.

It is best to make measurements from a transverse slice of the ventricles at mid-septal level (Fig. 12.2). The thickness of the septum and posterior wall of the left ventricle are recorded, along with the dimensions of the cavity. Right ventricular wall thickness is difficult because of the fatty infiltration from the epicardium and unless the wall is more than 1 cm thick seldom meaningful.

Assessment of ischaemic myocardial damage

The key to successful clinicopathological correlation is to take a 1 cm thick transverse slice through the short axis of both ventricles at mid-septal level. This passes through the body of the papillary muscles. The advantage of this approach is that the slice achieved is exactly analogous to the short axis, echocardiographic, magnetic resonance and isotope views used in life to assess the localisation of ischaemic changes and ventricular shape, and moreover allows any ischaemic myocardial damage to be exactly localised with respect to the region involved — antero-lateral, postero-septal etc — and thereby indicates the coronary artery likely to be involved. A very small minority of old or recent infarcts will not reveal themselves in a mid-septal slice but higher and lower slices can always be made later.

The infarct of more than 48 hours duration which has become well delineated with a red rim and a yellow centre causes no difficulties either of recognition or of topographical localisation. The use of enzyme staining methods does help in a number of ways and various techniques are available. They are used on a 1 cm thick fresh slice of myocardial tissue. The techniques depend on the presence of dehydrogenases in normal heart muscle and their loss in infarcted muscle. A range of variants of the technique are described; in some substrate is added to the incubation media improving the colour developed and enhancing the contrast between normal and ischaemic myocardium. Enzyme activity in the normal muscle is detected by a colour reaction developed with nitro blue tetrazolium.[5,6] These techniques are of some but limited value in detecting myocardial necrosis of less than 12 hours duration before naked-eye changes appear, but are of great use in delineating the margins of necrotic areas of 12–36 hours' duration and thus in aiding accurate descriptions of infarct shape. Any regional infarct should be classified as non-transmural or transmural, a distinction that is only accurate using enzyme methods. A further use of enzyme methods is in the accurate detection of widespread focal damage or diffuse subendocardial damage, for example after cardiac surgery. Enzyme methods should be used with caution in demonstrating infarction that is not visible macroscopically to some extent. The development of the colour reaction is not necessarily uniform in different parts of a normal myocardial slice and if the process is stopped before the full overall colour is developed a patchy appearance results. Interpretation of such uneven staining is difficult. On one hand it may indicate some enzyme loss and thus ischaemic damage; if the pattern fits the clinical expectation this interpretation may be valid. On the other hand even control hearts from road traffic deaths that are virtually instantaneous will develop the colour reaction at a slower rate in the subendocardial zone.

The detection of a regional area of infarction places the onus on the pathologist to identify the reason for a failure of perfusion in the arterial supply to that region. The cause should either be stated as thrombotic in relation to atheroma or, if not, accurate observations should be made on the artery indicating whether spasm or dissection are possibilities.

Examination of valves

Valve function can only be properly ascertained if the valve rings are kept intact. The mitral and tricuspid valves are first examined from the atria; if two fingers can be passed through the orifice no stenosis is present. At the same time the atrial appendages are checked for thrombosis. Regurgitation of the atrioventricular valves is far more difficult. Prolapse of mitral cusps or of ruptured papillary muscles is easily seen from the atria. Jet lesions on the atrial wall are also useful indicators of regurgitation. Apart from this all that can be done is to record abnormalities of the valve apparatus that could cause regurgitation. This is best done at the final stage of dissection when the atrioventricular valve rings are cut laterally to allow the ring circumference to be measured. While these ring dimensions are often taken, their value is limited and for practical purposes only values of 11 cm for the mitral and 14 cm for the tricuspid valve are unequivocal indicators of ring dilatation. Pressure fixation of the mitral valve in its closed position via a tube passed through the aortic valve, in which systemic pressure with formal saline is maintained, does produce good pictorial demonstrations of mitral incompetence, particularly with valve prolapse, but is too time-consuming for routine use. It is also unphysiological in that the mitral valve is not normally closed when the ventricle dilates in diastole. The fact that a normal mitral valve is so competent when the left ventricle is distended at systemic pressures indicates the considerable functional reserve built into the cusp structure.

The aortic and pulmonary valves are viewed from above. If a forefinger can be passed through the orifice stenosis is not present. The number of cusps, their shape, the shape of the orifice and the pattern of commissure fusion and calcification are all features which should be recorded to allow the pathogenesis of stenosis to be ascertained.

Incompetence is again the most difficult to assess. The valve is inspected from above and the relation between cusp and root area noted. Whether the commissures are normal is noted. Pressure fixation gives excellent demonstrations of regurgitation but is time-consuming. In the final stage of examining the heart the aortic ring circumference at the level of the commissures can be measured but is again of limited use. Figures above 11 cm are associated with regurgitation but this degree of root dilation is easily recognised from above and for purposes of demonstration it is better to keep the valve intact.

Examination of surgically excised valves

The examination of surgically excised valves is more dependent on macroscopic examination and recognition of the various combinations of commissural fusion, calcification and cusp morphology discussed in Chapter 5. Histological examination is an adjunct only to macroscopic examination. Random sections of valve material without a macroscopic examination are seldom of any use. Sections should be taken in the long axis of the cusp and assessment should be made of the factors such as fibrosis or calcification that are disturbing the normal architecture.

Examination of the coronary arteries

In common with the examination of other components of the heart the methods used depend on how comprehensive an answer is required.

The position of the coronary artery orifices should always be checked. A malleable blunt-ended probe 2–3 mm in diameter can be used to find the orifices even when the aortic valve has not been opened. If the probe slips in easily there is no ostial stenosis. At this stage the simplest way to proceed is to cut cross-sections across the coronary arteries at 3 mm intervals starting close to the aorta. The presence of high-grade stenosis is indicated to the naked eye by a pinpoint lumen. This corresponds to about 70% diameter stenosis. Lesser degrees of stenosis are often subjectively assessed by naked-eye examination but the reproducibility of such impressions is poor. With the high background level of atherosclerosis in Western populations it is always difficult to know the significance of single areas of high-grade stenosis or of multiple segments of less severe stenosis. The problem becomes particularly difficult if an autopsy report records 'moderate atherosclerosis' and legal questions on life expectancy emerge. It is advisable always to record the number of vessels with high-grade stenosis and the anatomical points at which stenosis occurs. Naked-eye examination of multiple cross-sections will show the presence or absence of thrombus and failure to find thrombus in regional infarction is more related to a failure to cut cross-sections of the relevant artery than failure to recognise thrombus with the naked eye.

This simple cross-sectional approach is however often limited by calcification. If cross-sections cannot be cut with a scalpel the pathologist has two options. A heavy pair of scissors can be used to cut the sections, but the ragged ends make the naked-eye assessment of stenosis even more difficult. The second option is to dissect the coronary arteries from the heart and decalcify the tissue. Which technique is adopted depends on the circumstances.

Opening the coronary arteries longitudinally has limited applications. It does show the presence or absence of atherosclerosis; the percentage of the intimal area occupied by plaques is a classic epidemiological tool used to compare populations. The technique of slitting the artery open is easy and quick but ensures that the exact degree of stenosis at any particular point will never be known.

More specialised methods of assessing coronary artery disease at autopsy exist. Post-mortem angiography (Chapter 3) produces pictures directly comparable to those obtained in life. A cannula is tied into each coronary artery orifice and a warm mixture of gelatine and barium sulphate is injected. The injection may be hand-controlled and barium is allowed to fill the artery until some resistance is felt; the pressure is then just maintained for a few minutes. Alternatively, various means of controlling the injection pressure are described. After filling the artery the cannula is removed, tying off the artery proximally. The heart is then cooled to solidify the injection media and can be fixed in formalin. X-ray pictures can either be taken of the entire heart or, to make the pictures less complex, the coronary arteries can be dissected from the main specimen and then decalcified prior to X-ray.

Another method of examining coronary arteries is by perfusion fixation of the aorta with formal saline at a pressure of 100 mmHg. The aortic valve closes and the coronary arteries are perfused. After perfusion for 24 hours with a recycling system in which the formalin draining from the coronary sinus is returned to the perfusion reservoir, the coronary arteries are dissected free from the heart, decalcified and then examined in serial cross-cuts at 3 mm intervals. This method, while time-consuming, allows very accurate measurements of the lumen cross-sectional area along the whole length of the artery, free from interference by calcium or collapse of the vessel to produce non-circular lumens. Examination of the cross-sections under a dissection microscope gives very striking visual images of the different type of plaque and of plaque disruption with thrombosis.

Correlation of clinical and pathological estimation of coronary stenosis

Clinicians and pathologists often assume that their estimates of the degree of stenosis agree. Nothing could be further from the truth. Clinicians measure the diameter of the lumen at a segment of stenosis and compare it with the diameter of a normal adjacent segment of artery. Pathologists, particularly when measuring stenosis from histological sections, compare the lumen diameter with the diameter of the vessel at that point. This introduces a major discrepancy because it ignores the remodelling and increase in vessel diameter that occurs with atherosclerosis (Fig. 12.2). The two data sets, however, converge at the highest grades of stenosis and for the pathologist perhaps the single most important observation is that if the lumen appears as a pinpoint it is significant stenosis. Pathologists can be less certain of the significance of plaques which appear to occupy half the cross-section of the artery.

A general scheme for examining the heart

When no specific objective exists for the examination of the heart and a routine method is needed the following (or close adaptations) is used by most cardiovascular pathologists.

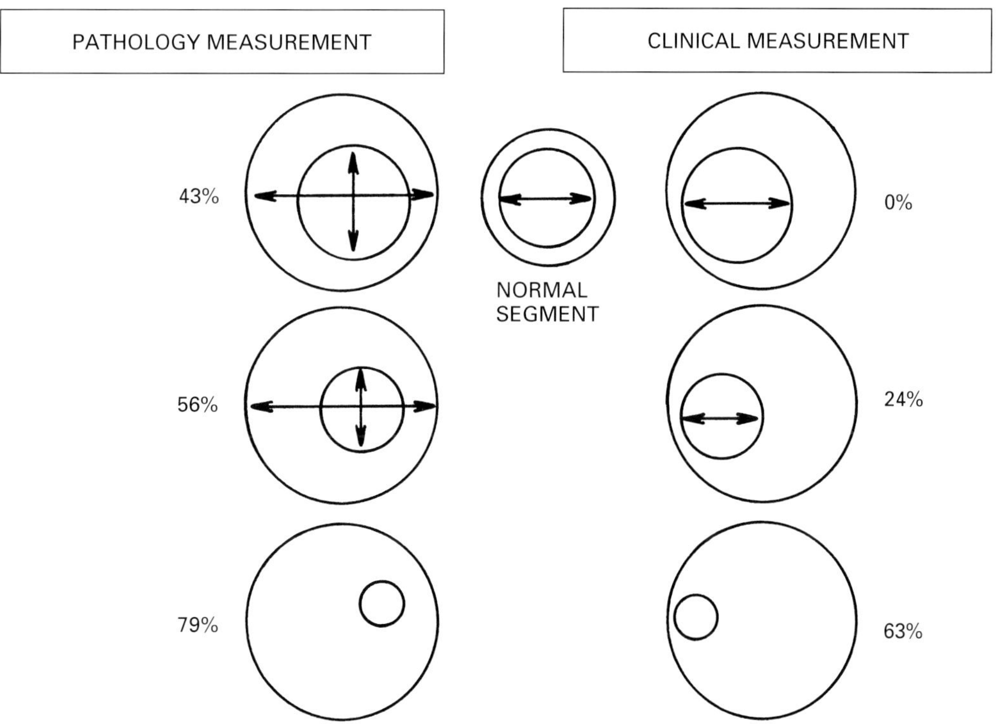

Fig. 12.2 Measurement of stenosis. In angiography the diameter of the lumen at a stenotic segment is compared to that of the closest segment of normal artery. Pathological methods based on histology compare the lumen size to that of the cross-section of the artery within the elastic lamina at the same point. The two methods only give identical values at very high-grade stenosis. Pathological measurements overestimate considerably at lower grades of stenosis.

1. Note any pericardial fluid with its nature, and comment if under pressure.

2. Remove heart intact by dividing pulmonary artery and aorta 3 cm above valves and dividing superior and inferior vena cava, followed by identifying and dividing four pulmonary veins.

3. Take a transverse slice 1 cm thick from across both ventricles at mid-septal level. Record any infarction (old or recent), its site and record if transmural. Record mural thrombi. Carry out enzyme study if indicated. Measure septal and posterior LV wall thickness and cavity diameter (mean of two planes) for left ventricle.

4. Open left atria (cut from a left to a right pulmonary vein) and right atrium (inferior vena cava to atrial appendage). Check atrial appendages for thrombus. Wash out post-mortem clot from left and right ventricles. Weigh whole heart. Record body weight.

5. Examine mitral and tricuspid valves from atria — record any abnormality.

6. Examine aortic and pulmonary valves from above. Check coronary artery orifices.

7. Make cross-sections across coronary arteries.

8. Take relevant histology blocks.

Autopsies after cardiac surgery

Autopsies for the purpose of audit of cardiac surgical procedures are never an easy exercise. Frequently the chest has been re-explored and Gelfoam has been packed around any potential bleeding point. It is all too easy to record Gelfoam as blood clot. Bleeding points may have been resutured and these autopsies should not be undertaken without access to the full clinical details.

The following points should be assessed.

Bleeding

Sudden bleeding in the first 48 hours after cardiac surgery comes from a variety of sources, including the sternal split, the division of pericardial adhesions, the atrial puncture and suture line sites, the insertion of grafts into the aorta, graft branch points and the aortic suture lines. Most cases will have been re-explored and the bleeding point resutured before the patient died. The suture lines will have been resewn, often over Teflon felt. If the case is re-explored and bleeding is found but the exact site is not identified the area is often packed with Gelfoam. In these circumstances the pathologist must not be embarrassed by also being unable to identify the bleeding point. In part diminished coagulation is responsible but if the surgeon cannot see a bleeding point when it is actually bleeding what chance does the pathologist have?

In most surgical centres the pericardium is left open after cardiac surgery and a drain is left in situ. Pathologists must therefore not expect to see tamponade and the subject has died of hypoperfusion and hypotension rather than external pressure on the heart. Sudden bleeding some days after pericardial and pleural drains have been removed often results in rapid death before the chest can be re-opened. Such disasters usually represent dehiscence of the aortic suture line due to suture breakage or a stitch cutting through the tissue. There is usually a noticeable gap in the edges of the aortotomy at either the bottom or the top of the suture line. The suture line should not be dissected further but kept to show the surgeon. Surgical practice varies as to whether the aortotomy sutures are interrupted or continuous and the surgeon who carried out the procedure is best placed to ascertain what went wrong.

Myocardial hypoperfusion injury

A major cause of mortality after cardiac surgery is acute myocardial damage sustained during the perioperative period. Many factors are concerned in this damage and include left ventricular hypertrophy, long bypass and arrest times, multiple procedures (e.g. valve plus vein grafts) and redo operations of all types. In an effort to sustain cardiac output inotropic sympathomimetic drugs, including noradrenaline and dopamine, as well as calcium infusions are often given. These drugs, while improving ventricular contraction, have a potential for perpetuating myocardial damage and many subjects have a prolonged postoperative course with increasing use of inotropic agents before finally dying.

The left ventricle at autopsy may be hypercontracted with a small cavity, or dilated. The cut surface is often partly haemorrhagic (Fig. 5.1) with a blotched appearance; enzyme studies are useful in showing a complete ring of myocardial necrosis in the subendocardial zone.

Histological examination shows patchy myocyte necrosis, often with a preponderance of the contraction band form of necrosis with an interstitial inflammatory response containing both polymorphs and macrophages. Regional rather than diffuse areas of necrosis always require explanation and are common in cases in which vein grafts have been inserted. If no coronary surgery has been carried out the coronary cannulation technique during the operation should be questioned. Where infusions of calcium have been used in order to maintain cardiac output and the patient survives some days, widespread calcification of dead myocardial muscle fibres may be seen.

Bypass graft patency

Most cases will have at least one arterial graft (internal mammary artery) and up to five saphenous vein grafts anastomosed to the aorta and inserted into the distal coronary arteries. Vein grafts are of large calibre and easily seen on the epicardium. Thrombotic occlusion leads to a solid expanded graft which is easily visible externally. Normal grafts are collapsed and empty. A cannula slipped into the aortic openings allows saline to be injected down the grafts to check flow into the distal native coronaries.

Localised regional infarction in the territory supplied by a thrombosed graft is common and easily explicable. Severe native coronary stenosis at or just distal to the vein graft anastomosis is the usual factor precipitating graft thrombosis and is also potentiated by low flow. Internal mammary or gastroepiploic artery grafts are usually very small and only admit a 1 mm probe immediately after surgery. They undergo flow-related dilatation with time and by 6 months may have a calibre equivalent to vein grafts. Patency can be confirmed by injection of saline. Regional areas of infarction in which either the arterial or venous graft to that area appear to be technically well carried out and patent are a not infrequent phenomenon at autopsy and more common with arterial grafts. In part spasm may be responsible but long manipulation times and refashioning of grafts are common associated factors. The manipulation of vein grafts that are severely diseased with atherosclerosis very readily leads to distal emboli of cholesterol and thrombi. Widespread small vessel occlusion within the myocardium may occur and is a cause of ischaemic damage at redo operations. In very severe diffuse coronary stenosis the insertion of vein grafts may be a 'final straw' which produces small regional areas of necrosis for which no clear reason can be found.

Prosthetic valves

The different types are considered in Chapter 5. In general the pathologist, whether faced with a valve in situ for a few days or one that has been in place for some years, must consider the following points.

Is there a para-prosthetic leak? Have the ring sutures cut through or broken, allowing the valve to tilt or be in an abnormal position?

Does the valve mechanically work? Has any part of the valve jammed or broken?

Is the ball, valve flap or disc moving freely?

Is there evidence of infection in the para-valve area?

Is there thrombus over the valve or its ring? Does thrombus encroach on the valve orifice?

Mitral and tricuspid prosthetic valves are relatively easy to examine from their respective atria. Aortic prosthetic valves are more difficult to see. The root of the aorta may be small and the best view is obtained by cutting the aorta transversely close to the valve itself. It is almost impossible to assess prosthetic valves which have not been displayed prior to fixation. It is heart-breaking for the professional cardiovascular pathologist to receive the entire thoracic contents unopened in a bucket of formalin and be expected to produce a meaningful opinion.

Histological examination of the heart

The heart is not a homogeneous organ from which random histological blocks will give the same information. Any particular pathologist should evolve a personal scheme which will allow each block to be recognised by its topography. In general the scheme involves taking blocks from the short axis slice of ventricles in the horizontal plane, sampling the full thickness of the septum, the anterolateral wall including the papillary muscles and the posterior wall. A block is taken vertically through the left atrium to the left ventricle through the posterior cusp of the mitral valve. In the right ventricle a block should be taken from the free wall of the right ventricular outflow. These six blocks, if normal for all practical purposes, exclude any myocarditis or cardiomyopathy.

Examination of the conduction system

There have to be good reasons to examine the conduction system given the technical effort that is involved. What are good reasons? One is where there is good clinical electrocardiographic evidence of rhythm or conduction abnormalities in life. In general conduction defects such as, for example, congenital heart block imply that there is anatomical disruption of the atrioventricular conduction system and as such are a fruitful area for clinicopathological correlation. The difficulty is that serial sections are needed to demonstrate what is a 'break in the wiring'. Pre-excitation, where conduction paths outside the atrioventricular system exist, and a range of complex A-V nodal tachycardias are areas in which further clinico-pathological studies may be rewarding but require a great deal of technical work to reconstruct large areas of tissue from serial sections. Such studies should be taken in association with the electrophysiologist, who can advise what areas of the heart to study. Considerable knowledge on the part of the pathologist in the variations that occur in the conduction system of normal hearts is needed. Atrial arrhythmias are associated with a wide range of morphological abnormalities and while it may be satisfying to show amyloid in the sinus node, the satisfaction must be balanced against the cost of the examination in time and effort.

It is in the area of sudden unexpected death that most controversy exists. Some cases will have had prior ECG studies and it is on what these show that the decision whether to study the conduction system depends. Others will have no prior ECG data and views differ on the value of a conduction system study. Some groups have made a speciality of describing, in an endless stream of case reports, minor morphological abnormalities in the conduction system which are confidently said to have caused death. The spectrum of these abnormalities, including AV nodal artery dysplasia, excessive subdivision of the AV bundle and anomalous nodal connections, all of which can be seen in control accidental death hearts, requires a critical appraisal of whether they are proved to be a cause of death. Others, like ourselves, feel that examination of the conduction system in unexplained death with a morphologically normal heart is seldom helpful.

Sino-atrial node

The sinus node or pacemaker of the normal functioning heart lies in the lateral and central portions of the junction between the superior vena cava and right atrium. The point at which the crest of the right atrial appendage crosses the root of the superior vena cava is a useful landmark. The node is a spindle-shaped mass of densely packed small myocytes lying in a rich fibrous stroma set around one or more central arteries. Trichrome stains delineate the node, because of its high content of connective tissue, and allow recognition that small myocytes with relatively scanty myofibrils are buried in the stroma.

Histological examination is most easily made if the superior vena cava is divided 1 cm above the sinocaval junction and a cuff of atria is removed. The resulting tube about 2–3 cm in length is opened longitudinally and the tissue is pinned out flat. The cut is made on the wall opposite to the atrial appendage, whose crest can be easily seen. When fixed the tissue is blocked in series of longitudinal cuts. The node lies in those blocks on and lateral to the crest of the appendage.

Atrioventricular node and conduction system

The AV node is a right atrial structure whose site just beneath the endocardium in the septum is easily recognised by certain key landmarks. The node is found at the apex of the triangle of Koch whose boundaries are the tendon of Todaro and the attachment of the septal cusp of the tricuspid valve. The base of the triangle is on the coronary sinus and its apex meets the central fibrous body. The node is examined (Fig. 12.3) by taking out a tissue block (A) that contains the triangle of Koch and sectioning in the vertical axis (right angles to septal cusp), starting posteriorly. The fewer blocks that are taken and the more exactly

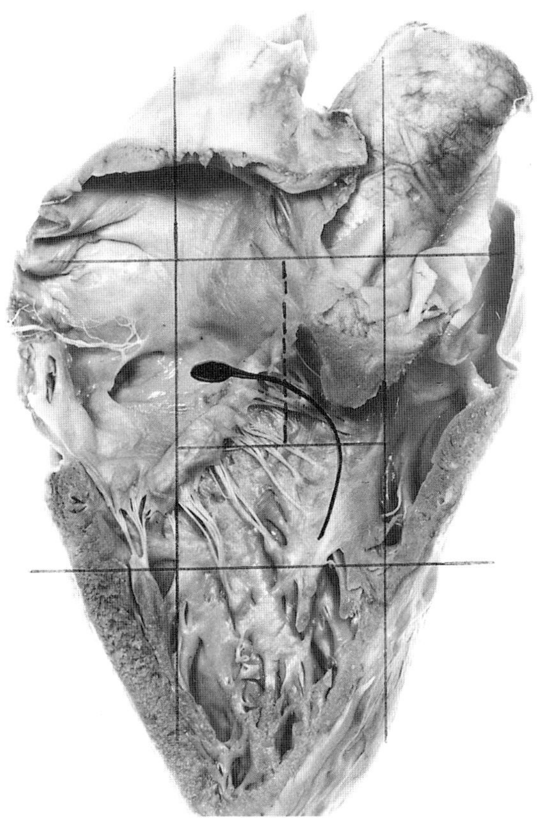

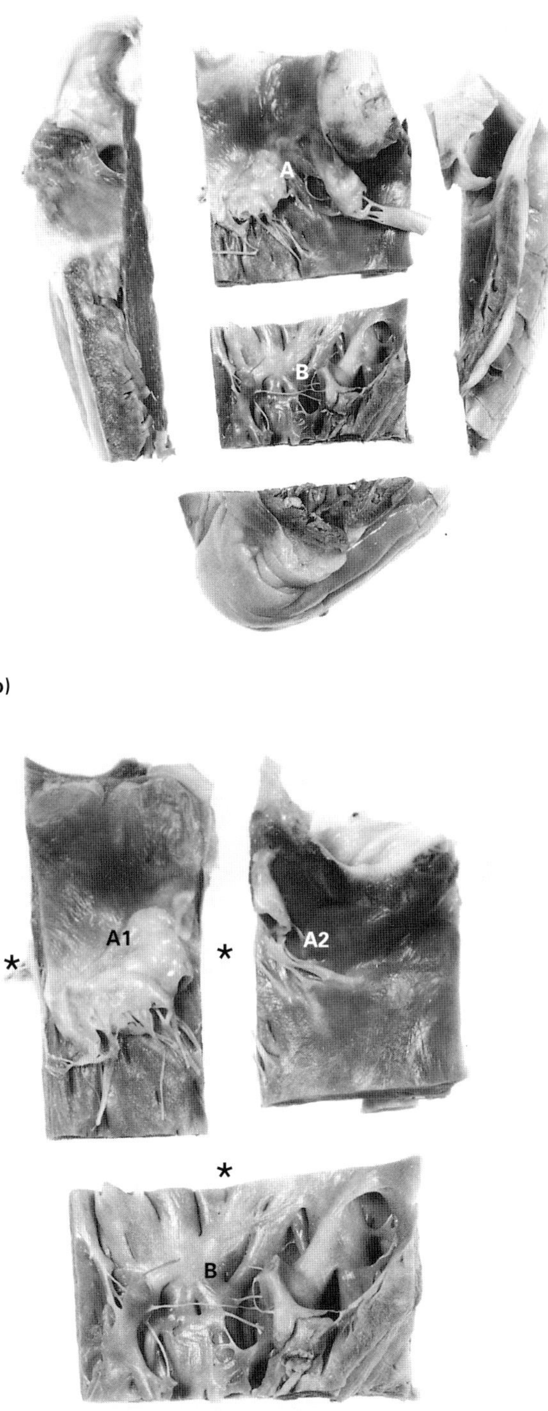

Fig. 12.3a,b,c Histological examination of the conduction system (**a**) The procedure starts with the interatrial and interventricular septa after removal of the lateral walls of the ventricles. The procedure is carried out from the right side. Vertical and lateral cuts are made to leave the conduction system isolated in two blocks. The vertical cuts are just anterior to the coronary sinus and along the junction between the inflow and outflow tracts of the ventricle. (**b**) The two central blocks (A and B) containing the conduction system. (**c**) Block A is divided into at least two portions with a vertical cut through the membranous septum. While it is ideal to keep the block numbers small the practical limitations of processing mean that most pathologists will divide A into at least 5 separate pieces. Sections are cut starting at the posterior aspect (*) of each block. Block B is sectioned in a plane at right angles to the long axis of the ventricular septum (*).

they are cut with parallel sides the more likely it is that a good reconstruction will be possible. As the sections are taken progressively more anteriorly the AV node, the penetrating bundle and bifurcating bundle appear in the sections. It is not practical to examine every section in a tissue block up to 4 cm in width. Most acceptable studies examine one in 50 while retaining unstained sections in between. Only sectioning this close allows connections between different muscle bundles to be established. On the other hand, if the objective is simply to confirm, for example, inflammatory involvement of the node in AV block due to ankylosing spondylitis, fewer sections are needed. Block B (Figure 12.3) is sectioned in a plane at right angles to that in A. It gives cross-sections of both bundle branches.

Table 12.4 Sudden death in ischaemic heart disease — mechanisms

Mechanism	Morphology	Probability of causal relation to death
Acute myocardial ischaemia	Coronary atheroma with stenosis and a) coronary thrombosis and acute infarction b) coronary thrombosis alone	Very high probability
Chronic ischaemic myocardial damage	Coronary atheroma with stenosis and a) macroscopic LV scars b) macroscopic LV scars with hypertrophy	Moderate to high probability
	c) No scars — LV hypertrophy (>500 g THW)	Moderate probability
Coronary stenosis alone	Coronary atheroma with stenosis — normal LV myocardium	Questionable probability depending on number of stenoses and the circumstances

Examination of the heart in sudden natural death

Examination of the heart is a key element in the elucidation of the cause of sudden natural death. Many pathologists face this task in carrying out work for HM Coroner. A sequential approach is best.

1. Is death really natural? In this respect the pathologist is heavily dependent on the police officers attached to the Coroner's office for detecting suicides and unnatural death.

2. Is death due to extracardiac causes? A wide range of extracardiac conditions can kill rapidly. Most are readily identified. The commonest causes are pulmonary emboli and aortic aneurysms of all types, including dissection.

3. Is death cardiac? Approximately 80% of sudden natural death is cardiac in origin and of this the greater part, in Western populations, is due to coronary atherosclerosis producing ischaemic heart disease. There is a high background level of atherosclerosis, particularly in males, and this may complicate the issue of whether coronary disease actually caused death. Sudden death in ischaemic heart disease is precipitated by ventricular fibrillation but there are several mechanisms by which this develops. The two main mechanisms are new acute myocardial ischaemia and chronic myocardial damage with fibrosis initiating ventricular tachycardias by re-entry. The pathologist should look for the features that indicate these mechanisms and can then give ischaemic heart disease as a cause of death with varying degrees of certainty that this is correct (Table 12.4). If coronary stenosis with a normal myocardium is capable of causing sudden death the mechanism is unclear. Ascription of death to coronary stenosis alone without thrombosis, infarction or myocardial sears should always be guarded.

4. Are any cardiac non-ischaemic conditions capable of producing sudden death present? Checks should be made for all the conditions listed in Table 12.5.

5. If no cause of death is apparent by this stage, recheck history and consider carrying out toxicological examination by consultation with HM Coroner. Certain conditions do seem to carry an inherent risk (albeit low) of sudden death and include epilepsy and chronic alcoholism. The heart is macroscopically and microscopically normal. The previous medical history of the subject should be reviewed and any family history of sudden death noted. History of previous syncopal attacks is strongly suggestive of cardiac arrhythmias. Examination of the conduction

Table 12.5 Non-atherosclerotic causes of sudden cardiac death

Vascular	Anomalous coronary artery anatomy Supra-aortic stenosis Coronary aneurysms/arteritis
Valvar	Aortic stenosis Mitral valve prolapse
Myocardial	Severe LV hypertrophy Dilated cardiomyopathy Hypertrophic cardiomyopathy Right ventricular dysplasia Myocarditis Sarcoid Idiopathic myocardial fibrosis Myocardial tumours
Conduction	Aneurysms of membranous ventricular septum Chronic AV block due to calcification Mesothelioma of AV node Pre-excitation — anomalous conduction pathway

system may be indicated but has a very low positive yield. In around 3% of what are highly likely to be totally natural sudden deaths even this detailed approach does not show a cause of death. What to do under these circumstances depends on the view of the individual Coroner. Some may hold an inquest, leading to a verdict of natural death — cause unknown. Other coroners will accept spontaneous cardiac arrhythmia as a natural cause of death for certification.

EXAMINATION OF CARDIAC BIOPSIES

The advent of cardiac transplantation led to the need for regular biopsies of the myocardium to manage rejection. Techniques for obtaining myocardial biopsies were developed which were relatively easy and risk-free. The techniques are now so widely available that cardiac biopsy for diagnosis of a range of diseases has become commonplace.

The biopsies are obtained by passing a bioptome into the right ventricle via the superior or inferior vena cava under radiological screening. The bioptome is impacted into the apex of the right ventricle or on to the interventricular septum and the jaws are closed. The tissue is retrieved by withdrawing the catheter, which can then be repassed to obtain multiple fragments up to 3 mm in diameter. The bioptome tends to lodge in the same position in the ventricle each time. Most operators try and avoid the free wall of the right ventricle due to the risk of perforation. Biopsies can be obtained from the left ventricle crossing the aortic valve from the femoral or brachial artery. It is usual to leave a sheath across the valve through which the bioptome is reintroduced several times.

The pathologist will usually receive up to eight fragments. Cardiac biopsies should be jointly planned by the clinician and pathologist to maximise the benefit. Under some circumstances one or more of the biopsies should be frozen or submitted for electronmicroscopy. The biopsies fixed in formalin are conventionally embedded and cut at several levels through the block. Each level should be stained by haematoxylin and eosin and a stain that demonstrates collagen, such as variations on the trichrome method. A band artefact due to the myocytes intensely contracting as an injury response to the crushing action of the bioptome is almost universal.

The reporting schedule should comment on the following features.

1. Is an endocardial surface present; if so is the endocardium of normal thickness? Thickened endocardium, occasionally with thrombus incorporated, is a feature of endomyocardial fibrosis (EMF). The operator may comment that biopsy was difficult to obtain due to the bioptome failing to gain bites of tissue without very firm wedging against the endocardium.

2. Is pericardium present? — up to 10% of right ventricular biopsies do contain epicardial fat. It is worth telling the clinician in order to allow the patient to be monitored closely but the vast majority of perforations cause no trouble other than minor pericarditis.

3. Record myocyte size, either as a subjective opinion or by formal measurement. Myocyte diameter is measured by taking the shortest diameter of a number of myocytes through the nucleus. The average biopsy will yield more than enough myocytes to randomly select 100 myocytes for measurement. Papers are often published in which far fewer myocytes are measured. If small numbers are counted the method of random selection has to be very rigorous. The diameter of

myocytes in right ventricular biopsies may reflect the right ventricular or the left ventricular myocardium or both. This is because the interventricular septum is essentially a component of the left ventricle. Distribution curves of the myocyte diameters often show that there may be major differences between different biopsies taken at the same time. The normal range for right ventricular myocytes is up to 12 μm, for the left ventricular myocytes up to 20 μm.

4. Record the amount and distribution of myocardial fibrosis. A wide range of stains, including Sirius red, elastic/Van Gieson and trichromes are used for this purpose, depending on individual preference. Subjective impressions have to be based on considerable experience of what is normal. Fibrosis may be seen either as an increase in coarse trabeculae or finer interstitial fibrosis or as large focal scars. Fibrosis surrounding individual myocytes is always abnormal and worth recording. Objective measurements of fibrosis are either dependent on visual point counting with a quantification grid or by use of quantifying microscopes automatically detecting the proportion of the field occupied by a particular colour. Considerable variation occurs in the normal values reported by different laboratories.

5. Myocyte hypertrophy should also be assessed by nuclear size. This is usually done subjectively but can be measured by nuclear area. Counting nuclear area is difficult due to the different planes in which nuclei are cut. It is best either to measure only round or oval nuclei, depending on preference. Once again each laboratory should establish its own range.

6. Assess interstitial cellularity. This is perhaps the most difficult subjective assessment. It is all too easy to mistake endothelial cell nuclei for lymphocytes. It is good practice always to identify interstitial cells by immunohistochemistry if an increase in number is suspected. We personally freeze one or two biopsies for this purpose rather than relying on immunohistochemical marking in paraffin-embedded material.

7. Consider if amyloid material is present. All the amyloid stains will work. We personally use Congo red under polarised light in sections cut somewhat thicker than usual (10–15 μm). Confirmation of amyloid by electron microscopy is desirable but it is very costly to embed every case. A good practice is to embed one biopsy for electronmicroscopy only if there is a high clinical suspicion of amyloid, e.g. a restrictive physiological pattern.

8. Reports exist which measure the medial-to-lumen ratio of small arteries. Very few vessels more than 50 μm external diameter will be present in any biopsy, making statistical correlation difficult. Many vessels of more than 100 μm external diameter show an artefact in which there is intussusception.

Indications for cardiac biopsy

Some indications are well established and can be more than justified by the benefit of a positive diagnosis to the patients. These include

- cardiac rejection detection
- assessment of the myocardium in Adriamycin therapy (EM obligatory)
- differential diagnosis of restrictive cardiomyopathy (EM desirable)
- tissue diagnosis in suspected myocarditis.

Other indications are less clear-cut and include

- diagnosis of dilated cardiomyopathy — possible diagnosis of persistent viral infection by in-situ hybridisation.

Cardiac biopsy has virtually no part to play in the diagnosis of hypertrophic cardiomyopathy or ischaemic heart disease. The interpretation of cardiac biopsies is very dependent on ischaemic damage having been previously excluded by coronary angiography.

REFERENCES

1. Hangartner J, Marley N, Whitehead A, Thomas A, Davies M. The assessment of cardiac hypertrophy at autopsy. Histopathology 1985; 9: 1295–1306.
2. Hudson R. Structure and function of the heart. In: Cardiovascular pathology. London: Edward Arnold, 1965; vol 1.
3. Kitzman D, Scholz D, Hagen P, Ilstrup D, Edwards W. Age-related changes in normal human hearts during the first 10 decades of life. Part II Maturity: a quantitative anatomic study of 765 specimens from subjects 20 to 99 years old. Mayo Clin Proc 1988; 63: 137–146.
4. Fulton R, Hutchinson E, Morgan-Jones A. Ventricular weight in cardiac hypertrophy. Br Heart J 1952; 14: 413–420.
5. Derias N, Adams C. Nitro blue tetrazolium test: early gross detection of human myocardial infarcts. Br J Exp Pathol 1978; 59: 254–258.
6. Anderson K, Popple A, Parker D, Sayer R, Trickey R, Davies M. An experimental assessment of macroscopic enzyme techniques for the autopsy demonstration of myocardial infarction. J Pathol 1979; 127: 93–98.

Index